FOURTH EDITION

AIDS/HIV
Reference Guide for
Medical Professionals

FOURTH EDITION

AIDS/HIV
Reference Guide for
Medical Professionals

Editors

JOHN L. FAHEY, MD

DIANA SHIN FLEMMIG, MPH

Center for Interdisciplinary Research in
Immunology and Disease (CIRID) at UCLA

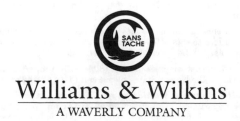

Williams & Wilkins
A WAVERLY COMPANY

BALTIMORE • PHILADELPHIA • LONDON • PARIS • BANGKOK
BUENOS AIRES • HONG KONG • MUNICH • SYDNEY • TOKYO • WROCLAW

Editor: Jonathan W. Pine, Jr
Managing Editor: Molly L. Mullen
Production Coordinator: Raymond E. Reter
Designer: Norman W. Och
Illustration Planner: Ray Lowman
Cover Designer: Wilma Rosenberger
Typesetter: Digitype, Waynesboro, Pa.
Printer & Binder: Port City Press, Inc., Baltimore, Md.

Every effort has been made to ensure that diagnostic and therapeutic recommendations, including drug dosage schedules, contained herein are accurate and in accord with the standards accepted at the time of publication. However, as new research and experience broaden our knowledge, changes in diagnosis and treatment occur. Therefore, the reader is advised to check current authoritative reference sources, including product information sheets, for each drug he or she plans to administer. With regard to drugs, the reader should be certain that changes have not been made in the recommended dose or in the contraindications. Opinions expressed herein are not necessarily those of the UCLA Center for Interdisciplinary Research in Immunologic Disease or The Regents of the University of California.

This publication was supported by Grant AI 15332 from the National Institute of Allergy and Infectious Diseases. Its contents are the sole responsibility of the authors and do not necessarily represent the official views of the National Institute of Allergy and Infectious Diseases.

Printed in the United States of America

Portions of this book originally appeared under the titles
AIDS Reference Guide for Medical Professionals © 1985 The Regents of the University of California
AIDS Reference Guide for Medical Professionals, Second Edition © 1986 The Regents of the University of California
AIDS/HIV Reference Guide for Medical Professionals, Third Edition © 1988 The Regents of the University of California

Library of Congress Cataloging-in-Publication Data

AIDS/HIV reference guide for medical professionals / editors, John L. Fahey, Diana Shin Flemmig — 4th ed.
    p. cm.
    Includes bibliographical references and index.
    ISBN 0-683-02960-6
    1. AIDS (Disease)—Handbooks, manuals, etc. 2. HIV (Viruses)—Handbooks, manuals, etc. I. Fahey, John L. II. Shin Flemmig, Diana
    [DNLM: 1. Acquired Immunodeficiency Syndrome. 2. Acquired Immunodeficiency Syndrome—therapy—United States—directories. 3. Community Health Services—United States—directories. WC 503 A2885 1996]
    RC607.A26A34734 1996
    DNLM/DLC
    for Library of Congress   95-52143
                                      CIP

The publishers have made every effort to trace the copyright holders for borrowed material. If they have inadvertently overlooked any, they will be pleased to make the necessary arrangements at the first opportunity.

To purchase additional copies of this book, call our customer service department at **(800) 638-0672** or fax orders to **(800) 447-8438.** For other book services, including chapter reprints and large quantity sales, ask for the Special Sales department.

Canadian customers should call **(800) 665-1148,** or fax **(800) 665-0103.** For all other calls originating outside of the United States, please call **(410) 528-4223** or fax us at **(410) 528-8550.**

Visit Williams & Wilkins on the Internet: **http://www.wwilkins.com** or contact our customer service department at **custserv@wwilkins.com.** Williams & Wilkins customer service representatives are available from 8:30 am to 6:00 pm, EST, Monday through Friday, for telephone access.

97 98 99 00
1 2 3 4 5 6 7 8 9 10

PREFACE

The world was unprepared for AIDS. Previously unknown, the human immunodeficiency virus (HIV-1) is a lethal pathogen that has now infected millions of persons throughout the world. Every subpopulation within every country has been affected by problems caused by HIV/AIDS in medical, ethical, legal, political, financial or social areas.

AIDS has responded poorly to the conventional medical and public health approaches, in part because of the complexity and unique features of the virus. Fifteen years after the identification of AIDS, there is no vaccine, and the benefits of medical therapies, although helpful in controlling complications, are transient. It is certainly hoped that vaccines and effective antiviral or immune restorative and immune maintenance therapies will be developed. An enormous amount of knowledge concerning the HIV epidemic has been accumulated rapidly by the medical, scientific, and behavioral community. Public health measures such as effective and comprehensive testing have reduced the spread of HIV by blood and blood products, and the ongoing education efforts directed toward individuals and communities have provided information and skills to alleviate fears and to reduce HIV transmission.

The purpose of this book is to provide a primary resource for all health care providers with clinical, laboratory, social, preventive, behavioral, epidemiologic, legal or personal interests in HIV/AIDS. It should meet most initial informational needs with references and resources to assist in making important decisions concerning HIV/AIDS.

The knowledge about HIV/AIDS is continually evolving, from an increasingly well-established information base. Clinical information and current therapies are covered in this text. Information about the virus, its components, and the host response is also outlined, along with a variety of counseling, behavioral, preventive, and legal issues relevant to the control of HIV transmission. In addition to knowledge, appropriate actions are required to limit the spread of AIDS, to care for HIV-infected individuals and to control HIV infection. It is hoped that this book will provide assistance to those individuals and institutions who desire the knowledge for the optimal contemporary response to HIV/AIDS.

John L. Fahey, MD
Diana Shin Flemmig, MPH

ACKNOWLEDGMENTS

Our sincere appreciation goes to those contributors and individuals who have given their time and expertise to this reference guide as well as the agencies who have supplied valuable resource information.

UCLA AIDS Institute
UCLA Center for Clinical AIDS Research and Education
CDC Public Information Service
Global Programme on AIDS, World Health Organization

CONTRIBUTORS

Martin M. Anderson, M.D., M.P.H.
Assistant Clinical Professor
Department of Pediatrics
Director, Adolescent Medicine Program
UCLA School of Medicine
Los Angeles, California

Pamela J. J. Boyer, M.D., Ph D.
Assistant Professor
Division of Maternal/Fetal Medicine
Department of Obstetrics & Gynecology
UCLA School of Medicine
Los Angeles, California

Yvonne J. Bryson, M.D.
Professor
Department of Pediatrics
UCLA School of Medicine
Los Angeles, California

Suzanne M. Donovan, M.D., M.P.H.
Assistant Professor
Division of Infectious Disease
Department of Medicine
Olive View-UCLA Medical Center
Los Angeles, California

Lewis Roy Eversole, D.D.S., M.S., M.A.
Professor and Chairman
Diagnostic Sciences
UCLA School of Dentistry
Los Angeles, California

John L. Fahey, M.D.
Professor
Department of Microbiology & Immunology
    and Medicine
Director, Center for Interdisciplinary
    Research in Immunology and Disease
UCLA School of Medicine
Los Angeles, California

Diana Shin Flemmig, M.P.H.
Director, Education and Prevention
Center for Interdisciplinary Research in
    Immunology and Disease
UCLA School of Medicine
Los Angeles, California

Donna Futterman, M.D.
Director, Adolescent AIDS Program
Associate Professor of Pediatrics
Albert Einstein College of Medicine
Montefiore Medical Center
Bronx, New York

Sheila Gillette, M.S.N., R.N.C.S.
Academic Coordinator
Department of Pediatrics
UCLA School of Medicine
Assistant Professor
UCLA School of Nursing
Los Angeles, California

Gary N. Holland, M.D.
Professor of Ophthalmology
UCLA School of Medicine
Director, UCLA Ocular Inflammatory
    Disease Center
Jules Stein Eye Institute
Los Angeles, California

Ann K. Johiro, R.N.C., M.N., F.N.P.
Research Nurse Practitioner
UCLA Center for Clinical AIDS Research
    and Education
Los Angeles, California

Peter Katona, M.D., F.A.C.P.
Chairman, Infection Control Committee
UCLA School of Medicine
Los Angeles, California

Douglas Longshore, Ph.D.
Associate Research Sociologist
Drug Abuse Research Center
UCLA Neuropsychiatric Institute
Los Angeles, California

Lesley MacArthur-Chang
Research Coordinator
UCLA Ocular Inflammatory Disease
    Center-Clinical Trials
Los Angeles, California

Steven A. Miles, M.D.
Associate Professor of Medicine
Division of Hematology and Oncology
UCLA School of Medicine
Clinic Director, UCLA Center for Clinical
  AIDS Research and Education
Los Angeles, California

Ronald T. Mitsuyasu, M.D.
Professor of Medicine
UCLA School of Medicine
Director, UCLA Center for Clinical AIDS
  Research and Education
Los Angeles, California

Pari Nishanian, Ph.D.
Assistant Research Immunologist
Center for Interdisciplinary Research in
  Immunology and Disease
UCLA School of Medicine
Los Angeles, California

Adeline Nyamathi, R.N., Ph.D., F.A.A.N.
Professor and Chair
Acute Care Nursing
UCLA School of Nursing
Los Angeles, California

Mary Jane Rotheram-Borus, Ph.D.
Professor, Division of Social Psychiatry
UCLA School of Medicine
Director, Clinical Research Center at UCLA
Los Angeles, California

Elyse J. Singer, M.D.
Associate Professor
Department of Neurology
UCLA School of Medicine
Research Physician
Veterans Administration Medical Center
West Los Angeles, California

Jorge Vargas, M.D.
Associate Professor
Division of Gastroenterology
Department of Pediatrics
UCLA School of Medicine
Los Angeles, California

Barbara R. Visscher, M.D., Dr.P.H.
Professor Emeritus
Department of Epidemiology
UCLA School of Public Health
Los Angeles, California

Lorenz Von Seidlein, M.D.
Fellow, Pediatric Infectious Disease
UCLA School of Medicine
Los Angeles, California

CONTENTS

CHAPTER / 1

EPIDEMIOLOGY AND HIV TRANSMISSION 1
Diana Shin Flemmig and Barbara R. Visscher

CHAPTER / 2

HIV COUNSELING AND TESTING 57
Diana Shin Flemmig and Ann K. Johiro

CHAPTER / 3

LABORATORY DIAGNOSIS AND EVALUATION OF
HIV INFECTION 75
John L. Fahey and Pari Nishanian

CHAPTER / 4

CLINICAL ASPECTS OF HIV INFECTION 97

CHAPTER / 5

WOMEN AND HIV INFECTION 215

CHAPTER / 11

ACRONYMS AND ABBREVIATIONS

ACOG   American College of Obstetricians and Gynecologists
Ab   antibody
ACTG   AIDS Clinical Trials Group
ACUS   atypical cells of undetermined significance
AFB   acid-fast bacillus
Ag   antigen
AHCPR   Agency for Health Care Policy and Research
AIDS   acquired immunodeficiency syndrome
AP   aerosol Pentamidine
AZT   azidothymidine
BCG   bacille Calmette-Guérin
bid   twice a day
biw   twice a week
BMT   bone marrow transplant
CBC   complete blood count
CDC   Centers for Disease Control
CIN   cervical intraepithelial neoplasia
CMV   cytomegalovirus
CNS   central nervous system
CPCRA   Community Programs for Clinical Research on AIDS
CSF   cerebrospinal fluid
CT   computerized tomographic (scan)
d4T   stavudine
ddC   2′, 3′-dideoxycytidine (zalcitabine)
ddI   2′, 3′-dideoxyinosine (didanosine)
DFA-TP   direct fluorescent antibody staining for *Treponema pallidum*
DOT   directly observed therapy
EBV   Epstein-Barr virus
ELISA   enzyme-linked immunosorbent assay
FDA   Food and Drug Administration
FTA-ABS   fluorescent treponemal antibody absorption
g or gm   gram
gp   glycoprotein
GI   gastrointestinal
G6PD   glucose-6-phosphate dehydrogenase
Hct   hematocrit
Hgb   hemoglobin
h   hour
HIV   human immunodeficiency virus
HPV   human papilloma virus
HSV   herpes simplex virus
HZV   herpes zoster virus
ID   intradermal
IFA   immunofluorescence antibody

IFN   interferon
IgG   immunoglobulin gamma
IL   interleukin
IL   intralesional
IN   intranasal
IM   intramuscular
IND   investigational new drug
INH   isoniazid
IV   intravenous
IVIG   intravenous immune gammaglobulin
kg   kilogram
LAS   Lymphadenopathy Syndrome
LIP   lymphoid interstitial pneumonitis
LP   lumbar puncture
m   month
ml   milliliter
mm   millimeter
mm³   cubic millimeter
MAI   *Mycobacterium avium intracellulare*
MAC   Mycobacterium Avium-Intracellular Complex
MACS   Multicenter AIDS Cohort Study
MDR-TB   multidrug-resistant tuberculosis
MHA-TP   microhemagglutination assay for *Treponema pallidum*
MRI   magnetic resonance imaging
NIAID   National Institute of Allergy and Infectious Diseases
NICHD   National Institute of Child Health and Human Development
NIH   National Institutes of Health
NLM   National Library of Medicine
OI   opportunistic infection
Pap   Papanicolaou (smear)
PCP   *Pneumocystis carinii* pneumonia
PCR   polymerase chain reaction
PID   pelvic inflammatory disease
PLWA   persons living with AIDS
PML   Progressive Multifocal Leukoencephalopathy
PPD   purified protein derivative
PO   by mouth
q   every
qd   every day
qod   every other day
qm   every month
RBC   red blood cell
RDA   recommended daily allowances
RPR   rapid plasma reagin
SC   subcutaneous

SIL squamous intraepithelial lesion
STD sexually transmitted disease
TB tuberculosis
tid three times daily
TMP-SMX trimethoprim-sulfamethoxazole
TPN total parenteral nutrition

TU tuberculin unit
VDRL Venereal Disease Research Laboratories
WB Western Blot
WHO World Health Organization
ZDV zidovudine
3TC lamivudine

CHAPTER 1

Epidemiology and HIV Transmission

Overview: Acquired Immunodeficiency Syndrome

The first cases of acquired immunodeficiency syndrome (AIDS) were described in homosexual men in the United States in 1981, and the etiologic agent, human immunodeficiency virus (HIV) was identified by 1983. The extensive spread of HIV appears to have begun in the late 1970s or early 1980s in the Americas, Australasia and Western Europe (1). AIDS has since reached epidemic proportions worldwide.

AIDS is the end-stage outcome caused by infection with the human immunodeficiency virus (HIV). The Centers for Disease Control (CDC) devised an AIDS case definition and classification system based on the presence of certain opportunistic infections and/or malignancies in the absence of other causes of immunodeficiencies. As knowledge of the natural history of HIV increased and in order to remain consistent with the clinical management of AIDS, the AIDS case definition has been expanded twice, in late 1987 and in 1993. The most recent revision of this system published in 1993 emphasized the importance of the CD4+ T-lymphocyte count in the categorization of HIV-related clinical conditions (2). Clinically, HIV infection should be described as a continuum of conditions associated with immune dysfunction, and is often described as HIV disease.

The virus is transmitted through sexual intercourse, contaminated blood and blood products, and perinatally from an infected mother to her infant. Activities which place an individual at risk for HIV infection include: sexual contact (heterosexual, homosexual, and bisexual); injecting drug use (IDU); receipt of contaminated blood and blood products (e.g. transfusion, hemophiliacs); and sexual contact with any of the above individuals. Children born to mothers infected with HIV are also at risk for acquiring infection. Mother-to-child transmission is thought primarily to occur during pregnancy and delivery, although there has been evidence to also suggest transmission through breast-feeding. There has been no epidemiological or laboratory evidence to suggest HIV is transmitted by casual contact (e.g. hugging, shaking hands), food, water, or mosquitoes.

Approved commercial blood testing for detection of HIV-1 antibodies has been available in the United States since 1985. A confirmed positive antibody test is considered as evidence of HIV infection, and the individual is considered capable of transmitting infection. If an infected individual is tested during the interval between HIV infection and development of antibodies (i.e., the "window period"), the individual will test negative for HIV antibody, even though transmission is possible because the virus is present. Seroconversion (i.e., the appearance of detectable HIV antibodies) occurs within eight weeks of infection for most individuals. Other methods used to detect HIV infection include gene amplification of HIV DNA or RNA sequences (e.g. polymerase chain reaction), HIV antigen testing, and HIV viral culture.

The time interval between infection and onset of clinical symptoms is long compared to other communicable diseases and varies among individuals. Some individuals have flu-like symptoms for a short time during the initial period of viral multiplication. The asymptomatic phase of disease ranges from a few months to greater than 12 years (3). Within 10 years following initial infection, approximately half will have developed symptoms. At present it seems that almost all HIV-infected persons will ultimately die of AIDS, but cohort studies have not yet demonstrated this (3). There are also individuals who have had long-term HIV infection without immunologic progression for 10 to 15 years (4–6). Factors which may influence the rate of progression to clinical illness include the strain of HIV, concurrent infections, age, human genetic factors, and other viral and/or host-specific factors. Antiretroviral therapy and therapy to prevent opportunistic infections in the HIV-infected patient is available. These agents include zidovudine (ZDV), dideoxyinosine (ddi), zalcitabine (ddc) stavudine (d4T), lamivudine (3TC), saquinavir, trimethoprim-sulfa, aerosolized pentamidine, and dapsone. Recently, a new class of AIDS drugs, protease inhibitors (e.g. ritonavir) has also been shown to extend life. The combination of protease inhibitors with current drugs may provide another treatment alternative to slow disease progression. Currently, there is no known method of eradicating the primary HIV infection. The average survival time after an AIDS diagnosis is one to three years; this may be influenced by exposure to opportunistic infections or access to health care (1).

Early identification of HIV infection in individuals is important for several reasons. The availability of therapies and preventive measures can delay disease progression and prevent opportunistic infections. In addition, education, counseling, as well as linking the HIV-infected individual to supportive networks can assist in maintaining good health, delaying onset of symptoms, and preventing transmission to others.

There are two serotypes of HIV currently recognized, HIV-1 and HIV-2. The predominant virus worldwide is HIV-1, although HIV-2 appears to have spread during the 1980s, principally in West Africa, with sporadic cases reported from East Africa, Europe, Asia and Latin America (1,7–8). The two viruses are similar in their modes of transmission and clinical manifestations, although HIV-2 may not be as easily transmissible and it appears progression from infection to disease is longer for HIV-2 (1,8).

There have been recent reports of severe immunodepression in the absence of HIV infection, raising concern of another undetected virus (9,10). Further investigations have demonstrated no links among these cases or any new immunodeficiency virus (9,10).

NOTE: The use of HIV in the book will refer to HIV-1 unless otherwise specified.

REFERENCES

1. Global Programme on AIDS. The HIV/AIDS Pandemic: 1994 Overview. WHO: Geneva;1994.
2. CDC. 1993 Revised Classification System for HIV Infection and Expanded Surveillance Case Definition for AIDS Among Adolescents and Adults MMWR 1993; 41/No RR-17.
3. CDC. 1993 Sexually Transmitted Diseases Treatment Guidelines. MMWR. 1993; 42(RR-1);1–44.
4. Buchbinder SP, Katz MH, Hessol NA, et al. Long-term HIV-1 infection without immunologic progression. AIDS 1994;8:1123–28.
5. Ho, DD. Long-term Nonprogressors. Xth International Conference on AIDS. 1994. (abstr PS-10).
6. Deacon NJ, Tyskin A, Solomon A, Smith K, Ludford-Menting M, Hooker DJ, et al. Genomic structure of an attentuated quasi species of HIV-1 from a blood transfusion donor and recipients. Science 1995;270:988–991.
7. CDC. Testing for antibodies to human immunodeficiency virus type 2 in the United States. MMWR 1992. 41:RR-12
8. O'Brien TR, George JR, Holmberg SD. Human immunodeficiency virus type 2 infection in the United States. JAMA. 1992;267:2775–2779.
9. CDC. Update: CD4+ T-Lymphocytopenia in persons without evident HIV Infection— United States. MMWR. 1992;41:578–579.
10. Smith DK, Neal JJ, Holmberg SD, et al. Unexplained opportunistic infections and CD4+ T-lymphocytopenia without HIV infection. NEJM 1993;328:373–9.

Global Aspects of HIV/AIDS

By mid-1995, over one million cumulative AIDS cases worldwide have been reported to the World Health Organization (WHO) Global Programme on AIDS (1). Allowing for under-diagnosis, incomplete reporting and reporting delay, and available HIV infection data worldwide, over 4.5 million AIDS cases in adults and children have been estimated to occur since the pandemic began (1). Africa accounts for over 70% of the estimated worldwide AIDS cases, followed by the USA (9%), the Americas (9%, excluding the USA), Asia (<6%), Europe (4%) and Oceania (<1%) (1). As of mid-1995, an estimated 18.5 million adults and 1.5 million children are HIV-infected worldwide. As depicted by Figure 1.1, people with HIV infections are also unequally distributed, with over 11 million in Africa (1). Evidence suggests that the prevalence of HIV infection may be stabilizing in certain areas such as developed regions of Australia, North America and Western Europe and possibly in high prevalence areas of East and Central Africa (2). HIV infections continue to increase disproportionately in the developing world, particularly in southern and central Africa and South Asia (1). Although the majority of new infections are still occurring in sub-Saharan Africa, the potential for an explosive increase in HIV infections exists in areas of Asia (2). The proportion of AIDS cases occurring in Asia increased from 1% in mid-1993 to 6% in mid-1994, primarily due to the rapid epidemic growth in South and South-East Asia (3).

Heterosexual intercourse is the predominant and increasing mode of HIV transmission worldwide, and the ratio of infected men to women is 3:2, (2). In industrialized countries, more men were initially affected by HIV as a result of transmission by male-to-male sexual contact or injecting drug use; however, the difference between the numbers of HIV-infected men and women is becoming smaller (2). The proportion of heterosexual transmission in industrialized countries is increasing and AIDS is now one of the predominant causes of death in young men and women (4). By the year 2000, WHO predicts that the number of new HIV infections among women will be equal to the number among men (2).

Global Patterns of HIV

Geographic variations in epidemiology, clinical symptoms, and distribution of different human retroviruses have been reported. There are four distinct epidemiological global patterns of infection and disease, based on the temporal spread of HIV and the associated risk behaviors (5). However, these patterns changed over time; a fourth epidemiologic pattern I/II emerged in the late 1980s. Although these classifications are not commonly used, they are sometimes referred to and are outlined below (5,6):

PATTERN I

Pattern I is found primarily in industrialized countries, including the United States, Mexico and Canada, many Western European countries, Australia, and New Zealand. Although not industrialized, areas of North Africa also exhibit pattern I. The extensive spread of HIV began in late 1970s and early 1980s. The male-to-female ratio is approximately 5–6:1 (2). Perinatal transmission is not common and the overall prevalence of HIV is less than 1%. Most cases occur among homosexual or bisexual males and injecting drug users (IDUs).

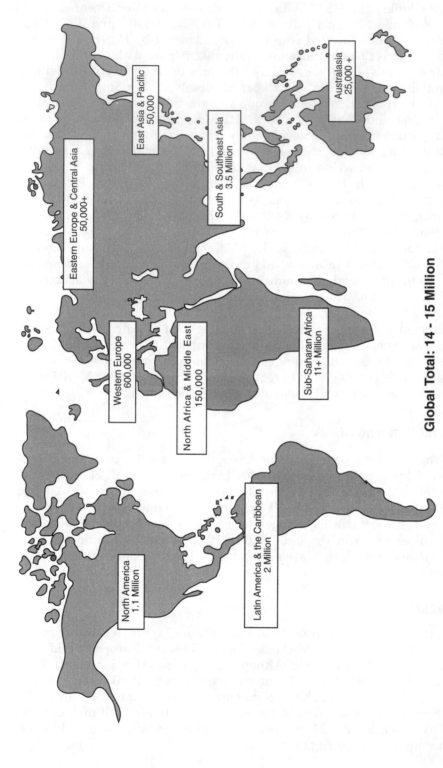

Global Total: 14 - 15 Million

Figure 1.1. Estimated distribution of total adult HIV infections from late 1970s/early 1980s to mid-1995. Source: Global Programme on AIDS. The Current Global Situation of the HIV/AIDS Pandemic, July 3, 1995. Geneva, Switzerland: World Health Organization, 1995.

PATTERN II

In Pattern II countries, heterosexual transmission accounts for most of the AIDS cases and the male-to-female ratio is approximately 1:1. Injecting drug use and homosexual transmission either occur rarely or not at all. Perinatal transmission is common, and transmission via contaminated blood/blood products is a factor in many countries. The national prevalence of HIV infections can exceed 1% and similar to pattern I countries, the extensive spread of HIV also began in the late 1970's. Pattern II countries include areas of sub-Saharan Africa and some Caribbean countries.

PATTERN I/II

Pattern I/II describes the epidemiologic pattern in Central and South America; the evolution from pattern I (initial AIDS cases primarily in homosexual/bisexual men and injecting drug users, recipients of HIV-contaminated blood or blood products) to pattern II (heterosexual transmission). The male-to-female ratio of HIV infection is decreasing, and the number of pediatric cases increasing. In pattern I/II areas, HIV began spreading extensively from the late 1970s to the early 1980s.

PATTERN III

In Pattern III countries, there are relatively few AIDS cases, which generally occur in people who travel to higher prevalence areas or who have had sexual contact with individuals from such areas. HIV was introduced in the mid- to late 1980s to pattern III countries, which include areas of Eastern Europe, North Africa, the Middle East, Asia and most of the Pacific, except for Australia and New Zealand.

Africa

The World Health Organization estimates more than 3 million adult AIDS cases have occurred in sub-Saharan Africa, accounting for more than two-thirds of the world total of AIDS cases (1). Approximately half to two-thirds of the cases infected in sub-Saharan Africa are in the East and Central area (2). Heterosexual transmission is the primary mode of transmission in this region (2). Perinatal transmission is a widespread problem, and transmission through receipt of contaminated blood and blood products accounts for a small proportion of total HIV infections (probably less than 10%) (2).

The pandemic is evolving, particularly in western and southern Africa. HIV has spread through Nigeria, with 1992 sentinel surveillance revealing HIV prevalence of 15% to 20% among some groups of female sex workers, and prevalence ranging from 0.5% to 22.1% in sexually transmitted disease (STD) clinics, and as high as 6% among pregnant women in one state. Data also suggest a threefold increase in HIV prevalence in women attending antenatal clinics in most regions of the Republic of South Africa between 1990 and 1992 (2). In Botswana, HIV prevalence greater than 20–30% has been observed among adults in major urban areas of Botswana (2).

North Africa and the Middle East

The few available studies suggest that HIV began to spread extensively in some parts of North Africa and the Middle East in the late 1980s (2). As of mid-1995, an estimated 150,000 adults are HIV infected in this region (1).

Eastern Europe and Central Asia

AIDS is still in an early phase in eastern Europe and the relative importance of the different transmission routes are not yet fully established (2). As of mid-1995, WHO estimated that there were over 50,000 cumulative HIV infections in Eastern Europe and Central Asia (1). Sexual transmission is believed to be the predominant route of HIV transmission in Eastern Europe (2). HIV prevalence among injecting drug users (IDUs) in Poland has been reported to be at least 10% since 1989 (2).

Localized outbreaks of HIV have occurred in infants and young children as a consequence of unsafe infection control practices. In the Russia Federation, several hundred children were infected through injections of medicines using shared syringes contaminated with HIV blood, and 1000 to 2000 children in Romania were infected through transfusions of unscreened blood, and possibly via the use of improperly sterilized or disinfected needles/syringes (2).

Asia and Southeast Asia

Japan, Singapore and Hong Kong have shown low prevalence rates, and the majority of HIV-infected persons are homosexuals (7,8). However, there is a rising prevalence rate among women, indicating that heterosexual transmission is becoming a factor (9,10).

The extensive spread of HIV began in South and Southeast Asia only in the mid- or late 1980s, but progression has been rapid. India and Thailand account for the majority of reported infections, with HIV spreading into specific populations in other parts of the region. Significant levels of HIV infection have been reported in Ho Chi Minh City, Vietnam; peninsular Malaysia, and Yunnan province, China (2). Between the late 1980s and 1992, HIV prevalence rates among IDUs in Bangkok, Thailand, Manipur, India and Yangon, Myanmar increased to 50% (2). Ten to thirty percent of IDUs in Yunan Province, China, have been found to be HIV infected. Because this province is contiguous with Southeast Asia, it is considered as part of the epidemic in Southeast Asia (11). Heterosexual transmission is increasing rapidly in certain groups. A rapid rise in HIV prevalence has been seen in Thailand among prostitutes and their clients and pregnant women (2,11,12). In 1991, median HIV prevalence rates of 21% were seen in female prostitutes, and

5.6% in people attending STD clinics (11). In India, HIV prevalence among STD patients in Pune, West India increased from 9% in 1991 to 17% in 1992 (11). Significant levels of HIV infection have been reported among female sex workers in several states of India, cities of Myanmar, and across Thailand, with HIV infection detected among female sex workers in Cambodia (2). 1992 data indicates HIV infection is spreading into Thailand's general population, with increasing HIV prevalence among military recruits and antenatal clinic attendees (2).

North America, Western Europe and Australasia

The predominant groups affected in these regions are men who have sex with men and injecting drug users (IDUs), as well as their sex partners. By mid-1995, over 1.7 million cumulative HIV infections are estimated to have occurred in this region (1) with over one million infections occurring in the United States alone (13).

HIV transmission patterns vary between and within these countries. In the eastern USA, up to 40% of persons with AIDS have been IDUs, while on the west coast, 90% of persons with AIDS are in men who have sex with men (2). Similarly, in northern Europe, homosexual/bisexual men account for more than 70% of the AIDS cases, whereas in southern Europe (particularly Spain and Italy), AIDS cases are primarily among IDUs (2,14). AIDS cases increased faster in the northern and central areas of Europe until 1987, but the spread of the epidemic has since been remarkably more rapid in southern Europe (14). The majority of cumulative AIDS cases in Europe have been reported from France, Spain and Italy (1).

While HIV incidence among homosexual men appears to be decreasing since the early to mid-1980s, HIV infection is increasing among IDUs, very young homosexual men, and heterosexuals in many areas (2,14). In both the USA and Western Europe, the proportion of new AIDS cases attributable to male-to-male sexual contact has been decreasing, while the proportion of cases attributed to IDU and heterosexual transmission is increasing (2). Heterosexual transmission of HIV increased during the late 1980s and early 1990s, particularly in urban populations with high rates of IDU and sexually transmitted diseases (2) [see Figure 1.2].

In Australia, HIV transmission is primarily attributed to sexual contact between men. Injecting drug use is reported in only a small proportion of persons with HIV and there is a low prevalence of HIV infection among IDUs. Heterosexual transmission appears to have been infrequent, possibly because of the low rate of HIV infection in IDUs (15).

Latin America and the Caribbean

As of mid-1995, there were an estimated 2 million cumulative adult HIV infections in Latin America and the Caribbean (1). The majority of AIDS cases from this region have been reported from Brazil, Mexico, Ar-

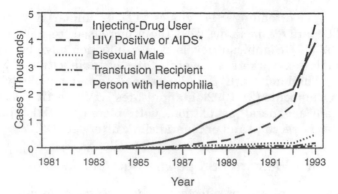

Figure 1.2. Number of AIDS cases attributed to heterosexual HIV transmission by partner's risk factor, United States, 1991–1993. *Partner's risk unknown or not reported. Source: Expanded AIDS surveillance case definition implemented. Source: CDC. Heterosexually acquired AIDS—United States, 1993. MMWR 1994;43:155–160.

gentina, Colombia, and Haiti (1). In Latin America, initial AIDS cases occurred among homosexual or bisexual men; however since the mid-1980s, there has been an increase in heterosexual transmission, primarily among bisexual men and their female partners, and female sex workers and their clients (2,11). Injecting drug use plays a variable role, but appears to be a growing problem in some areas. The prevalence of HIV infection among IDUs is reported to be high in Argentina (30% to 50%) and Brazil (20% to 60%) (2). The number of AIDS cases are increasing among women. In 1992, the male-to-female ratio of AIDS cases in Colombia was 5.3 compared to 75.0 in 1987 (17). Similarly in Mexico, this ratio declined from 25:1 in 1984 to 4:1 in 1990 (17).

Heterosexual transmission has been the primary mode of HIV transmission in the Caribbean (2). Heterosexual exposure accounts for 53% of all cases in the Dominican Republic, with a male-to-female ratio of 2.2:1 (18). A high proportion of AIDS cases are attributable to IDUs in Puerto Rico; although this is declining—from 70% of AIDS cases before 1988 to 59% in 1991 (19). Conversely, HIV infection acquired by heterosexual transmission is increasing from 5% of AIDS cases before 1988 to 18% in 1991 (19).

Global Projections

The WHO has made projections regarding the HIV/AIDS epidemic based on the current global data and recent epidemiological trends. However, WHO results are considered conservative, because WHO uses the lower limit of the estimated range (Table 1.1). By the year 2000, WHO projects a cumulative total of approximately 10 million adult AIDS cases, and 30–40 million HIV-infected adults and children worldwide; more than 90% of these infections will be in developing countries (2). WHO projects that the impact of AIDS in the 1990s will be greatest in large urban areas of sub-Saharan Africa, especially in Eastern and Central Africa (11). Currently one-fourth to one-third of all adults are

Table 1.1.

WHO Estimated and Projected HIV Prevalence in Adults by "Macro" Region

Region	Mid-1995 Estimated HIV prevalence[1]	2000 Projected HIV prevalence[2]
Australasia, Europe & North America	>1.2 million	1 million
Latin America & Caribbean	>1.5 million	>2 million
Africa	>8.5 million	>9 million
Asia	>3 million	8 million
Global Total	14–15 million	>20 million

[1]Total number of HIV-infected adults alive in mid-1995
[2]Total number of HIV-infected adults alive in the year 2000
Sources: World Health Organization Global Programme on AIDS. The Current Global Situation of the HIV/AIDS Pandemic. -WHO July 3, 1995. WHO:Geneva, 1995; World Health Organization Global Programme on AIDS. The HIV/AIDS Pandemic: 1994 Overview. WHO:Geneva, 1994.

HIV-infected in some cities of these regions so that expected population growth may be reduced more than 30% and the adult mortality tripled (11). WHO estimates that by the end of the 1990s, over 5 million children under 10 years of age will be orphans as a result of their mothers' HIV-related death (2). The proportion of new infections attributed to sexually active youths, especially in developing countries which have large numbers of young people, is likely to increase with time (2). Evidence of high incidence rates in young age groups compared to older cohorts in various countries indicates the urgent need for prevention programs directed towards youth.

REFERENCES

1. World Health Organization Global Programme on AIDS. The current global situation of the HIV/AIDS pandemic—July 3, 1995. World Health Organization: Geneva; 1995.
2. WHO Global Programme on AIDS. The HIV/AIDS Pandemic: 1994 Overview. World Health Organization: Geneva; 1995.
3. The Current Global Situation of the HIV/AIDS Pandemic—January 4, 1994. WHO Global Programme on AIDS. World Health Organization: Geneva; 1994.
4. Kallings LO. HIV Infection in the Nineties Vaccine. 1993;11:525–528.
5. Sato Paul A, Chin J, Mann JM. Review of AIDS and HIV infection: global epidemiology and statistics. AIDS 1989;3(suppl 1):S301–S307.
6. Mann JM, Chin J, Piot P, Quinn T. The international epidemiology of AIDS. Scientific American 1988;256:82–89.
7. Soda K, Fukutomi K, Hashimoto S, et al. Temporal trend and projection of HIV/AIDS epidemic in Japan. IX International Conference on AIDS Berlin 1993(abstr PO-CO8-2779).
8. Lee SS, Lim WL, Lee SH, et al. Epidemiology of HIV infection in Hong Kong—Analysis of the First 300 Cases. IX International Conference on AIDS Berlin 1993(abstr PO-CO8-2780).
9. Conferences Summary Report. VIII international conference on AIDS/III STD World Congress. Amsterdam, The Netherlands, July 19–24, 1992.
10. Chew SK. Trends in human immunodeficiency virus infection: Epidemiology in Singapore. Ann Acad Med Singapore 1993;22:142–145.
11. WHO Global Programme on AIDS. The HIV/AIDS Pandemic: 1993 Overview World Health Organization: Geneva; 1993.

12. Siriwasin W, Singhaneti S, Kaewchaiyo G, et al. Rapid rise in maternal HIV-1 sero-prevalence. IX International Conference on AIDS, Bangkok, Thailand, 1993(abstr PO-C08-2767).
13. CDC. HIV prevalence estimates and AIDS case projections for the United States: report based on a workshop. MMWR 1990; 29:30.
14. Serraino D, Franceschi S, Tirelli U, Monfardini S. The epidemiology of Acquired Immunodeficiency Syndrome and associated tumours in Europe. Ann Oncol 1992; 3:595–603.
15. Kaldor J. Epidemiological pattern of HIV infection in Australia. J Acquir Immune Defic Syndr 1993; 6(suppl 1):S1–S4.
16. Marino M, Castano LD, Suarez J, et al. Spread of HIV/AIDS to the female population in Colombia. IX International Conference on AIDS. Berlin June 1993. (abstr PO-C06-2720).
17. Mexico Ministry of Health: Boletin Mensual SIDA/ETS, 1990; 4:1017.
18. Garris I, Rodriguez EM, DeMoya EA, et al. AIDS Heterosexual Predominance in the Dominican Republic. J Acquir Immune Defic Synd 1991;4:1173–1178.
19. CDC. Heterosexual transmission of HIV—Puerto Rico: 1981–1991. MMWR 1992; 41:899–906.

United States

At the end of October 1995, over 500,000 persons had been reported with acquired immunodeficiency syndrome (AIDS) in the United States (1). Approximately one million people in the USA are estimated to be infected with HIV (2). In 1992 AIDS became the eighth leading cause of death in the United States (3) and national trends indicate that HIV infection/AIDS continues to cause an increasing proportion of all deaths in the United States, particularly among women, young adults age 25–44, adolescents, and racial/ethnic populations (1,4–8). There are also larger proportionate increases in reported AIDS cases among injecting drug users (IDUs) and their heterosexual partners, other persons infected through heterosexual contact, as well as among persons from the South and Midwest (1,6,7,9). The epidemiological trends reflect the evolving nature of the HIV epidemic in the United States, which consists of multiple epidemics in different regions and among different groups.

The AIDS surveillance case definition has been expanded twice, in late 1987 and again in 1993, to reflect the increased knowledge of the natural history of HIV and to be consistent with its clinical management (10,11). Following the 1993 expansion of the AIDS surveillance case definition to include all those with less than 200 CD4T cells/μL, the number of AIDS cases reported in 1993 significantly increased. However, this was a one-time and transient effect. The number of AIDS cases reported in 1994 declined compared to 1993 but remained substantially higher than in 1992 (12,13). Before 1993, trends in AIDS incidence were evaluated by examining the number of AIDS opportunistic illnesses (AIDS-OI) diagnosed per year or quarter (8). Since most HIV-infected persons become severely immunosuppressed before the onset of AIDS-OIs, the addition of the CD4 levels criteria temporarily distorted observed trends in AIDS incidence. Consequently CDC developed a procedure to estimate the incidence of AIDS-OIs among persons reported with AIDS

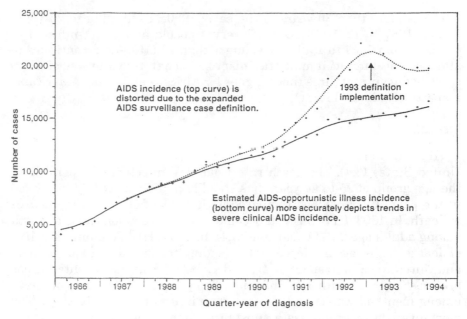

Figure 1.3. AIDS incidence, and estimated AIDS-opportunistic illness incidence (adjusting for delays in reporting) by quarter-year of diagnosis, January 1986 through June 1994, United States. Source: CDC. HIV/AIDS Surveillance Report. Year-end Edition. Atlanta GA: CDC. 1994:6(2).

based on the CD4 criteria (8). AIDS incidence and estimates of trends in AIDS-OIs from January 1986 through 1994 are shown in Figure 1.3.

Epidemiological Trends

Men having sex with men remains the major mode of exposure among AIDS cases (52%) in the United States, followed by injecting drug use (25%) and heterosexual contact (8%) (8). However, epidemiological trends demonstrate that the proportion of AIDS cases attributed to men who have sex with men is decreasing, while the proportion of cases attributed to injecting drug use (IDU) and heterosexual contact is increasing. The proportion of persons with AIDS infected through male-male sexual contact decreased from 64% during 1981–1987 to 45% during 1993–October 1995, periods corresponding to changes in the AIDS definition (1). During the same period, reported AIDS cases attributed to injecting drug use increased from 17% to 27%, and those attributed to heterosexual transmission increased from 3% to 10% (1). The increase in AIDS cases from IDU and heterosexual contact is reflected in the increase of cases reported for women; the proportion of AIDS cases among women increased from 8% during 1981–1987 to 18% during 1993–October 1995 (1). The number of pediatric AIDS cases are also projected to increase as it is closely associated with the epidemic in women (14). The estimated median age at the time of HIV infection in the United States has substantially declined (15). The median age at the time of HIV infection was more than 30 years in the early 1980s, decreasing to 25 years during 1987 to 1991 (15). One of every 4 people newly HIV-infected in the U.S. from 1987 to 1991 was younger than 22 (15). AIDS continues to affect ethnic and racial minorities disproportionately, with rates of AIDS cases being six and three times higher for African- and Latin-Americans, respectively, than whites (1).

Mortality

HIV infection is the eighth leading cause of death overall in the United States (3,4). The death rate from HIV infections for persons in the age group of 25 to 44 years has steadily and dramatically increased in the past 10 years when compared with rates of other leading causes of death. In 1993, HIV infection became the most common cause of death among adults age 25–44 years old (3,4). In 1994, HIV accounted for 19% of deaths in this age group, being the leading cause of death among men, and third among women (Figs. 1.4 and 1.5) (4). Large metropolitan areas are most affected with HIV infection, being the leading cause of death among men and women of this age group in a number of cities (5). The mortality in this group has a substantial impact on society because of the loss of productive years of life and the loss of parents from families with young children. HIV infection has become a leading cause of premature mortality, being in 1994 the fourth leading cause of years of potential life lost before age 65 (4).

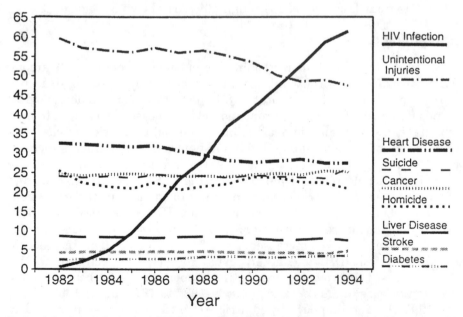

Figure 1.4. Death Rates (per 100,000 population) from leading causes of death among men aged 25–44 years, by year—United States, 1982–1994. National vital statistics based on underlying cause of death, using final data for 1982–1992 and provisional data for 1993–1994. Source: CDC. Update: Mortality Attributable to HIV Infection Among Persons aged 25–44—United States, 1994. MMWR 1996;45:121–125.

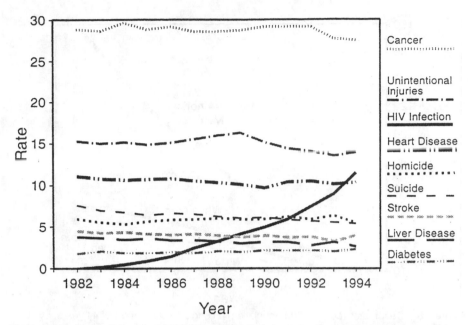

Figure 1.5. Death Rates (per 100,000 population) from leading causes of death among women aged 35–44 years, by year—United States, 1982–1994. National vital statistics based on underlying cause of death, using final data for 1982–1992 and provisional data for 1993–1994. Source: CDC. Update: Mortality Attributable to HIV Infection Among Persons aged 25–44—United States, 1994. MMWR 1996;45:121–125.

Among persons in this age group, HIV infection became the most common cause of death for African-American men in 1991, for all men (all racial/ethnic groups combined) in 1992, and for white men in 1994 (4). HIV-related mortality trends reflect the changes in the demographic patterns of HIV. Young adults of certain populations have been particularly affected with HIV death rates for women and African-American men increasing (Figure 1.6). Among males 25 to 44 years old, HIV infection was the leading cause of death for Whites and African-Americans in 1994 (4). Among females in the same age group, HIV infection was the fifth leading cause of death for whites, and the leading cause of death for African-Americans (4). Data available from 1991 for other ethnic/racial populations of this age group, reveal HIV infection as the leading cause of death for Latin American males, and the sixth leading cause of death for Asian/Pacific Islander and American Indians/Alaskan Native males (6). Among females in this age group, HIV infection was the third leading cause of death for Latin-Americans, seventh for American Indians/ Alaskan Natives, and ninth for Asians/Pacific Islanders in 1991 (6).

Geographical Distribution

Approximately 59% of AIDS cases reported in the United States and its territories through mid-1995 have been reported from New York, California, Florida, Texas and New Jersey (8). Rates of AIDS cases remain highest in the Northeast, Florida and Puerto Rico (8). Cities with the

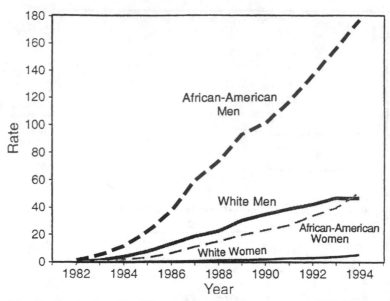

Figure 1.6.   Death rates (per 100,000 population) among persons aged 25–44 years, by sex, race (Data were unavailable for races other than white and black), and year—United States, 1982–1994. National vital statistics based on underlying cause of death, using final data for 1982–1992 and provisional data for 1993–1994. Source: CDC. Update: Mortality Attributable to HIV Infection Among Persons aged 25–44—United States, 1994. MMWR 1996;45: 121–125.

highest reported annual rates of AIDS include: San Francisco, CA (131 AIDS cases per 100,000 population); Miami, FL (147); New York, NY (125.6); Jersey City, NJ (161), and Ft. Lauderdale, FL (116) (8). AIDS annual rates in the United States reported for July 1994 through June 1995 are shown in Figures 1.7 and 1.8 (8). Although the majority of AIDS cases are predominantly in large metropolitan areas, the number as well as the rate of cases being reported from smaller cities and rural communities indicates a continuing increasing trend (1,8). Changing geographic patterns are reflected by the increases in cases occurring in the South and Midwest regions of the United States (1). The proportionate increases in reported AIDS cases from 1988–1992 to 1993–October 1995 for the South Midwest, Northeast, and West regions were 31%, 22%, 20%, and 15%, respectively (1).

Men Who Have Sex With Men (MSM)

Through mid-1995, males accounted for 86% of all AIDS cases, with male-to-male sexual contact accounting for 60% of cumulative AIDS cases among adults and adolescents (8). The large number of AIDS cases among men who have sex with men (MSM) reflect the rapid spread of HIV infection in the initial years of the epidemic. However, there has been a continuing decline in the proportion of AIDS cases among MSM in the United States (1,17,18). Significant changes have been reported among men participating in cohort and follow-up studies. In a San Francisco male cohort, the annual seroconversion rate peaked in 1982 (20%), but declined to less than 1% in 1987 (19,20). HIV infection and other STDs (a proxy marker for behaviors associated with sexual HIV transmission) have also been reported to decline among homosexual/bisexual men in some regions of the United States (7). The decline in new HIV infections began in the mid-1980s, and contribute to the recent slower rate of increase in AIDS cases among homosexual/bisexual men (21). Fewer sex partners, decrease in anal intercourse, and greater condom use have been correlated to declines

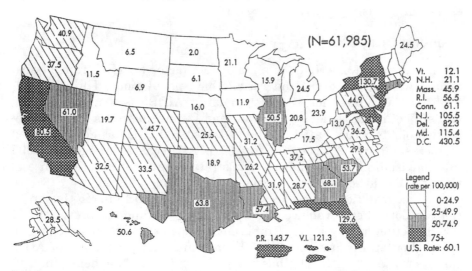

Figure 1.7. Male adult/adolescent AIDS annual rates per 100,000 population of AIDS cases reported July 1994 through June 1995, United States. Source: CDC. HIV/AIDS Surveillance Report. Mid-Year Edition. Atlanta, GA: CDC 1995:7(1).

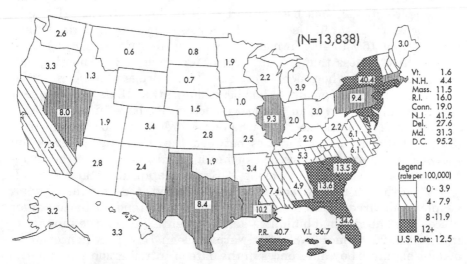

Figure 1.8. Female adult/adolescent AIDS annual rates per 100,000 population of AIDS cases reported July 1994 through June 1995, United States. Source: CDC. HIV/AIDS Surveillance Report. Mid-Year Edition, Atlanta GA: CDC; 1995–7(1).

in HIV rates (22–24). However, relapse from safer sex to riskier practices has been reported (25). There is also evidence that high-risk behaviors are being practiced by nonwhite homosexual/bisexual men, young homosexual/bisexual males, as well as homosexual men residing in small cities outside the epicenters (25–29). AIDS rates in rural metropolitan statistical areas (MSAs) (i.e., population less than 50,000) increased 69% from mid-1989 to mid-1994 (2.6 to 4.4 per 100,000 males ≥13 years), and increased 55% in areas with populations of 50,000–1 million (mid-1994 rate:10.2) (18). Areas with populations over 2.5 million reported the smallest 5-year percentage increase (19%) (18).

Injecting Drug Use

Injecting drug use (IDU) is a major risk factor for HIV transmission among women, children, and racial/ethnic populations. Through mid-1995 IDU accounted for 47% of cumulative AIDS cases among women, and 40% of all cases among African- and Latin-Americans (8). The proportion of AIDS cases attributed to heterosexual IDU has demonstrated an increasing trend, accounting for 25% of AIDS cases through mid-1995 (8). Longitudinal trends have demonstrated that the seroprevalence of HIV in IDUs in some areas is stable or decreasing (30–32).

The geographical differences in the rates of AIDS mirror the variations in both the prevalence of injecting drug use and the prevalence of HIV infection among IDUs in different groups or geographic areas (33). Throughout the course of the HIV epidemic, the proportion of AIDS cases associated with IDU has been higher in the Northeast than in other regions (32,33). The seroprevalence of HIV infection among IDUs in the U.S. is highest among drug users in New York City, the metropolitan areas in the Northeast and the Atlantic coast states including Florida, and Puerto Rico (32,34). HIV seroprevalence among IDUs outside the Northeast has been reported to be lower (6,31). HIV seroprevalence rates for IDUs enrolled in drug treatment programs have ranged from 15% to 40% in most cities along the Atlantic coast and in Puerto Rico to less than 7% in most other areas (32). "Shooting galleries" are places where people inject ("shoot") drugs with borrowed or rented injection equipment. It has been shown that IDUs who frequent shooting galleries, even in low-prevalence cities, have higher HIV infection rates compared to IDUs who do not frequent shooting galleries (35,36). Differing characteristics between the "shooting galleries" on the west coast and those in the Northeast may be a factor in the variation of HIV seroprevalence among IDUs geographically. "Shooting galleries" on the west coast tend to be small, and visited by relatively few people, compared to those in New York, which tend to be in larger places (e.g., abandoned buildings) and frequented by a large number of injectors (100 or more) (37–39). Variations in HIV prevalence might also be explained by differences in the date of introduction of virus into different communities, racial or socioeconomic factors, and different risk behaviors that promote transmission. Other factors may also be related to differences in sexual behaviors, needle-sharing practices or access to drug treatment.

Women

AIDS cases among women have increased rapidly in the United States since 1981, becoming the fourth leading causes of death in women of reproductive age in 1993 (16). Approximately 14% of cumulative AIDS cases reported in adults and adolescents are women; (8) with the proportion of cases among women increasing steadily since 1985 (16). During 1981–1987, females accounted for 8% of the AIDS cases; during 1993–October 1995 this proportion increased to 19% (1). Eighty-one percent of women with AIDS are of childbearing age (13–44 years) and approximately three-quarters of the cases are among African- and Latin-American women (8). In 1994, the rates for African- and Latin-American women were 16 and 7 times higher, respectively than those for white women (16). HIV infection in women of reproductive age has a direct consequence to AIDS in children; 90% of HIV-infected children have mothers with/at risk for HIV (8).

Most women with AIDS live in urban metropolitan areas, inject drugs (or have sex partners who do), are women of color, and are of reproductive age. Generally, AIDS is more prevalent among women residing in metropolitan counties than in other areas, with the most cases reported from large metropolitan areas in the Northeast (16,40,41). The concentration of injecting drug use in the Northeast cities may account for the disproportionate rates of HIV found in women in these geographical areas (40). National serosurveys of childbearing women demonstrated the highest HIV seroprevalence rates in New York, New Jersey, Florida, and Puerto Rico, areas which also report the greatest numbers of AIDS cases associated with injecting drug use (32,41–43). However, the proportion of women with AIDS reported in smaller cities and rural areas has been increasing (16,44).

Eighty-three percent of all AIDS cases among women are attributed to injecting drug use and heterosexual contact (8). Compared to males, a greater percentage of female adult cases are attributed to IDU (47% vs. 22% for males) (1). In addition, heterosexual contact is the only transmission category where the number of cases in women outnumber men (8). HIV transmission by heterosexual contact is closely linked to IDU, with approximately half of heterosexually acquired AIDS cases among women attributed to sexual contact with an IDU (8). Twelve percent of women with AIDS could not identify a risk for HIV infection (8); since many women and their health providers may be unaware of the woman's or her partners' risk for HIV infection, this may represent unrecognized heterosexual contact (45,46). Increased heterosexual transmission among some women may be attributed to the high rates of sexually transmitted diseases associated with the use of noninjecting drugs and with the exchange of sex for drugs, money, and personal items (47). Women who may have sex with other women may also be at risk for HIV infection if they inject drugs or have partners with high-risk behaviors (48).

Adolescents

Among young people age 15 to 24 years of age, HIV infection and AIDS is the sixth leading cause of death (49). By mid-1995, over 2,000 adolescents (ages 13 to 19) and 17,700 young adults (20–24 years of age) were reported with AIDS (8). Considering the long latency period associated with HIV disease, it is likely that young adults were infected as adolescents, and describe the risk behaviors for acquiring HIV infection as teens. Heterosexual contact plays a large role particularly for females, accounting for 53% of female adolescent cases (8). While the ratio for U.S. adults with AIDS is approximately 6 males to one female, the ratio is 3:1 for young adults, and 2:1 among adolescents (8). An even ratio of males to females with AIDS is generally considered an indication of heterosexual transmission. Although treatment for a hemophilia/coagulation disorder represents the most frequent mode of HIV transmission among adolescents (28%), HIV infection attributed to this mode of exposure has been virtually nonexistent, since the implementation of HIV screening of blood and blood products (1985) and heat treatment for clotting factors. Cases in this exposure category primarily represent persons who received blood products before 1985.

HIV exposures among adolescents vary by age, sex, and race/ethnicity. The majority of adolescents between ages 13 and 16 acquired HIV through exposure to blood or blood products, while injecting drug use and sexual activity are the primary routes of exposure for older adolescents with AIDS (17 to 19 years) (50). Cumulatively, hemophilia/coagulation disorder (43%) and male-male sexual contact (33%) are the primary exposure categories for male adolescents with AIDS (8). The most frequent modes of HIV transmission among female adolescents are heterosexual contact (53%) and injecting drug use (16%); 22% reported or identified no risk for HIV (8). HIV exposure categories vary by race among male adolescents; treatment for hemophilia/coagulation disorder accounts for a majority of AIDS cases among white male adolescents, whereas the majority of cases among African-Americans are attributed to male-male sexual contact and coagulation disorder and male-male sexual contact for Latin-Americans (50). For female adolescents of all racial groups, heterosexual contact transmission and IDU are the primary modes of HIV exposure (50).

Recent seroprevalence data indicate that a substantial number of adolescents are currently infected with HIV. These are based on population-based seroprevalence studies that include adolescents, e.g., military, Job Corps, Department of Defense, runaway centers, university health centers, and STD clinics (32,50). Relatively high HIV seroprevalence has been shown among female adolescents in several states. Adolescents initially identified as being at high risk of infection were homeless, gay, prostitutes, and injecting drug users. However, HIV is also concentrated among sexually active adolescents in large urban areas, and spreading to less urban areas. Adolescents living in urban areas with high sero-prevalence rates of HIV (particularly in the Northeast and the South) have higher infection rates probably because of the greater likelihood of encountering an infected partner (50).

However, HIV is also concentrated among sexually active adolescents in large urban areas, and spreading to less urban areas. Compared with the Northeast and the West, a higher proportion of AIDS cases among adolescents and young adults (ages 13–29 years), particularly cases resulting from IDUs, heterosexual contact, and men who have sex with men occurred in small (50,000–499,999 populations) metropolitan statistical areas (MSAs) and non-MSAs (rural areas) during 1993–October 1995 (1).

Children

Although pediatric cases account for less than 2% of the AIDS cases reported in the United States (8), AIDS has become a major cause of death among young children in some locations (51). In New York, HIV/AIDS was the leading cause of death among African- and Latin-American children ages 1 to 4 years (51,52). It is estimated that approximately 1,800 newly infected infants are born each year in the United States (41). Because most pediatric AIDS cases are attributed to perinatal infection (90%) (8) the number of children with AIDS in the United States will increase as HIV infection is increasingly reported among women of childbearing age. Of children born to mothers with or at risk for HIV, most mothers were exposed to HIV through IDU (41%) or heterosexual contact (33%) (8). Zidovudine therapy has been recommended for infected pregnant women and their newborns as an effective means for reducing the risk for perinatal HIV transmission (53).

Racial/Ethnic Minority Populations

Racial/ethnic minority populations accounted for 48% of adult (≥13 years) male AIDS cases, 76% of adult female cases, and 82% of pediatric cases through mid-1995 (8). The major modes of HIV exposure vary among racial/ethnic minorities. Among African- and Latin-American males, injecting drug use and male-male sexual contact are the major modes of transmission, while MSM accounts for the majority of AIDS cases among White, Asian/Pacific Islander, and American Indian/Alaska Native males (See Table 1.2). IDU and heterosexual contact are the major modes of exposures for racial/ethnic minority women, with the exception of Asian/Pacific Islander women, where heterosexual contact and receipt of blood transfusion, blood components or tissue were the primary modes of exposure (8).

While Asians/Pacific Islanders and American Indians/Alaskan Natives represent less than 1% of AIDS cases in the United States, (1) African- and Latin-Americans continue to be more severely affected than other racial/ethnic populations. Although African- and Latin-Americans represent 12% and 6% of the population in the U.S., respectively,

Table 1.2.

Percent of U.S. Adult/Adolescent AIDS Cases by Primary HIV Exposure and Ethnicity Reported Through June 1995

Exposure Category	African-American % of Male Cases	African-American % of Female Cases	Latin-American % of Male Cases	Latin-American % of Female Cases	Asian/Pacific Islander % of Male Cases	Asian/Pacific Islander % of Female Cases	White % of Male Cases	White % of Female Cases
Men who have sex with men (MSM)	40%	—	45%	—	78%	—	77%	—
Injecting drug use (IDU)	36%	50%	38%	45%	5%	18%	8%	43%
Men who have sex with men and IDU	8%	—	7%	—	3%	—	8%	—
Heterosexual contact	5%	33%	4%	44%	2%	44%	1%	37%
Receipt-blood transfusion blood comp, tissue	1%	2%	1%	3%	3%	21%	1%	10%
Risk not reported or identified	10%	15%	6%	7%	8%	16%	3%	9%
Cumulative AIDS cases	121,017	35,372	68,051	13,293	2,667	325	211,856	15,570

Source: CDC. HIV/AIDS Surveillance Report. Mid-Year End Edition. Atlanta GA: CDC. 1995;7(1).

they account for approximately 34% and 17% of persons with AIDS, respectively (8). Seventy-five percent of AIDS cases among women, and 81% of pediatric AIDS cases are among African- and Latin-Americans (8). The disproportionate rates of AIDS cases reported in African- and Latin-American reflect the higher rate of AIDS in African- and Latin-American IDUs, their sex partners and infants. Recent trends demonstrate that the rate of AIDS continues to increase disproportionately among African- and Latin-Americans compared to Whites (17,54). The increase is associated more with the rising number of AIDS cases attributed to heterosexual than with IDU transmission. From 1988 to 1991, the percent of reported AIDS cases reported associated with heterosexual transmission increased from 10.7% to 14.0% among African-Americans, and from 5.5% to 7.1% for Latin-Americans (54). During this same time period, history of IDU exposure among AIDS cases decreased from 41% to 39% for African-Americans, and 37% to 34% for Latin-Americans, (54). Among African- and Latin-Americans, AIDS incidence rates are 6 and 3 times higher than among Whites, respectively (1). African- and Latin-American women have cumulative incidence rates of AIDS that are 13 and 8 times, respectively, higher than those of white women (44). Nearly every serosurveillance survey has reported HIV seroprevalence to be substantially higher among African-Americans than Whites (32). Data from Latin Americans have been less consistent. HIV seroprevalence is similar to Whites in western states, while higher than Whites in the Atlantic coast states (32). Morality rates for HIV infection also reflect racial differences. The 1994 death rate from HIV infection (per 100,000 population) was almost four times as high for African-American men (177.9) as for White men (47.2) and nine times as high for African-American women (51.2) as for White women (5.7) (4).

Race and ethnic differences, themselves, are probably not risk factors for HIV transmission but are markers for underlying social, economic and cultural factors, and personal behaviors that affect health. Socioeconomic status is associated with morbidity and premature mortality in general. Unemployment, poverty and illiteracy are associated with decreased access to health education, prevention services and medical care, all of which result in increased risk for disease. Compared to Asians/Pacific Islanders (13%) and Whites (10%), a higher percentage of African-Americans (33%) and Latin-Americans (29%) lived below the federal poverty level, compared with Asians/Pacific Islanders (13%) and Whites (10%) (55). Rates of AIDS and modes of HIV exposure may vary greatly by geographic regions among and within racial/ethnic populations. Geographic and racial/ethnic differences relate directly to variations in the prevalence of HIV infection, the type and frequency of behaviors associated with HIV transmission, and the time that HIV was introduced into the specific communities; they relate indirectly to the social, economic, and cultural influences within those communities (6). The incidence of AIDS and distribution of HIV modes of exposure also varies among Asian/Pacific Islanders and Latin-Americans relative to their place of birth (6). In addition, a greater proportion of racial/ethnic populations may be initially classified as without a known risk for HIV because of unrecognized heterosexual exposures, diagnosis of AIDS at or near death, or language and cultural differences that make ascertaining risk more difficult (6).

Transfusion with Blood and Blood Products

Less than 2% of AIDS cases reported in the United States through mid-1995 have been attributed through receipt of blood, blood components, or tissue (8). The implementation of screening of blood and blood products for HIV antibody (in 1985), with procedures such as heat treatment of factor concentrates (in 1984), and self-deferral of blood donors, has resulted in decreases of AIDS cases among persons with hemophilia and among transfusion recipients. Most new cases of AIDS associated with receipt of blood, blood products, and tissues reflect HIV transmission before screening was available (56). There is still a very small risk of HIV infection from receipt of a blood transfusion, since units of blood may be tested for HIV antibody when there are no detectable antibodies by the screening test (e.g., during the window period, dilution of blood resulting from receipt of other transfusions).

The additional safety measure of screening all blood and plasma donations for HIV-1 p234 antigen recommended by the Food and Drug Administration (FDA) in August 1995 is expected to reduce the number of otherwise undetected infectious donations by approximately 25% per year.

Health Care Setting

There have been 46 documented occupational cases of HIV transmission in health care workers (HCWs) in the United States through mid-1995 (8). Health care workers are defined by the CDC as those persons, including students and trainees, who have worked in a health care, clinical or HIV laboratory setting at any time since 1978. Of these occupational exposures, 40 had percutaneous exposure, four with mucocutaneous exposure, one had both percutaneous and mucocutaneous exposures, and one had an unknown route of exposure (8). Most of the exposures were to blood from an HIV-infected person (41), with one to visibly bloody fluid, one to an unspecified fluid, and three to concentrated virus in a laboratory. Twenty of these HCWs have developed AIDS. There are 97 additional possible cases of occupational HIV transmission. These HCWs had no identifiable behavioral or transfusion risks; each reported percutaneous or mucocutaneous occupational exposures to blood or body fluids, or laboratory solutions containing HIV, but HIV seroconversion specifically resulting from an occupational exposure was not documented.

Transmission from a health care worker to patients has also been reported. An investigation of a Florida dentist with AIDS concluded that HIV was transmitted to six of his patients (57). However, it now appears that other modes of exposure to HIV has not been ruled out for these six persons. Lookback studies of patients treated by other infected health care workers have identified other HIV-infected patients who were treated by an infected HCW, but have not demonstrated the HCW as a source of infection (58).

REFERENCES

1. CDC. First 500,000 AIDS Cases—United States, 1995. MMWR 1995;44:849–853.
2. CDC. HIV prevalence estimates and AIDS case projections for the United States: report based on a workshop. MMWR 1990;29:30.
3. CDC. Update: Mortality attributable to HIV infection among persons aged 25–44 years—United States, 1991 and 1992. MMWR 1993;42:869–872.
4. CDC. Mortality Attributable to HIV infection/among persons aged 25–44 years—United States, 1994. MMWR 1996;45:121–125.
5. Selik RM, Chu SY, and Buehler JW. HIV infection as leading cause of death among young adults in US cities and states. JAMA 1993;269:2991–2994.
6. CDC. AIDS among racial/ethnic minorities—United States, 1993. MMWR 1994; 43:644–647, 653–655.
7. CDC. Update: Acquired Immunodeficiency Syndrome—United States, 1991. MMWR 1992;41:463–468.
8. CDC. HIV/AIDS Surveillance Report. 1995 Mid-year edition; 1995;7:1.
9. CDC. Heterosexually acquired AIDS—United States, 1993. MMWR 1994;43:155–160.
10. CDC. Revision of the CDC surveillance case definition for acquired immunodeficiency syndrome. MMWR 1987;36:(suppL 1).
11. CDC. 1993 Revised classification system for HIV infection and expanded surveillance case definition for AIDS among adolescents and adults. MMWR 1992;41(no. RR-17).
12. CDC. HIV/AIDS Surveillance Report. Year-end Edition 1994 6(2).
13. CDC. Update: Impact of the expanded AIDS surveillance case definition for adolescents and adults on case reporting—United States, 1993. MMWR 1994;43:160–1, 167–70.
14. CDC. Projections of the number of persons diagnosed with AIDS and the number of immunosuppressed HIV-infected persons—United States, 1992–1994. MMWR 1992;41(RR-18).
15. Rosenberg PS, Biggar RJ, Goedert JJ. Declining age at HIV infection in the United States. N Engl J Med 1994;330:789–90.
16. CDC. Update: AIDS Among Women-United States, 1994. MMWR 1995;44:81–84.
17. CDC. Update: acquired immunodeficiency syndrome—United States, 1994. MMWR 1995;44:64–67.
18. CDC. Update trends in AIDS among men who have sex with men—United States, 1989–1994. MMWR 1995;44:401–404.
19. Winkelstein W, Wiley JA, Padian NS, et al. The San Francisco Men's Health Study. Continued decline in HIV seroconversion rates among homosexual/bisexual men. Am J Public Health 1988;78:1472–1474.
20. Hessol NA, Lifson A, O'Malley PM, et al. Prevalence, incidence, and progression of human immunodeficiency virus infection in homosexual and bisexual men in hepatitis B vaccine trials, 1979–1988. Am J Epidemiol 1989;130:1167–1175.
21. Karon JM, Berkelman RL. The geographic ethnic diversity of AIDS incidence trends in homosexual/bisexual men in the United States. J Acquir Immune Defic Syndr 1991;4:1179–89.
22. Winkelstein W, Samuel M, Padian NS, et al. The San Francisco Men's Health Study. III. Reduction in human immunodeficiency virus transmission among homosexual/bisexual men, 1982–1986. Am J Public Health 1987;77:685–689.
23. Becker MH, Joseph JG. AIDS and behavioural change to reduce risk. Am J Public Health 1988;78:394–410.
24. Coutinho RA, van Griensven GJP, Moss A. Effects of preventive efforts among homosexual men. AIDS 1989;3(suppl 1):253–256.
25. Stall R, Ekstrand M, Pollack L, et al. Relapse from safer sex: the next challenge for AIDS prevention efforts. J Acquir Immune Defic Syndr 1990;3:1181–1187.
26. Hays RB, Kegeles SM, Coates TJ. High HIV risk taking young among young gay men. AIDS 1990;4(90):901–907.
27. Dean L, Meyer I. Rates of unprotected anal and oral sex in a cohort of young gay men in New York City, 1990–1991. IX International Conference of AIDS. Berlin, Germany, June 1993;(abstract PO-C12-2884).

28. Hirozawa AM, Givertz D, Lemp G, et al. Prevalence of HIV-1 among young gay and bisexual men in San Francisco and Berkeley, CA: The second young men's survey. IX International Conference of AIDS. Berlin, Germany, June 1993;(abstract PO-C12-2875).
29. Kelly JA, Lawrence JS, Brasfield TL, et al. AIDS risk behavior patterns among gay men in small southern cities. Am J Public Health 1990;80:416–417.
30. Moss AR, Vranizan K, Gorter R, et al. HIV seroconversion in intravenous drug users in San Francisco, 1985–1990. AIDS 1994;8:223–231.
31. Des Jarlais DC, Friedman SR, Novick DM, et al. HIV-1 infection among intravenous drug users in Manhattan, New York City, from 1977 through 1987. JAMA 1989; 261:1008–1012.
32. CDC. National HIV Serosurveillance Summary. Results through 1992. Volume 3. Atlanta, GA: U.S. Dept. Health and Human Services; 1994.
33. CDC. Update: Acquired immunodeficiency syndrome associated with intravenous-drug use—United States, 1988. MMWR 1989;38:165–170.
34. Hahn RA, Onorato IM, Jones TS, et al. Prevalence of HIV infection among intravenous drug users in the United States. JAMA 1989;261:2677–2684.
35. Chaisson RE, Bacchetti P, Osmond D, et al. Cocaine use and HIV infection in intravenous drug users in San Francisco. JAMA 1989;261:561–565.
36. Des Jarlais DC. The first and second decades of AIDS among injecting drug users. British J Addiction 1992;87:347–353.
37. Des Jarlais DC, Friedman SR, Strug D. AIDS and needle sharing within the IV drug use subculture. In Feldman DA, Johnson TM. eds. The social dimensions of AIDS: Methods and theory. New York: Praeger 1986;11–125.
38. Watters J. Observations on the importance of social context in HIV transmission among intravenous drug users. J Drug Issues 1989;19:9–26.
39. Longshore D, Anglin MD, Henson KD, Annon K. HIV transmission and risk behavior among drug users in Los Angeles County, 1993 Update. Los Angeles: UCLA Drug Abuse Research Center, 1993.
40. Caussy D and Goedert J. The epidemiology of human immunodeficiency virus and Acquired Immunodeficiency Syndrome. Seminars in Oncology 1990;17(3);244–250.
41. Gwinn M, Pappaioanou M, George JR, et al. Prevalence of HIV infection in childbearing women in the United States. JAMA 1991;265:1704–1708.
42. Sweeney PA, Onorato IM, Allen DM, et al. Sentinel surveillance of human immunodeficiency virus infection in women seeking reproductive health services in the United States, 1988–1989. Obstet Gynecol April 1992;79(4):503–510.
43. CDC. Update: Acquired immunodeficiency syndrome associated with intravenous-drug use—United States, 1988. MMWR 1989;38;165–70.
44. Ellerbrock T, Bush T, Chamberland M, et al. Epidemiology of women with AIDS in the United States, 1981 through 1990: a comparison with heterosexual men with AIDS. JAMA 1991;265:2971–2975.
45. Castro KG, Lifson AR, White CR, et al: Investigations of AIDS patients with no previously identified risk factors. JAMA 1988;259:1338.
46. CDC. Heterosexually acquired AIDS-United States, 1993. MMWR 1994;43:155–60.
47. Edlin BR, Irwin KL, Faruque S, et al. Intersecting epidemics: crack cocaine use and HIV infection among inner-city young adults. N Engl J Med 1994;331:1422–7.
48. Chu SY, Hammett TA, Buehler JW. Update: epidemiology of reported cases of AIDS in women who report sex only with other women, 1980–1991. AIDS 1992;6:518–9.
49. National Center for Health Statistics. Advance report of final mortality statistics, 1991. Monthly vital statistics report. Hyattsville, MD: Public Health Service 1993; 42(suppl 2).
50. Lindegren ML, Hanson C, Miller K, et al. Epidemiology of human immunodeficiency virus infection in adolescents, United States. Pediatr Infect Dis J 1994;13:525–35.
51. CDC. Mortality attributable to HIV infection/AIDS-United States, 1981–90. MMWR Jan 25 1991;40(3):41–44.
52. Chu Sy, Buehler JW, Oxtoby MJ, et al. Impact of the human immunodeficiency virus epidemic on mortality in children, United States. Pediatrics 1991;87:806–810.
53. CDC. Recommendations of the U.S. Public Health Service Task Force on the use of zidovudine to reduce perinatal transmission of human immunodeficiency virus. MMWR 1994;43:(no RR-11).
54. Dean HD, Fleming PI and Ward JW. Recent trends among black and hispanic adults with AIDS in the United States: 1988–1991. Abstract. Presented at the IX International Conference on AIDS, Berlin, Germany, June 1993.
55. Bureau of the Census. Poverty in the United States, 1992. Washington, DC: US De-

partment of Commerce, Economics and Statistics Administration, Bureau of the Census, September 1993.

56. Ward JW, Homberg SD, Allen JR et al: Transmission of HIV by blood transfusions screened as negative for HIV antibody. N Engl J Med 1988;318:473-8.

57. CDC. US public health service guidelines for testing and counseling blood and plasma donors for human immunodeficiency virus type 1 antigen. MMWR 1996;45:RR-2.

58. CDC. Update: Investigations of patients who have been treated by HIV-infected health-care workers. 1992;41(19):344-346.

Transmission of HIV

Sexual Transmission

MALE-TO-MALE TRANSMISSION

Since the first cases of AIDS were reported among homosexual men, AIDS attributed to male-to-male sex still accounts for the majority of AIDS cases (52%) (1) in the United States. However, the proportion of AIDS cases among men who have sex with men (MSM) and who are not injecting drug users (IDUs) is decreasing. A decline in the incidence of HIV infection, beginning in the mid-1980s, contributes to the current slower rate of increase in AIDS cases among MSM (2,3). The proportion of new AIDS cases attributed to male-to-male sexual contact decreased from 66% during 1981-87 to 45% during 1993-October 1995 (4). Reports of HIV infection and other sexually transmitted diseases (STDs) which are a proxy marker for behaviors associated with sexual HIV transmission have declined among homosexual/bisexual men in some regions of the U.S. (2,5) and may suggest a decline in high-risk sexual behaviors. However, the trend is not uniform geographically, and has not occurred among certain sub-populations. There has been a rapid increase in AIDS cases among MSM reported in the South (2,4), Midwest, (4) rural and smaller metropolitans areas (populations of 50,000-1 million) (4) as well as among young and racial/ethnic minority men (4). Unsafe behaviors by African and Latino homosexual and bisexual men, young gay males, gay males in small cities, as well as some relapse to unsafe behaviors by gay men in general have been reported (6-10).

Receptive anal intercourse with a high number of male sexual partners is the most important HIV risk factor among homosexual men (5,11-14). Other risk factors include: a high number of sexual partners, rectal trauma (e.g. fisting), rectal douching, history of anogenital rectal gonorrhea, and history of ulcerative STDs (e.g. syphilis, herpes simplex) (5,13-15). Although orogenital sex was initially thought to be associated with little or no risk of HIV transmission (14), recent evidence suggests that receptive oral sex is associated with a small risk (16-17). Factors which reflect the probability of encountering an infected sexual partner (e.g., sexual contact with partners from cities with high prevalence of AIDS, bathhouses, or sex clubs) have been also associated with sexual transmission (18,19).

HETEROSEXUAL TRANSMISSION

In the United States, heterosexual transmission accounts for only 8% of all AIDS cases, but accounts for 36% of the AIDS cases among women

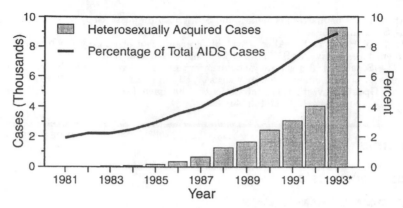

Figure 1.9 Number of AIDS cases attributed to heterosexual HIV transmission and percentage of total AIDS cases—United States, 1981–1993. *Implementation of expanded AIDS surveillance case definition in 1993. Source: Centers for Disease Control. Heterosexually Acquired AIDS—United States, 1993. MMWR 1994;43:155–160.

(1). The proportion and number of AIDS cases from heterosexual exposure is increasing steadily, and is the most rapidly increasing transmission category for women (See Figure 1.9). Between 1983 and 1994, the proportion of AIDS cases associated with heterosexual contact increased from 0.1% to 4% among men, and from 13% to 38% among women (21,22). In 1994, most heterosexually acquired AIDS cases were attributed to having sex with an HIV-infected partner whose risk was unspecified (58%) or with an injecting drug user (36%) (21).

Persons at highest risk for heterosexually transmitted HIV infection include adolescents and adults with multiple sex partners, those with sexually transmitted diseases (STDs) and heterosexually active persons residing in areas with a high prevalence of HIV infection among IDUs (20). The majority of AIDS attributed to heterosexual contact in the U.S. occur among racial/ethnic minorities. Increased rates of HIV infection through heterosexual contact have been associated with multiple sexual partners (23), receptive anal intercourse (24), and the presence of other STDs (e.g., syphilis), particularly those causing genital ulcers (25–29). Other nonulcerating STDs (e.g., gonorrhea, Chlamydia infections) have also been linked to heterosexual transmission (30–31). Other possible factors facilitating transmission include genital trauma and exposure to blood during intercourse (32). Lack of male circumcision, Chlamydia trachomatis infection, and use of the IUD and oral contraceptives have also been suggested to increase risk of HIV infection (18,19,30,33). Sexual transmission may more likely occur when the infected partner has advanced HIV disease (e.g., AIDS diagnosis, low CD4 count, presence of p24 antigen) (28,33). These surrogates for disease stage probably reflect greater viral burden and more virus in genital fluids, increasing the likelihood of transmission (28). Although not a direct cofactor, the use of alcohol or other recreational drugs often impairs judgment and may lead to unsafe sex. The use of crack (a smokable form of cocaine) is associated with increased sexual activity, exchange of sex for drugs or money, and increased rates of STDs.

FEMALE-TO-FEMALE TRANSMISSION

Reported cases to the CDC demonstrate that lesbians represent less than 1% of all cases, with the majority occurring among IDUs, and the remainder attributed to receipt of contaminated blood or blood products. Anecdotal cases suggest there has been transmission between women in association with traumatic sex (34,35) but male-to-female transmission may also occur among primarily lesbian women.

There is a lack of information regarding HIV risk factors among women who have sex with women. Only 2% female AIDS cases reported through September 1989 identified as being homosexual or bisexual (36). It has been estimated that 3% to 4% of all women in the U.S. may be homosexual or bisexual (37,38). Of the 164 cases of AIDS reported in exclusively homosexual women from June 1980–June 1991, 93% were attributed to IDU, and the remainder to blood transfusion (39). IDU was a reported risk factor for 79% of AIDS cases in bisexual women (103) from June 1980 through September 1989 (36). HIV seropositivity in lesbian women and bisexuals has been linked to IDU and heterosexual contact (37,38). Of women patients at a sexually transmitted disease clinic, those reporting same sex contact were much more likely than heterosexual women to engage in HIV-associated risk behaviors such as IDU, contact with high-risk male sex partners, and sex trading (40). Bisexual women were also more likely to be IIIV positive than homosexual or heterosexual women, and were more likely to exchange sex for money (40). This may be indicative of survival sex attributed to drug addiction, low income, low education levels or multiple-risk behavior syndrome (40). No clinical or statistical evidence of female-to-female transmission was reported among exclusively homosexual women (40).

PROTECTED SEX

Latex condoms provide an effective barrier against HIV transmission when used consistently and correctly (41,42). *In vitro* permeability tests of latex condoms to HIV-1 have demonstrated effectiveness in blocking its passage (13,42,43) and behavioral studies have shown that when used consistently and correctly, use of condoms reduces the risk of HIV among heterosexual couples, gay men, and commercial sex workers (13,33,42,44–46).

Consistent condom use during sexual intercourse among serodiscordant pairs (one HIV positive, one HIV negative) was associated with no HIV transmission in one study (33) and a 90% risk reduction in another (46).

REFERENCES

1. CDC. HIV/AIDS Surveillance Report. Mid-Year Edition. 1995 7(1). Atlanta, GA:CDC, 1995.

2. CDC. Update: Acquired Immunodeficiency Syndrome—United States, 1991. MMWR 1992;41:463–468.
3. Karon JM, Berkelman RK. The geographic and ethnic diversity of AIDS incidence trends in homosexual/bisexual men in the United States. J Acquir Immune Defic Syndr 1991;4:1179–1189.
4. CDC. First 500,000 AIDS Cases—United States, MMWR. 1995;44:849–853.
5. Winkelstein W, Lyman DM, Padian N, et al. Sexual practices and risk of infection by the human immunodeficiency virus: The San Francisco Men's Health Study. JAMA 1987;257:321–325.
6. Dean L, Gallaher P. Trends in sexual behavior practices of a panel of NYC gay men. IXth International Conference on AIDS 1993; (abstr PO-D06-3603). Berlin.
7. Koblin B.A, Taylor PE, Rubenstein P, et al. The effect of age on high-risk sexual behavior and HIV-I infection among gay men. IXth International Conference on AIDS, Berlin. 1993; (abstr PO-D06-3603).
8. Pagan R, Rios O, Pintado EA, et al. Sexual practices and attitudes among homosexual and bisexual men attending an inner city early intervention clinic in San Juan, Puerto Rico. IXth International Conference on AIDS. 1993; (abstr PO-D06-3598). Berlin.
9. Mays VM, Cochran SD. High risk HIV-related sexual behaviors in a national sample of U.S. black gay and bisexual men. IXth International Conference on AIDS. 1993; (abstr PO-C03-2613). Berlin.
10. Kelly JA, St Lawrence JS, Brasfield TL, et al. AIDS risk behavior patterns among gay men in small southern cities. Am J Public Health 1990;80:416–418.
11. Caussy D, Goedert J. The epidemiology of human immunodeficiency virus and acquired immunodeficiency syndrome. Seminars in Oncology 1990;17:244–250.
12. Kingsley L.A, Detels R, Kaslow R, et al. Risk factors for seroconversion to human immunodeficiency virus among male homosexuals: Results from the Multicenter AIDS Cohort Study. Lancet 1987;1:345–349.
13. Moss AR, Osmond D, Bacchetti P, et al: Risk factors for AIDS and HIV seropositivity in homosexual men. Am J Epidemiol 1987;125:1035–1047.
14. Cecares CF, van Griensven GJP. Male homosexual transmission of HIV-1. AIDS 1994;8:1051–1061.
15. Chmiel JS, Detels R, Kaslow RA, et al. Factors associated with prevalent human immunodeficiency virus (HIV) infection in the Multicenter AIDS Cohort Study. Am J Epidemiol 1987;126:568–577.
16. Samuel M, Hessol N, Shiboski S, et al. Factors associated with human immunodeficiency virus seroconversion in homosexual men in three San Francisco cohort studies, 1984–1989. J Acquir Immune Defic Syndr 1993;6:303–312.
17. Keet IPM, Albrecht van Lent N, Sanfort TEM, et al. Orogenital sex and the transmission of HIV among homosexual men. AIDS 1992;6:223–226.
18. Jeffries E, Willoughby KB, Boyko W, et al. The Vancouver lymphadenopathy—AIDS study: 2. Seroepidemiology of HTLV-III antibody. Can Med Assoc J 1985;132:1373–1377.
19. Melbye M, Biggar R, Ebbesen PE, et al. Seroepidemiology of HTLV-III antibody in Danish homosexual men: prevalence, transmission, and disease outcome. BJM 1984;289:573–575.
20. CDC. Heterosexually acquired AIDS—United States, 1993. MMWR 1994;43:155–160.
21. HIV/AIDS Surveillance Report. Year End Edition. 1994;6(2). Atlanta GA: CDC.
22. Holmes KK, Karon JM, Kreiss J. The increasing frequency of heterosexually acquired AIDS in the United States, 1983–88. Am J Public Health 1990;80:858–863.
23. CDC. The second 100,000 cases of acquired immunodeficiency syndrome—United States, June 1991—December 1991. MMWR 1992; 41:28–29.
24. Padian N, Marquis L, Francis D, et al. Male-to-female transmission of human immunodeficiency virus. JAMA 1987;258:788–790.
25. Glasel M. High-risk sexual practices in the transmission of AIDS. In DeVita VT, ed. AIDS: etiology, diagnosis, treatment, and prevention. 2nd ed. Philadelphia: JB Lippincott, 1988.
26. Cameron DW, Simonsen JN, D'Costa LJ, et al. Female to male transmission of human immunodeficiency virus Type 1: Risk factors for seroconversion in men. Lancet 1989;2:403–407.
27. Plummer FA, Simonsen JN, Cameron DW, et al. Cofactors in male-female sexual transmission of human immunodeficiency virus type 1. J Infect Dis 199;163:233–239.
28. Nolte S, Sohn MA and Koons B. Prevention of HIV infection in women. J Ob/Gyn 1993;2:128–134.

29. Padian N, Shiboski S, Jewell N. Female-to-male transmission of human immunodeficiency virus. JAMA 1991;266:1664–1668.
30. Greenspan A, Castro KG. Heterosexual transmission of HIV infection. SIECUS Report 1990;19:1–8.
31. Cameron DW, Padian NS. Sexual transmission of HIV and the epidemiology of other sexually transmitted diseases. AIDS 1990;4(suppl1): S99–S103.
32. Lifson AR. The epidemiology of AIDS and HIV infection. AIDS 1990;4(suppl 1): S23–S28
33. Saracco A, Musicco M, Nicolosi A, et al. Man-to-woman sexual transmission of HIV: Longitudinal study of 343 steady partners of infected men. AIDS 1993;6:497–502.
34. Marmor M, Weiss L, Lynden M, et al. Possible female-to-female transmission of human immunodeficiency virus. Ann Intern Med 1986;105:969.
35. Monzon OT, Capellan JM. Female-to-female transmission of HIV. Lancet 1987;1:40–1.
36. Chu SY, Buehler JW, Fleming PL, Berkelman RL. Epidemiology of reported cases of AIDS in lesbians, United States 1980–89. Am J Public Health. 1990;80:1360–81.
37. McCombs SB, McCray E, Wendell DA, Sweeney PA, Onorato IM. Epidemiology of HIV-1 infection in bisexual women. J Acquir Immune Defic Syndr. 1992;5:850–852 (in Bevier).
38. Petersen LR, Doll L, White C, Chus S, and the HIV Blood Donor Study Group. No evidence for female-to-female HIV transmission among 960,000 female blood donors. J Acquir Immune Defic Syndr 1992;5:853–855.
39. Chu SY, Hammett TA, Buehler JW. Update: epidemiology of reported cases of AIDS in women who report sex only with other women, United States, 1980–1991. AIDS. 1992;6:518–519.
40. Bevier PJ, Chiasson MA, Hefferman RT, Castro KG. Women at a sexually transmitted disease clinic who reported same-sex contact: their HIV seroprevalence and risk behaviors. Am J Public Health. 1995;85:1366–1371.
41. CDC. Update: Barrier protection against HIV infection and other sexually transmitted diseases. MMWR 1993;42:589–591, 597.
42. Keeling RP. HIV disease: Current concepts. J Counseling & Development 1993; 71:261–274.
43. CDC. Facts about condoms and their use in preventing HIV infection and other STDS. January 1995.
44. Padian NS. Prostitute women and AIDS epidemiology. AIDS. 1988;2:413–419.
45. European study group on heterosexual transmission of HIV. Comparison of female to male and male to female transmission of HIV in 563 stable couples. Br Med J 1992;304:809–813.
46. De Vincenzi I, and the European Study Group on Heterosexual Transmission of HIV. Heterosexual transmission of HIV in a European cohort of couples. IXth International Conference on AIDS. Berlin, June 1993. (abs WSC02-1).

Injecting Drug Use

Injecting drug use (IDU) is a major risk factor for HIV transmission in the United States, accounting for 25% of all AIDS cases (1). It is particularly significant among African- and Latin-Americans, women, and children. Once HIV is introduced into an area, the prevalence of HIV among injecting drug users (IDUs) can increase very rapidly (e.g., reaching above 50% in 2 years in Edinburgh) (2–4). Longitudinal trends have demonstrated that the seroprevalence of HIV in some areas is stable or decreasing (3–6).

The relationship between sexual behavior, sexually transmitted diseases (STDs), and the increase in cocaine use are factors in HIV transmission via drug use. The sharing of needles, syringes, and other drug paraphernalia is a major mode for HIV transmission among drug users and has been reported to be common (7). Frequency and patterns of injection practices may vary among IDUs and influence the risk of becoming infected. "Booting," the practice of drawing a small amount of blood back into the syringe prior to injection, facilitates transmission of any blood-borne infectious agent to the next person using the syringe or needle. The equipment used to prepare the drugs ("cooker") may also be contaminated with infected blood and when shared, facilitate HIV transmission. Frontloading is a syringe-mediated practice where the needle is removed from the recipient syringe (and the syringe pulled back) and replaced with a needle from a donor syringe; this allows solution to be transferred from the donor to the recipient syringe (8). This is practiced by IDUs using syringes with detachable needles (8). "Backloading," also a syringe-mediated method of drug sharing, has been recently described to increase risk for HIV transmission (8). The syringe is used to mix drugs and to give measured shares to other IDUs by squirting drug solution into the syringes of other IDUs. "Skin popping," in which drugs are inserted into a muscle or under the skin, may be practiced by some users. Once infected, an IDU can transmit HIV infection via: unsafe injection practices; sexually to his/her partner and, for women, perinatally to the unborn child.

Most information concerning drug-using behaviors in the U.S. has been obtained from drug users in treatment programs. Risk of HIV infection has been associated with the frequency of drug injection; frequency of sharing equipment; numbers of different needle-sharing partners; use of unsterilized needles; frontloading; backloading; use of "shooting galleries"; sharing of cookers; use of cocaine, or the combination of cocaine and heroin ("speedball"); receptive anal intercourse among men, and racial or ethnic minority status (7–17). The higher risk of HIV infection associated with injecting cocaine may be related to the more frequent daily injections due to its short half-life, and the highly addictive nature of this drug (18). Crack, a purified form of cocaine is smoked by inhaling the vapors given off when it is heated. Readily available and inexpensive, the use of crack cocaine has been identified as a risk factor for AIDS. Users of crack tend to have higher prevalence of syphilis, and engage in risky sexual behavior (e.g., having multiple partners, exchanging sex for drugs or money) and injecting practices (19,20). HIV prevalence among IDUs vary by geographic region, race and ethnicity, as well as drug-use and sexual behaviors (4,21). HIV seroprevalence surveys among IDUs in treatment centers reveal the highest rates in the Atlantic coast area and Puerto Rico (15%–40%) compared to rates generally below 7% elsewhere (4). HIV seroprevalence was higher among African-American than among white IDUs, although HIV seroprevalence among Latin-American IDUs was also generally higher than among Whites, this difference was largely due to the higher rates among Latin Americans in the Northeast (4).

Risky sexual behavior appears to contribute to a large proportion of HIV infection among some IDU populations. Studies have suggested that IDUs are likely to be men, sexually active, are unlikely to use condoms, and often have a partner who does not use drugs (22). The number of sexual partners is a risk factor for HIV infection, and is perhaps related to crack use. Alcohol use can also lead to disinhibition of behavior, resulting in unsafe sexual practices (5).

Once an IDU is infected, more rapid disease progression is associated with increasing age (23–25). Continued active drug use has not been shown to be a consistent factor in progression to AIDS (23–24,26–27).

REFERENCES

1. CDC. HIV/AIDS Surveillance Report. Mid-Year Edition, 1995;7(1), Atlanta, GA:CDC.
2. Robertson JR, Bucknall ABV, Welsby PD, et al. Epidemic of AIDS-related virus (HTLV-III/LAV) infection among intravenous drug abusers. Br Med J 1986;292:527–529.
3. Des Jarlais DC, Friedman SR, Novick DM, et al. HIV-1 infection among intravenous drug users in Manhattan, New York City, from 1977 through 1987. JAMA 1989; 261:1008–1012.
4. CDC. National HIV Serosurveillance Summary. Results through 1992. Vol. 3. Atlanta, GA:US Dept Health Human Services; 1994.
5. Moss AR, Vranizan K, Gorter R, et al. HIV seroconversion in intravenous drug users in San Francisco, 1985–1990. AIDS 1994;8:223–231.
6. Des Jarlais DC, Friedman SR, Sotheran JL, Wenston J, Marmor M, Yancovitz SR, et al. Continuity and change within an HIV epidemic. Injecting drug users in New York City, 1984 through 1992. JAMA 1994;271:121–127.
7. Chaisson RE, Bacchetti T, Osmond D, et al. Cocaine use and HIV infection in intravenous drug users in San Francisco. JAMA 1989;261:561–565.
8. Jose B, Friedman SR, Neaigus A, et al. Syringe-mediated drug-sharing (backloading): a new risk factor for HIV among injecting drug users. AIDS 1993;7:1653–1660.
9. Sasse H, Salmas S, Conti S, et al. Risk behaviors for HIV-1 infection in Italian drug users: report from a multicenter study. J Acquir Immune Defic Syndr 1989;2:486–496.
10. Vlahov D, Munos A, Anthony JC, et al. Association of drug-injection patterns with antibody to human immunodeficiency virus type 1 among intravenous drug users in Baltimore, Maryland. Am J Epidemiol 1990;132:847–856.
11. Chaisson RE, Moss AR, Onishi R, Osmond D, Carlson J. Human immunodeficiency virus infection in heterosexual intravenous drug users in San Francisco. Am J Public Health 1987;77:169–172.
12. Van de Hoek JA, Coputinho RA, Van Haastrecht JHA, van Zadelhoff AW, Goudsmit J. Prevalence and risk factors of HIV infections among drug users and drug-using prostitutes in Amsterdam. AIDS 1988;2:55–60.
13. Marmor M, Des Jarlais DC, Cohen H, et al. Risk factors for infection with human immunodeficiency virus among intravenous drug abusers in New York City. AIDS 1987;1:39–44.
14. Battjes RJ, Pickens RW, Haverkos HW, Sloboda Z. HIV risk factors among injecting drug users in five US cities. AIDS 1994;8:681–687.
15. Schoenbaum EE, Harter D, Selwyn PA, et al. Risk factors for human immunodeficiency virus infection in intravenous drug users. N Engl J Med 1989;321:874–879.
16. Wodak A and Moss A. HIV infection and injecting drug users: from epidemiology to public health. AIDS 1990;4(suppl1):S105–S109.
17. Vlahov D. HIV seroconversion studies among intravenous drug users. AIDS 1994;8:263–265.
18. Karan LD, Primary Care for AIDS and Chemical Dependence. West J Med 1990;152:538–542.
19. Edlin Br, Irwin K, Serrano Y, et al. The impact of cocaine smoking on injection practices of street recruited drug injectors. IX Conference of AIDS. Berlin, June 1993. (abstr P0–C15-2952).
20. Diaz T, Chu C, et al. Sexual practices among crack/cocaine users with AIDS: Supplement to HIV/AIDS Surveillance. IX Conference of AIDS. June 1993 (abstr PO-C15-2953). Berlin.
21. Hahn RA, Onorato IM, Jones TS, et al. Prevalence of HIV infection among intravenous drug users in the United States. JAMA 1989;18:2677–2684.
22. Brundage J.F. Epidemiology of HIV Infection and AIDS in the United States Dermatologic Clinics 1991;9:442–452.
23. Ronald PJM, Robertson JR, Elton RA. Continued drug use and other cofactors for progression to AIDS among injecting drug users. AIDS 1994;8:339–343.

24. The Italian seroconversion study. Disease progression and early predictors of AIDS in HIV-seroconverted injecting drug users. AIDS 1992;6:421–426.
25. Phillips AN, Lee CA, Elford J, et al. More rapid progression to AIDS in older HIV-infected people: the role of CD4+ T-cell counts. J Acquir Immune Defic Syndr 1991; 4:970–975.
26. Selwyn PA, Alcabes P, Hartel D, et al. Clinical manifestations and predictors of disease progression in drug users with human immunodeficiency virus infection. N Engl J Med 1992;327:1697–1703.
27. Phillips AN, Sabin CA, Mocroft A. Active drug injecting and progression of HIV infection. AIDS 1994;8:385–386.

Maternal-Fetal Transmission

Maternal-fetal (vertical) transmission is the primary mode of HIV transmission for children in the United States, accounting for approximately 90% of children with HIV (1). The mechanism and timing of vertical transmission is uncertain. HIV can be transmitted from mother to infant in utero, intrapartum, or postpartum by breast feeding. Since breast feeding is discouraged among HIV-infected women in the United States, the majority of infants here acquire HIV in utero or intrapartum. Evidence of HIV infection in the fetus has been shown from the early to late stages of pregnancy; virus has been detected in fetal and placental tissue in the first trimester (2,3), and isolated from the cord blood of infants at delivery (4). HIV transmission can also occur during delivery through exposure to maternal blood or genital tract secretions. Some studies have suggested cesarean section decreases the risk of HIV transmission, whereas others have shown no effect in rates compared to vaginal delivery (5–8). Although the efficiency of HIV transmission through breast-feeding is unknown, high levels of viremia and lack of neutralizing antibody in the mother may be associated with increased risk of transmission (9).

Not all infants born to HIV-infected mothers become infected. Observed rates of transmission have been variable, ranging from 14% in Europe, to 45% in Kenya (4–6,10). In the United States, HIV is transmitted to approximately 20% to 30% of babies born to HIV-infected pregnant women (9). Geographic variations in transmission rates have been attributed to a number of factors: virulence characteristics of the virus itself, inherent factors of the study population (e.g., advanced maternal disease), and obstetric or breast feeding practices (9). Research artifacts (e.g., incomplete follow-up, varying diagnostic precision) may also be a reason for the observed differences in rates.

A number of factors facilitating maternal-fetal transmission have been identified. Advanced HIV disease or low CD4 counts (i.e., less than 400), maternal p24 antigenemia, lack of maternal neutralizing antibody, placental membrane inflammation, and high CD8+ lymphocyte counts have been associated with increased rates of perinatal transmission (4,10–14). Premature infants and first-born twins (as compared to those second born) also appear to have a greater risk of HIV infection (7,15,16). In one study the presence of maternal anti-gp 120 was associated with a lower likelihood of transmission, but another study showed no correlation (17–19). Recently, it has been demonstrated that zidovudine administered during gestation and/or labor and delivery reduces

HIV transmission, even in women with low CD4 counts (13,20). Administration of ZDV to a selected group of HIV-infected women during pregnancy, labor, and delivery and to their newborns reduced the risk of perinatal HIV transmission by approximately two-thirds compared to mothers in the placebo group with minimal adverse effects (ACTG Protocol 076) (20). Consequently, recommendations regarding ZDV therapy for perinatal HIV transmission were developed by the Public Health Service (21) and ZDV use in this situation was approved by the Food and Drug Administration (22).

REFERENCES

1. CDC. HIV/AIDS Surveillance Report. Mid-Year Edition. Atlanta, GA: CDC 1995;7(1).
2. Jovaisas E, Koch MA, Schafer A, et al. Vertical transmission of HIV in a 20 week fetus. Lancet 1986;2:288,
3. Sprecher S, Soumenkoff G, Puissant F, et al: Vertical transmission of HIV in 15-week fetus. Lancet 1986;2:288.
4. Ryder R, Nsa W, Hassig S, et al. Perinatal transmission of the human immunodeficiency virus type 1 to infants of seropositive women in Zaire. N Eng J Med 1989; 320:1637–1642.
5. Blanche S, Rouzioux C, Guihard Moscato ML, et al. A prospective study of infants born to women seropositive for human immunodeficiency virus type 1. N Eng J Med 1989;320:1643–1648.
6. European Collaborative Study: Mother-to-child transmission of HIV infection. Lancet 1988:2;1039–1043.
7. European Collaborative Study. Risk factors for mother-to-child transmission of HIV-1. Lancet 1992;339:1007–1012.
8. Hutto C, Parks WP, Lai SH, et al. A hospital-based prospective study of perinatal infection with human immunodeficiency virus type 1. J Pediatr 1991;118:347–353.
9. Von Seidlein L, Bryson YJ. Maternal-fetal transmission of the human immunodeficiency virus type 1. Seminars in Pediatric Infectious Diseases 1994;5(1):78–86.
10. ACOG issues report on HIV infection in women. AFP Amer. Family Physician 1992;46(2):579–585.
11. Caussy D, Goedert J. The epidemiology of human immunodeficiency virus and acquired immunodeficiency syndrome. Seminars in Oncology 1990;17:244–250.
12. St Louis ME, Kamenga M, Brown C, et al. Risk for perinatal HIV-1 transmission according to maternal immunologic, virologic and placental factors. JAMA 1993; 269:2853–2859.
13. Boyer PJ, Dillon M, Navaie, M, et al. Factors predictive of maternal-fetal transmission of HIV-1: preliminary analysis of zidovudine given during pregnancy and/or delivery. JAMA 1994;271:1925–1930.
14. Scarlatti G, Albert J, Rossi P, et al. Mother-to-child transmission of human immunodeficiency virus type 1: Correlation with neutralizing antibodies against primary isolates. J Infect Dis 1993;168:207–210.
15. Goedert JJ, Duliege AM, Amos CI, et al. High risk of HIV-1 infection for first-born. The International Registry of HIV-exposed Twins. Lancet 1991;338:1471–1475.
16. Duliege AM, Amos CI, Felton S, et al. HIV-1 infection rate and progression of disease in 1st and 2nd born twins born to HIV infected mothers: hypothesis regarding in utero and perinatal exposures. IX International Conference AIDS, Berlin 1993; (abstr WS-C10-4).
17. Goedert JJ, Mendez H, Drummond JE, et al. Mother-to-infant transmission of human immunodeficiency virus type 1: Association with prematurity or low anti-gp120. Lancet 1989;2:1351–1354.
18. Rossi P, Moschese V, Broliden PA, et al. Presence of maternal antibodies to human immunodeficiency virus 1 envelope glycoprotein gp120 epitopes correlates with the uninfected status of children born to seropositive mothers. Proc Natl Acad Sci USA 1989;86:8055–8058.
19. Halsey NA, Markham R, Wahren B, et al. Lack of association between maternal antibodies to V3 loop peptides and maternal infant HIV-1 transmission. J Acquir Immune Defic Syndr 1992;5:153–157.

20. Connor EM, Sperling RS, Gelber R, et al. Reduction of maternal-infant transmission of human immunodeficiency virus type 1 with zidovudine treatment. N Engl J Med 1994;331:1173–1180.
21. CDC. Recommendations of the U.S. Public Health Service Task Force on the Use of Zidovudine to Reduce Perinatal Transmission of Human Immunodeficiency Virus. MMWR 1994;43 (No. RR-11).
22. CDC. US Public Health Service Recommendations for Human Immunodeficiency Virus Counseling and Voluntary Testing for Pregnant Women. MMWR 1995;44 (No. RR-7).

Blood Transfusion, Blood Products, and Organ Transplants

In the United States and most other developed nations, transmission of HIV by transfusion is extremely low. Self-deferral by potential donors who know they may be HIV-infected, improved donor interviewing about behaviors associated with risk for HIV infection, HIV *antibody* testing of all donated blood and plasma, increased sensitivity of contemporary HIV-antibody enzyme immunosorbent assays (EIAS), deferral of donors who test positive for HIV, hepatitis, human T-cell leukemia virus type 1 (HTLV-1), or syphilis, and the maintenance of donor-deferral lists of individual donors who have previously tested positive for HIV antibodies all contribute to the safety of the blood supply. Heat-treatment or other methods of viral inactivation for clotting factor concentrations also ensures protection of hemophiliacs. HIV transmission appears likely after receipt of HIV-infected blood; with over 90% of those receiving HIV-positive blood and cellular blood components becoming infected (1). Transmission appears to be very frequent with receipt of whole plasma and all cellular components, but not with most blood products other than clotting factor concentrates. Before HIV screening was available, 75% to 90% of those who received factor VIII concentrate became infected; only 30% of those receiving factor IX concentrate resulted in infection, although used in the same period (2). The risk of HIV transmission from various tissues is not known, although some organs and tissues clearly present a higher risk for HIV transmission than others (3). The risk of HIV transmission from a whole organ of an HIV-infected donor is almost 100%. There also appears to be a high risk for transmission from fresh-frozen, unprocessed bone, particularly if marrow elements and adherent tissue are not removed. There appears to be a lower risk for transmission from relatively avascular solid tissue, some of which is also processed by techniques which might inactivate HIV (4).

There are a small number of persons who become infected by receipt of blood, organs, and tissues from donors who are recently HIV-infected but seronegative (3–5). In these cases, a false-negative screening test result was caused either by multiple blood transfusions just prior to donation, resulting in the dilution of the anti-HIV antibody titer below a detectable level or HIV infection during the window period (4 to 26 weeks from the primary infection to seroconversion) (3,5). The risk of acquiring HIV infection through receipt of a unit of blood that tests negative for HIV antibody has been estimated to be about 26 per million, with other studies suggesting lower risks (6,7). In 1993, only approximately six per 100,000 blood donations collected by the American Red Cross tested positive for HIV antibody (8). In addition, only an estimated one in 450,000 to one in 660,000 donations per year (i.e., 18–27 donations) were infectious for HIV but were not detected by current screening tests (9). As an additional safety measure to maintain a safe blood supply, the Food and Drug Administration (FDA) recommended in August 1995 that all blood and plasma donations be screened for p24 antigen to reduce the risk for HIV infection for persons who receive donated blood or blood products (10). During the acute period of HIV infection, tests for p24 antigen can detect HIV infection earlier than antibody test (10); recent studies indicated that p24 screening reduces the infectious window period (11). Among the 12 million annual blood donations in the United States, p24-antigen screening is expected to remove four to six infectious donations that would not be identified by other screening tests (10). Donor screening for p24 antigen is considered as an interim measure by the FDA pending the availability of technology that would further reduce the risk for HIV transmission from blood donated during the infectious window period (10).

REFERENCES

1. Donegan E, Stuart M, Niland JC, Sacks HS, Azen SP, Dietrich SL, et al. Infection with human immunodeficiency virus type 1(HIV-1) among recipients of antibody-positive blood donations. Ann Intern Med 1990;113:733–739.
2. Caussy D, and Goedert J. The Epidmiology of Human Immunodeficiency Virus and Acquired Immunodeficiency Syndrome. Seminars in Oncology 1990;17:244–250
3. Simonds RJ, Holmberg SD, Hurwitz RL, et al. Transmission of human immunodeficiency virus type 1 from a seronegative organ and tissue donor. NEJM. 1992;326:726–732.
4. CDC. Guidelines for preventing transmission of human immunodeficiency virus through transplantation of human tissue and organs. MMWR. 1994, 43 (RR-8).
5. Patijn GA, Strengers PFW, Persijn HM. Prevention of transmission of HIV by organ and tissue transplantation. Transplant International 1993;6:165–172.
6. Ward JW, Holmberg SD, Allen JR, Cohn DL, Critchley SE, Kleinman SH, et al. Transmission of human immunodeficiency virus (HIV) by blood transfusions screened as negative for HIV antibody. N Eng J Med 1988;318:473–478.
7. Cumming PD, Wallace EL, Schorr JB, Dodd RY: Exposure of patients to human immunodeficiency virus through transfusion of blood products that test antibody negative. N Engl J Med, 1989;321:941–946.
8. CDC. National HIV serosurveillance summary: results through 1992. Vol 3. Atlanta, GA: US Department of Health and Human Services; 1994.
9. Lackritz EM, Satten GA, Aberle-Grasse J, et al. Estimated risk of transmission of the human immunodeficiency virus by screened blood in the United States. N Engl J Med 1995;333:1721–1725.
10. CDC. US Public Health Service Guidelines for Testing and Counseling Blood and plasma donors for human immunodeficiency virus type 1 antigen. MMWR 1996;45:RR-2.
11. Busch MP, Lee LLJ, Satten GA, et al. Time course of detection of viral and serologic markers preceding human immunodeficiency virus type 1 seroconversion:implications for screening of blood and tissue donors. Transfusion 1995;35:91–7.

Health Care Setting

Health care workers (HCW) and laboratory personnel are at risk for HIV infection if they work with or handle sharp instruments contaminated with the blood or other body fluids of an HIV patient. The greatest risk of HIV transmission in the health care setting is through needlestick accidents, as compared to intact skin or mucous membrane exposure to blood or other body fluids. HIV infection acquired following percutaneous injuries with instruments used on HIV-infected patients have resulted in an HIV seroconversion rate of 0.4% (1,2). These injuries often occur in emergency situations (e.g., resuscitation attempts) or surgery. Among HCWs with a percutaneous occupational exposure, an increased risk for HIV infection has been associated with an exposure which involve a large quantity of blood and if the source patient had terminal illness (with presumably high viral load) (3). The risk from mucosal and nonintact skin exposure appears to be much less than that with needlestick exposures; it is not zero but too low to be reliably estimated in studies performed to date (4). One assessment of health care workers exposed to HIV-infected blood estimated the risk for HIV transmission to be less than 0.1% for a single mucous-membrane exposure (5). Transmission by apparent skin contact over a prolonged period or with HIV-infected blood splashes has also been reported (4). A large prospective study evaluating cutaneous exposures detected no infections after 2712 instances of HIV exposure to intact skin (6).

HIV transmission from an HIV-infected dentist to six of his patients has been reported (7,8) but other identified risk factors could have been responsible, according to later reports. Follow-up of patients who underwent procedures by infected HCWs have been followed (9–11). Only one patient who had been treated by a surgeon was found to be infected, but had a risk behavior for HIV (i.e., injection drug user) (9). In other countries, inadequate infection control practices have resulted in the nosocomial spread of HIV to patients (e.g., via contaminated syringes and needles).

REFERENCES

1. Tokars JI, Marcus R, Culver DH, Schable CA, et al. Surveillance of HIV infection and zidovudine use among health care workers after occupational exposure. Ann Intern Med 1993;118:913–919.
2. CDC. Public Health Service statement on management of occupational exposure to human immunodeficiency virus, including considerations retarding zidovudine postexposure use. MMWR 1990;39(RR-1) whole pamphlet
3. CDC. Case-control study of HIV seroconversion in health-care workers after percutaneous exposure to HIV-infected blood—France, United Kingdom, and United States, January 1988–August 1994. MMWR 1995;44:929–933.
4. Caussy D, Goedert J. The epidemiology of human immunodeficiency virus and acquired immunodeficiency syndrome. Seminars in Oncology 1990;17:244–250.
5. Ippolito G, Puro V, De Carli G. The risk of occupational human immunodeficiency virus infection in health care workers: The Italian Study Group on Occupational risk of HIV infection. Arch Intern Med 1993;153:1451–1458.
6. Henderson DK, Fahey BJ, Willy M, et al. Risk for occupational transmission of human immunodeficiency virus type 1 (HIV-1) associated with clinical exposures. A prospective evaluation. Ann Intern Med 1990;113:740–746.
7. CDC. Investigations of patients who have been treated by HIV-infected health-care workers—United States. MMWR. 1993;42:329–331, 337.
8. Gooch B, Marianos D, Ciesielski C, et al. Lack of evidence for patient-to-patient transmission of HIV in a dental practice. JADA 1993;124:38–44.
9. Mishu B, Schaffner W, Horan JM, et al. A surgeon with AIDS; lack of evidence of transmission to patients. JAMA. 1990;264:467–470.
10. Armstrong FG, Miner JC, Wolfe WH. Investigation of a health care worker with symptomatic HIV infection: an epidemiologic approach. Military Med 1987;52:414–418.

11. Porter JD, Cruickshank JG, Gentle PH, et al. Management of patients treated by a surgeon with HIV infection. Lancet 1990;335:113–114.

HIV and the Environment

No environmentally mediated mode of HIV transmission has been documented. An extensive study performed on HIV survival in the environment found HIV to be recoverable by tissue-culture techniques one to three days after drying (1). However, the HIV samples used in laboratory studies are much more concentrated than normally found in the blood of HIV-infected persons (i.e., 100,000 times greater). Even though HIV could be detected for up to three days, the rate of inactivation was very rapid. CDC studies have shown that drying causes a 90–99% reduction in HIV concentration within several hours (2). In tissue-culture fluid, cell-free HIV could be recovered up to 15 days at room temperature, up to 11 days at 37 C (98.6°F) and up to one day if the HIV was cell-associated (2). Laboratory study results cannot be used to determine specific personal risks of infection because a similarly high concentration of virus is not found in human specimens or any place else in nature. In addition, no one has been HIV infected as a result of contact with an environmental surface. Moreover, HIV is unable to reproduce outside its living host (3), except under laboratory conditions, and cannot spread or maintain infectiousness outside its host. Current laboratory and epidemiologic data do not support HIV transmission by casual contact (without exposure to blood or body fluids) or insects (4–7).

REFERENCES

1. Resnik L, Veren K, Salahuddin SZ, Tondreau S, Markham PD. Stability and inactivation of HTLV-III/LAV under clinical and laboratory environments. JAMA 1986; 255:1887–91.
2. CDC. Recommendations for prevention of HIV transmission in health-care settings. MMWR 1987;36:(No.2S).
3. CDC. Facts about the human immunodeficiency virus and its transmission. Atlanta, GA: Centers for Disease Control, February 1993.
4. Webb PA, Happ CM, Maupin GO, et al. Potential for insect transmission of HIV: Experimental exposure of Cimex hemipterus and Toxorbynchites amboinensis to human immunodeficiency virus. J Infect Dis 1989;160:970–977.
5. Srinivasan A, York D, Bohan C. Lack of HIV replication in arthropod cells. Lancet 1987;1:1094–1095.
6. Jupp PG, Lyons SF. Experimental assessment of bedbugs (Cimex lectularius and Cimex hemipterus) and mosquitoes (Aedes aegypti formosus) as vectors of human immunodeficiency virus. AIDS 1987;1:171–4.
7. Castro KG, Lieb S. Jaffe HW, et al. Transmission of HIV in Belle Glade, Florida. Lessons for other communities in the United States. Science 1988;239:193.

Casual Contact

Concerns regarding HIV transmission via casual contact have been raised since HIV was isolated from many body fluids, including saliva, urine and tears. HIV nucleic acid—but not infectious HIV—has been detected in feces (1). HIV has not been shown to be transmitted through sharing of household items (e.g., glasses, towels, sheets, plates, toilet and bath facilities) which are likely to be soiled by saliva, urine, tears, and feces. A considerable body of literature indicates that household transmission in the absence of sexual or percutaneous exposure is rare.

Although contact with blood and other body substances can occur in households, HIV transmission is rare in this setting. Several studies of nonsexual, nonneedle-sharing household contacts of HIV-infected individuals in the United States and Europe have documented no evidence for HIV infection (2–5). Of 1167 household contacts who were followed in 17 studies, none were infected; the estimated rate of transmission from these reported studies was 0–.2 infections per 100 person-years (5). Cases of HIV transmission have been reported in households where: needles were shared for medical injections at home; there was mucocutaneous exposure to blood or other body substances during home health care in persons receiving care from or providing care to HIV-infected family members; and where there was presumably, although unrecognized contaminated blood contact between young children (6–11). In some cases, blood exposure might have occurred during nursing care but was not documented; however, skin contact with body secretions and excretions occurred. There have also been anecdotal cases that appeared to implicate transmission by close contact, although other exposure modes could not be excluded (6,7). A case of HIV transmission between hemophiliac brothers suggested that transmission most likely occurred during an episode of razor sharing (5). These incidents highlight the need to follow precautions which prevent contact with blood and body fluids in households and other settings.

REFERENCES

1. Levy JA. Pathogenesis of human immunodeficiency virus infection. Microbiol Rev 1993;57:183–289.
2. Friedland G, Kahl P, Saltzman B, et al. Additional evidence for lack of transmission of HIV infection by close interpersonal casual contact. AIDS 1990;4:639–644.
3. Friedland GH, Salthzman BR, Rogers MF, et al. Lack of transmission of HTLV-III/LAV infection to household contacts of patients with AIDS or AIDS-related complex with oral candidiasis. N Engl J Med 1986;314:344–349.
4. Rogers MF, White C, Sanders T, et al. Lack of transmission human immunodeficiency virus from infected children to their household contacts. Pediatrics 1990;84:210–214.
5. CDC. HIV transmission between two adolescent brothers with hemophilia. MMWR 1993;42:948–951.
6. Wahn V, Kramer H, Voit T, et al. Horizontal transmission of HIV infection between two siblings. Lancet 1986;2:694.
7. Koenig RE, Gautier T, Levy JA. Unusual intrafamilial transmission of human immunodeficiency virus. Lancet 1986;2:627.
8. Fitzgibbon JE, Gaur S, Frenkel, LD, et al. Transmission from one child to another of human immunodeficiency virus type 1 with a zidovudine-resistance mutation. N Engl J Med 1993;329:1835–1841.
9. CDC. HIV infection in 2 brothers receiving intravenous therapy for hemophilia. MMWR 1992;41:228–231.
10. CDC. Apparent transmission of human T-lymphotrophic virus type III/lymphadenopathy associated virus from a child to a mother providing health care. MMWR 1986;35:76–79.
11. CDC. Human immunodeficiency virus transmission in household settings—United States. MMWR 1994;43:347–356.

HIV Classification System and AIDS Case Definition for Adolescents and Adults

The Centers for Disease Control (CDC) revised the classification for HIV infection and expanded the case definition for AIDS surveillance in 1993; these are summarized here (1). The objectives of the new classification system were to simplify the classification and reporting process, to be consistent with standards of medical care for HIV-infected persons, to better categorize HIV-related morbidity, and to more accurately record the number of persons with severe HIV-related immunosuppression who are most affected by clinical conditions.

HIV Classification System for Adolescents and Adults

The 1993 CDC classification system for HIV-infected adolescents and adults emphasizes the importance of CD4+ T-lymphocyte testing in the clinical management of HIV-infected persons. The classification system was revised to include the CD4+ T-lymphocyte count as a marker for HIV-related immunosupression. This classification system categorizes persons on the basis of clinical conditions associated with HIV infection and CD4+ T-lymphocyte counts. The system, outlined in Table 1.3, is based on three ranges of laboratory categories (CD4+ T-lymphocyte counts) and three clinical categories, represented by a matrix of nine mutually exclusive categories.

Table 1.3.

1993 CDC Classification System for HIV Infection and AIDS Surveillance Case Definition for Adolescents and Adults

	Clinical Categories		
CD4+ Cell Categories	A Asymptomatic, Acute (Primary) HIV or PGL#	B Symptomatic, Not A or C Conditions	C AIDS Indicator Conditions *
≥500/mm³	A1	B1	C1
200−499/mm³	A2	B2	C2
<200/mm³	A3	B3	C3
AIDS indicator T-cell count			

Persons under Category C, as well as those with CD4+ lymphocyte counts of less than 200/μL (A3 or B3) are reportable as AIDS cases in the U.S. and Territories.
PGL = persistent generalized lymphadenopathy. Clinical category A includes acute (primary) HIV infection
* See Table 1.4
Adapted from CDC. 1993 Revised Classification System for HIV Infection and Expanded Surveillance Case Definition for AIDS Among Adolescents and Adults MMWR 1992;41:(No RR-17).

This system replaced the 1986 classification system which included only clinical disease criteria and was developed before the widespread use of CD4+ T-cell testing (2).

CRITERIA FOR HIV INFECTION IN PERSONS—13 YEARS AND OLDER

A person is considered HIV infected when he or she has:

- Repeatedly reactive screening tests for HIV-1 antibody (e.g., enzyme immunoassay) and who also have specific antibody identified by the use of supplemental tests (e.g., Western blot, immunofluorescence assay);
- Direct identification of virus in host tissues by virus isolation;
- HIV antigen detection; or
- A positive result on any other highly specific licensed test for HIV.

LABORATORY CATEGORIES

There are three designated lab categories of CD4+ T-lymphocyte counts per microliter of blood to guide clinical and/or therapeutic actions in the management of HIV-infected adolescents and adults. The revised HIV classification system also allows for the use of percentage of CD4+ T-cells (Appendix I). HIV-infected persons should be classified according to existing guidelines for medical management of HIV-infected persons (3,4). Therefore, the lowest accurate but not necessarily the most recent, CD4+ T-lymphocyte count should be used for classification purposes.

Category 1   ≥500 cells/μL
Category 2   200–499 cells/μL
Category 3   <200 cells/μL

CLINICAL CATEGORIES

There are three clinical categories for HIV infection and are defined as follows:

Category A

In category A, one or more of the conditions listed below occur in the adolescent or adult (13 years and older) with documented HIV infection. Conditions listed in categories B and C *must not* have occurred.

- Asymptomatic HIV infection
- Persistent generalized lymphadenopathy (PGL).
- Acute (primary) HIV infection with accompanying illness or history of acute HIV infection.

Category B

Category B comprises symptomatic conditions occurring in an HIV-infected adolescent or adult which are not included among conditions listed in clinical category C and which meet at least one of the following criteria: a) the conditions are attributed to HIV infection and/or indicative of a defect in cell-mediated immunity; or b) the conditions are considered by physicians to have a clinical course or management that is complicated by HIV infection. Examples of conditions in clinical category B include, but **are not limited to:**

- Bacillary angiomatosis
- Candidiasis, oropharyngeal (thrush).
- Candidiasis, vulvovaginal; persistent (>1 month duration), frequent, or poorly responsive to therapy
- Cervical dysplasia (moderate or severe) or cervical carcinoma in situ
- Constitutional symptoms, such as fever (38.5°C) or diarrhea lasting >1 month
- Hairy leukoplakia, oral
- Herpes zoster (shingles), involving at least two distinct episodes or more than one dermatome
- Idiopathic thrombocytopenic purpura
- Listeriosis
- Pelvic inflammatory disease, particularly if complicated by tubo-ovarian abscess
- Peripheral neuropathy

For classification purposes, Category B conditions take precedence over those in Category A. For example, someone previously treated for oral or persistent vaginal candidiasis (and who has not developed a Category C disease) but who is now asymptomatic should be classified in clinical Category B.

Category C

Category C includes the clinical conditions listed in the AIDS surveillance case definition (Table 1.4). Once a Category C condition has occurred, the person will remain classified in Category C.

1993 EXPANSION OF THE CDC SURVEILLANCE CASE DEFINITION FOR AIDS

The 1993 expansion of the AIDS surveillance case definition includes all adolescents and adults with HIV infection who have: CD4+ T-lymphocyte counts of less than 200 cells/μL, or a CD4+ percentage of less than 14. The 1993 expansion includes the addition of three clinical conditions—pulmonary tuberculosis (TB), recurrent pneumonia, and invasive cervical cancer—and retains the 23 clinical conditions in the 1987 AIDS surveillance case definition (5). The diagnostic criteria for AIDS-defining conditions included in the expanded surveillance definition are in Appendices I & II. This expanded definition requires laboratory con-

Table 1.4.
Conditions Included in the 1993 CDC AIDS Surveillance Case Definition

- Candidiasis of bronchi, trachea, or lungs
- Candidiasis, esophageal
- Cervical cancer, invasive*
- Coccidioidomycosis, disseminated or extrapulmonary
- Cryptococcosis, extrapulmonary
- Cryptosporidiosis, chronic intestinal (>1 month duration)
- Cytomegalovirus disease (other than liver, spleen, or nodes)
- Cytomegalovirus retinitis (with loss of vision)
- Encephalopathy, HIV-related
- Herpes simplex: chronic ulcer(s) (>1 month's duration); or bronchitis, pneumonitis, or esophagitis
- Histoplasmosis, disseminated or extrapulmonary
- Isosporiasis, chronic intestinal (>1 month duration)
- Kaposi's sarcoma
- Lymphoma, Burkitt's (or equivalent term)
- Lymphoma, immunoblastic (or equivalent term)
- Lymphoma, primary, of brain
- *Mycobacterium avium* complex or *M. kansasii,* disseminated or extrapulmonary
- *Mycobacterium tuberculosis,* any site (pulmonary* or extrapulmonary)
- *Mycobacterium,* other species or unidentified species, disseminated or extrapulmonary
- *Pneumocystis carinii* pneumonia
- Pneumonia, recurrent*
- Progressive multifocal leukoencephalopathy
- *Salmonella* septicemia, recurrent
- Toxoplasmosis of brain
- Wasting syndrome due to HIV

*Added in the 1993 expansion of the AIDS surveillance case definition
Adapted from CDC. 1993 Revised Classification System for HIV Infection and Expanded Surveillance Case Definition for AIDS Among Adolescents and Adults MMWR 1992;41:(No RR-17).

firmation of HIV infection in persons with CD4+ T-lymphocyte count of <200 cells/μL or with one of the added clinical conditions.

In the 1993 HIV classification system, persons in subcategories A3, B3, and C3 meet the immunologic criteria of the surveillance case definition, and those persons with conditions in subcategories C1, C2, and C3 meet the clinical criteria for surveillance purposes (Table 1.3). Conditions included in the 1993 AIDS surveillance case definition (1) are in Table 1.4.

REFERENCES

1. CDC. 1993 revised classification system for HIV infection and expanded surveillance case definition for AIDS among adolescents and adults. MMWR 1992;41:(No RR-17).
2. CDC. Classification system for human T-lymphotropic type II/lymphadenopathy-associated virus infections. MMWR 1986;25:334–339.
3. NIH. State of the art conference on AZT therapy of early HIV infection. Am J Med 1990;89:335–344.
4. CDC. Guidelines for the performance of CD4+ T cell determinations in persons with HIV infections. MMWR 1992;41(No RR-8):1–12.
5. CDC. Revision of the CDC Surveillance case definition for acquired immunodeficiency syndrome. MMWR 1987;36:1–155.

APPENDIX I
Equivalences for Absolute Numbers of CD4+ T-lymphocytes and CD4+ Percentage

Compared with the absolute CD4+ lymphocyte count, the percent of CD4+ T-cells of total lymphocytes (or CD4+ percentage) is less subject to variation on repeated measurements. However, data correlating natural history of HIV infection with CD4+ percentage have not been as consistently available as data on absolute CD4+ lymphocyte counts. Therefore, the 1993 classification system is based on CD4+ lymphocyte counts but allows for the use of the CD4+ percentages. However, it must be recognized that these suggested equivalences (Table I.1) may not always correspond with values observed in individual patients (1).

Table I.1.
Equivalences for Absolute Numbers of CD4+ T-lymphocytes and CD4+ Percentage

CD4+ T-cell Category	CD4+ Cells/μL	CD4+ Percentage (%)
1	≥500	≥29
2	200–499	14–28
3	<200	<14

The percentage of lymphocytes that are CD4+ T-cells Adapted from CDC. 1993 Revised Classification System for HIV Infection and Expanded Surveillance Case Definition for AIDS Among Adolescents and Adults MMWR 1992;41:(No RR-17).

APPENDIX II
Definitive Diagnostic Methods for Diseases Indicative of AIDS

Diseases	Diagnostic Methods
Cryptosporidiosis Isosporiasis Kaposi's sarcoma Lymphoma *Pneumocystis carinii* pneumonia Progressive multifocal leukoencephalopathy Toxoplasmosis Cervical cancer	Microscopy (histology or cytology)
Candidiasis	Gross inspection by endoscopy or autopsy or by microscopy (histology or cytology) on a specimen obtained directly from the tissues affected (including scrapings from the mucosal surface), not from a culture
Coccidioidomycosis Cryptococcosis Cytomegalovirus Herpes simplex virus Histoplasmosis	Microscopy (histology or cytology), culture, or detection of antigen in a specimen obtained directly from the tissues affected or a fluid from those tissues

(continued)

Diseases	Diagnostic Methods
Other mycobacteriosis Salmonellosis Tuberculosis	Culture
HIV encephalopathy (dementia)	Clinical findings of disabling cognitive or motor dysfunction interfering with occupation or activities of daily living, progressing over weeks to months, in the absence of a concurrent illness or condition other than HIV infection that could explain the findings. Methods to rule out such concurrent illness and conditions must include cerebrospinal fluid examination and either brain imagining (computed tomography or magnetic resonance) or autopsy.
HIV wasting syndrome	Findings of profound involuntary weight loss of >10% of baseline body weight plus either chronic diarrhea (at least two loose stools per day for ≥30 days), or chronic weakness and documented fever (for ≥30 days, intermittent or constant) in the absence of a concurrent illness or condition other than HIV infection that could explain the findings (e.g. cancer, tuberculosis, cryptosporidiosis, or other specific enteritis).
Pneumonia, recurrent	Recurrent (more than one episode in a 1-year period), acute (new x-ray evidence not present earlier) pneumonia diagnosed by both: a) culture (or other organism-specific diagnostic method) obtained from a clinically reliable specimen of a pathogen that typically causes pneumonia (other than *Pneumocystis carinii* or *Mycobacterium tuberculosis*), and b) radiologic evidence of pneumonia; cases that do not have laboratory confirmation of a causative organism for one of the episodes of pneumonia will be considered to be presumptively diagnosed.

Adapted from CDC. 1993 Revised Classification System for HIV Infection and Expanded Surveillance Case Definition for AIDS Among Adolescents and Adults MMWR 1992; 41:(No RR-17).

APPENDIX III
Suggested Guidelines for Presumptive Diagnosis of Diseases Indicative of AIDS

Diseases	Presumptive Criteria
Candidiasis of esophagus	a. Recent onset of retrosternal pain on swallowing; AND b. Oral candidiasis diagnosed by the gross appearance of white patches or plaques on an erythematous base or by the microscopic appearance of fungal mycelial filaments from a noncultured specimen scraped from the oral mucosa.
Cytomegalovirus retinitis	A characteristic appearance on serial ophthalmoscopic examinations (e.g. discrete patches of retinal whitening with distinct borders, spreading in a centrifugal manner along the paths of blood vessels, progressing over several months, and frequently associated with retinal vasculitis, hemorrhage, and necrosis). Resolution of active disease leaves retinal scarring and atrophy with retinal pigment epithelial mottling.

Diseases	Presumptive Criteria
Mycobacteriosis	Microscopy of a specimen from stool or normally sterile body fluids or tissue from a site other than lungs, skin, or cervical or hilar lymph nodes that shows acid-fast bacilli of a species not identified by culture.
Kaposi's sarcoma	A characteristic gross appearance of an erythematous or violaceous plaque-like lesion on skin or mucous membrane. (Note: Presumptive diagnosis of Kaposi's sarcoma should not be made by clinicians who have seen few cases of it.)
Pneumocystis carinii pneumonia	a. A history of dyspnea on exertion or nonproductive cough of recent onset (within the past 3 months); AND b. Chest x-ray evidence of diffuse bilateral interstitial infiltrates or evidence by gallium scan of diffuse bilateral pulmonary disease; AND c. Arterial blood gas analysis showing an arterial pO_2 of <70 mm Hg or a low respiratory diffusing capacity (<80% of predicted values) or an increase in the alveolar-arterial oxygen tension gradient; AND d. No evidence of a bacterial pneumonia.
Pneumonia, recurrent	Recurrent (more than one episode in a 1-year period), acute (new symptoms, signs, or x-ray evidence not present earlier) pneumonia diagnosed on clinical or radiologic grounds by the patient's physician.
Toxoplasmosis of brain	a. Recent onset of a focal neurologic abnormality consistent with intracranial disease or a reduced level of consciousness; AND b. Evidence by brain imaging (computed tomography or nuclear magnetic resonance) of a lesion having a mass effect or the radiographic appearance of which is enhanced by injection of contrast medium; AND c. Serum antibody to toxoplasmosis or successful response to therapy for toxoplasmosis.
Tuberculosis, pulmonary	When bacteriologic confirmation is not available, other reports may be considered to be verified cases of pulmonary tuberculosis if the criteria of the Division of Tuberculosis Elimination, National Center for Prevention Services, CDC, are used.

Adapted from CDC. 1993 Revised Classification System for HIV Infection and Expanded Surveillance Case Definition for AIDS Among Adolescents and Adults MMWR 1992;41:(No RR-17).

Classification System for HIV Infection in Children

In 1994, the Centers for Disease Control (CDC) revised the classification system for HIV infection in children under 13 years of age (1), replacing the pediatric classification system published in 1987 (1) to reflect the stage of the child's disease and establish mutually exclusive classification categories (Table 1.5). The 1994 classification system sum-

Table 1.5.
Pediatric Human Immunodeficiency Virus (HIV) Classification*

Immunologic Categories	Clinical Categories			
	N: No Signs/ Symptoms	A: Mild Signs/ Symptoms	B:[+] Moderate Signs/Symptoms	C:[+] Severe Signs/Symptoms
1. No evidence of suppression	N1	A1	B1	C1
2. Evidence of moderate suppression	N2	A2	B2	C2
3. Severe suppression	N3	A3	B3	C3

*Children whose HIV infection is not confirmed are classified by using the above grid with a letter E (for perinatally exposed) placed before the appropriate classification code (e.g., EN2)
[+]Both Category C and lymphoid interstitial pneumonitis in Category B are reportable to state and local health departments as acquired immunodeficiency syndrome.
Adapted from CDC. 1994 Revised Classification System for Human Immunodeficiency Virus Infection in children less than 13 years of age / Official Authorized Addenda: Human immunodeficiency virus infection codes and official guidelines for coding and reporting ICD-9-CM. MMWR. 1994;43 (RR-12).

marized here, classifies infected children into mutually exclusive categories according to three parameters: a) infection status; b) clinical status; and c) immunologic status. Once classified, an HIV-infected child cannot be reclassified to a less severe category even if the child's clinical or immunologic status improves. In addition, pediatric definitions for two acquired immunodeficiency syndrome-defining conditions (2) are described here.

Diagnosis of HIV Infection in Children

Diagnosing HIV infection in children born to HIV-infected mothers (Figure 1.10) is complicated by the presence of maternal anti-HIV IgG antibody, which crosses the placenta to the fetus. Although virtually all children born to HIV-infected mothers are HIV-antibody positive at birth, only 15%–30% are actually infected. In uninfected children, this antibody usually becomes undetectable by 9 months of age but occasionally remains detectable until 19 months of age. Therefore, standard anti-HIV IgG antibody tests cannot be used to indicate reliably a child's infection status before 18 months of age (3). Polymerase chain reaction (PCR) and virus culture are probably the most sensitive and specific assays for detecting HIV infection in children born to infected mothers (4–6). The use of these assays can identify approximately 30%–50% of infected children at birth and nearly 100% of infected infants by 3–6 months of age (7).

The standard p24 antigen assay is less sensitive than either virus culture of PCR, especially when anti-HIV antibody levels are high, because it fails to detect immune-complexed p24 antigen (8). However, modifica-

DIAGNOSIS: HIV INFECTED

a)   A child <18 months of age who is known to be HIV seropositive or born to an HIV-infected mother and:

- has positive results on two separate determinations (excluding cord blood) from one or more of the following HIV detection tests:
    - HIV culture,
    - HIV polymerase chain reaction (PCR),
    - HIV antigen (p24),

or

- meets criteria for acquired immunodeficiency syndrome (AIDS) diagnosis based on the 1987 AIDS surveillance case definition (10).

b)   A child 18 months of age or older born to an HIV-infected mother or any child infected by blood, blood products, or other known modes of transmission (e.g., sexual contact) who:

- is HIV-antibody positive by repeatedly reactive enzyme immunoassay (EIA) and confirmatory test (e.g., Western blot or immunofluorescence assay [IFA])

or

- meets any of the criteria in a) above.

DIAGNOSIS: PERINATALLY EXPOSED (PREFIX E)

A child who does not meet the criteria above who:

- is HIV seropositive by EIA and confirmatory test (e.g., Western blot or IFA) and is <18 months of age at the time of the test;

or

- has unknown antibody status, but was born to a mother known to be infected with HIV.

DIAGNOSIS; SEROREVERTER (SR)

A child who is born to an HIV-infected mother and who:

- has been documented as HIV-antibody negative (i.e., two or more negative EIA tests performed at 6-18 months of age or one negative EIA test after 18 months of age);

and

- has had no other laboratory evidence of infection (has not had two positive viral detection tests, if performed);

and

- has not had an AIDS-defining condition.

---

* This definition of HIV infection replaces the definition published in the 1987 AIDS surveillance case definition (10).

Adapted from CDC. 1994 Revised Classification System for Human Immunodeficiency Virus Infection in children less than 13 years of age / Official Authorized Addenda: Human immunodeficiency virus infection codes and official guidelines for coding and reporting ICD-9-CM. MMWR 1994;43 (RR-12).

Figure 1.10   Diagnosis of human immunodeficiency virus (HIV) infection in children.*

tion of the p24-antigen assay to dissociate immune complexes has increased its sensitivity in diagnosis HIV infection among children exposed to HIV (9). Other laboratory assays which are less commonly used (e.g., anti-HIV IgA and ELISPOT/ in vitro antibody production [IVAP]) and less sensitive than both PCR or virus culture, were not included in the algorithm for determining infection status. However, clinicians who determine a child's antiretroviral therapy on the basis of such assays may use them to classify the child as being infected.

Some children develop severe clinical conditions resulting from HIV infection before their infection status has been sufficiently established. For classification purposes, a child meeting the criteria for the 1987 AIDS case definition (10) should be considered HIV-infected—even in the absence of definitive laboratory assays.

Children born to mothers with HIV infection are defined as seroreverters (SRs) and are considered uninfected with HIV if they a) become HIV-antibody negative after 6 months of age, b) have no other laboratory evidence of HIV infection, and c) have not met the AIDS surveillance case definition criteria (Fig. 1.10). Sufficient data are unavailable to conclusively define a child who is uninfected on the basis of viral detection tests. However, in certain situations (e.g., clinical trials), negative viral detection tests may be used presumptively to exclude infection.

Immunologic Categories

Children are categorized by the severity of immunosuppression attributed to HIV infection. Although CD4+ T-lymphocyte counts are used in the adult classification system (11), the use of CD4+ counts to assess HIV-associated immunosuppression in children are complicated by several findings. Normal CD4+ counts are higher in infants and younger children than in adults and decline over the first few years of life (12–16). Children may also develop opportunistic infections at higher CD4+ levels than do adults (17–19). Data are insufficient to correlate CD4+ levels with disease progression at all age groups, although low age-specific CD4+ counts appear to correlate with conditions associated with immunosuppression in children (12,17,20,21). Therefore, despite the complications, classification based on age-specific CD4+ levels appears to be useful for describing the immunologic status of HIV-infected children.

There are fewer data available on age-specific values for CD4+ T-lymphocyte percent of total lymphocytes than for absolute counts; however, the CD4+ T-lymphocyte percent has less measurement variability than the absolute count (22). To establish the age-specific values of CD4+ percent that correlate with CD4+ count thresholds, the CDC collected data on selected clinical projects in the United States and Europe on both HIV-infected and uninfected children <13 years of age: nonparametric regression modeling was used to establish the CD4+ percent boundaries that best correlated with the CD4+ boundaries in the classification system.

Table 1.6.

Immunologic Categories Based on Age-Specific CD4+ T-Lymphocyte Counts and Percent of Total Lymphocytes

Immunologic Category	Age of Child					
	<12 months		1–5 Years		6–12 Years	
	μL	(%)	μL	(%)	μL	(%)
1. No evidence of suppression	≥1,500	(≥25)	≥1,000	(≥25)	≥500	(≥25)
2. Evidence of moderate suppression	750–1,499	(15–24)	500–999	(15–24)	200–499	(15–24)
3. Severe suppression	<750	(<15)	<500	(<15)	<200	(<15)

Adapted from CDC. 1994 Revised Classification System for Human Immunodeficiency Virus Infection in children less than 13 years of age / Official authorized Addenda: Human immunodeficiency virus infection codes and official guidelines for coding and reporting ICD-9-CM. MMWR. 1994;43 (RR-12).

The immunologic category classification (Table 1.6) is based on either the CD4+ T-lymphocyte count or the CD4+ percent of total lymphocytes. If both the CD4+ count and the CD4+ percent indicate different classification categories, the child should be classified into the more severe category. Repeat or follow-up CD4+ values that result in a change in classification should be confirmed by a second determination. Values thought to be in error should not be used. A child should not reclassified to a less severe category regardless of subsequent CD4+ determinations.

Clinical Categories

Based on signs, symptoms, or diagnoses related to HIV infection, children who are HIV-infected or perinatally exposed to HIV may be classified into one of four mutually exclusive clinical categories (Fig. 1.11). The clinical categories have been defined to provide a staging classification (e.g., the prognosis for children in the second category would be less favorable than for those in the first category). The four clinical categories are: Category N, not symptomatic; Category A, mildly symptomatic; Category B, moderately symptomatic; and Category C, severely symptomatic. In addition, children who have uncertain HIV-infection status are designated with a prefix E.

CATEGORIES N AND A

Category N includes children with no signs or symptoms considered to be the result of HIV infection or with only one of the conditions listed in Category A. Category N was separated from Category A partly because of the substantial amount of time that can elapse before a child

---

CATEGORY N: NOT SYMPTOMATIC

Children who have no signs or symptoms considered to be the result of HIV infection or who have only one of the conditions listed in Category A.

CATEGORY A: MILDLY SYMPTOMATIC

Children with two or more of the conditions listed below but none of the conditions listed in Categories B and C.
- Lymphadenopathy (≥ 0.5 cm at more than two sites; bilateral = one site)
- Hepatomegaly
- Splenomegaly
- Dermatitis
- Parotitis
- Recurrent or persistent upper respiratory infection, sinusitis, or otitis media

CATEGORY B: MODERATELY SYMPTOMATIC

Children who have symptomatic conditions other than those listed for Category A or C that are attributed to HIV infection. Examples of conditions in clinical Category B include but are not limited to:
- Anemia (< 8 gm/dL), neutropenia (<1,000/mm³), or thrombocytopenia (<100,000/mm³) persisting ≥30 days
- Bacterial meningitis, pneumonia, or sepsis (single episode)
- Candidiasis, oropharyngeal (thrush), persisting (>2 months) in children >6 months of age
- Cardiomyopathy
- Cytomegalovirus infection, with onset before 1 month of age
- Diarrhea, recurrent or chronic
- Hepatitis
- Herpes simplex virus (HSV) stomatitis, recurrent (more than two episodes within 1 year)
- HSV bronchitis, pneumonitis, or esophagitis with onset before 1 month of age
- Herpes zoster (shingles) involving at least two distinct episodes or more than one dermatome
- Leiomyosarcoma
- Lymphoid interstitial pneumonia (LIP) or pulmonary lymphoid hyperplasia complex
- Nephropathy
- Nocardiosis
- Persistent fever (lasting > 1 month)
- Toxoplasmosis, onset before 1 month of age
- Varicella, disseminated (complicated chickenpox)

CATEGORY C: SEVERELY SYMPTOMATIC
- Children who have any; condition listed in the 1987 surveillance case definition for acquired immunodeficiency syndrome (10), with the exception of LIP (Fig. 1.12)

Adapted from CDC. 1994 Revised Classification System for Human Immunodeficiency Virus Infection in children less than 13 years of age / Official authorized Addenda: Human immunodeficiency virus infection codes and official guidelines for coding and reporting ICD-9-CM. MMWR. 1994;43 (RR-12).

Figure 1.11.   Clinical categories for children with HIV infection.

manifests the signs or symptoms defined in Category B. In addition, more information during this early stage of disease can be ascertained by separating these two categories. For children who have uncertain HIV-infection status (prefix E), Categories N and A may help to distinguish those children who are more likely to be infected with HIV (23) (i.e., children in Category EA may be more likely to be infected than children in Category EN).

CATEGORY B

This includes all children with signs and symptoms thought to be caused by HIV infection but not specifically outlined under Category A or Category C. The conditions listed in Figure 1.11 are examples only; any other HIV related condition not included in Category A or C should be included in Category B. Anemia, thrombocytopenia, and lymphopenia have defined thresholds in the new classification system (23).

CATEGORY C

All AIDS-defining conditions except lymphoid interstitial pneumonitis (LIP) are included under this category (Figure 1.12). As the prognosis for children with LIP has been reported to be substantially better than that for children who have other AIDS-defining conditions (21,24,25), LIP has been separated from the other AIDS-defining conditions in Category C and placed in Category B.

Signs and symptoms related to causes other than HIV infection (e.g., inflammatory or drug-related causes) should not be used to classify children. For example, a child with drug-related hepatitis or anemia should not be classified in Category B solely because the conditions may be associated with HIV infection, whereas a child with anemia or hepatitis thought to be HIV-related should be classified in Category B. Because the criteria for diagnosing some conditions and determining whether a child's signs, symptoms, or diagnoses are related to HIV infection may not be clear in all cases, judgment of the clinicians and researchers using the classification system may be required.

CATEGORY C: SEVERELY SYMPTOMATIC*

- Serious bacteria infections, multiple or recurrent (i.e., any combination of at least two culture-confirmed infections within a 2-year period), of the following types: septicemia, pneumonia, meningitis, bone or joint infection, or abscess of an internal organ or body cavity (excluding otitis media, superficial skin or mucosal abscesses, and indwelling catheter-related infections)
- Candidiasis, esophageal or pulmonary (bronchi, trachea, lungs)
- Coccidiomycosis, disseminated (at site other than or in addition to lungs or cervical or hilar lymph nodes)
- Cryptococcosis, extrapulmonary
- Cryptosporidiosis or isosporiasis with diarrhea persisting >1 month
- Cytomegalovirus disease with onset of symptoms at age >1 month (at site other than liver, spleen, or lymph nodes)
- Encephalopathy (at least one of the following progressive findings present for at least 2 months in the absence of a concurrent illness other than HIV infection that could explain the findings): a) failure to attain or loss of developmental milestones or loss of intellectual ability, verified by standard developmental scale or neuropsychological tests; b)impaired brain growth or acquired microcephaly demonstrated by head circumference measurements or brain atrophy demonstrated by computerized tomography or magnetic resonance imaging (serial imaging is required for children <2 years of age); c) acquired symmetric motor deficit manifested by two or more of the following: paresis, pathologic reflexes, ataxia, or gait disturbance
- Herpes simplex virus infection causing a mucocutaneous ulcer that persists for > 1 month; or bronchitis, pneumonitis, or esophagitis for any duration affecting a child >1 month of age
- Histoplasmosis, disseminated (at a site other than or in addition to lungs or cervical hilar lymph nodes)
- Kaposi's sarcoma
- Lymphoma, primary, in brain
- Lymphoma, small, noncleaved cell (Burkitt's), or immunoblastic or large cell lymphoma of B-cell or unknown immunologic phenotype
- *Mycobacterium tuberculosis*, disseminated or extrapulmonary
- *Mycobacterium*, other species or unidentified species, disseminated (at a site other than or in addition to lungs, skin, or cervical or hilar lymph nodes)
- *Mycobacterium avium* complex or *Mycobacterium kansasii*, disseminated (at site other than or in addition to lungs, skin, or cervical or hilar lymph nodes)
- *Pneumocystis carinii pneumonia*
- Progressive multifocal leukoencephalopathy
- Salmonella (nontyphoid) septicemia, recurrent
- Toxoplasmosis of the brain with onset at >1 month of age
- Wasting syndrome in the absence of a concurrent illness other than HIV infection that could explain the following findings:
    - a) persistent weight loss >10% of baseline ;OR
    - b) downward crossing of at least two of the following percentile lines on the weight for age chart (e.g, 95th, 75th, 50th, 25th, 5th) in a child ≥1 year of age; OR
    - c) <5th percentile on weight-for-height chart on two consecutive measurements, ≥ 30 days apart PLUS
        - a) chronic diarrhea (i.e., at least two loose stools per day for ≥30 days) OR
        - b) documented fever (for ≥30 days, intermittent or constant)

---

*See the 1987 CDC AIDS surveillance case definition (10) for diagnosis criteria

Adapted from CDC. 1994 Revised Classification System for Human Immunodeficiency Virus Infection in children less than 13 years of age / Official authorized Addenda: Human immunodeficiency virus infection codes and official guidelines for coding and reporting ICD-9-CM. MMWR. 1994;43 (RR-12).

Figure 1.12.   Conditions included in clinical Category C for children infected with HIV.

Table 1.7.
Comparison of the 1987 and 1994 Pediatric HIV Classification Systems

1987 Classification	1994 Classification
P-0	PREFIX "E"
P-1	N
P-2A	A, B, and C
P-2B	C
P-2C	B
P-2D1	C
P-2D2	C
P-2D3	B
P-2E1	C
P-2E2	B
P-2F	B

Adapted from CDC. 1994 Revised Classification System for Human Immunodeficiency Virus Infection in children less than 13 years of age / Official authorized Addenda: Human immunodeficiency virus infection codes and official guidelines for coding and reporting ICD-9-CM. MMWR. 1994;43 (RR-12).

Translating the 1987 Pediatric HIV Classification Categories into 1994 Classification Categories

In most cases, categories from the 1987 pediatric HIV classification system can be translated into categories in the 1994 system (Table 1.7). Children previously classified as P2A are now classified in more than one category, reflecting the different prognoses for children with different conditions included in the P2A category (e.g., children who have wasting syndrome have a worse prognosis than those who have lymphadenopathy).

EFFECT ON THE AIDS SURVEILLANCE CASE DEFINITION FOR CHILDREN

As the classification system is used in conjunction with the AIDS case definition, the 1994 revision provides an opportunity to update certain features of the 1987 AIDS surveillance case definition for children <13 years of age (10). Although LIP falls under Category in the 1994 classification system, it continues to be reportable to state and local health departments (along with the conditions in Category C) as an AIDS-defining condition in children. Two changes in the definitions for other conditions follows:

HIV ENCEPHALOPATHY AND HIV WASTING

There are new definitions for HIV encephalopathy and HIV wasting (Fig. 1.12) which replace the definitions published in the 1987 AIDS surveillance case definition for children. The definition of HIV encephalopathy follows the recommendations of the American Academy of Neurology AIDS Task Force (26). Because this condition is complex, diagnosis may require neurologic consultation.

HIV INFECTION

The new definition of HIV infection (Fig. 1.10) replaces the definition for laboratory evidence of HIV infection in children used in the 1987 pediatric AIDS case definition. For children with an AIDS-defining condition that requires laboratory evidence of HIV infection, a single positive HIV-detection test (i.e., HIV culture, HIV PCR, or HIV antigen [p24]) is sufficient for a reportable AIDS diagnosis if the diagnosis is confirmed by a clinician.

REFERENCES

1. CDC. 1994 revised classification system for human immunodeficiency virus (HIV) infection in children less than 13 years of age. MMWR 1984;43:(RR-12).
2. CDC. Classification System for Human Immunodeficiency Virus (HIV) Infection in Children Under 13 Years of age. MMWR. 1987;36:225–235.
3. Simpson BJ, Andiman WA. Difficulties in assigning human immunodeficiency virus-1 infection and seroreversion status in a cohort of HIV-exposed children using serologic criteria established by the CDC and Prevention. Pediatrics 1994;93:840–842.
4. Krivine A, Firtion G, Cao L, Francoual C, Henrion R, Lebon P. HIV replication during the first weeks of life. Lancet 1992;339:1187–1189.
5. Rogers MF, Ou C-Y, Rayfield M, et al. Use of the polymerase chain reaction for early detection of the proviral sequences of human immunodeficiency virus in infants born to seropositive mothers. N Engl J Med 1989;320:1649–1654.
6. Burgard M, Mayaux M-J, Blanche S et al. The use of viral culture and p24 antigen testing to diagnose human immunodeficiency virus infection in neonates. N Engl J Med 1992;327:1192–1197.
7. Anonymous. Report of a consensus workshop, Siena, Italy, January 17–18, 1992: early diagnosis of HIV infection in infants. J Acquir Immune Defic Syndr 1992;5:1169–1178.
8. Rogers M, Ou, Kilbourne B, Schocehetman G. Advances and problems in the diagnosis of human immunodeficiency virus infection in infants. Pediatr Infect Dis J 1991; 10:523–531.
9. Miles SA, Baldern E, Magpantay L, et al. Rapid serologic testing with immune-complex-dissociated HIV p24 antigen for early detection of HIV infection in neonates. N Engl J Med 1993;328:297–302.
10. Revision of the CDC surveillance case definition for acquired immunodeficiency syndrome. MMWR 1987;36(suppl):1–15s.
11. CDC. 1993 Revised classification system for HIV infection and expanded surveillance case definition for AIDS among adolescents and adults. MMWR 1993;41 (RR-17).
12. Erkeller-Yuksel FM, Deneys V, Yuksel B, et al. Age-related changes in human blood lymphocyte sub-populations. J Pediatr 1992;120:216–222.
13. Denny T, Yogev R, Gelman R, et al. Lymphocyte subsets in healthy children during the first 5 years of life. JAMA 1992;267:1484–1488.
14. McKinney RE, Wilfert CM. Lymphocyte subsets in children younger than 2 years old: normal values in a population at risk for human immunodeficiency virus infection and diagnostic and prognostic application to infected children. Pediatr Infect Dis J 1992; 11:639–644.
15. The European Collaborative Study. Age-related standards for T-lymphocyte subsets based on uninfected children born to human immunodeficiency virus-1-infected women. Pediatr Infect Dis J 1995;11:1018–1026.
16. Waecker NJ, Ascher DP, Robb ML, et al. Age adjusted CD4+ lymphocyte parameters in HIV at risk uninfected children. Clin Infect Dis 1993;17:123–126.
17. Leibovitz E, Rigaud M, Pollack H, et al. *Pneumocystis carinii* pneumonia in infants infected with the human immunodeficiency virus with more than 450 CD4 T lymphocytes per cubic millimeter. N Engl J Med 1990;323:531–533.
18. Connor E, Bagarazzi M, McSherry G, et al. Clinical and laboratory correlates of *Pneumocystis carinii* pneumonia in children infected with HIV. JAMA 1991;265: 1693–1697.
19. Kovacs A, Frederick T, Church J, et al. CD4 T-Lymphocyte counts and *Pneumocystis carinii* pneumonia in pediatric HIV infection. JAMA 1991;265:1698–1703.

20. Butler KM, Husson RN, Lewis LL, et al. CD4 status and p24 antigenemia: are they useful predictors of survival in HIV-infected children receiving antiretroviral therapy. Am J Dis Child 1992;146:932–936.
21. de Martino M, Tovo PA, Galli L, et al. Prognostic significance of immunologic changes in 675 infants perinatally exposed to human immunodeficiency virus. J Pediatr 1991;119:702–709.
22. Raszka WV, Meyer GA, Waecker NH, et al. Variability of serial absolute and percent CD4+ lymphocyte counts in healthy children born to HIV-1 infected parents. Lancet 1994;13:70–72.
23. Caldwell B, Oxtoby M, Rogers M. Proposed CDC pediatric HIV classification system: evaluation in an active surveillance system (Abstract). IXth International Conference on AIDS, Berlin, June 7–11, 1993.
24. Tovo PA, deMartino M, Gabiano C, et al. Prognostic factors and survival in children with perinatal HIV-1 infection. Lancet 1992;339:1249–1253.
25. Blanche S, Tardieu M, Duliege AM, et al. Longitudinal study of 94 symptomatic infants with perinatally acquired human immunodeficiency virus infection. Am J Dis Child 1990;144:1210–1215.
26. Working Group of the American Academy of Neurology AIDS Task Force. Nomenclature and research case definitions for neurologic manifestations of human immunodeficiency virus-type 1 (HIV-1) infection. Neurology 1991;41:778–786.

CHAPTER 2

HIV Counseling and Testing

HIV counseling and testing are an important components of HIV prevention. Counseling and testing can increase self-perception of risk as well as assist individuals initiate behavior changes that reduce their risk of becoming infected or if infected, prevent transmission to others. Through counseling and testing, identification of HIV-positive persons enables early medical care, appropriate counseling, and referral to appropriate health, preventive, and social services. Early intervention, including medical evaluation, antiretroviral therapy and pharmacologic prophylaxis can enhance and prolong the life of HIV-positive individuals.

Essential components of HIV prevention counseling includes:

- Maintaining confidentiality of test results and other information.

- Providing information regarding the transmission and prevention of HIV.

- Providing a personalized risk assessment to facilitate a realistic perception of self-risk.

- Providing prevention counseling which helps the individual identify his or her risk behaviors and assists the individual initiate or maintain behavior change to reduce or eliminate his or her risk of HIV transmission or acquisition (i.e., a realistic risk reduction plan).

- Preparing the individual to receive, understand, and manage his or her test result.

- Providing the HIV antibody test result and based on that knowledge, assist the individual plan behavior change. Providing necessary referrals for psychosocial support, appropriate drug treatment services, necessary medical and preventive services. Discussing the responsibility of appropriate disclosure of serostatus (e.g., partner notification).

Risk reduction and prevention aspects are addressed separately *(See Risk Reduction and Prevention)*.

Risk assessment, counseling and testing information, and prevention should be individualized, with consideration of the cultural, educational, and lifestyle differences that are unique to each individual. The various aspects of testing and counseling will be considered in the following section.

Indications for HIV Counseling and Testing

Current guidelines recommend that HIV prevention counseling and voluntary testing be offered to individuals practicing behaviors which place them at risk for infection (1–10). A routine counseling and testing program should include a policy to offer these services to all patients, inform them when testing should be done, and explain the reasons for this recommendation. Except where testing is required by law (e.g., blood donors, immigrants, military recruits), individuals have the right to decline to be tested without being denied health care or other services (1).

The recommendation of HIV counseling and testing should be considered when persons report the following at-risk behaviors or circumstances (1–11):

- Individuals who consider themselves at risk.

- Men who have or have had sex with other men.

- Individuals who have a history (past or current) of injecting drug use (IDU), including steroids.

- Individuals who have a history of sexually transmitted disease (past or current).

- Individuals with multiple sexual partner (past or currently).

- Individuals who exchange sex for drugs or money.

- Individuals who use crack. (The use of "crack" cocaine is associated with increased sexual activity and the exchange of sex for drugs. Most mood-altering drugs are also associated with behavior changes that can cause a decrease in preventive behavioral practices.)

- Individuals who have lived in or come from countries where heterosexual transmission of HIV is prevalent.

- Individuals who received blood components or transfusions between early 1978 to mid-1985.

- Hemophiliacs.

- Sexual partners of individuals with or at risk for HIV infection (e.g., IDU, bisexual).

- Sexually active individuals who are living or have lived in high HIV prevalence areas.

- History of survival sex (i.e., sex in exchange for housing, food, clothes, or money).

- History of body piercing or tattooing with nonsterile equipment.

- Individuals with a recent diagnosis of tuberculosis (TB) or suspicion of TB. (A high prevalence of HIV infection has been shown among patients with tuberculosis. All patients with tuberculosis should be routinely counseled and tested for HIV antibody.)

- Individuals presenting with clinical signs and symptoms of HIV infection. Clinical signs and symptoms include: generalized lymphadenopathy; unexplained dementia; chronic, unexplained fever or diarrhea; unexplained weight loss; tuberculosis; also shingles, persistent or recalcitrant dermatologic conditions; sexually transmitted diseases; persistent herpes, or chronic candidiasis.

- Presence of any illness which a positive HIV test result might alter the recommended diagnostic evaluation, treatment or follow up.

- Women of childbearing age. All women of childbearing age (usually ages 15–44) should be routinely counseled and offered voluntary HIV testing, regardless of whether they are pregnant (4–11).

In addition to women presenting with the above behaviors or circumstances, testing and counseling should also be offered to the following women (4,7,12):

- Mothers who have delivered HIV-infected children.

- Women artificially inseminated since 1979 (unless donor was screened for HIV).

- Women who present with signs or symptoms of HIV infection. Gynecological indicators include (4,7):

- Persistent or recurrent vaginal candidiasis.

- Recurrent (more than 2 episodes within 6 months) of severe genital herpes simplex.

- Genital ulcer diseases (e.g., syphilis, chancroid, lymphogranuloma venereum).

- Condyloma acuminatum recalcitrant to conventional therapy or involving multiple sites.

- Abnormal pap smear with moderate-to-severe cervical dysplasia, or invasive carcinoma.

- Recurrent or persistent pelvic inflammatory disease despite appropriate nonsurgical treatment.

- Pregnant women. Because specific medical interventions are available which prevent perinatal transmission and in order to offer these interventions in a timely and effective manner, the U.S. Public Health Service (PHS) recommends routine HIV counseling and voluntary testing to all pregnant women, regardless of the prevalence of HIV infection in their community or their risk for infection (11).

Considerations When Recommending Testing

There have been adverse reactions reported following the receipt of an HIV test result. These include depression, increased risk-taking behavior, and suicidal attempts. It is important to assess the coping skills of the individual and the social support available to the person prior to testing. Reasons to consider against testing include pressure from a family member, significant other, or agency to share the test results; indications that a positive test might result in termination from medical or chemical dependence treatment, or emotional instability (13,14). For chemically dependent persons, HIV testing must occur after withdrawal is stabilized and preferably when the person is emotionally stable (13).

REFERENCES

1. CDC. Guidelines for counseling and antibody testing to prevent HIV infection and AIDS—Public Health Service. MMWR 1987;36:509–515.
2. Kassler WJ, Wu AW. Addressing HIV infection in office practice. Primary Care 1992;19:19–33.
3. Rutherford GW, Oliva GE, Grossman M. Guidelines for the control of perinatally transmitted human immunodeficiency virus infection and care of infected mothers, infants and children. West J Med 1987;147:104–108.
4. ACOG issues report on HIV infection in women. Special medical report. Am Fam Physician 1992;46:579–585.
5. NYC Department of Health: Guidelines for physicians in HIV counseling and testing and related documents. New York, N.Y.: NYC Department of Health, Bureau of Public Health Education, 1989.
6. Anastos K, Palleja SM. Caring for women at risk of HIV infection. J Gen Inter Med 1991;6(Jan/Feb Suppl):S40–S46.

7. Allen MH and Marte C. HIV infection in women: presentation and protocols. Hosp Pract 1992;27:155–162.
8. CDC. 1993 Sexually transmitted diseases treatment guidelines. MMWR 1993;42 (RR-1).
9. CDC. Recommendations for assisting in the prevention of perinatal transmission of human T lymphotropic virus type II/lymphadenopathy associated virus and acquired immunodeficiency syndrome. MMWR 1985;34:721–731.
10. Anderson MM, Morris RE. HIV and adolescents. Pediatric Annals 1993;22:436–446.
11. CDC. US Public Health Service Recommendations for human immunodeficiency virus counseling and voluntary testing for pregnant women. MMWR 1995;44 (RR-7).
12. Poole L. HIV infection in women. In: Cohen PT, Sande MA, Volberding PA , eds. The AIDS knowledge base. Waltham Mass: The Medical Publishing Group 1990:4.29–1–4.29–10.
13. Karan LD. Primary Care for AIDS and chemical dependence. Addiction Medicine West J Med 1990;152:538–542.
14. Hein K. AIDS in adolescence. J Adolesc Health Care 1989;10:10S–35S.

Risk Assessment

In conjunction with a complete medical history, a risk assessment will help determine whether an individual should be counseled with respect to risk reduction and HIV testing. Risk assessment assists in identifying an individual's behaviors that place him or her at risk for HIV infection. Assessing a patient's risk of HIV exposure includes direct and specific questioning regarding blood product exposures, sexual practices, and drug use. Although the clinician should be able to discuss frankly the risk of HIV infection, discussing sexual and drug behavior is difficult for many individuals and physicians. The following highlights recommendations regarding assessing risk for HIV exposure in an individual (1–15).

Introducing the Risk Assessment to the Patient

It is important to justify why questions on sexual and drug history are being asked of the patient. Opening statements should emphasize that specific questions about lifestyle and sexual behaviors are being asked of *all* patients in order to explore what behaviors may place them at risk for certain medical conditions, including HIV infection (7–9). It should be explained that this type of history is important in preventing disease and assessing health, and the patient reassured that this type of history is taken from all patients. Signs and symptoms of HIV infection should also prompt a risk assessment; these include unexplained fever, night sweats, weight loss, cough, dyspnea, or diarrhea of more than two weeks' duration (2). The presence of unexplained oral thrush; hairy leukoplakia; recurrent or chronic perianal herpes infection; and anemia, neutropenia, or thrombocytopenia should also necessitate a risk assessment (2). Explaining to the patient that although the symptoms may be indicative of other illnesses, an in-depth history may help identify any possible risk to certain diseases.

Issues concerning privacy and confidentiality should also be addressed to reassure the patient, and to facilitate honest disclosure of sensitive issues. A code system might be used to enter the information in the medical record (8). Acknowledge that the questions surround sensitive issues and give the patient permission not to answer questions that make him/her feel too uncomfortable. An example of an introductory statement may be, "I am going to ask some personal questions that I ask all my patients (7). There are certain medical conditions such as hepatitis, sexually transmitted diseases, and HIV infection that are related to sexual and drug practices (13). I believe these questions are important so I can take care of you appropriately. I realize that the nature of these questions may be sensitive, so please let me know if you do not wish to answer any of them. Everything you tell me will remain confidential."

Assessing Risk

A risk assessment should determine whether the patient is sexually active, and if so,

- the number of sexual partners (casual and steady) and sexual activities (including vaginal, anal, and oral sex, both receptive and insertive activities, condom use);
- having sex with persons at risk for HIV (e.g. injection drug user);
- whether substances such as alcohol, cocaine, etc., are used in connection with sexual activity;
- a history of any sexually transmitted diseases (STDs), and/or having sex with persons who have STDs, especially genital lesions
- birth control (pregnancy prevention) methods.

A drug history, including alcohol use, should also be included in the risk assessment. In-depth questioning may be necessary as risk behaviors are identified (e.g., if an individual reports multiple partners, specific questions regarding risk behaviors of partners might be solicited).

INTERVIEWING CONSIDERATIONS

The interview style and terminology should be tailored to suit the comfort of the individual patient and physician. The physician must be sure that the patient understands the terminology, and if possible, should use language that the patient relates to. Depending on the age, cultural background, and educational level of the patient, the terminology used may vary; descriptive terms may need to be used (e.g., "Do you engage in anal sex?" versus "When you have sex do you insert your penis into a person's anus [butt] or does someone insert his penis into your anus [butt]?")(8) Questions should be nonjudgmental and open-ended (questions that require more than a yes or no answer) to determine the patient's risk of HIV infection. The sexual orientation of the patient is less important than the specific sexual practices in which the patient is involved. Many men who may have had sex with men do not perceive themselves at risk, or being homosexual/bisexual. In one survey, 37% of men had at least one male-male sexual experience in their lifetime (16). Assumptions regarding sexual activity because of age, being handicapped, or marital status should not be made. Being married does not always equate to being monogamous or heterosexual, just as being elderly, adolescent, or handicapped does not exclude sexual activity.

When asking questions, a nonjudgmental attitude should be maintained as much as possible. The importance of body language, voice inflections and reactions may reveal underlying judgment and biases that words, themselves, do not. Questions should be solicited in a professional and systematic manner. Directing the interview as a conversion, exchanging information rather than as a question-and-answer session has also been suggested (15). If the clinician is somewhat embarrassed and shy in asking the questions, the patient may feel reluctant to answer. The phrasing of questions should be a consideration, with avoidance of biased questioning (e.g., "You don't use drugs, do you?"). "Do you have sex, or have you ever had sex?" is more neutral than "You don't have sex, do you?" People who have experienced sexual activities with a person of the same sex (even once) may not identify with a given category, especially a stigmatized one. Questions should focus on the aspect of risky behavior, "Have you ever had sex with men, women or both?" rather than being in a "risk" group, "Are you heterosexual, homosexual, or bisexual?" Depending on the risks identified, questions concerning sexual practices might include: "How often do you use a condom when you have sexual intercourse?" "Have you ever had gonorrhea, herpes, genital ulcers, or any other sexually transmitted diseases?" or "Have you ever exchanged sex for money or drugs?" If the patient has had sex, raising the patient's awareness to the risk of STDs, HIV, and the importance of safer sex is essential.

SUBSTANCE USE

Discussing drug use and chemical dependency with patients may also be difficult. When taking a drug history, it is especially important to be nonjudgmental. Given that injection drug use (IDU) is illegal in the United States, patients may be reluctant to answer questions truthfully unless they trust the interviewer. It may be less threatening to start with questions concerning alcohol and tobacco use, over-the-counter and prescription drugs, etc. "Have you ever used drugs bought from or given to you by a nonmedical source?" is more direct and less threatening than asking about "street or illicit drugs." Casual, social or experimental use of injection drugs even once can result in exposure to HIV and no one should be ruled out. A history of substance use should include the type of substance(s) used (e.g., opiate, stimulates, alcohol, etc.); routes of administration; and patterns of use (e.g., duration, frequency and amount) (12). Asking when the substance was last used can help define recent use (12). If injection drugs were ever used, questions regarding needle sharing, and disinfection of needles and "works" (e.g., equipment) should be asked. Treatment history and potential medical and social complications should be investigated (e.g., history of hepatitis, STDs, drug treatment program, etc.) (12). Tattooing and use of anabolic steroids are frequent practices, especially among youth and questions should be asked about them. Any drug use, including alcohol, or cocaine, can impair judgment and lead to unsafe behaviors. Users of crack have a higher incidence of HIV infection, usually acquired through unsafe sex (13). If the individual has a history of drug use, the topic of the risk of HIV transmission may then be broached and risk reduction discussed.

Based on the assessment of an individual's risk for HIV, healthy behaviors can be reinforced and/or recommendations behavior change discussed. If appropriate, the individual should be given prevention counseling and offered voluntary HIV testing. Assessing an individual's risk for HIV can lead to early identification and therapy of HIV-infected persons, and provide an opportunity for education and specific risk reduction strategies for persons practicing at-risk behaviors.

REFERENCES

1. American Medical Association. HIV blood test counseling: AMA physician guidelines. Chicago: American Medical Association, 1988.
2. Antoniskis D, Sattler FR, Leedom JL. Importance of assessing risk behavior for AIDS. Postgrad Med 1988;83:138–152.
3. Blais FX. How to recognize patients at risk or infected with HIV. JAOA 1992; 92(2):234–235.
4. DeHovitz JA and Sadovsky R. Initial clinical assessment and management of HIV infection. Primary Care 1992;19:35–56.
5. Filardo TW. Obtaining a sexual history (letter). AFP American Family Physician 1990;41:7769–7770.
6. Jewell ME and Jewell GS. How to assess the risk of HIV exposure. Am Fam Physician 1989;40(1):153–161.
7. Johnson MC. Taking sexual histories: now it's essential. Iowa Med 1988;78:118–120.
8. Kassler WJ, Wu AW. Addressing HIV infection in office practice. Primary Care 1992;19:19–33.
9. Makadon HJ. Assessing HIV infection in primary care practice. J Gen Int Med 1991;6: S2–S11.
10. Nolte S, Sohn MA, and Koons B. Prevention of HIV infection in women. JOGNN-J of Obstet Gynec Neonat Nurs 1993;2:128–134.
11. Rinaldi RC, Henning JC. HIV Blood Test Counseling (AMA Physician Guidelines). KMA Journal 1989;87:375–377.
12. Selwyn PA, O'Connor PG. Diagnosis and treatment of substance users with HIV infection. Primary Care 1992;19:119–156.
13. Owen WF Jr. The clinical approach to the male homosexual patient. Med Clin North Am 1986;70:499–535.
14. CDC. HIV counseling, testing, and referral: standards and guidelines. Atlanta, GA: US Department of Health and Human Services, Public Health Service, CDC, 1994.
15. Anglin TM. Interviewing guidelines for the clinical evaluation of adolescent substance abuse. Pediatric Clin North America 1987;34:381–398.
16. Kinsey AC, Pomeroy WB, Martin CE. Sexual behavior in the human male. Philadelphia: WB Saunders, 1948:610–666.

Counseling for HIV Antibody Testing

Whether HIV testing is recommended based on a risk assessment or medical finding, or requested by the individual, an HIV-testing program should include the following services:

- Obtaining informed consent for testing (preferably written).
- Providing pretest counseling information and education, including a risk reduction plan, and making a return appointment to receive the test result.
- Informing patients of test results and providing posttest counseling, making referrals as appropriate.

General Considerations

Counseling should be client-centered, i.e., counseling which is interactive and responsive to the individual's needs (1). The focus is to develop prevention goals and strategies together with the individual, rather than simply to provide information. The ability to listen to the individual enables the provision of education specific to each person's needs as well as realistic risk reduction options. Individuals should be encouraged to express their feelings, concerns and to ask questions. Counseling should be tailored to each person's behavior, circumstances and needs. Information should be age-, educational-, and cultural-specific, and terminology understandable, incorporating appropriate slang and street terms as necessary. The following summarizes published guidelines concerning HIV counseling (1–18).

Pretest Counseling Information

The time before the antibody test is given is an opportunity to provide general education about HIV, the antibody test and its implications; to assess an individual's risk for HIV; to discuss risk reduction measures (e.g., safer sex, safer needle use); and to assess the individual's support systems and coping mechanisms. Education should be given to all patients, whether they decide to be tested or not. Written materials can enhance counseling sessions and a telephone number should be given if the patient has any further questions. It is important that pretest counseling prepare the individual to receive and manage his or her test result; patients have been shown to cope better with test results if they are prepared and informed by counseling prior to HIV testing (19,20). The type of information given during counseling will be directed by an individual's understanding of HIV transmission and meaning of HIV antibody test result. It is therefore important to ascertain an individual's knowledge regarding HIV and discuss the issues which are appropriate and relevant in detail. Pretest counseling may include the following aspects:

1. The reason for taking the test.
    If the individual is requesting the test, it is important to know why the person wants to take the test. The individual should be directly asked why he/she needs to be tested. This provides an opportunity to review any behaviors which place the individual at risk of acquiring HIV infection, and to discuss HIV prevention and activities which lower the risk of HIV transmission.

2. Defining HIV and AIDS and clarifying the difference between the two.

HIV is a virus which causes the immune system to become suppressed and causes AIDS (acquired immunodeficiency syndrome). A person with HIV infection can be asymptomatic and appear healthy for several years. AIDS refers to the stage of HIV infection when an individual is diagnosed with certain opportunistic infections or shows certain laboratory results which define AIDS. It is important that the individual understand that a person with HIV infection does not necessarily have AIDS.

3. The modes of HIV transmission.

If necessary, the modes of HIV transmission which place an individual at risk should be discussed in detail and any misconceptions concerning transmission clarified (e.g., HIV is not transmitted by mosquitos, hugging, sneezing, sharing glasses, etc.) It is important to facilitate an accurate perception of HIV risk for those who are unaware or uninformed.

4. Defining the HIV antibody test.

The antibody test is not a test for AIDS, but is a test to detect the presence of antibodies to HIV. When a person is infected by a virus, the body's white blood cells normally begin to react to infection by producing antibodies. Antibodies can therefore be used to indicate whether or not a person has been infected by a virus. A positive test result indicates a person is infected with the virus, but is not diagnostic of AIDS.

5. Explaining the meaning of a negative test.

A negative result indicates that no antibodies to HIV were detected. A negative test may mean either that the person is not HIV infected or was so recently infected that the test did not detect infection. Antibodies may not have yet developed if exposure to the virus was recent (especially less than three months). It takes from 6 weeks to 6 months to seroconvert following exposure to HIV. Therefore, a negative test does not guarantee that a person is uninfected, particularly if the individual has engaged in at-risk behaviors within the last 6 months.

6. Explaining the meaning of a positive test result. *A positive preliminary screening test (e.g., ELISA) should never be indicated as a positive HIV test to a patient (21). A person is considered to HIV infected only after an enzyme immunoassay screening test is repeatedly positive and is validated by another test such as the Western blot.*

A positive result indicates that the person is infected with HIV and is infectious, i.e., he/she has the ability to transmit HIV to others by sexual contact, sharing of injection drug needles, sharing of blood products, or (if the individual is a woman) to her unborn child. It should be explained that although a person with HIV can appear and feel healthy, he/she is able to transmit HIV to another person. He/she should be advised to take precautionary steps to prevent the spread of the virus.

7. Discussing the possibilities of indeterminate results.

   An indeterminate test result is possible for a noninfected person, or it can represent a stage in the progression of HIV disease. Persons should be retested to determine true antibody status approximately 6 weeks from the date of the inconclusive test. Persons are considered to be negative for antibodies to HIV if their Western Blot test results continue to be consistently indeterminate for at least 6 months in the absence of any known risk behaviors, clinical symptoms or other findings (22).

8. Risk reduction.

   Review those behaviors that place the individual at risk for HIV and discuss the ways that behaviors can be changed to reduce risk (e.g., safer sexual and drug use practices). Develop a risk reduction plan together with the individual. Persons with behavioral risk for HIV should be advised not to donate blood and not to use the blood bank as a means for periodic HIV testing. *(See Risk Reduction and Prevention.)*

9. Preparing the individual for the test result.

   The stress related to waiting for test results and possible reactions to learning a positive result (e.g., depression and anxiety) should be discussed: How does the individual plan to cope while waiting for the test results? The individual's coping mechanisms and support system should be assessed—how does the individual generally react to stressful situations? What does the individual expect the test results to be? If seronegative, what would the individual do differently? How would the individual react if given a positive result? If the test is positive, who could the individual confide in that would be supportive and keep the information confidential? How would the individual tell his or her partners? This gives the individual an opportunity to think about these issues in advance and prepare for a possible positive HIV test. A positive HIV test is emotionally traumatic, and the clinician should be aware of potential problems. Suicide risk and previous psychiatric problems should be assessed. If there is a history of psychiatric problems, the appropriateness of HIV testing should be discussed. The individual should be allowed to express whether he/she can handle a positive test result and encouraged to ask questions. The option to defer testing should be given if the individual needs to consider it further or discuss it with others. Persons who decline HIV testing must not be denied needed medical care or provided suboptimal care.

10. Assisting the individual in making a decision about testing.

   The potential benefits and risks of HIV testing should be discussed. Benefits of being tested include identifying HIV-infected individuals who might benefit from early prophylaxis, motivating behavior change to reduce risk of future infection, alerting women considering pregnancy or breast feeding, decreasing anxiety for high and low risk individuals. Being identified as HIV-infected can cause psychological, social, and economic changes. The disadvantages of being tested and/or being HIV-positive include discrimination and stigmatization in employment, housing, insurance, and personal relationships (14,23). The decision to be tested is the patient's own.

11. Discussing the confidentiality of test results in relation to office/clinic procedures.

This includes where results are to be recorded and procedures for release of information, local and state reporting requirements of positive results, and accessibility of test results to insurers, employers, other health care providers, and social contacts. Discuss potential benefits of anonymous testing (where the person is identified only by number). Individuals who do not want to be tested in the office should be referred to an anonymous testing site. The availability of anonymous services may encourage individuals at risk who would otherwise be reluctant to do so to seek services.

12. Informed Consent.

Obtain an informed consent (written) before voluntary testing is conducted. An informed consent requires that the provider give the patient sufficient information so she or he can make an informed decision (local statutes pertaining to adults and minors should be consulted).

13. Establishing a plan to give and discuss test results.

Ensure that the individual understands what will occur during his/her visit to receive the test results. The individual should be encouraged to identify someone with whom she or he can discuss the test, and to bring a supportive person (not children) and/or partner to the postcounseling session. The individual should be asked to identify his/her plans in the 24 hours immediately after receiving the test result.

Posttest Counseling

DISCLOSURE OF TEST RESULTS & COUNSELING

Since many individuals are anxious and eager to learn the test result, disclosure is best done at the beginning of the posttest session in a direct manner. The result should always be done in person, and preferably by the same person who conducted the pretest counseling. The individual should be ensured that test results and other information provided will remain confidential. After the result is disclosed, the individual should be encouraged to express his/her feelings and reactions. The clinician should be prepared for a wide range of emotional reactions when the test result is given. The ability of the individual to cope may depend on a number of factors: level of understanding regarding HIV infection and testing; the individual's age, sex, and sexual orientation; physical and mental health; available support system; acknowledgment of previous HIV exposure; perception of partner acceptance; beliefs with respect to religion and health care; if testing was voluntary (versus mandatory), and the setting which the information is given (14,19,24).

The individual's understanding of the test results should be assessed and the individual asked what the result means to him/her. For both seronegative and seropositive individuals, risk reduction practices should be emphasized. The risk reduction plan developed during pretest counseling should be reviewed and modifications recommended based on the HIV test result. Uninfected persons should be assisted to initiate and sustain behavior changes that reduce their risk of becoming HIV-infected. For seropositive individuals, the implications of a positive test should be clarified, the immediate needs for services and support (e.g., medical, financial, preventive, psychosocial) determined, and appropriate referrals given. A follow-up appointed shortly after the initial session may be helpful to reassess the patient's emotional status and repeat any information that the individual may not have been able to absorb.

HIV-NEGATIVE TEST RESULT

Counseling sessions for HIV-negative individuals are another opportunity to provide education. The information content will be similar to the pretest counseling, with emphasis placed on risk reduction measures specific to the individual. The need for retesting should be assessed. If exposure to HIV has been recent (less than 6 months) or the individual continues to practice at-risk behaviors, a repeat test is recommended; retesting should be scheduled approximately 6 months following the last episode of high risk behavior.

Patients should understand that a negative test provides no protection from HIV. A negative result can provide an incentive to adopt safer behaviors to protect oneself from infection. Risk reduction and intended behavior change should be discussed.

HIV-POSITIVE TEST RESULT

How the results are disclosed will set the tone and foundation for the patient's acceptance, knowledge base and attitudes regarding his/her own HIV status, and initiates the ongoing relationship between the provider and patient (14).

Because the emotional impact of learning about a positive HIV test result often prevents an individual from absorbing other information (1), additional counseling sessions and follow-up telephone calls may be required. Disclosure of a positive result is often distressing, with individual's reactions ranging from denial to anger, fear, and remorse. It may be helpful to repeat the individual's remarks and concerns and label his/her underlying feelings. Clinical depression is common among those testing positive for HIV. If the individual expresses any suicidal ideation, this should be explored in detail; any concrete plan for a suicide attempt should prompt an immediate psychiatric consultation. The individual's supportive network should be identified, and if possible, a specific supportive person identified to whom he or she could tell the result.

Ensure that the individual understands the meaning of the positive test result. The spectrum of illness, as well as prognosis should be discussed. It is important to convey the perspective that HIV infection is a chronic illness rather than an acute disease (25). Early initiation of prophylactic agents has been demonstrated to help prolong longevity and improve the quality of life. Available treatment options to delay disease progression should be discussed and a comprehensive care plan for continuing medical care and psychological support developed. The postcounseling session should introduce the individual to the available HIV-related health care and social support services and systems. The individual's immediate medical, preventive and psychosocial needs should be assessed and the appropriate referrals given (e.g., follow-up medical services, enrollment into drug and alcohol abuse treatment programs, HIV support groups, etc.)

Risk reduction should be highlighted to help the individual prevent HIV transmission to others and to stay healthy. Further HIV exposure should be avoided since repeated reinfection with HIV can accelerate the progress of the disease toward AIDS (7). Basic blood and body fluid precautions should be discussed. The individual should also be told not to donate blood, semen, or body organs; and not to share personal hygiene items (e.g., razors, toothbrushes). Signs and symptoms of HIV disease should be taught and the benefits of health maintenance (e.g., nutrition, food safety) discussed. Counseling issues specific to women such as risk of perinatal transmission and treatment opportunities are addressed separately *(See Women and HIV Infection)*.

Issues related to appropriate disclosure of serostatus to others should also be discussed *(See also Disclosure of HIV Status)*. This involves all of the circumstances in which others should be informed of the client's HIV infection status and requires consideration of local and state laws, client confidentiality and the need to inform others. Disclosure to health care providers and current and subsequent sex- and needle sharing-partners is important. The reasons for partner notification should be explained and the individual encouraged to notify their partners and refer them for counseling and testing. Individuals may require assistance on the methods of informing persons who need to know. For example, concerning partner notification, discuss how the individual plans to tell his/her sex- or needle partner the news; this may include role-playing as well rehearsing anticipated scenarios and reactions.

REFERENCES

1. CDC. HIV counseling, testing and referral: standards and guidelines. Atlanta, GA: Department of Health and Human Services, Public Health Service. 1994.
2. CDC. Technical guidance on HIV counseling. MMWR 1993;42 (RR-2).
3. Nolte S, Sohn MA, and Koons B. Prevention of HIV infection in women JOGN 993;2:128–134.
4. Friedman LS, Goodman E. Adolescents at risk for HIV infection. Primary Care 1992; 19:171–190.
5. Kassler WJ, Wu AW. Addressing HIV infection in office practice. Primary Care 1992; 19:19–33.
6. New York City Department of Health. A woman's guide to AIDS. New York, N.Y.: New York City Department of Health, 1989.
7. Anderson MM, Morris RE. HIV and adolescents. Pediatric Annals. 1993;22:436–446.
8. Moroso G, Holman S. Counseling and testing women for HIV. NAACOG's Clinical Issues in Perinatal and Women's Health Nursing 1990;1:10–20.
9. Rinaldi RC, Henning JC. HIV blood test counseling. AMA Physician Guidelines. KMA Journal 1989;87:375–377.

10. Tuomala R. Human immunodeficiency virus education and screening of prenatal patients. Obstetrics and Gynecology Clinics of North America 1990;17:571–583.
11. CDC. Public Health Service Guidelines for counseling and antibody testing to prevent HIV infection and AIDS. MMWR 1987;36:509–515.
12. Massachusetts Department of Health. Guidelines for physicians and health care providers on HIV counseling, testing, and early treatment. Boston, MA: Massachusetts Department of Health, Feb 1990; Pub no. 16202-52-20,000-2-90 CR.
13. Anastos K, Palleja SM. Caring for women at risk of HIV infection. J Gen Int Med 1991;6(suppl):S40–S46.
14. El-Sadr W, Oleske JM, Agins BD, et al. Evaluation and management of early HIV infection. AHCPR Publication No. 94-0572 Rockville, MD: Agency for Health Care Policy and Research, Public Health Service, US Department of Health and Human Services, January 1994.
15. Makadon HJ. Assessing HIV infection in primary care practice. J Gen Int Med 1991;6(suppl):S2–S11.
16. AMA. HIV Blood Test Counseling: AMA Physician Guidelines. Chicago. AMA, 1988.
17. CDC. 1993 Sexually Transmitted Diseases Treatment Guidelines. MMWR 1993;42 (RR-1).
18. CDC. Recommendations for HIV testing services for inpatients and outpatients in acute-care hospital settings. MMWR 1993;42(RR-2):1–6.
19. Brown S, Barton S, Cutland D, et al. A study of disclosure of HIV antibody positive status: relationship to use of services and need for support [abstract S.C.652]. Int Conf AIDS; Jun 20–23, 1990:252.
20. Futterman D, Hein K. Medical care of HIV-infected adolescents. AIDS Clin Care 1992; 4:95–8.
21. Sherer R. Physician use of the HIV antibody test. JAMA. 1989;259:264–265.
22. CDC. Interpretation and use of the western blot assay for serodiagnosis of human immunodeficiency virus type 1 infections. MMWR 1989;38(S-7):1–7.
23. Lo B, Steinbrook RL, Cooke M et al. Voluntary screening for human immunodeficiency virus (HIV) infection: weighing the benefits and harms. Ann Intern Med 1989; 110:727–733.
24. O'Dell V. Fear of rejection: patients' reluctance to disclose HIV diagnoses AIDS. 1988 2:484–485.
25. Spiegel L, Mayers A. Psychosocial aspects of AIDS in children and adolescents. Pediatric Clinics of North America 1991;38:153–167.
26. CDC. Sexually transmitted diseases treatment guidelines. MMWR 1993;42 (RR-1).

Disclosure of HIV Status

Patient Disclosure to Individuals and Agencies

The provider should discuss the advantages and disadvantages of patients' disclosing their HIV status to others. Although disclosure of HIV infection may permit enhanced benefits in some states and increased support (e.g., significant others, family, etc.), it may also result in discrimination, loss of employment, loss of child custody, loss or reduction of health benefits, or rejection by a potential employer or significant other (1). There is also the potential for domestic violence within relationships where one or both partners are HIV infected (2). Domestic violence may occur in all types of relationships: heterosexual, homosexual, and parent-child (1).

Individuals should be advised to inform their health care providers (e.g., dentists, physicians) of their serostatus. In addition, they should be advised and encouraged to inform their sex- and needle-sharing partners of their HIV status, so that partners can be counseled and tested for HIV. The patient can either notify his/her partner directly or with a health care provider's immediate assistance, or through referral to health department partner notification programs. Health departments in all states will notify partners at the request of the patient; the index patient remains anonymous when public health officials notify contacts (3,4). Partner notification for HIV infection is highly confidential and varies from state to state.

Disclosure of a Child's HIV Status by Parent/Guardian

It has been recommended that providers assist parents and guardians in making decisions regarding disclosure of HIV infection to the infected child or adolescent and other family members (1). Disclosure may not be necessary for a very young or asymptomatic child. As the child becomes older or symptomatic, it is advisable to discuss the diagnosis with the child; by early adolescence, youths should be informed of their HIV infection (1). Problems which may occur following disclosure of status to a child or adolescent may include inadvertent disclosure to others, as well as feelings of depression or withdrawal by the youngster (5). Disclosure to infected children usually begins around the age of 5 but may vary, depending on the developmental stage. Disclosure is an ongoing process which often requires additional support services to help the family and child to cope. The provider can assist by educating parents and guardians and assist in securing available support services in anticipation of disclosure (6).

Provider Disclosure to Agencies

Providers should know their federal, state and local HIV reporting requirements and inform patients of the extent and limits of confidentiality of test results (1). Currently, all states and the District of Columbia require reporting of patients meeting the CDC surveillance case definition of AIDS (7). Current HIV infection reporting requirements for all states (1) are listed in Table 2.1.

Information concerning the State's mandatory or voluntary HIV reporting requirements should be provided to patients before testing. Patients should also be informed that once a diagnosis of AIDS is determined, the patient must be reported to the State health department and also reported anonymously to the CDC (7). Both tuberculosis and syphilis, (which may occur in HIV-infected patients) are also reportable in all jurisdictions; such reporting will trigger disclosure of limited information to a health department.

CONFIDENTIALITY AND LIMITATIONS

Maintaining patient confidentiality and any limitations regarding that should be discussed with the patient. The provider's record-keeping system should be appropriate and the system explained to the patient. Care should be taken to avoid inadvertent disclosure which could result in potential discrimination. The patient should be aware that AIDS may

Table 2.1.
Reporting Requirements for HIV Infection in the United States

Anonymous	Not Required	
Georgia	Alaska	Massachusetts
Iowa	California	Nebraska
Kansas	Connecticut	New Mexico
Kentucky	Delaware	New York
Maine	Florida	Pennsylvania
Montana	Hawaii	Vermont
New Hampshire	Louisiana	Washington
Oregon	Maryland[a]	District of Columbia
Rhode Island		
Texas		

By Name		
Alabama	Mississippi	South Carolina
Arizona	Missouri	South Dakota
Arkansas	Nevada	Tennessee
Colorado	New Jersey[b]	Utah
Idaho	North Carolina	Virginia
Illinois	North Dakota	West Virginia
Indiana	Ohio	Wisconsin
Michigan	Oklahoma	Wyoming
Minnesota		

Adapted from El Sadr W, Oleske JM, Agins BD et al. AHCPR Publication No. 94-0572. 1994:188.
[a]Requires reports of symptomatic HIV infection by name
[b]Implemented January 1992
All states require reporting AIDS cases by names at the state/local level as of 3/1/93.

be entered as a cause of death on the death certificate; consequently others may become aware of the diagnosis.

DUTY TO WARN

Legal implications regarding disclosure of HIV infection focuses on the ethical balance between patient confidentiality and the "duty to warn." The duty to warn involves the professional obligation to disclose a patient's status by a provider or agency to others potentially at risk of infection. This duty to warn may be most applicable to primary care physicians, who often have knowledge about a patient's social and family relationships (4). The CDC advises that the decision to invoke the duty to warn measure should be a last resort—applicable only in cases in which all efforts to persuade the patient to disclose positive test results to those who need to know have failed (4). Case law relating specifically to this dilemma and HIV is still limited (7).

REFERENCES

1. El-Sadr W, Oleske JM, Agins BD et al. Evaluation and management of early HIV infection. Clinical Practice Guideline No. 7 AHCPR, Publication No. 94-0572. Rockville, MD: Agency for Health Care Policy and Research, Public Health Service, US Department of Health and Human Services, January 1994.
2. Worth D. Sexual decision making and AIDS: why condom promotion among vulnerable women is likely to fail. Stud Fam Plann 1989;6:297–307.

3. Kassler WJ, Wu AW. Addressing HIV infection in office practice. Primary Care 1992;19:19–33.
4. CDC. 1993 Sexually Transmitted Diseases Treatment Guidelines. MMWR. 1993. 42 (RR-1).
5. Lipson M. What do you say to a child with AIDS? Hastings Center Report 1993; Mar–Apr:6–12.
6. Boland M, Tasker M, Evans P, Keresztes J. Helping children with AIDS: the role of the child welfare worker. Public Health 1987;23:23–29.
7. CDC. 1993 Revised classification system for HIV infection and expanded surveillance case definition for AIDS among adolescents and adults. MMWR 1992;41(RR-17).

CHAPTER 3

Laboratory Diagnosis and Evaluation of HIV Infection

After recognition of AIDS as a new disease in 1981 and description of its clinical features, the most significant advance was the identification of the causative virus, now termed Human Immunodeficiency Virus (HIV-1). Infection with HIV-1 leads to immune deficiency and, ultimately, the opportunistic infections and neoplasia that represent the clinical manifestations of AIDS. Recognition of the virus permitted development of serologic tests for antibody to it. Detection of the antibody has been essential in diagnosis and epidemiologic characterization of the spread of HIV infection. Serum antibody measurements, however, are not very useful for determining the course of infection. Furthermore, because the time for advancement to clinical AIDS averages about 10 years, reliance on the clinical signs and symptoms of AIDS has not pro-

---

Table 3.1.
Laboratory Tests Used in the Diagnosis and Staging of HIV Infection/AIDS

DIAGNOSIS
    Antibodies to HIV
        ELISA assays
        Western blot
        Immunofluorescence and other tests
STAGING
    Viral Quantitation
        p24 Antigen: Free and total serum (immune complex dissociated) levels
        HIV RNA in plasma
        HIV DNA
        Infectious virus
    CD4 T Cell Quantitation
        Flow cytometry:
            –CD4 percentage (% of total lymphocytes)
            –CD4 number (also requires WBC and differential counts for lymphocyte quantification).
        Alternative methods (non-flow cytometric) for CD4 quantitation
    Immune System Activation Measurements
        Serum (soluble) components
            Beta-2 microglobulin
            Neopterin
            Other serum components
        Serum cytokines
        Phenotypic markers of activation on lymphocytes (HLA-DR, CD38)
SPECIAL TESTING
    Specific Immunity to HIV
        Antibodies and Cell-mediated Immunity
    Lymphoid Tissue Changes

vided sufficient information for following the course of infection or for planning therapy.

Because there is a wide range to the course of disease, markers indicating the extent of disease activity are important in making decisions for assessing therapies. Laboratory markers used to assess disease course and stage (Table 3.1) are generally based on knowledge of the pathogenesis of the disease. The major aspects of the pathogenesis of HIV disease are (a) HIV infection of CD4 T cells and monocytes/macrophages with viral replication, (b) specific antiHIV immune responses, both humoral and cellular, (c) deficiency in CD4 T cell number, (d) immune dysregulation characterized by extensive activation throughout all components of the immune system, and (e) impaired immune function. Quantitative assessments of all these parameters are potentially important.

Diagnosis of HIV Infection

Detecting Serum Antibodies to HIV

The principal means for identifying HIV infection is the detection of antibodies to HIV. These antibodies usually appear within two to three months after initial exposure to the virus, but may take as long as six months to appear. These antibodies are generally IgG class, although IgM and IgA antibodies may also be detected early in the course of HIV infection. The antibody levels rise rapidly after their initial appearance and the high levels are maintained until advanced stages of disease. A fall in serum HIV antibody levels is often associated with fall in the CD8 T cells and other evidence of deteriorating immune functions.

The HIV genome includes 3 structural genes, env (envelope) for both gp 120/160 and gp41; gag (core) antigens, p55, p24 and p17 card pol (polymerase) p64, p51 and p32. Each may elicit antibodies.

ELISA TESTING

Many commercial kits are available for accurate detection of antibodies to HIV infection. These usually contain antigens to the most common immunogenic proteins of the HIV virus. They include gp41, p24, p17 and gp120/160. Total antibody levels over a sensitive threshold are considered to be positive.

WESTERN BLOT IDENTIFICATION OF SPECIFIC ANTIBODIES

To assure specificity of the antibodies detected by ELISA, a second method is required to confirm the existence of HIV infection. The most commonly used is the Western blot technique (1). This is an electrophoretic technique for separating the various antigens of HIV with special emphasis on gp41 and p24 as well as p17 and gp120/160. Antibodies to other HIV components may be present also, including nef, TAT and other HIV proteins, such as reverse transcriptase. The detection of these later antibodies is not necessary for the diagnosis of HIV infection. Presence of antibodies to at least two protein (from different genes) are usually required to confirm the diagnosis. The most common are antibodies to p24, gp41 and gp120/160.

Early in the course of HIV infection, antibodies to gp24 or gp41 may dominate and additional antibodies have not yet developed. As a result, the Western blot can not be considered as positive until at least two of the major groups of antibodies have developed.

In some other diseases, antibodies may develop that crossreact with HIV peptides. In these situations, however, the full pattern of crossreactions is not found. Thus, a Western blot can serve to distinguish a false positive ELISA test from existence of true HIV-1 infection. Fortunately, in the United States, the occurrence of false-positive ELISA tests is relatively rare.

OTHER METHODS FOR DETECTING ANTIBODIES TO HIV

Immunofluorescent techniques are commonly used in laboratories where the Western blot is not readily performed. These tests have worked satisfactorily as confirmatory test methods. Methods used in detecting antibodies to HIV are discussed in detail elsewhere (2,3).

QUALITY CONTROL

Quality control requires periodic testing with known positive and known negative samples. Testing, also, should be done with dilutions of seropositive serum to bring the antibodies to the level that is barely detectable by the most sensitive tests. If the laboratory has employed sensitive technology with appropriately trained personnel, very few seropositive samples will be missed. The laboratory should not rely, however, on only strongly positive sera for reference testing. Testing organizations also should make available sera from sources that provide potentially false-positive tests so as to ascertain the quality of both the primary and confirmatory procedures.

POTENTIAL PROBLEMS

HIV-2 is relatively uncommon in the United States, however, the antigens may crossreact and cause positive tests with many of the ELISA tests used for HIV-1. Specific tests for HIV-2 have become available as well as truly specific HIV-1 ELISA kits. Also, a carefully done Western blot can be used to distinguish the HIV-2 peptides from HIV-1.

Antibody may be absent or at very low levels early in HIV infection, especially during the viremic stage or as viremia is beginning to subside. Thus, there is a period early in infection when HIV infection exists but no antibodies have been formed, or the levels are too low to be detected, or one of the antibodies may have become dominant and not be sufficient to establish the diagnosis clearly. In these circumstances, taking of another blood sample is needed, e.g., a fresh sample of blood should be obtained (rather than retesting the same sample repeatedly) to see if the patient has developed more HIV-specific antibodies.

It is worth remembering that in the terminal stage of disease, the amounts of antibodies can be relatively low and might be missed by insensitive tests. Such a finding indicates a premorbid stage of illness.

HIV Antibody Detection in Other Body Fluids

Serum or plasma tests are the standard means of detecting antibodies to HIV infection and establishing HIV diagnosis. Testing of other body fluids, however, is being developed with encouraging results. Antibodies to HIV can be detected in oral fluids (saliva/oral mucosal transudates) (4). The levels are less than 1% of the levels in serum, but, can be detected by sensitive ELISA methodology. These methods have been shown to have high sensitivity and specificity in tests conducted both in the United States and in many other countries, including Tanzania, Thailand, Brazil, and elsewhere (4,5). It is possible in the future that these tests will be more commonly used when issues concerning confidentiality, counseling, follow-up, etc. have been resolved.

Urines of HIV-infected individuals also contain specific antibodies. These can be detected by appropriate ELISA tests (6). The urine tests also have been validated in studies in a number of countries. General application of HIV diagnosis by antibody detection in these other body fluids can be expected. Guidelines for satisfactory testing procedures and guidance for follow-up are being developed.

REFERENCES

1. CDC. Interpretive criteria used to report Western Blot results for HIV-1 antibody testing—United States. MMWR 1991;40:692–695.
2. Davey RT, Lane HC. Laboratory methods in the diagnosis and prognostic staging of infection with human immunodeficiency virus type 1. Rev Infect Dis 1990;12:912–930.
3. Saag MS. AIDS testing now and in the future. In Sande MA, Volberding PA, eds. Medical Management of AIDS, 4th Edition. Philadelphia: Harcourt Brace Jovanovich, Inc. 1995;65–88.
4. Frerichs RR, Htoon MT, Eskes N, Lwin S. Comparison of saliva and serum for HIV surveillance in developing countries. Lancet 1992;340:1496–1499.
5. Tamashiro H, Constantine NT. Serological diagnosis of HIV infection using oral fluid samples. Bull WHO 1994;72:135–143.
6. Connell JA, Parry JV, Mortimer PP, Duncan RJS, McLean KA, Johnson AM, Hambling MH, Barbara J, Farrington CP. Preliminary report: Accurate assays for anti-HIV in urine. Lancet 1990;335:1366–1369.

Staging and Prognosis

Three major categories of laboratory measurements for staging and prognosis are currently in use: CD4 T cell decrease, immune activation and viral load. These, and several additional pathogenetically relevant measurements, are described here.

CD4 T Cell Deficiency

The HIV-1 virus has a specific affinity for the CD4 molecule. Thus the virus gains preferential entry to CD4 T cells. (Because monocytes have low levels of the CD4 molecule they also become infected). The CD4 T cell population is specifically reduced and functionally impaired in HIV infection. Finally, the level of CD4 T cells is an important parameter of HIV infection and AIDS. For these reasons accurate measurements of CD4 T cell levels are important to evaluation of HIV infection.

CD4 T cell numbers can vary on serial measurements as much as plus or minus 25%. Thus serial testing and confirmatory measurements of CD4 T cell changes are needed to determine what the approximate level is for this important immune cell component. The principal difficulties lie in biologic factors and in the variabilities of the total white blood cell count (WBC) and differential cell counting used to determine the total number of lymphocytes. The flow cytometric determination of CD4 T cell percentage (of total lymphocytes) is less variable. Thus measurements should be recorded both as (a) CD4 number and (b) CD4 percentage.

FLOW CYTOMETRY MEASUREMENTS

The major points emphasized in carrying out flow cytometry are: use of whole blood collected in EDTA; use of suitable reagents and a well-calibrated machine; and determination that the overall procedure regularly yields consistent results both within the normal range and for samples with low or high CD4 T cell levels (1). Blood samples may be stored 24 hours but not longer than 30 hours. They may be shipped by long distance delivery but care must be taken to protect them during transit, so that the samples are not frozen during shipment in the winter or subjected to remarkable increases in temperature in the summer.

Quantitative determinations of white blood cell total and differential counts are needed to determine lymphocyte number in the peripheral blood, which is required for the determination of the CD4 T cell number. The WBC and differential counts introduce major variability into CD4 T cell measurements. Furthermore, visual counting of cells in a hemocytometer is far more variable than measurements made by standard machine procedures. In addition to the technological issues, biologic factors can also influence the number and distribution of lymphocytes in the peripheral circulation. Unfortunately, these many factors can impact directly on the final CD4 T cell values even though flow cytometry is very well controlled.

Percentage of CD4 T cells (rather than numbers) has been suggested as a means of avoiding the problems inherent in the WBC and differential counts needed to calculate absolute lymphocyte numbers (2). This percent, however, is itself dependent on variables, e.g., the CD8 T cell level and the level of other lymphocytes such as B cells and NK cells in the circulation. The circulating NK cells can increase markedly following exercise or during acute psychological stress. Changes in these other cell populations can influence the numbers of total cells in the lymphocyte pool and, thus, impact on the CD4 T cell percentage. Furthermore, most clinicians are oriented to normative data and stratification factors based on CD4 T cell numbers, but do not have similar reference points for CD4 percentages. On balance it is useful to have CD4 T cell data reported both as percentage of total lymphocytes and as numbers of CD4 cells. In this way, possible changes in CD4 T cells over time can be better evaluated.

QUALITY CONTROL AND POTENTIAL PROBLEMS

Quality control (QC) procedures, based on testing of several seronegative and seropositive blood samples shipped at monthly intervals, were introduced in the multicenter AIDS studies sponsored by NIAID, including the Multicenter AIDS Cohort Study (MACS) and the AIDS Clinical Trials Group (ACTG). These demonstrated that all laboratories did not report the same values for identical samples. Substantial effort was required to determine whether procedural steps, reagents, technician skill or supervisor knowledge needed corrective action. Occasionally, equipment differences were responsible. Because patients move from one place to another, test results should be comparable. In national studies where data is pooled, the information should be in the same framework if it is to be useful. Frequent testing is required to determine if a laboratory is consistent in measurements of samples within and outside the normal ranges. An example of the hazard of omitting a comprehensive QC program is seen in one of the ACTG studies in which the relationship of CD4 T cell level to clinical benefit is reported to be from zero to 37% (3). Furthermore, the cost of poor performance was seen in an unpublished analysis which indicated that a correlation of 24 to 35% was seen using data from laboratories that showed evidence of the best quality performance. In contrast, little or no correlation was seen when data was used from those laboratories with the poorest reproducibility in a quality control program. Such detailed quality assurance projects are rarely carried out but, certainly, are likely to benefit the field.

Diurnal variation is a normal process reflecting redistribution of lymphocytes within and among vascular compartments. The normal levels of circulating CD4 T cells as well as several other lymphocytes change substantially during a 24-hour cycle. These changes reflect the influence of glucocorticoids, since an increase in serum glucocorticoid levels is associated with reduced blood concentration of lymphocytes including CD4 T cell levels. The practical implications of this knowledge is to be sure that serial testing of individuals occurs at the same time of day. Having individuals come in the late afternoon on some occasions and in the morning at other times will certainly cause a variation in the blood level of CD4 T cells from diurnal differences alone.

Physicians, patients and laboratory personnel should all be aware that variation in test results can be caused by changes in procedure, substandard laboratory performance, reagent or machine failures and by biologic factors, some of which can be controlled. Patients are generally very concerned about changes in CD4 T cell levels and laboratories must maintain good quality programs to be certain that substantial changes do not reflect changes in procedure or technology and do accurately reflect changes in disease status.

ALTERNATIVE METHODS OF CD4 QUANTITATION

Because of the expenses and technical requirements for flow cytometry and the fact that flow cytometry is not now and is not likely to be readily available in many parts of the world, alternative methods for measuring CD4 have been explored. A number of these are described in a recent publication from the WHO (4).

Assessments of these procedures are underway at the present time. In general, in the hands of skilled operators, they agree quite well with the flow cytometry results. However, it is clear that the methods require careful pipetting at certain stages of the procedure in order to maintain reproducibility. Also, the methods may be less accurate with lower CD4 T cell levels (under 100/mm^3). Generally, the alternative methods do not require highly specialized equipment and should be feasible in many situations where flow cytometry is not readily available. Alternative methods have other advantages. They reduce expenses and make possible the direct measurement of CD4 T cells without the additional WBC and differential counts.

FUNCTIONAL IMMUNE DEFICIENCY

Reduced proliferation in response to stimulation (by mitogens or microbial antigens) has been documented in HIV infection (5). This may occur before the CD4 cell number is markedly reduced and reflects disordered function. Although these tests are used in clinical research, they are not likely to be widely used for clinical evaluation because of limited availability, substantial variability, cost, and absence of national quality assurance programs. In related testing, stimulated peripheral blood lymphocytes can produce and release cytokines. The production of cytokines is also reduced in HIV infection, but these tests have similar limitations to proliferation testing.

Immune System Activation and Dysregulation

Initial studies of the immune system changes in HIV/AIDS concentrated on defining the features of immune deficiency. However, immune activation was later appreciated as a major feature of HIV pathogenesis (Table 3.2). Furthermore, the level of immune activation relates closely to the course of illness (6) and transiently returns toward normal with introduction of antiretroviral therapy. Abnormal activation probably contributes in major ways to pathology of HIV infection, e.g., neoplasia, HIV production and immune malfunction.

Table 3.2.
Indicators of Immune Activation or Dysregulation

Serum	Phenotypic Antigen	Function of PBMC[a]
Beta-2 microglobulin Neopterin	Antigen increases HLA-DR CD 38	Impaired proliferation response to antigens or mitogens Altered cytokine production

[a]PBMC: periphoral blood mononuclear cells

SERUM SOLUBLE MARKERS

Measurements of serum β2-microglobulin (β2M) or neopterin are the easiest means of assessing the level of immune system activation in HIV infection. Serum neopterin and β2M (6,7,8) are the most thoroughly investigated of the markers with the best documentation of a strong relationship to prognosis. Soluble CD8 antigen is also elevated in HIV infection and the changes correlate with those of β2M and neopterin (9). Increased serum IgA levels are also prognostic in HIV infection (6). There are also many other soluble components increased during HIV infection.

Increased production (and elevated serum levels) of β2M and neopterin are caused by increased activation throughout the immune system due to elevated production of stimulatory and proinflammatory cytokines. Neopterin production in macrophages is induced largely by IFN-γ. β2M production by T and B cells is induced by several cytokines (10).

The serum levels of these components represent the sum of cytokine activity and other stimulatory activity in the immune system. They reflect the total activity in all lymphoid tissues, blood and bone marrow. Furthermore, they are stable on storage or shipment and can be tested in a batch manner and at less expense than testing by flow cytometry.

The serum markers of activation which change in HIV infection have been shown to be largely independent of the CD4 T cell changes (6). Thus, they provide information separate from that obtainable by CD4 T cell measurements.

CYTOKINES AND SOLUBLE CYTOKINE RECEPTORS

Immune cell activation involves production of cytokines and increased expression of cytokine receptors. However desirable as measurement of serum cytokines might first appear, there are practical limitations. A plethora of receptors result in low and often undetectable levels of cytokines in the serum. Furthermore, some cannot be readily detected in serum or their levels are near the detection limits of current methodologies. Test accuracy suffers. However, with advancing HIV disease the serum levels of TNF-alpha and IL-6 (proinflammatory cytokines) increase (11). Of the activation cytokines, IFN-γ is elevated but IL-2 has not been regularly detectable (12). Data on serum levels of IL-10, IL-4, and IL-12, important regulatory cytokines, have been difficult to obtain.

Cytokine gene expression also reflects immune activation and can be evaluated by the measurement of cytokine specific messenger RNA (mRNA) in the cells of the immune system. Present methodologies require either a very large number of cells for direct quantitation or amplification by PCR methodologies. Directional changes in HIV infection have been documented, e.g., increase in TNF-α and IL-6 and IFN-γ RNA and decreased IL-2 and approximately normal IL-4 mRNA levels in PBMC (12). The IL-2 mRNA decrease appeared to be due to substantial reduction in the number of CD4 cells, which are the principal source of IL-2. At the present time, cytokine measurements are not included in routine evaluations of HIV infection. Perhaps in the future, focus on a few cytokines will enable a more precise definition of this aspect of HIV immunopathology.

PHENOTYPIC CHANGES ON PERIPHERAL BLOOD LYMPHOCYTES

Many changes in phenotypic antigens on peripheral blood lymphocytes have been described in HIV infection (1). Activation occurs in all the peripheral blood lymphoid populations (CD4, CD8, NK and B cells) as well as macrophages. The loss of CD4 T cells and the increases in CD8 lymphocytes in HIV infection are well known. Increased expression of CD38 and HLA-DR on CD8 and CD4 T cells occurs with immune activation and in HIV infection. Some phenotypic antigens are decreased, including CD45RA and CD25 (IL-2 receptor-alpha chain). These changes are "associated with HIV infection" but for the most part, a quantitative measure of their hazard in the disease progression has not been determined. The phenotypic changes on CD8 T cells have been of special interest, because of the hope that some phenotypic change would be closely associated with the appearance of (or loss of) protective cellular immunity against HIV infection. The goal of substituting phenotypic change for function measurement, however, has not been achieved. Thus, the assessment of additional phenotypic antigens on CD4 or CD8 lymphocytes remains a research procedure.

Virus Quantitation

The detection and quantitation of the virus can contribute to diagnosis, staging of HIV infection and may contribute to prognosis and evaluation of therapies. In the very early stages of HIV infection, before antibodies develop, any method for detecting whole HIV, virus RNA or HIV proteins such as p24 antigens, etc. can be very useful in this period when infection is suspected but antibody has not yet appeared (13).

Many virologic methods have been used to detect and quantify HIV. Generally these methods could be divided into three groups: viral culture methods, nucleic acid hybridization and amplification techniques and methods of p24 antigen quantitation. Differences in viral load associated with various stages of disease have been described and support the general assumption that higher viral load has a poorer prognosis. However, wide ranges in viral load are also found in various stages, and the relative value (in quantitative terms) of most of these measurements in relation to patient prognosis (relative hazard of progression to AIDS) has not yet been established.

SERUM p24 ANTIGEN: FREE AND TOTAL SERUM LEVELS

Presence of viral proteins and specifically HIV core p24 antigen in serum, plasma or cell culture supernatants is considered as evidence of HIV infection. The p24 antigen assay is the simplest, the fastest and the least expensive virologic detection method. Briefly, the assay utilizes sandwich-type antigen capture ELISA technique. Wells of microtitre plates or polystyrene beads are coated with antibody to p24 antigen. Then the sample (serum, plasma or culture supernatant), pretreated with detergent for disruption of viral particles, is added to the plate or beads. After incubation, the unbound material is washed out. A second antibody to p24, linked to an enzyme, is then added. If p24 is present in the sample, an enzymatic colorimetric reaction is developed that can be quantified by spectrophotometric measurement.

Using this direct p24 ELISA assay, the free (unbound to antibody) p24 antigen level was first detected in the serum. Most of the research work published before 1992 in clinical studies utilized methods that detected only free p24 antigen. The major limitation of free p24 antigen was that most people with asymptomatic HIV infection did not have detectable levels of free p24 antigen in their serum (6). Even a third of the people with a diagnosis of AIDS, did not have free p24 antigen. Thus, this measure was not available in most patients with asymptomatic HIV infection and was of limited use. Furthermore, when study patients were preselected for presence of p24 antigen, they were more likely to have more advanced or more rapidly progressing forms of disease.

p24 Antigen can be present in the serum but totally bound to antibody, as was pointed out by Nishanian and colleagues (14). They dissociated the p24 antigen-antibody immune-complexes with an acid pretreatment of serum samples that inactivated the antibodies and made the antigen available to a direct p24 assay. They showed that antigen positivity, in the direct assay but with low pH pretreatment is significantly higher (50.6%) than without pretreatment (12.4%) of sera from an asymptomatic population. p24-positive Individuals have serum p24 antigen which is either free or bound to antibody as immune complexes or in a combination of both bound and free states. The terms total (free plus bound) serum p24 antigen or ICD (immune complex-dissociated) p24 antigen are commonly used for this measurement.

ICD p24 assay probably is more useful as a prognostic marker for disease progression than for diagnostic purposes, but it is useful in the diagnosis of neonatal HIV infection (15). It may be particularly valuable in a population with earlier stages of the disease, in which the frequency of detectable p24 by the direct assay is lower than in patients with more advanced disease stage. In recent recommendations of an ACTG committee, (16) a sustained 50% fall in ICD p24 concentration is considered a positive response to therapy. A rise after initially falling ICD p24 may indicate emergence of antiviral resistance to the drug. Other HIV antigens have been detected in the serum also, but p24 has been the principal one used to evaluate disease stage and response to therapy.

QUANTITY OF VIRUS IN CELLS

Viral isolation from blood cells, body fluids or tissue is a direct evidence of HIV infection. The most commonly used method for viral isolation is the PBMC coculture technique. Patients' PBMC are harvested by gradient separation of heparinized blood and cocultured with healthy donor PHA-stimulated PBMC in media containing IL-2. Culture supernatant is periodically collected and tested for either HIV p24 antigen or reverse transcriptase. Successful recovery of virus by culture may reflect patient viral load. Culture positivity and the time to positivity of a specimen may be used as a rough measure of viral burden. The results of cell culture assay are associated with the stage of disease: asymptomatic patients have significantly lower viral load than symptomatic ones.

QUANTITY OF VIRUS IN PLASMA

The quantity of cell-free infectious virus in patient plasma (plasma viremia) is determined by the quantitative plasma culture assay, which is similar in design to the quantitative PBMC culture assay. Coombs et al. (17) reported that plasma viremia is a measure for disease progression and is a more accurate predictor than the presence of p24 antigen in plasma.

POLYMERASE CHAIN REACTION (PCR) TECHNIQUES

A promising area of research for early diagnosis and for quantitation of HIV involves detection and quantitation of HIV nucleic acid (RNA or DNA) sequences by gene amplification techniques, such as PCR. This powerful technique can amplify target DNA sequences (or cDNA as a product of reverse transcribed RNA) that exist in extremely small quantities (e.g., one copy per 106 cells). PCR efficiently supplies hybridization probes with very high specific activity that are capable of detecting very small amounts of HIV. Thus, PCR enables the development of detection methods that are adaptable to clinical studies and potentially can be automated.

Blood PBMC are usually tested by PCR, although successful detection of proviral DNA sequences in plasma, body fluids and lymphoid tissue has been reported (18).

Since its introduction, the PCR technique has had rapid and extensive development with wide application to the qualitative and quantitative detection of HIV nucleic acids. However, there are technical problems associated with PCR, and to insure accuracy, it is highly recommended that all labs performing this assay participate in a quality assurance program. Although quantitative PCR measurements have been made in comparison to external or internal controls, there is no available standardized assay at this time.

Much of viral RNA is defective and nonpathogenic and, thus may not reflect infectious virus production, which poses problems in evaluating its measurements. Replicating virus can be detected by endpoint dilution methods for infective virus. These methods are labor-intensive and are likely to be used only in special research studies.

Assays using PCR or branched DNA (bDNA) signal amplification methods were developed and used for measurement of HIV RNA in plasma (19). Several studies have demonstrated an association between levels of plasma RNA and stage of HIV disease and clinical progression. However there are still unresolved issues such as the effect of the biological variability, the variability of reverse transcription step, the effect of processing and storage condition on genomic RNA stability, etc. At this time, a standardized quantitative RNA PCR assay is not available.

QUALITATIVE HIV CHARACTERIZATION

Recently some strains of virus have been found to induce syncytia with cultures of cell line MT-2 or with PBMC. There was an initial proposition that syncytium-forming viral strains were associated with more aggressive disease and that a change from syncytium-negative to -positive features was associated with more rapid disease progression, but such ideas have been modulated with experience.

Analyses of viral isolates from clinical trials have demonstrated the phenomena of reduced drug susceptibility for HIV, emergence of drug resistant HIV phenotypes and decline of therapeutic effectiveness. A temporal correlation between emergence of resistant virus and an increase in viral load (free p24 and plasma viremia) has been found for mononucleoside RT (reverse transcriptase) inhibitors and ZDV (20). Resistance to antiretroviral therapy is likely to be a factor in a decline of therapeutic effectiveness.

POTENTIAL PROBLEMS

As noted above, the high prevalence of defective virus may obscure and confound measurements of infectious HIV quantity. Virus mutation may change the viral pathogenic properties. Furthermore, viruses may escape from serologic or cellular specific immunity but these changes may not be reflected in the assessments described above. Detailed viral characterization can indicate which forms of mutation lead to viral escape from immune surveillance. These methods, however, are not clinically feasible in most circumstances. Furthermore, patients may harbor multiple variants of HIV and those which grow well will be characterized. Viral evaluation is a subject of continuing investigation in relation to the course of the illness.

Table 3.3.
Relationship of Immunologic Markers of HIV Infection

	Related				Unrelated
	A	B	C	D	
Serum markers	sIL-2R	Neopterin			
		β2M			
		sCD8			
Lymphoid phenotypic antigens		CD38	CD45RA	HLA-DR	CD57
			leu 8		CD11b
					CD71

Four serum markers and seven lymphoid phenotypic markers of immune activation were studied. The closely related measurements are in group B (increased serum neopterin, β2M, sCD8, and CD38). Less closely related markers are the increased sIL-2R in group A, and the reduction of CD45RA and leu 8 in group C. HLA-DR increase is more distantly related. No correlations were found with CD11b, CD57, and CD71 phenotypic antigens.

Bass H, Nishanian P, Fahey JL, et al. Immune changes in HIV infection: Significant correlations of markers. Clin Immunol Immunopath 1992;64:63–70.

Correlation Between Markers

Markers are needed which can contribute distinctive information to prognosis and to evaluation of antiretroviral therapy. Comparison of markers is important to determine the most significant (and independent) markers. Groups of markers which are closely correlated and provide essentially similar prognostic information have been identified (Table 3.3). Work is under way now to determine the relationship between viral levels and markers of immune activation or immune deficiency. Selection of representative markers from within groups will help to focus testing and allow combinations of markers to increase the power of evaluation. For example, the combination of CD4 and antibody response (21) and of CD4 and neopterin (or β2M) measures, e.g., of immune deficiency and of activation has been proposed (22).

Immune-based therapy such as specific immune enhancers or inhibitors or vaccines, presents additional responsibilities. Measures of the effects of therapy on essential components of the immune system are needed to determine the immunological effects of therapy. In addition, measures of general immune competence and of specific immunity to HIV infection are important in this context, as well as in staging disease.

Specific Immunity to HIV

There is substantial evidence that the immune response to HIV infection is responsible, at least in part, for limiting the amount of virus and pathology induced by HIV. Two modes of specific immunity, humoral (antibody) and cellular have been investigated to determine what factors are most relevant. For the most part, serum antibody levels have not been found to relate closely to prognosis, at least in the earlier stages of disease.

ANTIBODIES—NEUTRALIZING OR ENHANCING

Neutralizing antibodies on *in vitro* testing, reduces the infectivity of HIV for susceptible cell lines in tissue culture. Neutralizing antibodies are fairly easily demonstrated (23). Unfortunately no strong relationship has been confirmed between the level of neutralizing antibody and the course of illness.

Enhancing antibodies are the functional opposite of neutralizing antibodies. They increase the infectivity of virus for target cells in vitro and can be demonstrated in most patients (24). Their in vivo significance remains to be determined. Finally, the levels of specific HIV antibodies generally have not been found to relate to the course of disease.

CELL-MEDIATED IMMUNITY

Substantial attention has been devoted to measurements of cell-mediated immunity (CMI) to HIV because this is the principal means of controlling many viral infections. Cellular immunity has been identified where HIV infection is not advanced, but is usually not identifiable in later stages of disease (25). Furthermore, CMI has been found in some persons with substantial exposure to HIV infection but who have not become infected (26). This supports the possibility that CMI is significant in prevention as well as control of HIV infection.

Most measurements of cellular immunity have focused on the cell surface antigens of the gp120 viral surface protein because most of the vaccine trials have utilized these peptides for immunization. Cellular immunity against gp41, p17 and other non-surface components of the viruses is also being explored. The methods, however, are expensive and require skilled technical personnel. Furthermore, testing in each person is individualized to assure that testing is specifically directed to HIV antigens and not to histocompatibility antigen. Each patient's B cells must be grown in culture and transfected with HIV antigen-bearing vectors.

Immunity is most readily detected and increased in stages of disease when there is no rapid progression and the CD4 T cell reduction is minimal, e.g., before there is substantial deficiencies of the immune function. CMI evaluations, however, are currently research procedures and are not generally applicable in clinical care situations.

Staging of HIV Infection and Prognosis

GENERAL

Once diagnosis of HIV infection is established, the major uses of laboratory testing are (a) for staging of infection, (b) decision to start treat-

Table 3.4.
CD4 T Cell Levels as Indicators of Clinical Stage

CD4 - over 500×10^6/L - Unlikely to be symptomatic
CD4 - under 500 - Candidate for anti-retroviral therapy
CD4 - under 200 - Candidate for prophylactic antibiotics
CD4 - under 50 - Increased hazard of death

ment, (c) evaluation of treatment and (d) evaluation of vaccines. Laboratory measures are particularly important in the many years during which there are no clinical symptoms. Staging of advanced HIV infection is done by clinical parameters and include persistent fever, weight loss, frequent or restricted opportunistic infections (not sufficient to qualify for AIDS) and reduced overall capacity to maintain normal activities.

Staging of HIV infection has focused primarily on measurement of the CD4 T cell number. Reduced CD4 T cells are a principal measure of pathology and appear to be central to the disease process and its consequences. Several CD4 levels have been established as having clinical significance (See Table 3.4). CD4 levels below 500×10^6/L have been recommended as an indicator for the institution of antiretroviral therapy. Useful guidelines for decisions regarding prophylactic antibodies for opportunistic infection have been developed based on the occurrence of opportunistic infections and the cut-off was set at CD4 levels at 200×10^6/L. Of course, opportunistic infections and Kaposi's sarcoma do occur with CD4 levels above 200 but much less commonly than below 200. Furthermore, studies in institutions with substantial attention to control of opportunistic infection have shown that the patients rarely die with CD4 levels above 50×10^6/L.

What markers are used for staging and prognosis of HIV infection? How good are they? CD4 T cell level, the principal marker used for HIV infection, is only fairly good. In the prediction of occurrence of AIDS in individuals with HIV infection, the CD4 number has some use and is improved by adding other measures of the immunopathology of HIV infection, including serum neopterin levels (or β2M in homosexually active men) or serum p24 antibody levels or measures of viral load, e.g., p24 antigen or viral measurements. However, because of the broad availability of flow cytometry in the Northern hemisphere, CD4 T cell levels have come to be relied on extensively in relation to HIV staging and decisions regarding therapy. It can be expected that as other measures are evaluated, they will be added to or substituted for CD4 flow cytometry, especially in portions of the world where this technology can not be readily obtained.

SPECIAL POPULATIONS

Infants and Children

Infants normally have many more CD4 T cells (and lymphocytes) than do adults (27). The level at one year is about 4000×10^6/L. The CD4 values gradually fall during childhood to near adult levels. The normal range of CD4 T cell levels is wide and infants with HIV infection may not show CD4 levels below the normal range. Other parameters of disease can be used, however, to assess disease activity. Elevated serum activation markers are indicative of HIV infection (28). Patients with higher levels have poorer prognosis (28).

Detection of virus in the blood during the first months of life is useful in establishing the occurrence of HIV infection during the time when the antibodies from the mother are still present and serologic diagnosis can not be made (15). The characteristics of HIV infection in infants and children are considered elsewhere in this volume in more detail.

Intravenous Drug Users (IVDUs)

The significance of some laboratory data on immune activation appears to differ in HIV+ IVDU from HIV+ homosexually active men. Most of the laboratory data acquired in HIV infection in the United States have been obtained in homosexually-active Caucasian men. Intravenous drug users, however, have been extensively studied in the southern portions of Europe and several locations in the United States and found to have elevated serum activation markers (29,30). The elevation of β2M in IVDU was found to have less prognostic significance than in HIV+ homosexually-active populations. The concurrence of these findings in several different countries indicates that the marker, β2M, may be of limited value in the IVDU population.

The lack of specificity of β2M measurements may be due to the variable existence of other factors (infections) which increase β2M in the population to such an extent that the increases due to HIV are less clearly evident. Serum neopterin, however, was also measured in some of the IVDU studies and found to be a valid marker of activation and to contribute information in addition to that provided by CD4 measurements.

Co-Existence of Other Infections that Elevate Serum Activation Markers

Tuberculosis increases levels of β2M (31). Initial reports (32) have indicated that patients with an overall elevation in β2M that is attributed to both active tuberculosis and to HIV infection, have a poorer prognosis than those patients with lesser β2M increase, or who have HIV infection alone (without TB). Likely, the same factors causing the increases in activation markers (presumably, increased cytokine production) are also contributing to disease progression. The serum activation marker levels appear to reflect the sum of combined pathology in individual patients.

LYMPHOID TISSUE CHANGES

A great deal of pathology induced by HIV occurs in lymphoid tissues where CD4 and other lymphoid cells are generated and/or removed (33). Indeed, the principal sites of HIV pathology are likely to be lymphoid tissues rather than the peripheral blood. The lymph nodes in patients with advanced disease show disorganized structure and changes from the normal pattern of distribution of T and B cells. Individuals with little or no fall in CD4 T cells may show normal lymphoid architecture and low viral content. Although lymphoid biopsy has not yet been recommended to stage disease or to evaluate therapy, current investigations should provide more definitive information relevant to future clinical application.

Indirect information on the processes occurring in lymphoid tissues throughout the body, not just in lymph nodes, can be obtained by serum or plasma analyses for lymphoid cell metabolic products and the regulatory cytokines. Measurement of neopterin as a product of interferon-gamma action on monocytes and macrophages and of β2M as a marker of activation with the T and B cells system and other markers are readily available. Phenotypic characterization of the circulating lymphoid cells, also, offer opportunities to assess dysfunction, activation and apoptosis in an accessible lymphoid cell system that is in a dynamic relationship with lymphoid tissues.

REFERENCES

1. Giorgi JV, Cheng HL, Margolick JB, et al. Quality control in the flow cytometric measurement of T-lymphocyte subsets. Clin Immunol Immunopathol 1990;55:173–186.
2. Taylor JMG, Fahey JL, Detels R, Giorgi JV. CD4 percentage, CD4 number and CD4:CD8 ratio in HIV infection: Which to choose and how to use. J Acq Immun Def Synd 1989;2:114–124.
3. Choi S, Lagakos SW, Schooley RT, Volberding PA. CD4 lymphocytes are an incomplete surrogate marker for clinical progression in persons with asymptomatic HIV infection taking zidovudine. Ann Intern Med 1993;118:674–680.
4. Tamashiro H. Report on WHO Workshop on flow cytometry and alternative methodologies for CD4 lymphocyte determinations. AIDS 1994;8:1–4.
5. Lane HC, Depper JM, Greene WC, Whalen, G, Waldmann TA, Fauci AS. Quantitative analysis of immune function in patients with the acquired immunodeficiency syndrome: evidence for a selective defect in soluble antigen recognition. N. Engl. J. Med 1985;313:79–84.
6. Fahey JL, Taylor JMG, Detels R, Hofmann B, Melmed R, Nishanian P, Giorgi JV. The prognostic value of cellular and serological markers in infection with human immunodeficiency virus type 1. N Engl J Med 1990;322:166–172.
7. Fuchs D, Hausen A, Reibnegger G, Werner ER, Dierich MP, Wachter H. Neopterin as a marker for activated cell-mediated immunity: application in HIV infection. Immunol Today 1988;9:150–155.
8. Moss AR. Predicting who will progress to AIDS. Br Med J 1988;297:1067–1068.
9. Nishanian P, Hofmann B, Wang Y, Jackson AL, Detels R, Fahey JL. Serum soluble CD8 molecule is a marker of CD8 T-cell activation in HIV-1 disease. AIDS 1991;5:805–812.
10. Hofmann B, Bass H, Nishanian P, Faisal M, Figlin RA, Sarna GP, Fahey JL. Different lymphoid cell populations produce varied levels of neopterin, 2-microglobulin and soluble IL-2 receptor when stimulated with IL-2, interferon-gamma or tumor necrosis factor-alpha. Clin Exp Immunol 1992;88:548–554.
11. Aziz N, Nishanian P, Martinez-Maza O, et al. Related and unrelated cytokine changes in HIV infection. Proc Intern Symp Clin Immunol 1995;in press.
12. Fan J, Bass HZ, Fahey JL. Elevated IFN-γ and decreased IL-gene expression are associated with HIV infection. J Immunol 1993;151(9):5031–5040.
13. Saag MS. AIDS testing. In Sande MA, Volberding PA, ed. Medical Management of AIDS, 4th Edition. Philadelphia: WB Saunders, 1995;65–88.
14. Nishanian P, Huskins KR, Stehn S, Detels R, Fahey JL. A simple assay demonstrates that HIV p24 antigen is present as immune complexes in most sera from HIV-infected individuals. J Infect Dis 1990;162:21–28.
15. Miles SA, Balden E, Magpantay L, Wei L, Leiblein A, Hofheinz D, Toedter G, Steihm RE, Bryson Y. California Pediatric AIDS Consortium: Rapid serologic testing with immune-complex-dissociated HIV p24 antigen for early detection of HIV infection in neonates. N Eng J Med 1993;328:297–302.

16. Hammer S, Crumpacker C, D'Aquila, R, Jackson B, Lathey J, Livnat D, Reichelderfer P. Use of virologic assays for detection of human immunodeficiency virus in clinical trials: Recommendations of the AIDS clinical trials group virology committee. J Clin Microbiol 1994;31:2557–2564.

17. Coombs RW, Collier AC, Allain JP, Nikora B, Leuther M, Gjerset GF, Corey L. Plasma viremia in human immunodeficiency virus infection. N Engl J Med 1989;321: 1626–1631.

18. Arens M. Use of probes and amplification techniques for the diagnosis and prognosis of human immunodeficiency virus (HIV-1) infections. Diag Microbiol Infect Dis 1993; 16:165–172.

19. Hsiang JL, Myers LE, Hollinger BY, Henrard D, Hooper CJ, Kokka R, Kwok S, Rasheed S, Vahey M, Winters MA, McQuay LJ, Nara PL, Reichelderfer P, Coombs RW, Jackson JB. Multicenter evaluation of quantification methods for plasma human immunodeficiency virus type 1 RNA. J Infect Dis 1994;170:553–562.

20. Mohri H, Singh MK, Ching WTW, Ho D. Quantitation of zidovudine-resistant human immunodeficiency virus type 1 in the blood of treated and untreated patients. Proc Natl Acad Sci USA 1993;90:25–29.

21. Sheppard HW, Ascher MS, McRae B, Anderson RE, Lang W, Allain JP. The initial immune response to HIV and immune system activation determine the outcome of HIV disease. J Acq Immun Def Syndr 1991;4:704–712.

22. Fahey JL, Taylor JMG, Detels R. Is there a better index of HIV disease status than just CD4 T cell levels? Proc IX Intl Conference on AIDS Berlin, June 1993;1:45.

23. Ho DD, Rota TR, Hirsch MS. Antibody to lymphodenopathy-associated virus in AIDS. N Engl J Med 1985;312:649–650.

24. Homsy I, Meyer M, Levy JA. Serum enhancement of HIV infection correlates with disease in HIV-infected individuals. J Virol 1990;64:1437–1440.

25. Walker BD, Chakrabarti S, Moss M, et al. HIV-specific cytotoxic lymphocytes in seropositive individuals. Nature 1987;328:345–348.

26. Rowland-Jones S, Sutton J, Ariyoshi K, et al. HIV-specific cytotoxic T cells in HIV-exposed but uninfected Gambian women. Nature Med 1995;1:59–64.

27. Sison AV, Campos JM. Laboratory methods for early detection of human immunodeficiency virus type 1 in newborns and infants. Clin Micro Reviews 1992;238–247.

28. Watehi R, Stiehm ER, Fahey JL, et al. Serum neopterin is a better predictor of disease severity than 2M in pediatric HIV infection. In: Pediatric AIDS and HIV Infection: Fetus to Adolescent 1994;5:226–231.

29. Munoz A, Vlahor D, Solomon L, et al. Prognostic indicators for development of AIDS among intravenous drug users. J Acquir Im Defic Sydromes 1993;5:694–700.

30. Fuchs DN, Hausen A, Hengster P, et al. Is T-cell activation an unfavorable sign in IV-drug addicts infected with HIV Cancer? Detection and Prevention 1988;12:277–282.

31. Ogawa T, Uchida H, Kusumoto H, et al. Increase in TNF and IL-6 secreting cells in peripheral blood from subjects infected with M tuberculosis. Infect Immun 1991; 59:3021–3025.

32. Wallis RS, Vjecha M, Amir-Takmossele M, et al. Influence of tuberculosis on HIV: Enhanced cytokine expression and elevated 2M in HIV-associated tuberculosis. J Infect Dis 1993;167:43–48.

33. Pantaleo G, Graziosi C, Damres JF, Butini L, Montroni M, Fox CH, Orensteim JM, Kotelp DP, Fauci AS. HIV infection is active and progressive in lymphoid tissue during the clinical latent stage of disease. Nature 1993;362:355–358.

Evaluation of Therapy

NUCLEOSIDE ANALOGS

The evaluations of therapy initially relied on the expensive endpoints of clinical parameters and survival. Surprisingly, CD4 T cell measurements were found not to relate very well to the clinical benefit of zidovudine in relatively asymptomatic patients with CD4 T cell levels under 500 in the ACTG 019 study (1). Interestingly, the value of the test related directly to the performance of the test laboratories in a stringent quality control program. In the best performing labs, CD4 T cell change accounted for 25% to 34% of the clinical benefit observed. CD4 measurements in the poorest performing labs had little if any relation to clinical benefit. Clearly, quality control of laboratories doing CD4 quantification is of great importance. Evaluation of additional surrogate markers, particularly those reflecting activation and specific immunity as well as viral activity in relation to the effects of antiretroviral therapy is needed.

IMMUNE-BASED THERAPIES

Immune-based therapies are directed toward (a) restoring immune competence, (b) interfering with excessive immune activation or (c) inducing specific antiHIV immunity. Immune-based therapies clearly require evaluation of relevant immune parameters to indicate that the intervention has affected the immune system. Quantitative measures of specific HIV immunity and general immune parameters will be needed and the duration of effects will be important.

Immune-based therapies are generally directed at augmentation of deficient components of the immune system or at reduction of specific activation within the immune system. Inhibitors of immunity are frequently directed at specific cytokines, such as TNF-α, which are produced in excessive amounts. Assessments of such treatments, however, need to include several parameters because of the interlocking nature of cytokine actions.

Research with immune-based therapies is a broad field. Some forms of therapy may be most effective early in disease when the effective resistance to HIV may be prolonged. In more advanced disease, they may require combination with at least partially effective antiretroviral treatments.

REFERENCES

1. Choi S, Lagakos SW, Schooley RT, Volberding PA. CD4 lymphocytes are an incomplete surrogate marker for clinical progression in persons with asymptomatic HIV infection taking zidovudine. Am Intern Med 1993;118:674–680.

Summary and Prospects in the Future

Measures of immune deficiency (especially CD4 T cell level), of immune activation (serum neopterin and β2M) as well as viral load have been developed. Many have been or are being evaluated in relation to prognosis and in hopes they will assess the clinical benefit induced by therapy.

Presently, a small number can be used advantageously. The present dependence on CD4 T cell measurements emphasizes the importance of this marker. However, it is an incomplete means of assessing stage and prognosis and of evaluating therapy, so there is a need to advance beyond sole reliance on it. Further, it should be expected that several markers (such as CD4, activation markers and viral load) measuring different aspects of the disease can be combined advantageously for assessment of disease and therapy. Other measures that are relevant to disease course have been identified and shown to provide information separate from CD4. Thus, combination of measurements reflecting different aspects of disease should be more valuable than single markers.

Measurements to be used include (a) quantification of virus, (b) the level of CD4 T cells, (c) immune activation and dysregulation markers and (d) quantification of representative protective immunity, probably cell-mediated immunity. Additional measures are likely to be proposed. Currently, several of these measurements, such as functional tests, are difficult and expensive. It can be expected that as the value of specific markers is documented, testing procedures will become simpler and more widely available.

Vaccine programs require laboratory evaluations for several purposes: (a) establishment of the frequency and level and duration of both antibody and cellular immunity elicited by the vaccines, (b) detection of HIV infection in vaccinated individuals, and (c) evaluation of the course of HIV infection in vaccine recipients versus controls. The hope is that vaccine will reduce the occurrence of HIV infection and prolong the course of illness. The fear is that the vaccine may accelerate the course of HIV infection in some individuals. There is the additional need to make quantitative comparisons of the value of different vaccines. Laboratory parameters of HIV infection are essential to all these areas.

CHAPTER 4

Clinical Aspects of HIV Infection

Spectrum of Illness, Disease Staging, and Natural History

Definition of AIDS

Acquired immunodeficiency syndrome (AIDS) has been defined as the occurrence of life-threatening opportunistic infections, malignancies, neurologic diseases, and other specific illnesses in patients with human immunodeficiency virus (HIV) infection and/or with CD4 counts less than $200/mm^3$. The Centers for Disease Control (CDC) have established specific disease criteria for defining AIDS in both adults and children. These criteria (Table 4.1) has most recently been updated in 1993 to include asymptomatic individuals with CD4 counts less than $200/mm^3$ and to include a number of diseases which are believed to occur at higher frequency in individuals with HIV infection (1). A few of these newly added diseases in adults include recurrent or multiple bacterial infections, the HIV wasting syndrome, mycobacterium tuberculosis, and cervical carcinoma (1,2). The pediatric AIDS case definition includes multiple or recurrent serious bacterial infections, lymphoid interstitial pneumonitis, and progressive neurologic diseases.

It must be stressed that the CDC definition is a surveillance definition that was established to track the incidence of this disease and the relative occurrence of diseases that are likely to occur in severely immunosuppressed individuals. The general availability of HIV serologic tests and CD4 enumeration has allowed more precise identification of patients with HIV infection and determination of patients with severe immune compromise. In parts of the world where CD4 enumeration is

Table 4.1.

CDC Surveillance Case Definition for AIDS

I. HIV Status of Patient Is Unknown or Inconclusive

If laboratory tests for HIV infection were not performed or gave inconclusive results and patient had no other cause of immunodeficiency listed in IA (see below), a definitive diagnosis of any disease listed in IB (see below) indicates AIDS.

  A. *Causes of immunodeficiency that disqualify a disease as an indication of AIDS in the absence of laboratory evidence of HIV infection*

    1. The use of high-dose or long-term systemic corticosteroid therapy and other immunosuppressive/cytotoxic therapy within three months before the onset of the indicator disease.
    2. A diagnosis of any of the following diseases within three months after diagnosis of the indicator disease: Hodgkin's disease, non-Hodgkin's lymphoma (other than primary brain lymphoma), lymphocytic leukemia, multiple myeloma, any other cancer of lymphoreticular or histiocytic tissue, or angioimmunoblastic lymphadenopathy.
    3. A genetic (congenital) immunodeficiency syndrome or an acquired immunodeficiency syndrome that is atypical of HIV infection, such as one involving hypogammaglobulinemia.

  B. *Diseases that indicate AIDS (requires definitive diagnosis)*

    1. Candidiasis of the esophagus, trachea, bronchi, or lungs.
    2. Cryptococcosis, extrapulmonary.
    3. Cryptosporidiosis with diarrhea persisting for more than one month.
    4. Cytomegalovirus disease of an organ other than the liver, spleen, or lymph nodes in a patient older than one month.
    5. Herpes simplex virus infection causing a mucocutaneous ulcer that persists longer than one month; or herpes simplex virus infection causing bronchitis, pneumonitis, or esophagitis for any duration in a patient older than one month.
    6. Kaposi's sarcoma in a patient younger than 60 years.
    7. Lymphoid interstitial pneumonia or pulmonary lymphoid hyperplasia (LIP/PLH complex) in a patient younger than 13 years.
    8. Lymphoma of the brain (primary) affecting a patient younger than 60 years.
    9. *Mycobacterium avium* complex or *M. kansasii* disease, disseminated (at a site other than or in addition to the lungs, skin, or cervical or hilar lymph nodes).
    10. *Pneumocystis carinii* pneumonia.
    11. Progressive multifocal leukoencephalopathy.
    12. Toxoplasmosis of the brain in a patient older than one month.

II. Patient Is HIV Positive

Regardless of the presence of other causes of immunodeficiency (see IA, above), in the presence of laboratory evidence of HIV infection, any disease listed in IB (see above) or in IIA or IIB (see below) indicates a diagnosis of AIDS. In addition, beginning in 1993, all HIV-positive adults and adolescents with CD4+ T-cell counts less than 200/mm^3 or with pulmonary tuberculosis, recurrent pneumonia, or invasive cervical carcinoma should also be included in the AIDS case definition.

  A. *Diseases that indicated AIDS (requires definitive diagnosis)*

    1. Bacterial infections, multiple or recurrent (any combination of at least two within a two- to four-year period), of the following types in a patient younger than 13 years: septicemia, pneumonia, meningitis, bone or joint infection, or abscess of an internal organ or body cavity (excluding otitis media or superficial skin or mucosal abscesses) caused by *Haemophilus, Streptococcus* (including pneumococcus) or other pyogenic bacteria.
    2. Coccidioidomycosis, disseminated (at a site other than or in addition to the lungs or cervical or hilar lymph nodes).
    3. Histoplasmosis, disseminated (at a site other than or in addition to the lungs or cervical or hilar lymph nodes).
    4. HIV encephalopathy.
    5. HIV wasting syndrome.
    6. Isosporiasis with diarrhea persisting for more than one month.
    7. Kaposi's sarcoma at any age.
    8. Lymphoma of the brain (primary) at any age.
    9. *M. tuberculosis* disease, extrapulmonary (involving at least one site

(continued)

Table 4.1.— *continued*

CDC Surveillance Case Definition for AIDS

outside the lungs, regardless of whether there is concurrent pulmonary involvement).

10. Mycobacterial disease caused by mycobacteria other than *M. tuberculosis,* disseminated (at a site other than or in addition to the lungs, skin, or cervical or hilar lymph nodes).

11. Non-Hodgkin's lymphoma of B cell or unknown immunologic phenotype and the following histologic types: small noncleaved lymphoma (Burkitt's or non-Burkitt's) or immunoblastic sarcoma.

12. *Salmonella* (nontyphoidal) septicemia, recurrent.

B. *Diseases that indicate AIDS (presumptive diagnosis)*

1. Candidiasis of the esophagus.
2. Cytomegalovirus retinitis, with loss of vision.
3. Kaposi's sarcoma.
4. Lymphoid interstitial pneumonia or pulmonary lymphoid hyperplasia (LIP/PLH complex) in a patient younger than 13 years.

5. Mycobacterial bacteria (acid-fast bacilli with species not identified by culture), disseminated (involving at least one site other than or in addition to the lungs, skin, or cervical or hilar lymph nodes).
6. *P. carinii* pneumonia.
7. Toxoplasmosis of the brain in a patient older than one month.

III. Patient Is HIV Negative

With laboratory test results negative for HIV infection, a diagnosis of AIDS for surveillance purposes is ruled out unless:

A. All the other causes of immunodeficiency listed in 1A (see above) are excluded; and
B. The patient has had either of the following:

1. *P. carinii* pneumonia diagnosed by a definitive method.
2. A definitive diagnosis of any of the other diseases indicative of AIDS listed in IB (see above) and a CD4+ helper-inducer T cell count of less than 400/mm³.

---

not as readily available, clinical diagnoses, in conjunction with serologic tests for HIV, are used to define patients with AIDS and to track the spread of this epidemic. Refinements in the surveillance definition of AIDS is anticipated as the epidemic matures and as more precise prognostic indicators for disease stage and progression are established (e.g., HIV viral load measures).

Classification System for HIV Disease

The CDC has proposed the following classification system for HIV-infected adolescents and adults (1). This system is based on three ranges of CD4 T-cell counts and three clinical categories and can be represented by a matrix of nine mutually exclusive categories (Table 4.2).

The three designated CD4 T-cell count categories are: category 1—500 or more cells/mm³; category 2—200 to 499 cells/mm³; and category 3—fewer than 200 cells/mm³. CD4 enumeration should be done by an experienced laboratory with established quality assurance procedures. The lowest accurate CD4 T-cell count prior to initiation of therapy should be used for classification purposes.

The clinical categories of HIV infection are as follows:

Category A: This category includes the occurrence of one or more of the conditions listed below in a patient with documented HIV infection. Conditions listed in categories B and C must not have occurred.

1. Asymptomatic HIV infection.
2. Persistent generalized lymphadenopathy.
3. Acute (primary) HIV infection with accompanying illness or history of acute HIV infection.

Category B. This category consists of symptomatic conditions in any HIV-infected adolescent or adult that are not included in the AIDS surveillance case definitions (e.g., clinical category C) and that meet at least one of the following criteria:

1. Conditions are attributed to HIV infection or are indicative of a defect in cell-mediated immunity.
2. The conditions are considered by a physician to have a clinical course or management that is complicated by HIV infection. Some examples of conditions in clinical category B include, but are not limited to, the following:
   a. Bacillary angiomatosis.
   b. Bacterial endocarditis, meningitis, pneumonia, or sepsis.
   c. Candidiasis, oropharyngeal (i.e., thrush).
   d. Candidiasis, vulvovaginal that is persistent, frequent, or poorly responsive to therapy.
   e. Cervical dysplasia that is severe.
   f. Constitutional symptoms, such as temperature greater than 38.5°C or diarrhea lasting longer than 1 month.
   g. Hairy leukoplakia
   h. Herpes zoster (i.e., shingles) involving at least two distinct episodes or more than one dermatome.
   i. Immune thrombocytopenic purpura.
   j. Listeriosis.
   k. Nocardiosis.
   l. Peripheral neuropathy.

Table 4.2.

CDC Classification System for HIV Infection

| | Clinical Categories | | |
| | A
Asymptomatic,
PGL, or Acute | B | C |
CD4 Cell Categories	HIV Infection	Symptomatic (not A or C)	AIDS Indicator Condition
1. >500/mm^3 (≥29%)	A1	B1	C1
2. 200–499/mm^3 (14–28%)	A2	B2	C2
3. <200/mm^3 (<14%)	A3	B3	C3

From CDC. 1993 revised classification system for HIV infection. MMWR 1992;41:961.

Table 4.3.
Indicator Conditions in Case Definition of AIDS

Candidiasis of esophagus, trachea, bronchi, or lungs
Cervical cancer, invasive[a,b]
Coccidioidomycosis, extrapulmonary[a]
Cryptococcosis, extrapulmonary
Cryptosporidiosis with diarrhea for >1 month
Cytomegalovirus or any organ other than liver, spleen or lymph nodes
Herpes simplex with mucocutaneous ulcer for >1 month or bronchitis, pneumonitis,
  esophagitis
Histoplasmosis, extrapulmonary[a]
HIV-associated dementia: disabling cognitive and/or motor dysfunction interfering with
  occupation or activities of daily living
HIV-associated wasting: involuntary weight loss of >10% of baseline plus chronic diarrhea
  (≥2 loose stools/day for ≥30 days) or chronic weakness and documented enigmatic fever
  for ≥30 days
Isosporosis with diarrhea for >1 month
Kaposi's sarcoma in patient younger than 60 (or older than 60[a])
Lymphoma of brain in patient younger than 60 (or older than 60[a])
Lymphoma, non-Hodgkin's of B cell or unknown immunologic phenotype and histology
  showing small, noncleaved lymphoma or immunoblastic sarcoma
M. avium or *M. kansasii,* disseminated
M. tuberculosis, disseminated[a]
M. tuberculosis, pulmonary[a,b]
Nocardiosis[a]
P. carinii pneumonia
Pneumonia, recurrent-bacterial[a,b]
Progressive multifocal leukoencephalopathy
Salmonella septicemia (nontyphoid), recurrent[a]
Strongyloidosis, extraintestinal
Toxoplasmosis of internal organ

From CDC. 1993 revised classification system for HIV infection. MMWR 1992;41:961.
[a]Requires positive HIV serology.
[b]Added in the revised case definition 1993.

Category C: This category includes any condition listed in the CDC surveillance case definition for AIDS that occurs in an HIV-infected adult or adolescent (Table 4.3). All of these conditions are strongly associated with severe immune deficiency, have an increase incidence in HIV-infected individuals compared to uninfected individuals, are generally rare in the absence of immune suppression, and can cause serious morbidity or mortality.

The most severe clinical condition that has been diagnosed should be used to establish the HIV classification, regardless of the patient's current clinical condition. For example, a patient who was previously treated for oral or vaginal candidiasis and who is now asymptomatic should be classified in clinical category B.

Natural History of HIV Infection

As described in the section on disease mechanisms, the pathogenic process for the development of AIDS in patients with HIV infection involves a progressive deterioration of host immunity and consequent occurrence of clinical diseases as a result of HIV infection. A graphic representation of the natural history of HIV infection in an individual is shown in Figure 4.1. In this model, successful infection with HIV results in an initial burst of HIV viral replication and infection of many CD4 T-lymphocytes and monocytes, which is followed within a few weeks by the generation of a host immune response against the virus that reduces the rapid replication of cell-associated virus (3,4). This is reflected by a decrease in measured HIV viral load in the peripheral blood, although continued viral replication occurs in lymphoid tissues of the reticuloendothelial system. CD4 counts initially fall as a result of HIV-induced cell lysis, with the CD4 count stabilizing at a somewhat lower level than normal as a result of rapid homeostatic repletion of CD4 cells by the host. Several studies have shown that a large proportion of lymphocytes in lymph nodes and other lymphoid tissues are infected with HIV, but that replication of the virus may proceed at various rates in individuals and can be modulated by the host's immune response. Over time, continued viral replication results in a gradual decline in CD4 counts which often results in the development of opportunistic infections and other AIDS-defining diseases. The time course over which this process occurs varies from individual to individual, but the median estimated time from infection to clinical symptoms generally exceeds 10 years in untreated patients (4,5).

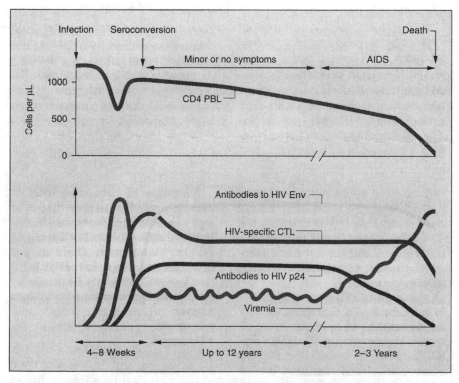

Figure 4.1. Infection with HIV elicits a protective immune response that may persist for 12 years or more. But progressive immune dysfunction usually eventually predisposes the host to a number of opportunistic infections, malignancies, and other diseases characterized as AIDS. (PBL, peripheral blood lymphocytes; Env, envelope protein; CTL, cytotoxic T lymphocytes.) (Adapted with permission from Science, © 1993.)

Table 4.4.
Stages in HIV Disease

	CD4 Count Range	Duration
Acute infection	1000–750	1–4 weeks
Asymptomatic	750–200	2–15+ years
Early symptomatic	500–100	1–5+ years
Late symptomatic	50–200	1–4+ years
Advanced disease	50–0	0–2+ years

CD4 count ranges and durations are quite variable. Numbers are provided to give general ranges for each of these stages of HIV disease.

HIV disease can be viewed as a continuum of progressively diminishing cellular immunity (Table 4.4). Acute HIV infection is often associated with flu-like or mononucleosis-like illness that typically occurs within a few weeks of initial exposure to HIV. A long asymptomatic phase averaging between 2–15+ years follows in which the patient has no signs or symptoms of illness. During this time, patients may display varying degrees of T-cell immune deficiency but are otherwise without clinical symptoms. Early symptomatic HIV infection that may occur at CD4 counts typically between 100–500 cell/mm^3 foretells the beginning of more severe cellular immune deficiency. Patients develop several diseases suggestive of immune deficiency, but they are not defined as AIDS (category B). These diseases, which were previously part of what was termed the AIDS-related complex (ARC), occur 3 or more years after initial acquisition of HIV infection and may recur several times in sequence over a period of 1–5 years. Early clinical studies suggested that patients with HIV symptoms had a high likelihood of progression to AIDS within a short period of time.

Late symptomatic disease with CD4 counts < 200/mm^3 or with *Pneumocystis carinii* pneumonia or candida esophagitis is often the first manifestation of clinical AIDS. The spectrum of diseases that manifest as the initial clinical presentation of AIDS has changed over the years in the U.S. as a result of earlier detection of HIV infection and the more widespread use of prophylactic antibiotics and antiretroviral drugs (Table 4.5). Thus, many patients with HIV infection will not develop an opportunistic infection until their CD4 counts fall below 50–100 cell/mm^3, at which time they would be considered in the late or advanced stages of HIV disease. In these stages, patients often present with life-threatening opportunistic infections, malignancies, or neurologic disorders that may be fatal. The use of prophylactic antibiotics, multi-drug antiretroviral regimens, close clinical monitoring, a high index of suspicion for signs of opportunistic diseases, and aggressive treatment once these diseases are recognized has resulted in a longer life expectancy and better quality of life for patients with advanced stage AIDS.

Table 4.5.
Correlation of CD4 Cell Count and AIDS Complications

CD4 Strata	Complication
>500/mm³	Persistent generalized lymphadenopathy
	Candida vaginitis
	Guillain-Barré syndrome
	Polymyositis
	Aseptic meningitis
200–500/mm³ (also seen with CD4 counts <200/mm³ as well)	Pneumococcal pneumonia
	Pulmonary tuberculosis
	Thrush
	Zoster
	Cryptosporidiosis, self-limited
	Cervical intraepithelial neoplasia
	Kaposi's sarcoma
	B cell lymphoma
	Anemia
	Idiopathic thrombocytopenic purpura
	Mononeuritis multiplex
	Oral hairy leukoplakia
<200/mm³ (usually < 100/mm³)	*P. carinii* pneumonia
	Disseminated or chronic herpes simplex
	Miliary or extrapulmonary tuberculosis
	Candida esophagitis
	CNS lymphoma
	Wasting
	HIV-associated dementia
	Peripheral neuropathy
	Cryptococcosis
	Disseminated histoplasmosis and coccidioidomycosis
	Chronic cryptosporidiosis
	Microsporidiosis
	Disseminated/chronic herpes simplex
<50/mm³	Disseminated *M. avium*
	CMV retinitis

From Bartlett JG. The Johns Hopkins Hospital Guide to Medical Care of Patients with HIV Infection, 5th ed. Baltimore: Williams & Wilkins, 1995:18.

Acute HIV Infection

Acute HIV infection has been described as an infectious, mononucleosis-like syndrome that develops 3 weeks to 3 months after initial exposure to HIV (6–8). It is characterized by the sudden onset of fevers, sweats, myalgias, arthralgias, headaches, sore throat, diarrhea, fatigue, malaise, a generalized lymphadenopathy, and a macular erythematous trunkle rash which may last from 3–14 days. After the acute phase has passed, other viral sequelae may occur, such as aphthous ulceration, exacerbation of seborrhea or psoriasis, recurrence of herpes simplex, and rarely rhabdomyolysis, acute renal failure, and mesangioproliferative glomerulonephritis. Lethargy and depression may persist for up to 3 months. Most patients are seronegative at the time of acute illness, but usually seroconvert within 2 months. Acute HIV infection should be considered in any high-risk patient who presents with an illness similar to mononucleosis. It should be noted, however, that the absence of such a clinical syndrome should not be taken as evidence of non-HIV infection.

Early Symptomatic Disease

Early symptomatic HIV disease, which previously was termed ARC, includes patients who have symptoms suggestive of impaired cellular immunity but who do not meet CDC's criteria for AIDS (9,10). Such conditions may include persistent generalized lymphadenopathy, recurrent fevers, night sweats, malaise, oral or vaginal candidiasis, oral hairy leukoplakia, recurrent herpes zoster outbreaks (i.e., shingles), dermatitis, seborrhea, and immune thrombocytopenia.

Late Symptomatic HIV Disease

Diseases associated with late-stage HIV infection and AIDS are listed in Table 4.5 (11). These illnesses affect just about every organ system in the body and can present with protean clinical manifestations. A listing of the various clinical syndromes, pathologic agent, and major clinical manifestation of disease is given in Table 4.6.

Clinical manifestations of selected disease states associated with HIV are given in following chapters; however, a few areas deserve special emphasis: One of the most direct clinical effects of HIV infection is on the nervous system. The brain appears to be a privileged sanctuary for HIV replication after infected monocytes and macrophages transport HIV across the blood-brain barrier. Various neurologic syndromes may be directly ascribable to HIV (Table 4.7) (12–14). AIDS encephalopathy or AIDS dementia complex is characterized by a progressive dementia, psychomotor retardation, focal motor abnormality, and behavioral changes. Pathologically, a diffuse leukoencephalopathy with enlargement of the cortical sulci and ventricles is seen. Clinical changes are often seen on magnetic resonance imaging (MRI) studies in HIV-infected patients who have no overt evidence of neurologic dysfunction (15). Up to ⅔ of patients with AIDS may have clinical manifestations of AIDS encephalopathy in the advanced stages of their disease. Workup to exclude central nervous system infections, neurosyphilis, progressive multifocal leukoencephalopathy, and B-cell lymphoma must be performed prior to establishing this diagnosis.

Other abnormalities which may arise from the direct effect of HIV include an enteropathy characterized by malabsorption (16); esophageal and oral aphthous ulcerations (17,18); focal and segmental glomerulosclerosis and other renal abnormalities often accompanied by proteinuria (19–20); congestive cardiomyopathy (21); thyroid dysfunction (22,23); wasting syndrome, which may be due to HIV-induced cytokines as well as hypogonadism; rheumatologic disorders (24) ranging from Reiter's syndrome and psoriatic arthritis to vasculitis, polymyositis, and Sicca syndrome resembling Sjögren's; biologic false-positive test for syphilis (25); amyloidosis (26); a syndrome mimicking systemic lupus

Table 4.6.

Infectious Complications of AIDS

	Infecting Organism	Type of Infection
Viruses	Cytomegalovirus	Penumonia, disseminated infection, retinitis, encephalitis, gastrointestinal ulcerations
	Epstein-Barr virus	Important pathogenic factor in B cell lymphoproliferative disorders and Burkitt's lymphoma, oral hairy leukoplakia
	Herpes simplex virus	Recurrent severe localized infection
	Papovavirus	Progressive multifocal leukoencephalopathy
	Varicella-zoster virus	Localized or disseminated infection
Fungi	*Aspergillus*	Invasive pulmonary infection with potential for dissemination
	Candida albicans	Mucocutaneous infection, esophagitis, disseminated infection
	Coccidioides immitis	Disseminated infection
	Cryptococcus neoformans	Meningitis, disseminated infection
	Histoplasma capsulatum	Disseminated infection
	Petriellidium boydii	Pneumonia
	Pneumocystis carinii	Pneumonia, retinal infection
Protozoa	*Cryptosporidium*	Enteritis
	Isospora belli	Enteritis
	Toxoplasma gondii	Encephalitis
Mycobacteria	*Mycobacterium avium-intracellulare*	Pulmonary, extrapulmonary, or disseminated infection
	M. tuberculosis	Pulmonary, extrapulmonary, or disseminated infection
	Atypical mycobacteria (e.g., *M. kansasii, M. haemophilum*)	Pulmonary, extrapulmonary, or disseminated infection
Bacteria	*Haemophilus influenzae* type b	Pneumonia, disseminated infection
	Legionella	Pneumonia
	Listeria monocytogenes	Bacteremia, meningitis, meningoencephalitis
	Norcardia	Pneumonia, disseminated infection
	Pseudomonas aeruginosa	Bacteremia, pneumonia
	Salmonella	Gastroenteritis, disseminated infection
	Streptococcus pneumoniae	Pneumonia, disseminated infection

From Rubin RH. AIDS. In: Scientific American Medicine, Infectious Disease Section XI, 1993:11.

erythematosus; presence of antinuclear and anticardiolipin antibodies and a variety of other autoimmune diseases such as immune thrombocytopenia (27), thrombotic thrombocytopenic purpura (28), lymphoid interstitial pneumonitis (29), endocrine dysfunctions (30), and an increased incidence of allergic reactions to medications such as trimethoprim-sulfamethoxazole. These latter diseases may be a reflection of immune activation induced by HIV and loss of normal immunologic controls resulting in autoimmune phenomena and a higher incidence of atypical antibody formation (31).

Table 4.7.
Neurologic Disorders Associated with HIV Infection

Neurologic Disorder	Prevalence (%)	Clinical Features	Histopathologic Features
Subacute encephalitis	90	Cognitive deficits, memory loss, psychomotor slowing, pyramidal tract signs, ataxia, weakness, depression, organic psychosis, incontinence, myoclonic seizures	Gliosis, myelin pallor, microglial nodules, perivascular inflammation, focal demyelination, multinucleate giant cells
Peripheral neuropathies Chronic distal symmetric polyneuropathy	10–50	Painful dysesthesias, numbness, paresthesias, weakness, autonomic dysfunction	Demyelination, axonal loss, mild inflammation
Chronic inflammatory demyelinating polyneuropathy		Weakness, sensory deficits, mononeuropathy multiplex, cranial nerve palsies, hyporeflexia or areflexia, cerebrospinal fluid pleocytosis	Marked inflammation, demyelination with secondary axonal loss
Vacuolar myelopathy	11–22	Gait ataxia, progressive spastic paraparesis, posterior column deficits, incontinence	Vacuolar degeneration of lateral and posterior columns
Aseptic meningitis	5–10	Headache, fever, meningeal signs, cranial nerve palsies, cerebrospinal fluid pleocytosis	

From Rubin RH. AIDS. In: Scientific American Medicine, Infectious Disease Section XI, 1993:9.

Pediatric Manifestation of HIV/AIDS

HIV-infected infants are typically asymptomatic at birth. Although variable, the average age of onset of symptoms suggestive of severe immune deficiency in newborn infants ranges from 5–10 months (32). Few infants who acquire HIV at birth remain asymptomatic beyond the 3rd year of life (33).

The principal signs and symptoms of pediatric HIV infection are listed in Table 4.8 (34). Many of these are non-specific. Lymphadenopathy, hepatomegaly, and failure to thrive are the most frequent presenting manifestations of HIV infection. Repeated common infections in young infants, e.g., recurrent *Haemophilus influenzae* infections, should arouse suspicion about underlying HIV infection. Certain clinical disease states are highly suggestive of HIV infection. Foremost among these is lymphocytic interstitial pneumonia (LIP) which occurs in 35–40% of children with AIDS (29,35). Children have nodular peribronchial lymphoid infiltrates and often hilar adenopathy. Diagnosis of LIP is made histologically, and it is important to exclude other forms of lung pathology. Salivary gland enlargement is also a unique manifestation of HIV in childhood. Other manifestations of HIV infection can include cardiomyopathy, hepatitis, pancreatitis, thrombocytopenia, and hemolytic anemia. Encephalopathy is also common and may cause developmental delay and loss of already acquired developmental milestones (36). Neurologic disease progression may be slow or rapid. Computed tomography (CT) scans show brain atrophy, ventricular enlargement, attenuation of white matter, and calcification of basal ganglia. The

---

Table 4.8.
Principal Signs and Symptoms of Pediatric AIDS

Failure to thrive
Diarrhea
Frequent otitis media
Frequent other common pediatric infections
Invasive or disseminated infections
Thrush
Opportunistic infections
Lymphocytic interstitial pneumonia
Skin diseases (*Candida* and seborrhea)
Parotid swellings
Neurologic involvement
Developmental delay
Loss of attained milestones
Dementia
Encephalopathy
Acquired or congenital microcephaly
Lymphadenopathy
Hepatosplenomegaly
Cardiomyopathy
Chronic eczematoid rash

From Grossman M, Sande MA, Volberding PA, eds. Pediatric AIDS. In: The Medical Management of AIDS, 3rd ed. Philadelphia: WB Saunders, 1992: 445.

Table 4.9.

CDC Classification System for HIV Infection in Children Under 13 Years of Age

Class	Symptom
P-0	Indeterminate infection in children <15 mo old
P-1	Asymptomatic infection
Subclass A	Normal immune function
Subclass B	Abnormal immune function
Subclass C	Immune function not tested
P-2	Symptomatic infection
Subclass A	Nonspecific findings
Subclass B	Progressive neurologic disease
Subclass C	Lymphoid interstitial pneumonitis
Subclass D	Secondary infectious diseases including opportunistic infections
Subclass E	Secondary cancers
Subclass F	Other diseases possibly due to HIV infection

From Centers for Disease Control, MMWR 1987;36:225–236.

most common opportunistic infection is *Pneumocystis* pneumonia which occurs in approximately 50% of children with AIDS. Other infectious diseases include *Mycobacterium avium* and candida infections (37). Children with vertically transmitted HIV infection generally have a very poor prognosis. Median survival time after diagnosis is approximately 9–12 months (38). The classification system for HIV-infected children is given in Table 4.9 (39).

The management of children with HIV infection involves a multidisciplinary approach that should include the physician, development specialist, social services, psychiatric and emotional support teams, and the family or foster care providers (40). Close attention to primary care with diligent observation for life-threatening infections and serious AIDS-related complications must be maintained. Nutritional support is important, as are timely immunization (41) and prophylaxis for opportunistic infections. Rapid diagnostic evaluation for fever and cough must be undertaken, and treatment initiated rapidly for both bacterial and/or opportunistic pathogens. Because of significant immunoglobulin deficiency in children with HIV, some clinicians favor monthly administration of intravenous immunoglobulin as an additional prophylactic measure to prevent bacterial infections (42). The use of antiretroviral therapy has also increased life expectancy of children with HIV infection and should be offered to children with established HIV infection (43). Clinical studies evaluating combination antiviral therapy and other measures to treat and prevent complications of AIDS are under evaluation by the AIDS Clinical Trials Group.

Additionally, it is important to provide general supportive care for the HIV-infected child and his or her caregiver. Financial as well as social and educational support and encouragement for these children should be provided. Education for adolescents and older children with HIV to prevent the further spread of HIV infection should also be provided and begun during childhood. Counseling for adolescents regarding maintenance of good health habits, avoidance of alcohol and other toxic substances, and the use of prophylactic measures to prevent spread of HIV and other sexually transmitted diseases should also be provided. Aspects of HIV infection in children and adolescents are discussed in detail elsewhere (*See Pediatric AIDS* and *Adolescents and HIV Infection*).

Summary

The clinical manifestation of disease in patients with HIV infection and AIDS are quite varied and present formidable diagnostic and therapeutic challenges for the clinician. The natural history of HIV disease follows from an understanding of the viral and immunopathogenesis of this disease, and the stages of HIV infection reflect the progression of immune deterioration. HIV itself can affect a number of organ systems in the body, resulting in specific clinical disease manifestations. HIV can also induce a severe immune deficiency that allows the occurrence of severe and life-threatening opportunistic and other infections and malignancies. The challenge for patients infected with HIV and their caregivers is to minimize the progressive immunologic damage caused by HIV over time and to prevent and treat complications of HIV and AIDS quickly and effectively when they occur.

ACKNOWLEDGMENT

Supported in part by grants from the State of California, Universitywide Task Force on AIDS to the UCLA AIDS Clinical Research Center (CC95-LA-194) and USPHS NIH grants AI-27660, CA70080, and RR-00865.

REFERENCES

1. Centers for Disease Control. 1993 revised classification system for HIV infection and expanded surveillance case definition for AIDS among adolescents and adults. MMWR 41:961, 1992.
2. Chang SW, Kate MH, Hernandez SR. The new AIDS case definition: implications for San Francisco. JAMA 267:973, 1992.
3. Weiss RA. How does HIV cause AIDS? Science 260:1273–1279, 1993.
4. Fauci AS. Multifactorial nature of human immunodeficiency virus disease: implications for therapy. Science 262:1011–1018, 1993.
5. Rubin RH. Acquired immunodeficiency syndrome. In: Scientific American Medicine, section, XI:1–24, 1993.
6. Cooper DA, Gold J, MacLean P, et al. Acute AIDS retrovirus infection: definition of a clinical illness associated with seroconversion. Lancet 1:537, 1985.
7. Ho DD, Sarngadharan MG, Resnick L, et al. Primary human T-lymphotropic virus type III infection. Ann Intern Med 102:800, 1985.
8. Del Rio C, Soffer O, Widell JL, et al. Acute human immunodeficiency virus infection temporally associated with rhabdomyolysis, acute renal failure, and nephrosis. Rev Infect Dis 12:282, 1990.
9. Fauci AS, Masur H, Gelmann EP, et al. The acquired immunodeficiency syndrome: an update. Ann Intern Med 102:800, 1985.
10. Valle S-L, Saxinger C, Ranki A, et al. Diversity of clinical spectrum of HTLV-III infection. Lancet 1:301, 1985.
11. Bartlett JG. The Johns Hopkins Hospital Guide to Medical Care of Patients with HIV Infection, 5th ed. Baltimore: Williams & Wilkins, 1995.
12. Gabuzda DH, Hirsch MS. Neurologic manifestations of infection with human immunodeficiency virus: clinical features and pathogenesis. Ann Intern Med 107:383, 1987.
13. Dalakas M, Wichman A, Sever J. AIDS and the nervous system. JAMA 261:2396, 1989.
14. McArthur JC. Neurologic manifestations of AIDS. Medicine (Baltimore) 66:407, 1987.

15. Sönnenborg A, Sääf J, Alexius B, et al. Quantitative detection of brain aberrations in human immunodeficiency virus type 1-infected individuals by magnetic resonance imaging. J Infect Dis 162:1245, 1990.

16. Greenson JK, Belitsos PC, Yardley JH, et al. AIDS enteropathy: occult enteric infections and duodenal mucosal alternations in chronic diarrhea. Ann Inter Med 114:366, 1991.

17. Rabeneck L, Popovic M, Gartner S, et al. Acute HIV infection presenting with painful swallowing and esophageal ulcers. JAMA 263:2318, 1990.

18. Bach MC, Howell DA, Valenti AJ, et al. Aphthous ulceration of the gastrointestinal tract in patients with the acquired immunodeficiency syndrome (AIDS). Ann Intern Med 112:465, 1990.

19. Rao TKS, Friedman EA, Nicastri AD. The types of renal disease in the acquired immunodeficiency syndrome. N Engl J Med 316:1062, 1987.

20. Glassock RJ, Cohen AH, Danovitch G, et al. Human immunodeficiency virus (HIV) infection and the kidney. Ann Intern Med 112:35, 1990.

21. Calabrese LH, Proffitt MR, Yen-Lieberman B, et al. Congestive cardiomyopathy and illness related to the acquired immunodeficiency syndrome (AIDS) associated with isolation of retrovirus from myocardium. Ann Intern Med 107:691, 1987.

22. LoPresti JS, Fried JC, Spencer CA, et al. Unique alterations of thyroid hormone indices in the acquired immunodeficiency syndrome (AIDS). Ann Intern Med 110:970, 1989.

23. Grunfeld C, Feingold KR. Metabolic disturbances and wasting in the acquired immunodeficiency syndrome. N Engl J Med 327:329, 1992.

24. Kaye BR. Rheumatologic manifestations of infection with human immunodeficiency virus (HIV). Ann Intern Med 111:158, 1989.

25. Rompalo AM, Cannon RO, Quinn TC, et al. Association of biologic false-positive reactions for syphilis with human immunodeficiency virus infection. J Infect Dis 165:1124, 1992.

26. Cozzi PJ, Abu-Jawdeh GM, Green RM, et al. Amyloidosis in association with human immunodeficiency virus infection. Clin Infect Dis 14:189, 1992.

27. Karpatkin S, Nardi MA, Humes KB. Immunologic thrombocytopenic purpura after heterosexual transmission of human immunodeficiency virus (HIV). Ann Intern Med 109:194, 1988.

28. Leaf AN, Laubenstein LJ, Raphael B, et al. Thrombotic thrombocytopenic purpura associated with human immunodeficiency virus type 1 (HIV-1) infection. Ann Intern Med 109:194, 1988.

29. Suffredini AF, Ognibene FP, Lack EE, et al. Nonspecific interstitial pneumonitis: a common cause of pulmonary disease in the acquired immunodeficiency syndrome. Ann Intern Med 107:7, 1987.

30. Aron DC. Endocrine complications of the acquired immunodeficiency syndrome. Arch Intern Med 149:330, 1989.

31. Farizo KM, Buehler JW, Chamberland ME, et al. Spectrum of disease in persons with human immunodeficiency virus infection in the United States. JAMA 267:1798, 1992.

32. Blanche S, Ramzioux C, Muscato M-LG, et al. A prospective study of infants born to women seropositive for human immunodeficiency virus type 1. N Engl J Med 320:1643–1648, 1989.

33. Johnson JP, Nair P, Hines SE, et al. Natural history and serologic diagnosis of infants born to HIV infected women. Am J Dis Child 143:1147–1153, 1989.

34. Grossman M. Pediatric AIDS. In: Sande MA, Volberding PA, eds. Medical Management of AIDS, 3rd ed. Philadelphia: W.B. Saunders Company, 1992:452–464.

35. Ognibene FP, Masur H, Rogers P, et al. Nonspecific interstitial pneumonitis without evidence of *Pneumocystis carinii* in asymptomatic patients infected with human immunodeficiency virus (HIV). Ann Intern Med 109:874, 1988.

36. Belman A, Diamond G, Dickson D, et al. Pediatric acquired immunodeficiency syndrome. Neurologic syndrome. Am J Dis Child 142:29–35, 1988.

37. Falloon J, Eddy T, Wiener L, Pizzo P. Human immunodeficiency virus infection in children. J Pediatr 114:1–30, 1989.

38. Prober CG, Gershon AA. Management of newborns and infants born to HIV seropositive mothers. Pediatr Infect Dis J 10:684–695, 1991.

39. CDC. Classification system for human immunodeficiency virus (HIV) infection in children under 13 years of age. MMWR 36:225–236, 1987.

40. Pizzo PA, Wilfert CM. Treatment considerations for children with human immunodeficiency virus infection. Pediatr Infect Dis J 9:690, 1990.

41. CDC. Immunization of children infected with human immunodeficiency virus: supplementary ACIP statement. MMWR 37:181–183, 1988.

42. National Institute of Child Health and Human Development Intravenous Immunoglobulin Study Group. Intravenous immunoglobulin for the preventing of bacterial infections in children with symptomatic human immunodeficiency virus infection. N Engl J Med 325:73–90, 1991.
43. McKinney RE, Maha MA, Connor EM, et al. A multicenter trial of oral zidovudine in children with advanced immunodeficiency virus disease. N Engl J Med 324:15, 1018–1025, 1991.

Therapy of HIV Spectrum Diseases

The management of patients with human immunodeficiency virus (HIV) disease involves not only an understanding of the pathophysiology of HIV infection and knowledge of recent advances in the medical management of acquired immunodeficiency syndrome (AIDS)-related complications, but also requires a sensitivity to the psychological, social, and public health ramifications of AIDS on the patient and his or her family and community. This section will focus on the medical evaluation and treatment of HIV and its related complications. Healthcare providers are cautioned to be sensitive to the fact that HIV is almost invariably a progressive disease that is often fatal and can cause considerable morbid consequences. These may include dementia, debilitating diarrhea, emaciation, and impairment of other bodily functions that can result in not only significant physical impairment but may also affect the individual's body image and ability to socialize normally. The medical tragedy of AIDS is also compounded in many situations by social stigmatization and social isolation. This, along with concerns over the cost of medical care and loss of ability to work and other important socially defining connections, makes living with AIDS particularly difficult and psychologically distressing. Health providers need to be compassionate, sensitive, and aware of these other issues facing most individuals with HIV and AIDS. Resources for patient services including financial assistance, social service organizations, and clinical trials are available in many areas from community-based organizations, local academic institutions, and special entitlement programs often administered through regional public health departments. Patients and providers should be aware of these resources available to them.

Diagnostic Evaluation

As discussed in *Spectrum of Illness, Disease Staging, and Natural History,* patients with HIV infection may present with various manifestations of their infection based on the stage of their illness and their exposure to specific infectious pathogens. The average time from acute HIV infection to serious complications, in the absence of antiretroviral therapy, is approximately 10 to 11 years (1). There is considerable variation, however, and many patients have stable CD4 counts and remain asymptomatic for many years (2). Patients should be aware that despite current limitations of treatment, therapy for HIV will clearly delay progression of the disease and may permit access to new and potentially more effective treatments in the future (3). The diagnostic evaluation of patients with HIV involves an awareness of specific complications likely at each stage of HIV infection as well as thorough physical and laboratory evaluations and a high index of suspicion for complications of HIV and AIDS.

PHYSICAL EXAMINATION

The physical examination of patients with HIV infection should focus on anatomical sites that are likely to show significant changes and may prove useful in the management of patients with HIV. Especially important are lymph node evaluation, fundoscopic examination, oral cavity examination, careful skin examination, abdominal examination for hepatosplenomegaly, genital examination for STDs, pelvic examination for women, and neuropsychological testing. Several components of the standard evaluation should be emphasized.

Neurologic Evaluation

The neurologic examination should include an evaluation for HIV-associated dementia that can occur in 20 to 30% of patients almost exclusively in late stages of HIV disease. Early symptoms of cognitive defects include problems with concentration and memory. Early subjective evidence of motor dysfunction includes imbalance; incoordination or difficulty with complex motor tasks; and difficulties with verbal responses, sequencing of items, psychomotor integrative capabilities, and performance under time pressure. Physical findings may include hyperreflexia, ataxia, and problems with rapid alternating movements. Neuroradiographic scans usually show cerebral atrophy with or without abnormalities in white matter.

Ophthalmologic Evaluation

While a variety of ophthalmologic abnormalities may be detected on standard examination, cytomegalovirus (CMV) retinitis is one of the more common findings and complicates the course of about 20% of advanced-stage patients with AIDS. Initial lesions are often in the periphery and may not be easily visualized by routine fundoscopic examination; therefore, a dilated examination is often required. AIDS patients with CMV retinitis have a mean CD4 count of around 20 cells/mm^3, with only 1% having counts above 100 cells/mm^3. Therefore routine ophthalmologic evaluation at 4 to 6 month intervals are recommended for patients with CD4 counts below 100 cells/mm^3.

Gynecologic Evaluation

Women with HIV infection have a high rate of gynecologic complications, including recurrent and refractory vaginal candidiasis as an early manifestation of HIV and a higher incidence of cervical dysplasia. A high association has been noted between declining CD4 counts and the occurrence of cervical dysplasia and cervical carcinoma in women with HIV infection. In addition, pelvic inflammatory disease appears to be more common and, perhaps, more severe in women with HIV infection (4). The CDC recommends a gynecologic examination and Pap smear at initial evaluation and repeat testing approximately every 6 months. Findings of an abnormal Pap smear should be followed by colposcopy and biopsy to detect early cervical intraepithelial neoplasia or invasive cervical carcinoma. Women with HIV infection also need specialized counseling regarding the HIV testing and care of their children and the risk of perinatal HIV transmission during pregnancy *(See Women and HIV infection)*.

NUTRITIONAL ASSESSMENT

Nutritional assessment is important not only because wasting is a common feature of late-stage disease, but also because metabolic requirements may be higher in patients with late-stage or advanced HIV disease as a result of HIV and related complications. Cachexia may be due to HIV-induced cytokine production, hypogonadism, or malnutrition. Reduced intake due to depression, dementia, anorexia, nausea, oral or esophageal lesions, or drug interactions may contribute to weight loss. A thorough medical evaluation should be performed for patients with significant weight loss and, if no readily reversible cause is found, then consultation with a nutritionist and/or the use of appetite stimulants and nutritional supplements would be appropriate. The value of prolonged parenteral hyperalimentation has not been established and, therefore, should be reserved for patients with devastating protein and caloric malnutrition due to gastrointestinal malabsorption such as that which occurs with uncontrollable cryptosporidiosis. Promising results have been reported with recombinant human growth hormone at a substantial financial cost, however.

The frequency of physical evaluations in patients with HIV disease will vary by stage of disease, severity of illness, and associated complications and their treatment. For patients with asymptomatic HIV infection and stable CD4 counts, routine visits with CD4 enumeration can be done at visits of approximately 3 to 4 month intervals. Patients with symptomatic disease may be seen every 1 to 2 months with more frequent visits during the course of their diagnostic evaluation and initiation of treatment. Visits for late-stage and/or advanced patients with AIDS will depend on the likelihood of developing complications of their treatment or disease and whether or not patients may be managed at home through care programs.

LABORATORY TESTING

The usual laboratory tests for known HIV-positive individuals are designed to establish the stage of disease, to identify potential pathogens that may influence treatment or prophylaxis, and to determine the general health status of the individual. Specific tests performed frequently in AIDS patients are as follows.

Complete Count (CBC)

This is a standard component of the initial evaluation of any patient and is especially important in patients with HIV infection because of the high incidence of anemia, leukopenia, and thrombocytopenia that are common complications of HIV and its treatment. The frequency of this testing depends on the stage of illness and the medications of the patient.

CD4 Cell Count

This is an important test for any patient with HIV infection to establish the stage of disease and to provide guidance for differential diagnoses of patients' complaints. It may also influence therapeutic decisions regarding antiretroviral therapy and prophylaxis for opportunistic infections. Standardization of the methodology for CD4 cell enumeration should be established as well as a range of normals for each laboratory. There is substantial intrapatient variability in results of this test due to diurnal variation, intercurrent illness, as well as the reagents and method for conducting the enumeration. Marked variation in laboratory results reflects the fact that the absolute CD4 count represents the product of three variables: the white blood cell count, percent lymphocytes, and percent lymphocytes bearing the CD4 receptor. The average within subject coefficient of variation for CD4 count has been shown to be around 25% in quality control assessments performed by the AIDS Clinical Trials Group (ACTG). Some clinicians prefer to utilize the CD4 percentage because this reduces the variation to one measurement. Corresponding CD4 counts with CD4 percentages are as follows:

CD4 Cell Count	Percent CD4
>500	>29
200–500	14–28
<200	<14

Medical conditions that can cause a decrease in CD4 counts include a variety of both acute and chronic opportunistic infections such as CMV, tuberculosis, and bacterial infections. Immune activation, such as after immunization or recent viral infections and corticosteroids, may induce profound decreases in CD4 counts. Pregnancy, physical and psychological stress, and the age of adult individuals have little effect on CD4 counts.

Serum Chemistry Panel

This test is a routine part of any initial evaluation but is of little use in routine evaluation of the healthy HIV-infected individual. For patients receiving medication or who have symptomatic disease, screening chemistry panels may be useful in providing early clues to organ system impairment and/or early toxicity from treatments.

Syphilis Serologies

Screening tests venereal disease research lab (VDRL) or reactive plasmin reagent (RPR) should be performed with the initial evaluation of any HIV-infected individual and repeated annually in patients who are sexually active. Both false-negative and false-positive tests have been reported in patients with HIV, but these are rare. Patients with positive screening tests should have a confirmatory fluorescent treponemal antibody absorption test, and all patients who are found to be positive should undergo a lumbar puncture to exclude latent neurosyphilis.

Hepatitis Serology

Hepatitis serologies are useful in patients with elevated liver function tests as well as in those with normal values. Hepatitis B testing may help identify individuals who may benefit from hepatitis B vaccination. Patients with abnormal liver function studies also need further evaluation to exclude active viral hepatitis infection with either hepatitis B-virus (HBV) or hepatitis C-virus (HCV). The appropriate tests are HBV surface antigen (HBsAg) and antibodies to HCV (anti-HCV).

Toxoplasmosis Serology

This test is useful in identifying patients with latent infection who may be candidates for prophylaxis when their CD4 count is below 100 cells/mm^3 and to assist in the subsequent evaluation of CNS disease in patients undergoing evaluation for CNS lesions. The seroprevalence of toxoplasmosis antibodies in the United States is 10 to 30% and the sensitivity of the tests for CNS toxoplasmosis is 85 to 90%. Patients with negative tests on initial evaluation should have a repeat serology performed if toxoplasmosis encephalitis is suspected.

PPD Skin Tests

The CDC recommends routine testing for all patients with purified protein derivative (PPD), using the standard Mantoux test, 5TU units with interpretation at 48 to 72 hours. Anergy testing should also be performed at the same time with at least two other skin test antigens. Patients with positive PPD of any degree of induration should be considered for prophylactic TB therapy.

Pap Smear

The CDC recommends gynecologic examination with pelvic examination and Pap smear in women with HIV infection at initial evaluation and every 6 to 12 months. Patients with a history of human papilloma virus (HPV) infection or previously abnormal Pap smears should have repeat testing every 6 months. Individuals with evidence of cervical dysplasia should be referred to a gynecologist for colposcopy and biopsy.

Women with HIV infection have an eight to tenfold higher incidence of cervical dysplasia than age-matched non-HIV-infected women. Recurrence rate of cervical intraepithelial neoplasia after standard therapy is also higher, and, therefore, frequent testing after local treatment for dysplasia should be performed.

Chest X-ray

A chest x-ray is recommended as a baseline assessment for all patients with HIV, both to detect asymptomatic tuberculosis and as a baseline for future evaluation of pulmonary symptoms.

Treatment

VACCINATION

Currently, recommended routine vaccinations for patients with HIV include annual influenza vaccine and pneumococcal vaccine. Other vaccines that can be considered include hepatitis B vaccine, hemophilus influenza B, and vaccines needed for foreign travel. All single-dose vaccinations should be given as early as possible after diagnosis of HIV infection to obtain optimal immune response to the vaccine when the CD4 count is highest. In general, live viral or bacterial vaccines should be avoided, although killed or inactivated vaccines are considered safe. Although there is some concern that vaccination may be associated with increased HIV replication, annual influenza vaccine and other indicated vaccinations are still recommended because the consequence of an acute influenza or other viral infection can be quite detrimental to patients with HIV infection.

PROPHYLACTIC MEDICATIONS

Recommendations for prophylaxis for various opportunistic infections have undergone considerable evaluation and refinements over the past several years. Current recommendations for prophylaxis of standard opportunistic infections in patients with AIDS is given in Table 4.10. A few infections, however, should be emphasized.

Tuberculosis

A medical history including an assessment of previous tuberculosis infection, history of exposure to *Mycobacterium tuberculosis,* and past treatment or preventive therapy should be elicited from all HIV-infected individuals. The risk of TB infection should also be assessed for each patient including predisposing conditions (e.g., household contacts, country of origin, homelessness, alcoholism, substance abuse, history of incarceration, or residence in a congregated living situation). The health and social conditions that may affect an individual's ability to complete a course of therapy should also be assessed (e.g., failure to keep appointments, mental illnesses, substance abuse, homelessness, or alcoholism).

Table 4.10.

Antimicrobial Prophylaxis of Opportunistic Infections

Disease	Indications	Preferred Regimen	Comment
Tuberculosis	PPD + (≥5 mm induration) Prior positive PPD High-risk exposure	INH 300 mg/day + pyridoxine 50 mg/day (S0.60/mo)	Efficacy established Alternative is rifampin 600 mg/day × 12 mo
P. carinii pneumonia	Prior PCP CD4 < 200 Thrush or FUO	TMP-SMX 1 DS/day	Efficacy established: cost effective, reduced morbidity and mortality Alternatives: dapsone 100 mg/day, regimens for toxoplasmosis (see below) or aerosolized pentamidine 300 mg/mo
Toxoplasmosis	CD4 < 100 *plus* positive serology (IgG)	TMP-SMX 1 DS/day	Efficacy established Main issue is use of alternative regimens in patients with TMP-SMX intolerance: dapsone 50 mg/day + pyrimethamine 50 mg/wk + leucovorin 25 mg/wk or dapsone 200 mg/wk + pyrimethamine 75 mg/wk + leucovorin 25 mg/wk
M. avium	CD4 < 75	Rifabutin 300 mg/day	Efficacy established Most breakthrough cases involve rifabutin-sensitive strains of *M. avium* Concerns are resistance of TB to rifampin (not established), cost, and drug interactions Clarithromycin 500 mg po bid may be more effective, but breakthrough disease usually involves clarithromycin = resistant strains Azithromycin 500 mg tiw
Cytomegalovirus	CD4 < 50	Oral ganciclovir 1000 mg po tid	Efficacy shown in one study Concerns are cost, promotion of ganciclovir resistance, and conflicting study results
Deep fungal infection	CD4 < 100	Fluconazole 200 mg/day	Efficacy established for prevention of cryptococcosis and *Candida* esophagitis (and thrush) Concerns are cost, lack of evidence for prolongation of survival, and promotion of infection with azole-resistant *Candida* spp.

From Bartlett JG. The Johns Hopkins Hospital Guide to Medical Care of Patients with HIV Infection, 5th ed. Baltimore: Williams & Wilkins, 1995:47.

Clinical history and physical examination of the patient should focus on symptoms suggestive of TB such as cough, hemoptysis, fevers, night sweats, and weight loss.

It should be noted that this complication often occurs relatively early in the course of HIV disease with the average CD4 count in newly detected cases being 200 to 300 cells/mm³. Additionally, up to 30 to 50% of cases of TB in HIV-infected patients are primary tuberculosis rather than reactivation of latent disease (5). Detection is often delayed because of atypical clinical features and a high rate of false-negative PPD skin tests (40% in HIV-infected patients compared to 10% in those without HIV infection). Atypical features of tuberculosis in HIV include lower lobe infiltrates, infrequent cavitary disease, more mediastinal adenopathy, and a high rate of extrapulmonary disease, especially lymph node and meningeal involvement. The rate of anergy to PPD is inversely correlated with CD4 counts, with the majority of patients with CD4 counts under 100 being anergic on routine skin testing (6).

Patients who are PPD positive or who have a history of positive PPD without adequate hemoprophylaxis, as well as those who are high-risk contacts of persons with active tuberculosis, should receive INH prophylaxis (7). Those with no evidence of active disease should receive INH with vitamin B_6 for 12 months. Alternative regimens have also been proposed, although the relative effectiveness and the complication rates of these alternative regimens have not been fully established.

Pneumocystis carinii Pneumonia (PCP)

PCP is the most common AIDS-defining diagnosis and is a major cause of death in patients with AIDS. Risk of PCP in patients with prior PCP is 60 to 70% (8) and for those with CD4 cell counts below 100 cells/mm³, 44% per year. A routine secondary prophylaxis is recommended for all patients who have had PCP previously, and primary prophylaxis is recommended for those who have not had PCP but are at increased risk as defined by CD4 counts <200 cells/mm³. Alternatively, an HIV-infected individual who is demonstrating a rapid decline in CD4 counts may benefit from initiating PCP prophylaxis at somewhat higher CD4 counts (e.g., <250 cells/mm³). Patients who are on systemic corticosteroids or who have oral candidiasis or other constitutional symptoms with declining CD4 counts may also benefit from PCP prophylaxis. Treatment should continue for the lifetime of the patient.

Specific prophylactic regimens for PCP are given in Table 4.10 and may include trimethoprim-sulfamethoxazole (TMP-SMX), dapsone, dapsone plus pyrimethamine, and aerosolized pentamidine.

Toxoplasmosis

Nearly all toxoplasmosis cases in patients with HIV infection in the U.S. appear to be relapses of latent infection as indicated by a previously positive baseline serologic test for *T. gondii*. The seroprevalence rate of *T. gondii* in the U.S. is 10 to 30% with a seroconversion rate of approximately 1% per year. The 1-year risk of toxoplasmosis in seropositive individuals with CD4 counts below 100 is 20 to 30%, and 75% of cases occur in patients with CD4 counts below 50.

While there are no prospective trials demonstrating the benefit of TMP-SMX as prophylaxis for toxoplasmosis, several retrospective analyses of this drug in PCP prophylaxis trials have shown consistent benefit in reducing the incidence of toxoplasmosis in treated individuals. In five such studies involving over 1800 participants, the rate of toxoplasmosis with TMP-SMX was less than 1% compared to 3 to 12% in controls (9). Alternative prophylaxis treatments include dapsone plus pyrimethamine on a daily or weekly basis.

Mycobacterium avium Complex (MAC)

The risk of disseminated MAC in patients with AIDS is 40 to 50% with median CD4 counts in these patients of 20 cells/mm^3 (10). The risk of MAC in patients with CD4 counts above 100 is quite low. Prospective placebo-controlled trials of rifabutin in patients with CD4 counts under 200 have demonstrated >70% efficacy of this drug in preventing MAC bacteremia in patients receiving this drug. There is also substantial experience with clarithromycin in the treatment of MAC and preliminary results suggest the efficacy of this drug as a prophylaxis for MAC as well. Azithromycin is also active against MAC and is being evaluated as a potential prophylactic drug for this infection. Current recommendations are to treat HIV-infected patients with CD4 counts <80 cells/mm^3 with either rifabutin, clarithromycin or possibly azithromycin.

Cytomegalovirus (CMV)

CMV is a major cause of multi-organ system disease in late stage HIV infection. CMV retinitis is a frequent vision-threatening complication seen in 15 to 25% of patients with AIDS. CMV may also be responsible for cases of esophagitis, colitis, enteritis, radiculitis, encephalitis, hepatitis, and adrenalitis in patients with AIDS. The occurrence of CMV retinitis requires lifetime maintenance therapy after acute treatment.

A recent controlled study of oral ganciclovir in patients with HIV infection and CD4 counts of <100 cells/mm^3 has shown that the rate of disseminated CMV disease was lower in patients receiving oral ganciclovir than in placebo recipients (11). A second study, however, failed to show a statistically significant decrease in CMV infection in oral ganciclovir recipients. In both studies, no survival benefit was demonstrated, although trends favored ganciclovir recipients. Oral ganciclovir has recently been approved by the FDA for use as a prophylactic agent for CMV in those with CD4 counts <100. Further evaluation of this agent will be needed in view of the relatively high cost and higher incidence of myelosuppression seen in treated individuals.

Fungal Infections

While the frequency of mucocutaneous candidal infection is high in patients with HIV, the use of prophylactic antibiotics for fungi in AIDS is targeted to prevent the occurrence of "deep fungal infections." The life-time risk of candida esophagitis in patients with AIDS is 17%, for cryp-tococcosis 5 to 10%, and for histoplasmosis and coccidioidomycosis 20% in endemic areas. These infections are typically seen in patients with CD4 counts <100 with most seen in those with CD4 counts <50.

A prospective prophylactic study of fluconazole versus clotrimazole in patients with CD4 counts <200 has shown a statistically significant re-duction in deep fungal infection in fluconazole recipients with the major benefit seen in patients with CD4 <100. Most invasive fungal infections occurred with CD4 counts <50.

Drug treatment for AIDS-associated infections are summarized in Table 4.11.

Antiretroviral Therapy

Significant advances have been made in the area of antiretroviral therapy for patients with HIV infection in the past few years. At the time of this writing, five nucleoside analog drugs (zidovudine, didano-sine, zalcitabine, stavudine, and lamivudine) and three protease in-hibitor (saquinavir, ritonavir, indinovir) have been approved by the FDA for treatment in patients with HIV. Recent studies have confirmed the clinical advantage of using combination therapy over monotherapy in antiretroviral-naive as well as in experienced patients. Additional clini-cal studies evaluating various two- and three-drug combinations are in progress. The use of peripheral blood viral load measures to assess the antiretroviral efficacy of these drugs will allow more rapid evaluation of these regimens in various populations. Correlation of antiretroviral ac-tivity with both CD4 responses and clinical outcome should provide im-portant information on the relative contribution and importance of the antiviral effects of these drugs and the indirect effect of increased CD4 counts in preventing HIV disease progression and prolonging life. Addi-tionally, more information on the use of viral load markers in the man-agement of antiretroviral therapy for individual patients with HIV will be forthcoming in the next few years.

Decisions regarding the immediate initiation or deferral of antiretro-viral therapy in individual patients should be made jointly with the pa-tient following a discussion of the risks and benefits of treatment. Anti-retroviral therapy with the nucleoside analog zidovudine (ZDV, formerly azidothymidine, AZT) has been shown to be effective as monotherapy in delaying disease progression and increasing the survival as in patients with advanced HIV disease. In patients with asymptomatic HIV infec-tion, however, randomized controlled study of ZDV monotherapy failed to demonstrate significant differences in rates of clinical disease pro-gression or in survival at 3 years' follow-up, although improvements in CD4 counts were seen after 1 year of treatment (12). At this time, no clinical study has clearly demonstrated clinical benefits for early use of zidovudine (or other antiretroviral agents) for asymptomatic individuals with CD4 counts >500/mm^3. HIV viral suppression with combination antiretroviral drugs and/or sequential modification in treatment regi-

Table 4.11.
Drug Treatment for AIDS-Associated Infections

Condition	Standard Treatment		Alternative Treatment	
	Drug	Dosage	Drug	Dosage
P. carinii pneumonia	TMP-SMX	15 mg/kg/day po or IV in 3 or 4 doses × 21 days	Pentamidine	3–4 mg/kg IV daily × 21 days
			Trimetrexate	45 mg/m² IV daily × 21 days
			+ Folinic acid	20 mg/m² po or IV q6h × 21 days
			Dapsone	100 mg po daily × 21 days
			+ Trimethoprim	5 mg/kg po tid × 21 days
			Atovaquone suspension	750 mg po bid × 21 days
			Primaquine	15 mg base po daily × 21 days, or
			+ Clindamycin	600 mg IV qid × 21 days, or 300–450 mg po qid × 21 days
	± Prednisone	40 mg po bid, days 1–5 20 mg po bid, days 6–10 20 mg po daily, days 11–21		
Toxoplasmosis	Pyrimethamine + Sulfadiazine	50–100 mg po daily 1–1.5 g po q6h	Pyrimethamine + Clindamycin	50–100 mg po daily 450–600 mg po or 600–1200 mg IV qid
Chronic Suppressive Therapy	Pyrimethamine ± Sulfadiazine	25–50 mg po daily 500 mg to 1 g po q6h	Pyrimethamine + Clindamycin	50 mg po daily 300 mg po qid
Cryptosporidiosis	Paromomycin	500–750 mg po qid		
Candidiasis Oral	Nystatin solution or tablets	500,000 to 1,000 000 units 3–5 ×/day	Fluconazole	100–200 mg po daily
			Itraconazole	200 mg po daily
			Ketoconazole	200 mg po daily
			or Clotrimazole troches	10 mg po 5 ×/day
Esophageal	Fluconazole	100–200 mg po daily × 1–3 wks	Itraconazole	200 mg po daily
			Ketoconazole	200–400 mg po daily × 2–3 wks
			Amphotericin B	0.3 mg/kg IV daily × 7 days

continued

Table 4.11.— *continued*
Drug Treatment for AIDS-Associated Infections

Condition	Standard Treatment		Alternative Treatment	
	Drug	Dosage	Drug	Dosage
Coccidioidomycosis	Amphotericin B	0.5–1 mg/kg IV daily	Fluconazole	400–800 mg po daily
Chronic Suppressive Therapy	Amphotericin B	1 mg/kg weekly	Itraconazole Fluconazole	400 mg po daily 200 mg po bid
Cryptococcosis	Amphotericin B	0.3–1 mg/kg IV daily	Fluconazole	400–800 mg po daily
Chronic Suppressive Therapy	Fluconazole	200 mg po daily	Amphotericin B	0.5–1 mg/kg IV weekly
Histoplasmosis	Amphotericin B	0.5–0.6 mg/kg IV daily	Itraconazole	200 mg po bid
Chronic Suppressive Therapy	Itraconazole	200 mg po bid	Amphotericin B	0.5–0.8 mg/kg IV weekly
Cytomegalovirus Retinitis, Colitis, Esophagitis	Ganciclovir	5 mg/kg IV q12h × 14–21 days	Foscarnet	60 mg/kg IV q8h or 90 mg/kg IV q12h × 14–21 days
Chronic Suppressive Therapy	Ganciclovir	5 mg/kg IV daily or 6 mg/kg IV 5×/wk or 1 g po tid	Foscarnet	90–120 mg/kg IV daily
Herpes Simplex Virus Primary or Recurrent	Acyclovir	200–800 mg po 5×/day	Foscarnet	40 mg/kg IV q8h × 21 days
Secondary Prophylaxis	Acyclovir	400 mg po bid	Foscarnet	40 mg/kg IV daily

Condition	Drug	Dose
Varicella-zoster, primary or disseminated	Acyclovir	10 mg/kg IV q8h × 7–14 days
	Foscarnet	40 mg/kg IV q8h
Dermatomal zoster	Acyclovir	800 mg po 5×/day × 7–10 days
	Famciclovir	500 mg po q8h × 7 days
	Foscarnet	40 mg/kg IV q8h
Syphilis		
Primary, secondary, latent	Benzathine Penicillin	2.4 million units IM
	or Doxycycline	100 mg po bid × 14 days
	or Erythromycin	500 mg po qid × 14 days
	For all stages:	
	Amoxicillin	2 g po tid × 14 days
	+ Probenecid	500 mg po tid × 14 days
	or Doxycycline	200 mg po bid × 21 days
	or Ceftriaxone	1 g IM daily × 5–14 days
	or Benzathine PCN	2.4 million units IM weekly × 3 doses
	+ Doxycycline	200 mg po bid × 21 days
Late latent	Benzathine PCN	2.4 million units IM weekly × 3
	or Doxycycline	100 mg po bid × 28 days
Neurosyphilis	Aqueous PCN G	12–24 million units/day IV × 10–14 days
	or Procaine PCN	2.4 million units IM daily × 10 days
	+ Probenecid	500 mg po bid × 10 days
Tuberculosis	Isoniazid	300 mg po daily
	+ Rifampin	600 mg po daily
	+ Pyrazinamide	15–25 mg/kg po daily
	+ Ethambutol	15–25 mg/kg po daily
	or Streptomycin	15 mg/kg IM daily
Disseminated *M. avium* Complex	Clarithromycin	500 mg po bid
	or Azithromycin	500 mg po daily
	+ one or more of the following:	
	Ethambutol	15–25 mg/kg daily
	Clofazimine	100–200 mg daily
	Ciprofloxacin	750 mg bid
	Rifabutin	300–450 mg po daily

From Med Lett 1995;37(959):90–91.

mens based on viral load over time may ultimately result in better HIV control, delayed disease progression, and possibly increases in survival. At this time, however, treatment is recommended only for individuals with CD4 counts <500 cells/mm^3 (13). The initiation of antiretroviral therapy for patients with CD4 counts >500 may be appropriate, but will require individual decision by the physician and patient after discussion and evaluation of all currently available clinical and laboratory data.

Alteration in treatment regimens, once initiated, will depend on tolerance of the individual to the initial treatment, occurrence of clinical disease progression that may indicate loss of efficacy, fall in CD4 counts, or increase in HIV viral load. Precise recommendations for use of CD4 and viral load measures have not been fully established, although guidelines are currently in the process of being developed. It should be noted, however, that day-to-day variation in absolute CD4 counts, as well as in HIV viral load, may occur as a result of diurnal variation, concurrent illnesses, immunization or other immune stimulants, or assay variability. The stability of CD4 counts and viral load measures should be validated by promptly repeating these tests prior to recommending changes in antiretroviral therapy. In general, however, a significant fall in CD4 count of >5 to 6% per year or an increase in HIV viral load above 100,000 copies/mL would generally trigger a change in antiretroviral therapy.

For patients on ZDV monotherapy, the addition of a second nucleoside analog (e.g., ddI, ddC, or 3TC) or a switch to an alternative monotherapy (e.g., ddI, ddC, or d4T) would be appropriate. Patients who are intolerant of ZDV may be switched to an alternative monotherapy or, preferably, to an alternative combination antiretroviral regimen that does not have the same toxicity. Patients who develop neutropenia or anemia as the major intolerance to zidovudine, if they continue to have clinical benefit from this treatment, may alternatively continue on zidovudine with the addition of erythropoietin and/or a myeloid hematopoietic growth factor (e.g., G-CSF or GM-CSF) to correct the cytopenia.

Recent results from two major prospective clinical trials of combination antiretroviral therapy versus monotherapy (ACTG 175 and the European/Australian Delta study) have shown an advantage for combination nucleoside analog therapy (ZDV + ddI and ZDV + ddC) over monotherapy with ZDV in both ZDV-inexperienced and naive individuals with CD4 counts between 200 to 500 cells/mm^3 (14). For ZDV-experienced individuals, clinical improvement was also seen in those switched to ddI monotherapy in the ACTG 175 study. These studies would suggest that combination antiretroviral therapy can provide clinical advantages over monotherapy in AIDS patients. The recent development of three drug antiretroviral regimens, including a protease inhibitor, and the use of combination regimens that may have differential effects on the susceptibility of resistant strains of HIV (e.g., AZT plus 3TC) may show ever greater clinical benefits and effects on inhibiting HIV viral replication and/or increasing CD4 counts (15).

Currently approved nucleoside analog drugs for the treatment of HIV are given in Table 4.12 and are briefly described below. HIV therapy using protease inhibitors are addressed separately.

Table 4.12.
Nucleoside Analog Therapies for HIV

	Zidovudine (AZT, ZDV)	Didanosine (ddI)	Zalcitabine (ddC)	Stavudine (d4T)	Lamivudine (3TC)
Indications: FDA labeling	Retrovir[R] FDA: CD4 < 500 Expert panel: CD4 count <500/mm³ with symptoms or CD4 count <200/mm³. Asymptomatic patients with CD4 counts 200–500/mm³: optional	Videx[R] FDA: Advanced HIV infection + prolonged prior therapy with AZT or advanced infection + AZT intolerance or significant clinical or immunologic deterioration during AZT treatment	HIVID[R] FDA: Monotherapy for advanced HIV infection + intolerance or progression with AZT or combined with AZT in selected patients with CD4 < 300/mm³	Zerit[R] FDA: Advanced HIV infection + intolerance to approved therapies with proven benefit or significant clinical or immunologic deterioration with these therapies	Epivir[R] FDA: Combination therapy with zidovudine as initial or subsequent HIV therapy
Usual dose (oral)	200 mg tid	(Tablet form) >60 kg: 200 mg bid <60 kg: 125 mg bid	0.75 mg tid	>60 kg: 40 mg bid <60 kg: 30 mg bid	150 mg bid
Minimum effective dose Oral bioavailability	300 mg/day 60%	200 mg/day (powder) Tablet: 40% Powder: 30%	Not studied 85%	Not studied 86%	Not studied 86%
Serum half-life Intracellular half-life CNS penetration (% serum levels)	1.1 hr 3 hr 60%	1.6 hr 12 hr 20%	1.2 hr 3 hr 20%	1.0 hr 3.5 hr 30%	3–6 hr 12 hr 10%
Elimination	Metabolized to AZT glucuronide (GAZT); renal excretion GAZT.	Renal excretion 50%	Renal excretion 70%	Renal excretion 50% unchanged	Renal
Major toxicity	Bone marrow suppression: anemia and/or neutropenia. Subjective complaints	Pancreatitis Peripheral neuropathy	Peripheral neuropathy Stomatitis	Peripheral neuropathy Pancreatitis	Headache, malaise, nausea, diarrhea, minimal myelosuppression

Modified from Bartlett JG. The Johns Hopkins Hospital Guide to Medical Care of Patients with HIV Infection, 5th ed. Baltimore: Williams & Wilkins, 1995:57.

ZIDOVUDINE (ZDV, AZIDOTHYMIDINE, AZT, RETROVIR) INDICATIONS

Current indications for ZDV are symptomatic HIV infection with CD4 count <200 cells/mm³ or asymptomatic HIV infection with CD4 count <500 cells/mm³. ZDV has been proven superior to ddI and ddC as initial monotherapy for patients with HIV (16). Improved tolerance, prolonged duration of action, and delayed emergence of resistance have been seen when treatment is initiated in earlier stages of HIV disease. Delay in clinical disease progression and improvement in survival have been seen in patients with late, symptomatic, or advanced-stage HIV disease.

Dosage

The standard dose of ZDV is 600 mg/day administered as two 100 mg tablets, three times a day. Benefit in terms of CD4 count preservation has been seen with doses as low as 300 mg/day in patients with CD4 cell counts of 200 to 500 cells/mm³; however, this dosage is recommended only for patients who cannot tolerate ZDV in standard dosage (17). Patients with HIV-associated dementia and those with immune thrombocytopenic purpura may benefit from higher doses of ZDV, e.g., 1000–1200 mg/day.

Side Effects

The major objective side effect of ZDV is marrow suppression resulting in anemia and granulocytopenia. Patients who begin ZDV therapy should have a CBC performed 2 weeks after initiating therapy and monthly thereafter for 3 months and then every 3 months. ZDV can cause macrocytosis with an increase in mean corpuscular volume and red cell distribution width. Common side effects include nausea, headache, insomnia, fatigue, myalgia, and abdominal pain. Myelosuppression is dose dependent and increases with the duration of treatment and with progressive HIV disease. The use of recombinant erythropoietin and granulocyte colony-stimulating factor may alleviate problems with cytopenias induced by ZDV. A less common side effect is myopathy with muscle pain and increased CPK levels which usually correct when the drug is discontinued. Most patients with this side effect have received ZDV therapy for more than 1 year. Elevations in liver function tests, occasional hepatomegaly, and lactic acidosis have been seen in a few cases with this and other nucleoside analogs.

Clinical Efficacy

The benefit of ZDV therapy has been documented in patients with HIV infections and CD4 counts below 500 cells/mm³ and is not race, gender, or risk factor dependent (18–20). Statistically significant delays in disease progression and improvement in survival have been seen in patients with AIDS and advanced symptomatic disease. Delay in HIV disease progression has been seen in at least one study (ACTG 019) in asymptomatic individuals with CD4 counts below 500/mm³ (20). Recent studies of combinations of ZDV with other nucleoside analogs have shown synergistic inhibition of HIV replication and greater improvements in CD4 counts and suppression of HIV viral load when compared to ZDV monotherapy in both previously treated and antiretroviral-naive individuals (21–23). Combinations of AZT with 3TC have shown continued sensitivity to AZT after development of specific 3TC resistance (184 mutation) in HIV isolates possessing a 215 ZDV resistant mutation (15). The clinical superiority of this combination over ZDV alone has been demonstrated in several randomized clinical studies (24).

DIDANOSINE (DDI, DIDEOXYINOSINE, VIDEX)

Indications

Didanosine is inferior to zidovudine as initial monotherapy for patients with HIV, but has been shown to be superior to continued ZDV in those previously treated with ZDV for 8 or more weeks (25). Didanosine has been recommended for use in patients who are intolerant or who experience clinical progression on zidovudine or whose CD4 counts have continued to fall with ZDV therapy. In vitro sensitivity studies have shown synergistic anti-HIV activity with ZDV and ddI and no evidence of cross resistance between ZDV and ddI. The combination of ZDV plus ddI has been shown to be superior to ZDV alone in patients who have had prior ZDV therapy with regard to overall survival (ACTG 175).

Dosage

Didanosine is currently available as chewable tablets, buffered powder, and solution. The bioavailability of the powder is somewhat less, so a higher dose is generally indicated. The drug should be taken on an empty stomach. Dosing with tablets must include two tablets taken simultaneously to provide sufficient buffer. Current recommended starting doses based on weight and preparation are as follows:

Weight	Tablets	Buffered Powder
≥60 kg	200 mg bid	250 mg bid
<60 kg	125 mg bid	167 mg bid

Side Effects

Studies of didanosine have shown that toxicity is dose related. The most serious side effects of ddI are pancreatitis in 5 to 9% and peripheral neuropathy in 5 to 12%. Patients who develop abdominal pain, nausea, vomiting, or elevated amylase levels should have therapy suspended and be closely monitored for further clinical evidence of pancreatitis. Approximately 6% of cases of pancreatitis are fatal. Didanosine is contraindicated in patients with a prior history of pancreatitis and in concurrent use with alcohol or other medications that can cause pancreatitis.

Peripheral neuropathy appears to be related to the cumulative dose of the drug and may present as paresthesias or painful neuropathy involving, primarily, hands and feet. Diarrhea can occur in up to 34% of patients, primarily those using the powdered formulation, and has been ascribed to the osmotic effect of the buffer. The high sodium and magnesium content of the tablet and powder may also be problematic in patients with renal failure or congestive heart failure. Other side effects include myelosuppression, hepatic failure, cardiomyopathy, and lactic acidosis. Drug interactions have also been found with other medications, and, therefore, drugs such as ketoconazole, dapsone, tetracycline, and quinalones should not be given within 2 hours of ddI dosing.

ZALCITABINE (DDC, DIDEOXYCYTIDINE, HIVID)

Indication

Zalcitabine as monotherapy or in combination with zidovudine has been approved for use in patients who have progressed or become intolerant to ZDV monotherapy. A study comparing ZDV monotherapy to ddC monotherapy and to combination ZDV plus ddC in ZDV-experienced patients with advanced HIV infection (ACTG 155) showed no clear advantage of the combination over either monotherapy, except in a subset of patients with CD4 counts between 150–300 cells/mm^3. A more recent randomized study comparison of ZDV to combination therapy (ACTG 175) did show a survival advantage of ZDV plus ddC over ZDV alone in antiviral-naive patients and also showed other clinical benefits of the combination in ZDV-experienced patients (14). A study in advanced patients with HIV infection (CPCRA 002) showed equivalence of ddI and ddC monotherapy in patients previously treated with ZDV (26).

Dosage

The standard dose of ddC is 0.75 mg as a single tablet, orally, three times a day. The drug does not need to be given on an empty stomach.

Side Effects

The major toxicity of ddC is peripheral neuropathy which is characterized by paresthesias or pain in the extremities, particularly the hands and feet. This side effect is dose related and seen in 12 to 15% of patients. The drug should be discontinued when symptoms develop. Resolution can be expected in a majority of patients. Other side effects include aphthous ulcers of the oral cavity, stomatitis, and pancreatitis in about 1% of patients. Patients with prior history of pancreatitis or those taking other medications that can induce pancreatitis should avoid zalcitabine.

STAVUDINE (D4T, ZERIT)

Indications

Stavudine is indicated in patients with advanced HIV disease who are intolerant of alternative antiretroviral therapy (e.g., ZDV, ddI, and ddC) or who have experienced significant clinical or immunologic deterioration while receiving these drugs (27–29). A randomized study of continued ZDV versus switching to d4T in patients who have previously received zidovudine showed superiority of d4T in terms of clinical disease progression and CD4 count. Studies evaluating ZDV plus d4T are currently in progress.

Dosage

The usual dose of d4T in patients who weigh ≥60 kg is 40 mg orally, two times a day; and for patients who weigh <60 kg, it is 30 mg orally, two times a day. Capsules need not be taken on an empty stomach

Side Effects

The major side effect of stavudine is peripheral neuropathy, which is dose related, and observed in 15 to 20% of patients at the 40-mg twice-a-day dosage. The use of d4T with other nucleoside analogs, which can induce peripheral neuropathy (e.g., ddI or ddC), is not recommended. Less common side effects include pancreatitis in 0.5 to 1.0%, drug-induced hepatitis, and rare cases of neutropenia and lactic acidosis.

LAMIVUDINE (3TC, EPIVIR)

Indications

Lamivudine has recently been approved for use in combination with zidovudine in patients who are tolerant of ZDV (30). The drug is not recommended for use as monotherapy due to the rapid rate of resistance development to monotherapy with 3TC (31). Additionally, patients who are intolerant or who have progressed on other nucleoside analogs and who can tolerate zidovudine may benefit by switching to the combination of ZDV plus 3TC (15). The effectiveness of other combinations of nucleoside analogs with 3TC is currently under investigation.

Dosage

The standard dosage of lamivudine is 150 mg orally, twice daily along with zidovudine at a dose of 200 mg orally, twice daily. The drugs may be administered together and need not be taken on an empty stomach.

Side Effects

The drug appears to be very well-tolerated with minimal side effects. Occasional headaches, fatigue, mild myelosuppression, and gastrointestinal intolerances have been seen.

COMBINATION THERAPIES

Several large randomized comparison studies of combination therapies have recently been reported and have demonstrated the superiority of combination nucleoside analogs over zidovudine monotherapy. ACTG 175 compared ZDV monotherapy to ddI monotherapy and to combinations of ZDV plus ddI and ZDV plus ddC in patients with CD4 counts between 200 and 500/mm^3. In patients who were antiretroviral naive, both combination regimens were superior to zidovudine monotherapy in delaying progression of AIDS, in maintaining CD4 counts, and in survival. Among ZDV-experienced patients, ddI monotherapy, as well as combinations of ZDV plus ddI or ZDV plus ddC, were superior to continued ZDV monotherapy in maintaining CD4 counts with the analysis suggesting greater survival and duration of disease-free progression with ZDV plus ddI or ddI monotherapy (14).

In the European/Australian Delta studies, ZDV was compared to ZDV plus ddI and ZDV plus ddC in either ZDV-naive (Delta 1) or ZDV-experienced individuals (Delta 2) with CD4 counts between 50 and 350 mm^3. Among ZDV-naive patients, combination therapy with either ZDV plus ddI or ZDV plus ddC was superior to ZDV alone in terms of disease progression and survival. Among ZDV-experienced patients (Delta 2), no advantage was seen to either combination regimen with regard to progression rate or survival when compared to ZDV monotherapy. The reason for the lack of any significant clinical advantage to the use of combination regimens in previously treated patients in the Delta 2 study, compared to the advantage of using ZDV plus ddI or switching to ddI monotherapy in this group of patients as seen in the ACTG 175 study, is unclear. A third study, the Nu Combo study of the Community Programs for Clinical Research on AIDS (CPCRA) comparing ZDV to ZDV plus ddI or ZDV plus ddC in advanced patients with CD4 counts $<200/mm^3$ will hopefully provide additional information regarding this subset of patients.

Zidovudine Plus Acyclovir

Several clinical studies of the combination of acyclovir with zidovudine have shown a survival advantage to the combination over zidovudine alone. This antiviral combination has been studied in six trials to date, four of which were prospective and controlled and two observational. Three studies showed a survival advantage and one a delay in CD4 decline, while two showed no such advantage (32–34). The proposed mechanism by which acyclovir may improve survival in AIDS is unclear. One possibility, however, is that acyclovir may have inhibitory effects on CMV or other DNA viruses that may delay occurrence of symptomatic illness and improve survival or that may decrease any stimulatory effects these infections may have on HIV replication. While controversial, the routine use of acyclovir in patients with early or late symptomatic disease is favored by many clinicians. Close observation for side effects of acyclovir in patients with more advanced HIV disease is indicated to avoid adverse drug-drug interactions and development of hepatic and other toxicities.

Use of Zidovudine to Reduce Perinatal Transmission of HIV

A randomized study to determine the efficacy of ZDV in reducing vertical transmission of HIV (ACTG 076) demonstrated the usefulness of zidovudine in the late stages of pregnancy and during delivery (35). The regimen utilized in ACTG 076 is as follows:

Before delivery: ZDV (100 mg, 5 times daily) initiated at 14 to 34 weeks of gestation and continued throughout pregnancy.

During labor: Intravenous ZDV (2 mg/kg for one hour, followed by 1 mg/kg until delivery).

For the infant: ZDV orally (ZDV syrup at 2 mg/kg, every 6 hours) for the first 6 weeks of life, beginning 8 to 12 hours after delivery.

Based on the findings of ACTG 076, the U.S. Public Health Service has issued the following recommendations (36,37):

1. For pregnant women with CD4 counts >200 and who have not received extensive prior antiretroviral therapy, the full ACTG 076 regimen should be utilized.
2. For pregnant women with CD4 counts <200 and with minimal history of prior antiretroviral therapy, ZDV should be recommended for the women's own health and the full ACTG 076 regimen should be utilized.
3. For pregnant women with a history of extensive prior zidovudine or other antiretroviral therapy, the ACTG 076 regimen should be carefully considered with the understanding that ZDV resistant strains of HIV may be present and alternative antiretroviral agents may be considered.
4. For pregnant women who are in labor and who have not received prior antiretroviral therapy, the intrapartum and neonatal components of ACTG 076 regimen should be offered.
5. For infants who are born to HIV-infected women who did not receive prenatal or intrapartum ZDV therapy, the postpartum component of ACTG 076 should be offered, if it can be initiated within 24 hours of delivery.

Monitoring for hematologic and hepatic side effects of ZDV should be done during treatment and women with CD4 counts <200 should also receive PCP prophylaxis.

ACKNOWLEDGMENT

Supported in part by grants from the State of California Universitywide Task Force on AIDS to the UCLA AIDS Clinical Research Center (CC-95-LA-194) and USPHS NIH grants AI-27660, CA-70080, and RR-00865.

REFERENCES

1. Rutherford GW, Lifson AR, Hessol NA, Darrow WW, et al. Course of HIV–1 infection in a cohort of homosexual and bisexual men—an 11-year follow-up study. Brit Med J 301:1183–1188, 1990.
2. Learmont J, Tindall B, Evans L, Cunningham A, et al. Long-term symptomless HIV-1 infection in recipients of blood products from a single donor. Lancet 340: 863–867, 1992.
3. Graham NMH, Zeger SL, Park LP, Vermund SH, et al. The effects on survival of early treatment of human immunodeficiency virus infection. N Engl J Med 326:1037–1042, 1992.
4. Carpenter CCJ, Mayer KH, Stein MD, Leibman BD, et al. Human immunodeficiency virus infection in North American women—experience with 200 cases and a review of the literature. Medicine 70:307–325, 1991.
5. Daley CL, Small PM, Schecter GF, Schoolnik GK, et al. An outbreak of tuberculosis with accelerated progression among persons infected with the human immunodefi-

ciency virus—analysis using restriction-fragment length polymorphisms. N Engl J Med 326:231–235, 1992.

6. Jones Be, Young SMM, Antoniskis D, Davidson PT, et al. Relationship of the manifestations of tuberculosis to CD4 cell counts in patients with human immunodeficiency virus infection. Am Rev Resp Disease 148:1292–1297, 1993.

7. Jordan TJ, Lewit EM, Montgomery RL, Reichman LB. Isoniazid as preventive therapy in HIV-infected intravenous drug abusers—a decision analysis. JAMA 265:2987–2991, 1991.

8. Fischl MA, Parker CB, Pettinelli C, Wulfsohn M, et al. A randomized controlled trial of a reduced daily dose of zidovudine in patients with the acquired immunodeficiency syndrome. N Engl J Med 323:1009–1014, 1990.

9. Bartlett JG. The Johns Hopkins Hospital Guide to Medical Cases of Patients with HIV Infection, 5th ed. Baltimore: Williams & Wilkins, 1995.

10. Nightingale SD, Byrd LT, Southern PM, Jockusch JD, et al. Incidence of *Mycobacterium avium intracellulare* complex bacteremia in human immunodeficiency virus positive patients. J Inf Dis 165:1082–1085, 1992.

11. Spector SA, et al. Second National Conference on Human Retroviruses, ASM. Washington DC, January 1995, abstract 2.

12. Aboulker JP, Babiker A, Darbyshire JR, et al. Concorde: MRC/ANRS randomized double-blind controlled trial of immediate and deferred zidovudine in symptom-free HIV infection. Lancet 343:871–880, 1994.

13. Sande MA, Carpenter CC, Cobbs CG, Holmes KK, Sanford JP. Antiretroviral therapy for adult HIV-infected patients. Recommendations from a state-of-the-art conference. NIAID State-of-the-art Panel on Anti-Retroviral Therapy for Adult HIV-infected Patients (see comments). JAMA 270:2583–2589, 1993.

14. Hammer S, et al. Interscience Conf Antib Antimicro Chemo, ASM. San Francisco, CA, October 1995, late breaker session.

15. Larder BA, Kemp SD, Harrigan PR. Potential mechanism for sustained antiretroviral efficacy of AZT–3TC combination therapy. Science 269:696–699, 1995.

16. Merigan TC, Skowron G, Bozzette S, et al. Circulating p24 antigen levels and responses to dideoxycytidine in human immunodeficiency virus (HIV) infections. A phase I and II study. Ann Intern Med 110:189–194, 1989.

17. Collier AC, Bozzette S, Coombs RW, et al. A pilot study of low-dose zidovudine in human immunodeficiency virus infection. N Engl J Med 323:1015–1021, 1990.

18. Fischl MA, Richman DD, Grieco MH, et al. The efficacy of azidothymidine (AZT) in the treatment of patients with AIDS and AIDS-related complex. A double-blind, placebo-controlled trial. N Engl J Med 317:185–191, 1987.

19. Fischl MA, Richman DD, Hansen N, et al. The safety and efficacy of zidovudine (AZT) in the treatment of subjects with mildly symptomatic human immunodeficiency virus type 1 (HIV) infection. A double-blind placebo-controlled trial. The AIDS Clinical Trials Group. Ann Int Med 112:727–737, 1990.

20. Volberding PA, Lagakos SW, Koch MA, et al. Zidovudine in asymptomatic human immunodeficiency virus infection. A controlled trial in persons with fewer than 500 CD4-positive cells per cubic millimeter. N Engl J Med 322:941–949, 1990.

21. Montaner JS, Schechter MT, Rachlis A, Gill J, Beaulieu R, Tsoukas C, et al. Didanosine compared with continued zidovudine therapy for HIV-infected patients with 200 to 500 CD4 cells/mm³. A double-blind, randomized, controlled trial. Canadian HIV Trials Network Protocol 002 Study Group. Ann Int Med 123:561–571, 1995.

22. Collier AC, Coombs RW, Fischl MA, Skolnik PR, Northfelt D, Boutin P, et al. Combination therapy with zidovudine and didanosine compared with zidovudine alone in HIV-1 infection. Ann Int Med 119:786–793, 1993.

23. Fischl MA, Stanley K, Collier AC, Arduino JM, Stein DS, Feinberg JE, et al. Combination and monotherapy with zidovudine and zalcitabine in patients with advanced HIV disease. The NIAID AIDS Clinical Trials Group. Ann Int Med 122:24–32, 1995.

24. Eron J, Katlama C, et al. Second National Conference on Human Retroviruses, ASM. Washington DC, January 1995, abstracts 31–36.

25. Kahn JO, Lagakos SW, Richman DD, et al. A controlled trial comparing continued zidovudine with didanosine in human immunodeficiency virus infection. N Engl J Med 327:581–587, 1992.

26. Abrams DI, Goldman AI, Launder C, Korvick JA, Neaton JD, Crane LR, et al. A comparative trial of didanosine or zalcitabine after treatment with zidovudine in patients with human immunodeficiency virus infection. The Terry Beirn Community Programs for Clinical Research on AIDS. N Eng J Med 330:657–662, 1994.

27. Peterson EA, Ramirez-Ronda CH, Hardy WD, Schwartz R, Sacks HS, Follansbee S, et al. Dose-related activity of stavudine in patients infected with human immunodeficiency virus. J Inf Dis 171(suppl 2):S131–S139, 1995.

28. Skowron G. Biologic effects and safety of stavudine: overview of phase I and II clinical trials. J Inf Dis 1995;171(suppl 2):S113–117, 1995.
29. Murray HW, Squires KE, Weiss W, Sledz S, Sacks HS, Hassett J, et al. Stavudine in patients with AIDS and AIDS-related complex: AIDS clinical trials group 089. J Inf Dis 171(suppl 2):S123–130, 1995.
30. van Leeuwen R, Katlama C, Kitchen V, Boucher CA, Tubiana R, McBride M, et al. Evaluation of safety and efficacy of 3TC (lamivudine) in patients with asymptomatic or mildly symptomatic human immunodeficiency virus infection: a phase I/II study. J Inf Dis 171(5):1166–1171, 1995.
31. Schuurman R, Nijhuis M, van Leeuwen R, Schipper P, de Jong D, Collis P, et al. Rapid changes in human immunodeficiency virus type 1 RNA load and appearance of drug-resistant virus populations in persons treated with lamivudine (3TC). J Inf Dis 171(6):1411–1419, 1995.
32. Cooper DA, Pehrson PO, Pedersen C, Moroni M, Oksenhendler E, Rozenbaum W, et al. The efficacy and safety of zidovudine alone or as cotherapy with acyclovir for the treatment of patients with AIDS and AIDS-related complex: a double-blind randomized trial. European-Australian collaborative group. AIDS 7(2):197–207, 1993.
33. Youle MS, Gazzard BG, Johnson MA, Cooper DA, Hoy JF, Busch H, et al. Effects of high-dose oral acyclovir on herpesvirus disease and survival in patients with advanced HIV disease: a double-blind, placebo-controlled study. European-Australian Acyclovir Study Group. AIDS 8(5):641–649, 1994.
34. Stein DS, Graham NM, Park LP, Hoover DR, Phair JP, Detels R, et al. The effect of the interaction of acyclovir with zidovudine on progression to AIDS and survival. Analysis of data in the Multicenter AIDS Cohort Study. Ann Int Med 121(2):100–108, 1994.
35. Connor EM, Sperling RS, Gelber R, Kiselev P, Scott G, O'Sullivan MJ, et al. Reduction of maternal-infant transmission of human immunodeficiency virus type 1 with zidovudine treatment. Pediatric AIDS Clinical Trials Group Protocol 076 Study Group. N Engl J Med 331(18):1173–1180, 1994.
36. Rogers MF, Mofenson LM, Moseley RR. Reducing the risk of perinatal HIV transmission through zidovudine therapy: treatment recommendations and implications. J Am Med Wom Assn 50(3–4):78–82, 93, 1995.
37. Centers for Disease Control and Prevention. Zidovudine for the prevention of HIV transmission from mother to infant. MMWR 43:285–287, 1994.

Protease Inhibitors—A New Approach to HIV Therapy

Protease inhibitors are a new class of potent anti-HIV drugs which work in a different part of the virus cycle than do nucleoside analogs. Nucleoside analogs (e.g. zidovudine, lamivudine, didanosine, zalcitabine, stavudine) inhibit the enzyme reverse transcriptase which is necessary to produce new virus. Protease inhibitors bind to the viral enzyme protease which is essential for the maturation of viral particles. HIV encodes protease to cleave large viral proteins into its various smaller components for assembly into a mature and infectious viral particle late in the virus life cycle. In the presence of protease inhibitors, the accumulation of large proteins results in virus particles that are reduced in their infectious capacity.

Studies of protease inhibitors indicate a wide variance in potency and duration of antiviral activity. Protease inhibitors currently licensed by the Food and Drug Administration (FDA) are saquinavir, ritonavir, and indinavir (Table 4.13). In general, ritonavir and indinavir appear to be the more potent protease inhibitors, largely because of the poor absorption of the current formulation of saquinavir. There is however, a new formulation with improved absorption in current trials. Ritonavir is the only agent reported so far to reduce the complications of AIDS and death. The potency of the protease inhibitors alone, and in combination

Table 4.13.

FDA Licensed Protease Inhibitors

	Saquinavir	Ritonavir	Indinavir
Trade Name	Invirase	Norvir	Crixivan
Indications: FDA Labeling	Advanced HIV in combination with other nucleoside analogs	HIV when therapy is warranted in combination or as monotherapy	HIV when antiretroviral therapy is indicated
Usual Dose	600 mg t.i.d. with food	600 mg b.i.d. with food	800 mg t.i.d. on an empty stomach
Minimum Effective Dose	600 mg t.i.d.	600 mg b.i.d.	800 mg t.i.d.
Serum half-life	12 hours	3–5 hours	1.8 hours
Elimination	1% urine 88% feces	11% urine 86% feces	<20% urine 80% feces
Major Toxicities	Nausea, diarrhea, fever, headache, abdominal pain, neutropenia, increase in AGT/AST and phosphorus, decrease in potassium and calcium	Increase in triglycerides, nausea, diarrhea, anorexia, abdominal pain, taste perversion, circumoral paresthesia, peripheral paresthesia, asthenia, increase in uric acid, AST/ALT, and GGT	Increase in indirect bilirubin, increase in ALT/AST, nephrolithiasis, nausea, headaches, abdominal pain diarrhea, insomnia, taste changes, back pain, flank pain

with nuceloside analogues suggests a shift in the goal of antiretroviral therapy.

Previously, CD4 counts were used to direct treatment; however, a longer period was necessary to determine if a person responded to treatment. Monitoring viral load appears to be a more accurate way to predict the course of HIV infection than CD4 cells. Monitoring viral load will be an earlier indicator of drug failure; within two weeks of initiating an effective therapy, viral load will decline. Most drugs have their maximal effect at 4 weeks.

Saquinavir

As a single agent at 1800 mg/day, Saquinavir has negligible effects (0.4 log reduction) on plasma HIV RNA levels in zidovudine-experienced patients; this is due to the poor oral absorption (approximately 4% of the drug). A new formulation of saquinavir with improved absorption is currently in trials. However, the combination of saquinavir/zalcitabine and saquinavir/zidovudine/zalcitabine (ACTG 229) have been associated with decreases in viral load in PBMC cultures. At doses of 3600 and 7200 mg/day (2 and 4 times the recommended dose), plasma HIV RNA is reduced to 0.9 to 1.2 log and is associated with increases of 80 to 120 CD4+ cells/μL. The most common reported side effects with use of saquinavir have been nausea, diarrhea, and abdominal bloating.

Ritonavir

As a single agent in zidovudine-experienced patients, ritonavir at 1200 mg/day is associated with sustained decreases in plasma HIV RNA levels of more than 2 logs and increases in excess of 80 CD4+ cells/μL for more than 24 weeks. Ritonavir is the only agent reported so far to reduce the complications of AIDS-related infections and death. In a placebo-controlled trial in late-stage patients (median CD4+ = 18 cells/μL), ritonavir at 600 mg bid decreased mortality and AIDS-related complications by 50%. Peak reduction in plasma HIV RNA level was 1.3 log at 2 weeks and was associated with a peak increase in CD4+ cell count of 47 plus/minus 5 μL at 16 weeks. In some instances these increases were accompanied by improved immunologic function, skin test reactivity, and clearance of opportunistic infections and malignancies. Most common side effects with use of ritonavir are hypertriglyceridemia, nausea, diarrhea, and circumoral paresthesia.

Indinavir

As a single agent at 800 mg tid in zidovudine-naive patients, indinavir is associated with decreases of more than 2 logs in plasma HIV RNA levels lasting more than 24 weeks. Increase in bilirubin, increase in incidence of kidney stones, and abdominal pain have been reported to be common side effects with use of indinavir.

Combination of Indinavir/Zidovudine/Lamivudine

A combination of indinavir, zidovudine, and lamivudine in zidovudine-experienced patients resulted in a decline of 2.0 logs in plasma HIV RNA levels and a median increase of 146 CD4+ cells/µL at 24 weeks. This combination resulted in >80% of patients with undetectable virus RNA by 12 weeks.

Resistance to Protease Inhibitors

Viral resistance has been demonstrated for all protease inhibitors. There does not appear to be any single mutation that confers high-level resistance. Rather, the accumulation of multiple mutations around the active site appears to impart resistance. Resistance to indinavir appears to impart resistance to all members of the protease inhibitor family; resistance to saquinavir and ritonavir does not appear to impart broad class resistance. Despite cross resistance between inhibitors, there is a scientific rationale for the use of these agents in combination. Ritonavir inhibits cytochrome p450 function, which is the principal metabolic pathway for other protease inhibitors. In animal models, the simultaneous administration of ritonavir with other protease inhibitors results in a dramatic prolongation of the plasma levels of other protease inhibitors, including saquinavir and indinavir.

Shift in the Goal of Antiretroviral Therapy

The tremendous potency of the protease inhibitors suggests a shift in the goal of antiretroviral therapy. The new goal is to lower the virus load as much as possible, preferably to undetectable levels to forestall resistance. Physicians might begin treatment with multiple drugs much earlier in the course of the disease, especially if tests indicate patients have high levels of virus in their bodies. The ascent of combination therapy also raises a variety of questions, such as which combinations of drugs are most effective for which patients or when combination therapy should be started. These issues must be addressed in clinical trials that compare various drug combinations for safety and efficacy.

SUGGESTED READING

Cameron B, Heath-Chiozzi M, Kravcik S, et al. Prolongation of life and prevention of AIDS in advanced HIV immunodeficiency with ritonavir (abstract). Program and Abstracts of the Third Conference on Retroviruses and Opportunistic Infections, Washington, DC. Alexandria, VA: Infectious Disease Society of America for the Foundation for Retrovirology and Human Health, 1996. Abstract LB6a, p. 162.

Collier AC, Coombs RW, Schoenfeld DA, Bassett R, et al: Extended treatment with saquinavir (SAQ), zidovudine (ZDV) and zalcitabine (ddC) vs. SAQ and ZDV vs ddC and ZDV (abstract). Program and Abstracts for the 35th Interscience Conference on Antimicrobial Agents and Chemotherapy, San Francisco. Washington DC: American Society for Microbiology, 1995, Abstract I173.

Danner SA, Carr A, Leonard JM, et al. A short-term study of the safety, pharmacokinetics, and efficacy of ritonavir, and inhibitor of HIV-1 protease. N Engl J Med. 1995; 333:1528–1533.

Emini E. HIV-1 protease inhibitors (abstract). Program and Abstracts of the Third Conference on Retroviruses and Opportunistic Infections, Washington, DC. Alexandria, VA: Infectious Disease Society of America for the Foundation for Retrovirology and Human Health, 1996. Abstract L1, p. 166.

Gulick R, Mellors J, Havlir D, et al. Potent and sustained antiretroviral activity of indinavir (IDV) in combination with zidovudine (ZDV) and lamivudine (3TC) (abstract). Program and Abstracts of the Third Conference on Retroviruses and Opportunistic Infections, Washington, DC. Alexandria, VA: Infectious Disease Society of America for the Foundation for Retrovirology and Human Health, 1996. Abstract LB7, p. 162.

Heath-Chiozzi M. Leonard J, Henry D, et al. Anti-HIV activity and lymphocyte surrogate marker response dynamics to ritonavir therapy in advanced HIV immunodeficiency (abstract). Program and Abstracts of the Third Conference on Retroviruses and Opportunistic Infections, Washington, DC. Alexandria, VA: Infectious Disease Society of America for the Foundation for Retrovirology and Human Health, 1996. Abstract LB6b, p. 162.

Markowitz M, Saag M, Powderly WG, et al. A preliminary study of ritonavir, an inhibitor of HIV-1 protease, to treat HIV-1 infection. N Engl J Med. 1995;333:1534–1539.

Hematologic Aspects

Hematologic abnormalities are widely recognized and have significant clinical importance in the management of patients with human immunodeficiency virus (HIV) infection. Impaired hematopoiesis, immune mediated cytopenias, and altered coagulation profiles have been described in HIV-infected individuals. These abnormalities may occur as the result of HIV infection itself, as a sequela of HIV-related opportunistic infections or malignancies, or as a consequence of therapies used to treat HIV infection and associated conditions. This section will review the clinical manifestations, etiology, diagnosis, and treatment of common hematologic problems encountered in patients with HIV infection.

Anemia

Anemia is a common finding in patients with HIV infection. In one study of patients receiving no myelosuppressive medications, 8% of asymptomatic HIV-seropositive patients, 20% of patients with acquired immunodeficiency syndrome (AIDS)-related conditions (ARC), and 71% of patients with AIDS were anemic. Anemia tends to worsen throughout the course of HIV infection, and patients with lower CD4 counts are more frequently anemic than patients with higher CD4 counts. The anemia associated with HIV infection is usually normochromic and normocytic, although both anisocytosis and poikilocytosis occur. Rouleaux formation may be seen, usually resulting from the polyclonal hypergammaglobulinemia that is present in HIV-infected individuals. Iron stores and ferritin are frequently increased as they are acute phase reactants that are often increased in chronic disease states. Although hemolytic anemia is unusual in HIV-infected individuals, there is an increased incidence of positive direct antiglobulin tests. These antibodies may react with specific red cell antigens or may be anti-phospholipid antibodies.

There are a number of possible etiologies of anemia in patients with HIV infection (Table 4.14). HIV infection alone may produce anemia in some patients. Studies of immunoreactive serum erythropoietin levels in HIV-infected patients have shown that levels of this hormone is often

Table 4.14.
Causes of Cytopenia in Patients with HIV Infection

Infections
  HIV
  B19 *Parvovirus*
  Mycobacterium avium complex (MAC)
  Mycobacterium tuberculosis (MTB)
  Cytomegalovirus
  Histoplasma capsulatum
  Coccidioides immitis
  Cryptococcus neoformans
  Pneumocystis carinii
Medications
  Zidovudine
  Ganciclovir
  Dapsone
  Trimethoprim-sulfamethoxazole
  Sulfadiazine
  Pyrimethamine
  Amphotericin B
  5-Flucytosine
  Antineoplastics
Tumors
  Non-Hodgkin's lymphoma

low for a given degree of anemia suggesting that insufficient production of erythropoietin may be one cause of anemia in this setting. Other studies have suggested that soluble factors in the serum of HIV-infected patients may inhibit hematopoiesis or that direct infection of bone marrow progenitor cells may also play a role in inducing anemia or other hematologic abnormalities in AIDS.

Medications are another common cause of anemia in HIV-infected patients. In the original phase II clinical trial demonstrating the efficacy of zidovudine in patients with AIDS, 34% of zidovudine-treated subjects developed significant anemia after 6 weeks of therapy. Thirty-one percent of zidovudine-treated subjects also required blood transfusions while receiving the drug. Subsequent studies have demonstrated that anemia is less common with a reduced dosage of zidovudine and occurs less frequently in patients with earlier stage disease.

Effective treatment for zidovudine-induced anemia is available in the form of recombinant human erythropoietin. Several randomized double-blind placebo controlled studies have demonstrated that recombinant human erythropoietin at a dose of 100 units/kg by intravenous bolus infusion or subcutaneous injections can reduce the transfusion requirements whose endogenous serum level of erythropoietin was less than 500 IU/L.

Other antimicrobial and antineoplastic agents used for the treatment or prophylaxis of HIV-related conditions may also cause anemia. Dapsone, which is used for the treatment or prevention of *Pneumocystis carinii* pneumonia, may cause a methemoglobinemia as well as general myelosuppression. Chemotherapy for AIDS-related non-Hodgkin's lymphoma or Kaposi's sarcoma may also cause significant myelosuppression.

Infections with *Mycobacterium avium* complex (MAC) is another common cause of anemia in AIDS patients. This infection, which is diagnosed in up to 18% of patients with AIDS, can cause widely disseminated bacteremia often involving the bone marrow. In this situation, anemia tends to occur out of proportion to other cytopenias. One study examining the relationship between MAC bacteremia and transfusion requirements showed that patients with a positive blood culture for MAC had a relative risk of 5.23 (p<0.001) of receiving a blood cell transfusion compared to patients with negative blood cultures.

Several reports have also highlighted the role of B19 parvovirus infection and the development of anemia in AIDS patients. B19 parvovirus has been recognized as a cause of severe chronic anemia in immunocompromise patients including the induction of pure red cell aplasia in some individuals. Parvovirus DNA can be detected in the serum and/or bone marrow of patients with severe anemia. Parvovirus infection has also been associated with varying degrees of pancytopenia in AIDS patients as well. The anemia of parvovirus infection can be alleviated with infusions of immunoglobulin.

Other conditions associated with HIV can cause anemia as a result of direct involvement of the bone marrow (Table 4.14). Tuberculosis, histoplasmosis, cryptococcosis, pneumocystosis, and non-Hodgkin's lymphoma can all infiltrate the bone marrow while causing anemia or pancytopenia.

Finally, gastrointestinal bleeding should also be considered in the evaluation of any HIV-infected patient with anemia. HIV-related infections such as cytomegalovirus colitis and malignancies such as Kaposi's sarcoma and non-Hodgkin's lymphoma can produce clinically-significant bleeding.

Granulocytopenia and Granulocyte Functional Defects

Granulocytopenia is also commonly encountered in patients with HIV infection. Low granulocyte counts typically reflect toxicities of therapies for HIV infection or associated conditions. In patients with more advanced HIV disease and profound immunodeficiency, low granulocyte counts have also been seen and attributed to HIV infection itself.

The pathogenesis of granulocytopenia in patients with HIV infection is multifactorial. An autoimmune mechanism involving antigranulocyte antibodies and impaired granulopoiesis has been postulated to account for granulocytopenia in some patients, but the clinical importance of these observations has not been clearly established. Infections, malignancies, and any infiltrative process involving the bone marrow may produce granulocytopenia. Drug toxicity, however, remains the primary cause of granulocytopenia in patients with HIV infection.

Zidovudine is probably one of the more common causes of low granulocyte counts in patients with HIV. Despite the relatively high frequency of zidovudine-induced granulocytopenia, there has been a relatively low observed risk of bacterial infection perhaps due to the relative brief duration of granulocytopenia prior to dose reduction or drug discontinuation. Ganciclovir therapy for symptomatic cytomegalovirus infection is another common cause of granulocytopenia in patients with AIDS. Other medications that are frequently associated with granulocytopenia include trimethoprim-sulfamethoxazole, pentamidine, and antineoplastic chemotherapy. The availability of recombinant granulocyte colony-stimulating factor (G-CSF)and recombinant granulocyte macrophage colony stimulating factor (GM-CSF) has allowed continued administration of high dose antibiotics and chemotherapy for patients with complications of AIDS, although their effect in improving clinical outcome and survival is still debatable.

Qualitative functional defects of granulocytes in patients with HIV infection have been noted in several in vitro studies. Defective chemotaxis, deficient degranulation responses, ineffective phagocytosis, and intracellular killing of pathogens have all been reported. The clinical importance of these observations has not been clearly established. These defects can be corrected transiently in vivo with the administration of recombinant myeloid hematopoietic growth factors.

Thrombocytopenia

Thrombocytopenia is frequently associated with HIV infection. In the Multicenter AIDS Cohort Study, among 1500 HIV seropositive individuals without AIDS, 6.7% had platelet counts below 15,000 cells/mm^3 on at least one visit.

There are a number of possible etiologies of thrombocytopenia in patients with HIV infection, including immune-mediated destruction, thrombotic thrombocytopenic purpura, impaired hematopoiesis, and toxic effects of medications. In other instances, thrombocytopenia is a isolated hematologic abnormality associated with normal or increased numbers of megakaryocytes in the bone marrow, and, therefore, presents as the clinical syndrome of immune thrombocytopenic purpura (ITP).

IMMUNE THROMBOCYTOPENIC PURPURA (ITP)

The first cases of HIV-associated ITP in homosexual men were reported in 1982. Subsequently, ITP was reported in narcotics addicts, hemophiliacs, transfusion recipients, and children with HIV infection. ITP is now recognized as a condition that is clearly associated with HIV infection.

HIV-related ITP is most often an early manifestation of HIV infection occurring before the development of other AIDS-defining conditions. CD4 counts in reported series of patients with HIV-ITP have averaged between 300–600 cells/mm^3. HIV-related ITP, therefore, has been included within group II in the Center for Disease Control's classification of HIV-related illnesses.

Several hypotheses have been advanced to explain the mechanism of HIV-related ITP. One theory holds that circulating immune complexes are nonspecifically deposited on platelet membranes, which result in reticuloendothelial clearance. Another hypothesis states that a specific IgG antiplatelet antibody binds to a 25-kilodalton antigen on the platelet membrane, resulting in platelet destruction. In addition to increased platelet destruction, thrombocytopenia in HIV-infected patients may be worsened by impaired ability of the host to produce platelets in sufficient numbers.

Ultrastructural analysis of bone marrow megakaryocytes from patients with HIV-related ITP have demonstrated structural abnormalities. HIV RNA has also been shown to be expressed in these megakaryocytes by in situ hybridization. It is possible that direct infection of megakaryocytes by HIV may also impair platelet production and contribute to thrombocytopenia.

A diagnosis of ITP requires exclusion of other causes of low platelet production or increased peripheral destruction of platelets. Bone marrow biopsy should be performed to exclude marrow infiltrator processes or other reasons for decreased platelet production. Splenic sequestration resulting from liver disease, thrombotic thrombocytopenic purpura, and disseminated intravascular coagulation should also be excluded. The finding of platelet-associated immunoglobulin or immune complexes strengthens the diagnosis of HIV-related ITP, but it is neither sufficient nor necessary for the diagnosis.

Treatment of HIV-related ITP parallels the treatment used for ITP in the non-HIV setting. Treatment with corticosteroids, splenectomy, cytotoxic agents, IV immune globulin infusions, anti-RhD globulin, danazol, plasmapheresis over protein-A column, and alpha interferon have all been used with varying degrees of success.

A randomized, placebo-controlled, double-blind study of zidovudine in patients with HIV-related ITP showed a marked increase in platelet count over an 6-week period with zidovudine therapy, but no change with placebo treatment. The dose of zidovudine studied was 2 grams/day for 2 weeks followed by 1 gram/day for 6 weeks. Similar results have been seen with didanosine in uncontrolled studies. Treatment of HIV-related ITP should probably be reserved for patients with clinically significant symptoms such as recurrent epistaxis, gingival or subconjunctival bleeding, or gastrointestinal hemorrhage. Therapy is also recommended for hemophiliacs with HIV-related ITP because of the substantial morbidity and mortality associated with bleeding in this group. All patients should receive standard antiretroviral therapy and, if immediate reversal of thrombocytopenia is indicated, intravenous immunoglobulin with corticosteroid therapy is effective over the short term. Other treatments for ITP should be reserved for the refractory, symptomatic patient.

Thrombotic Thrombocytopenic Purpura

Thrombotic thrombocytopenic purpura (TTP) is a clinical syndrome characterized by fever, neurologic dysfunction, renal dysfunction, microangiopathic hemolytic anemia, and thrombocytopenia. The diagnosis is supported by the findings of hyaline microvascular thrombi in tissue biopsy specimens. An abnormal interaction between platelets and endothelium is thought to be responsible for the clinical and pathologic findings of TTP. Plasma exchange is generally accepted as standard therapy for TTP, although plasma infusions, plasmapheresis, antiplatelet drug therapy, corticosteroids, and splenectomy have all been used with varying degrees of success.

Whether the incidence of TTP is increased in HIV infection remains to be proven; however, the diagnosis must be considered in seropositive or at-risk patients presenting with combinations of symptoms suggestive of this diagnosis. As most HIV-infected patients with TTP appear to have relatively well-preserved immune function, a good response to plasma infusion or exchange transfusion can be expected in most patients. Prompt diagnosis and appropriate therapy are essential.

Hemostatic Abnormalities

Prolonged activated partial thromboplastin times (aPTT) are occasionally detected in patients with HIV infection. Antiphospholipid antibodies have generally been detected in these patients. Antiphospholipid antibodies, including lupus anticoagulants and anticardiolipin antibodies, have been detected in a variety of disorders. These IgG or IgM antibodies are directed against phospholipid moieties and, therefore, interfere in vitro with the action of thromboplastin used in the aPTT tests. Antiphospholipid antibodies are rarely associated with clinical bleeding. These antibodies have been detected in 20 to 60% of HIV-infected patients. No associated thrombotic or hemorrhagic tendencies have been noted and, thus, no treatment is required.

Bone Marrow Changes

Bone marrow biopsies of patients with HIV infection are generally normocellular to moderately hypercellular with normal proportions of myeloid and erythroid progenitors. In advanced stages of HIV disease, however, the marrow can be hypocellular with fatty atrophy. Megakaryocytes are usually normal in number except in ITP where their number is increased. Mild plasmacytosis is commonly seen with the plasma cells generally arranged around small blood vessels. The plasmacytosis probably reflects nonspecific B cell activation or antigenic stimulation by various infectious agents. Mild reticulin fibrosis is often seen and may be present in as many as 50 to 75% of biopsy specimens.

In many HIV-infected patients, subtle myelodysplastic changes are found particularly in developing erythroid, myeloid and megakaryocytic cells. These features include megaloblastic maturation in the myeloid and erythroid series plus occasional binucleation or bizarre-shaped nucleii in red cell precursors. Less commonly, hypogranulation and pseudo Pelger-Huet changes in the myeloid series and small or hypolobulated megarkaryocytes are present.

Lymphoid infiltrates consisting of generally small mature lymphocytes can be seen, as well as scattered phagocytic histiocytes that are typically seen in the large stages of AIDS. Hemophagocytosis is not usually associated with constitutional symptoms, liver dysfunction, coagulation abnormalities, hepatosplenomegaly, or lymphadenopathy commonly encountered in other virus-associated hemophagocytic syndromes.

Granulomas are also occasionally seen and consist of small poorly-formed clusters of histiocytes and lymphocytes. The presence of granuloma is typically associated with mycobacterial or fungal infections in over two-thirds of patients. Special stains for mycobacterium and yeast should be performed on these patients. Mycobacterial and fungal cultures should also be obtained at the time of bone marrow biopsy if clinical symptoms warrant them.

Summary

Hematologic abnormalities are among the most frequent sequelae of HIV infection. A number of pathogenic mechanisms have been identified that account for these findings. Toxicities of medications as well as a variety of infectious diseases, neoplasms, and autoimmune phenomena may be responsible for these abnormalities. Hematopoietic growth factors can correct some of the abnormalities seen in these patients and would permit the continued use of essential therapies whose applications would be otherwise limited due to their toxicities.

ACKNOWLEDGMENT

Supported in part by grants from the State of California, Universitywide Task Force on AIDS to the UCLA AIDS Clinical Research Center (CC95-LA-194) and USPHS-NIH grants AI-27660, CA-70080, and RR00865.

SUGGESTED READING

ANEMIA

Fischl M, Galpin JE, Levine JD, et al. Recombinant human erythropoietin for patients with AIDS treated with zidovudine. Ann Intern Med 322:1488, 1990.

Frickhofen N, Abkowitz JL, Safford M, et al. Persistent B19 parvovirus infection in patients infected with human immunodeficiency virus type 1: a treatable cause of anemia in AIDS. Ann Intern Med 113:926, 1990.

Jacobson MA, Peiperl L, Volberding PA, et al. Red blood cell transfusion therapy for anemia in patients with AIDS and ARC: incidence, associated factors, and outcome. Transfusion 30:133, 1990.

Perkocha LA, Rodgers GM. Hematologic aspects of human immunodeficiency virus infection: laboratory and clinical considerations. Am J Hematol 29:94, 1988.

Richman DD, Fischl MA, Grieco MH, et al. The toxicity of azidothymidine (AZT) in the treatment of patients with AIDS and AIDS-related complex. N Engl J Med 317:192, 1987.

Spivak JL, Barnes DC, Fuchs E, Quinn TC. Serum immunoreactive erythropoietin in HIV-infected patients. JAMA 261:3104, 1989.

Toy PTCY, Reid ME, Burns M. Positive direct antiglobulin test associated with hyperglobulinemia in acquired immunodeficiency syndrome. Am J Hematol 19:145, 1985.

Walker RE, Parker RI, Kovacs JA, et al. Anemia and erythropoiesis in patients with the acquired immunodeficiency syndrome and Kaposi sarcoma treated with zidovudine. Ann Intern Med 108:372, 1988.

Zon L, Groopman J. Hematologic manifestations of the human immunodeficiency virus. Semin Hematol 25:208, 1988.

GRANULOCYTOPENIA

Baldwin CG, Gasson JC, Quan SG, et al. GM-CSF enhances neutrophil function in AIDS patients. Proc Natl Acad Sci USA 85:2763, 1988.

Ellis M, Gupta S, Galant S, et al. Impaired neutrophil function in patients with AIDS or AIDS-related complex: a comprehensive evaluation. J Infect Dis 158:1268, 1988.

Miles SA, Mitsuyasu RT, Moreno J, Baldwin G, Alton NK, Souza L, Glaspy JA. Combined therapy with recombinant granulocyte colony-stimulating factor and erythropoietin decreases hematologic toxicity from zidovudine. Blood 77:2109–2117, 1991.

Murphy MF, Metcalfe P, Waters, AH, et al. Incidence and mechanism of neutropenia and thrombocytopenia in patients with human immunodeficiency virus infection. Br J Haematol 66:337–40, 1987.

Murphy P, Lane HC, Fauci AS, et al. Impairment of neutrophil bactericidal capacity in patients with AIDS. J Infect Dis 158:627, 1988.

Shaunak S, Bartlett JA. Zidovudine-induced neutropenia: are we too cautious? Lancet 1:91, 1989.

Valone FH, Payan DG, Abrams DI, Goetzl EJ. Defective polymorphonuclear leukocyte chemotaxis in homosexual men with persistent lymph node syndrome. J Infect Dis 150:267, 184.

THROMBOCYTOPENIA

Caron D, Jacobson D, Walsh C. Hematologic findings in HIV infection. In: Wormser GP, ed. AIDS and Other Manifestations of HIV Infection, 2nd ed. New York: Raven Press, 1992:455–461.

Karpatkin S, Nardi M. On the mechanism of thrombocytopenia in hemophiliacs multiply transfused with AHF concentrates. J Lab Clin Med 111:441–448, 1988.

Leaf AN, Laubenstein LJ, Raphael B, Hochster H, Baez L, Karpatkin S. Thrombotic thrombocytopenic purpura associated with human immunodeficiency virus type 1 (HIV-1) infection. Ann Intern Med 109:194–197, 1988.

Swiss Group for Clinical Studies in AIDS. Zidovudine for the treatment of thrombocytopenia associated with HIV. Ann Intern Med 109:718–721, 1988.

Walsh C, Krigel R, Lennette E, et al. Thrombocytopenia in homosexual patients. Ann Intern Med 103:542–545, 1985.

Walsh C, Nardi M, Karpatkin S. On the mechanism of thrombocytopenic purpura is sexually active homosexual men. N Engl J Med 311:635–639, 1984.

Zucker-Franklin D, Cao Y. Megakaryocytes of HIV infected individuals express viral RNA. Proc Natl Acad Sci USA 86:5595, 1989.

HEMOSTATIC ABNORMALITIES

Bloom EJ, Abrams DI, Rodgers G. Lupus anticoagulant in the acquired immunodeficiency syndrome. JAMA 256:491–493, 1986.

Cohen AJ, Philips TM, Kessler CM. Circulating coagulation inhibitors in the acquired immunodeficiency syndrome. Ann Intern Med 104:175–180, 1986.

Cohen H, Mackie IJ, Anagnostopoulos N, et al. Lupus anticoagulant, anticardiolipin antibodies, and human immunodeficiency virus in haemophilia. J Clin Pathol 42:629, 1989.

Gold JE, Haubenstock A, Zalusky R. Lupus anticoagulant and AIDS [Letter]. N Engl J Med 314:1252–1253, 1986.

Kaye BR. Rheumatologic manifestations of infection with human immunodeficiency virus (HIV). Ann Intern Med 111:158–167, 1989.

Love PE, Santoro SA. Antiphospholipid antibodies: anticardiolipin and the lupus anticoagulant in systemic lupus erythematosus (SLE) and in non-SLE disorders. Ann Intern Med 112:682, 1990.

Stimmler MM, Quismorio FP, McGehee WG, et al. Anticardiolipin antibodies in the acquired immunodeficiency syndrome. Arch Intern Med 149:1833, 1989.

Neoplastic Aspects

A tumor develops in approximately 40% of all patients with AIDS during the course of their illness. These cancers are not only an immediate cause of death in some patients, but are also a source of considerable morbidity in many others. As treatment for human immunodeficiency virus (HIV) and related opportunistic infections improve, longer survival of HIV-infected patients is anticipated, and increasing numbers of patients with neoplasia are expected.

Aids-related Kaposi's Sarcoma

EPIDEMIOLOGY

Kaposi's sarcoma (KS) is the most common tumor associated with acquired immunodeficiency syndrome (AIDS). It is seen in approximately 17% of gay men with AIDS and 1 to 5% of other persons with HIV infection in the United States. Kaposi's sarcoma, as a proportion to all AIDS-defining diagnoses, is less frequent among IV drug users and higher in parts in Africa where Kaposi's sarcoma is endemic in the non-HIV infected population. Among U.S. AIDS cases, the proportion of patients with Kaposi's sarcoma has declined from the beginning of the AIDS epidemic, possibly as a result of changes in high-risk sexual behavior among gay men and as a result of more widespread use of antiretroviral drugs.

ETIOLOGY AND RISK FACTORS

The finding that Kaposi's sarcoma has declined among patients with AIDS in parallel with the declining incidence of sexually transmitted diseases among gay men supports the theory that a sexually transmitted agent may be involved in the development of AIDS-related Kaposi's sarcoma (AIDS-KS). Recently, sequences of a gamma human herpes virus, termed the KS-associated herpes virus (KSHV) or the human herpes virus #8 (HHV8), have been found in high frequency in Kaposi's sarcoma tissue from patients with AIDS. These viral sequences that are homologous to the herpes saimari virus have been identified in greater than 90% of KS biopsies from HIV-infected and uninfected individuals, but not in uninvolved tissues from the same patient or normal controls. The exact role of KSHV in KS pathogenesis has not been fully established and it is unclear whether this virus is directly transforming or may have secondary effects in the development of this tumor.

Other environmental and host factors including HIV-induced cytokines (Table 4.15), AIDS-associated infections, the host hormonal milieu, and antiretroviral therapy may induce or suppress the development of this tumor and alter its growth. The high male-to-female ratio among

Table 4.15.

Cytokines and Other Factors That Can Increase Growth of Kaposi's Sarcoma

Exogenous	Endogenous
TNF-α	IL-6
IL-6	IL-1β
Oncostatin M	bFGF
TGF-α	TGF-β
Tat protein	PDGF
Androgens	GM-CSF
Corticosteroids	

TNF-α = tumor necrosis factor-α; IL-6 = interleukin-6; TGF-α = transforming growth factor-α; Tat = transactivating protein; IL-1 = interleukin-1; bFGF = basic fibroblast growth factor; TGF-β = transforming growth factor-β; PDGF = platelet-derived growth factor; GM-CSF = granulocyte-macrophage colony-stimulating factor.

U.S. AIDS patients with Kaposi's sarcoma and the recent finding that pregnant female nude mice cannot sustain the growth of Kaposi's sarcoma tumors in vivo suggest the possibility that female sex hormones may confer some protection from this tumor or, conversely, that male sex hormones may help induce the development of KS.

CLINICAL PRESENTATION OF KAPOSI'S SARCOMA

The clinical manifestations of Kaposi's sarcoma in patients with AIDS are variable and range from small innocuous-looking cutaneous lesions to symptom-producing visceral or oral lesions. Lesions typically begin as macular and papular lesions that progress to placque-like or nodular tumors. Lesions vary in size and shape but are generally nonpuritic and painless. The color of lesions range from brown to pink to deep purple (Figure 4.2) and they can be found on any body surface but seem to have a predilection for the upper body and head and neck areas. Kaposi's sarcoma may be the presenting sign of HIV disease or a secondary manifestation of AIDS. Lesions that appear after the occurrence of opportunistic infection often have a more aggressive clinical course.

Kaposi's sarcoma lesions may be cosmetically disfiguring and may also carry significant social stigmatization that often exceed any actual physical impairment. Dermal and lymphatic infiltration with tumor can cause edema of the extremity, genitals, and periorbital areas and may be complicated by local skin breakdown and bacterial cellulitis. Lesions on the feet can cause pain and difficulty walking. Oral lesions are often asymptomatic but can produce pain, difficulty swallowing, gingival bleeding, and dental displacement. Gastrointestinal involvement with Kaposi's sarcoma is seen in up to 50% of patients and may occasionally cause obstruction, bleeding, or enteropathy. Pulmonary KS, usually presenting as dyspnea without fever, may be severely debilitating and often fatal if not treated. Bone marrow and central nervous system involvement with KS are exceedingly rare.

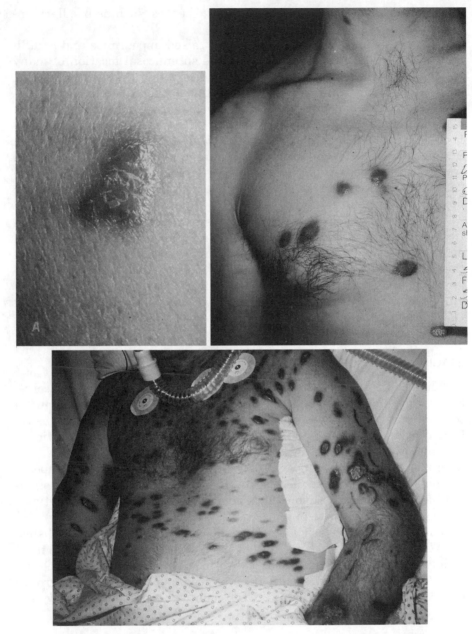

Figure 4.2   Kaposi's sarcoma lesions.

SCREENING AND DIAGNOSIS

The diagnosis of Kaposi's sarcoma is made by biopsy and histologic examination of a skin lesion, and excised lymph node or biopsy of other tissue, or by presumptive diagnosis based on the bronchoscopic or endoscopic appearance of visceral lesions. Although most Kaposi's sarcoma lesions are readily recognized, early lesions may be difficult to diagnose and are occasionally confused with other diseases, such as bacillary angiomatosis.

Gastrointestinal KS has a typical red, raised appearance and is difficult to diagnose by biopsy because of the submucosal location of many lesions. Pulmonary KS typically has radiographic findings of diffuse, reticular-nodular infiltrates and sometimes pleural effusion. Bronchoscopy may reveal extensive endobronchial involvement with tumor. The definitive diagnosis requires transbronchial or open lung biopsy, although transbronchial biopsies often yield negative results. Thalium and, more recently, technetium-99m scanning may help differentiate KS from other pulmonary diseases. Kaposi's sarcoma has been found to be thalium and technetium avid, whereas lymphoma and infection are more typically gallium avid.

The typical pathologic lesion of Kaposi's sarcoma involves proliferation of aberrant vascular structures lined by abnormal, spindle-shaped endothelial cells with extravasated erythrocytes and leukocytes within these structures. The putative tumor cell is a spindle cell that lies between the vascular structure and is believed to be of mesenchymal origin. Several endothelial cell markers also stain positive for KS including *Ulex europaeus* and EN-4. The tumor also stains positive in factor VIIIa, CD-34, and alpha-actin.

STAGING AND PROGNOSIS

While clinical presentation and extent of disease do not seem to correlate with tumor progression, several retrospective studies have shown a correlation of survival with the degree of T cell immune deficiency as reflected by the absolute number of T helper cells. Prior opportunistic infections or the presence of symptoms such as fever, night sweats, and weight loss also carry a poor prognosis. Patients who develop Kaposi's sarcoma or whose tumors accelerate after an opportunistic infection often have a more aggressive clinical course. Pulmonary involvement also generally carries a worse prognosis.

A uniform tumor classification system has not yet been established for AIDS-KS. Several staging systems have been proposed. The one most widely used presently is proposed by the AIDS Clinical Trials Group (ACTG), which segregates patients into good or poor prognostic groups based on tumor characteristics, CD4 count, and symptomatology (the TIS system). (Table 4.16)

MEDICAL MANAGEMENT

Treatment of AIDS-KS involves an individualized approach. Factors to consider in the development of a treatment plan include extent and location of lesions, presence of tumor-associated symptoms (e.g., pain, bleeding, edema), the presence of other AIDS-defining illnesses, the patient's tolerance of medications, and the desire of the patient for treatment. Patients with symptomatic disease or life-threatening visceral involvement require prompt, cytoreductive therapy with one or more chemotherapeutic drugs. Even without extensive disease, the disfigure-

Table 4.16.
Staging Classification for AIDS-Related Kaposi's Sarcoma[a]

	Good Risk (0) (All of the Following)	Poor Risk (1) (Any of the Following)
Tumor (T)	Confined to skin and/or lymph nodes and/or minimal oral diseases	Tumor-associated edema or ulceration; extensive oral KS[b]; gastrointestinal KS, KS in other non-nodal viscera
Immune system (I)	CD4 cells $\geq$ 200/μL	CD cells < 200/ μL
Systemic illness (S)	No history of opportunistic infection or thrush; no "B" symptoms;[c] performance status $\geq$ 70 (Karnofsky)	History of opportunistic infection and/or thrush; no "B" symptoms present; performance status < 70 (Karnofsky); other HIV-related illness (e.g., neurologic disease, lymphoma)

From Krown SE, Metroka C, Wernz JC. Kaposi's sarcoma in the acquired immunodeficiency syndrome: a proposal for uniform evaluation, response, and staging criteria. J Clin Oncol 1989;7:1201.
[a]Patients are assigned a disease state $T_x I_x S_x$ where X corresponds to the risk designation (0 or 1) for each risk category.
[b]Minimal oral disease on non-nodular KS confined to the palate.
[c]"B" symptoms: unexplained fever, night sweats, >10% involuntary weight loss, or diarrhea persisting more than 2 weeks.

ment and emotional distress of having these visual reminders of AIDS may mandate treatment for psychological reasons. For patients with asymptomatic indolent lesions, aggressive treatment is not generally indicated but can provide significant psychological benefits. These patients may derive substantial benefits from investigational therapies directed at HIV infection, interrupting the pathogenesis of Kaposi's sarcoma, and/or restoring immune competence.

Local treatment includes cryotherapy, intralesional chemotherapy, topical agents, and local radiation therapy and can induce good local control of tumors. Both alpha-interferon and cytotoxic chemotherapy are effective as systemic treatments in patients with more extensive or symptomatic disease. Chemotherapy with agents such as bleomycin, doxorubicin, etoposide, vinblastine, or vincristine singly or as part of combination regimens is effective in controlling tumors including those with very extensive disease and severe immunodeficiency. The use of hematopoietic growth factors with myelosuppressive treatments such as alpha-interferon and combination chemotherapy has facilitated the administration of these drugs. The overall treatment of Kaposi's sarcoma is in evolution with a number of newer approaches and new agents being evaluated in clinical trials.

ALPHA-INTERFERON

The first treatment licensed for use in AIDS-KS was recombinant alpha-interferon. Tumor responses have been seen in approximately 30% of all patients treated with alpha-interferon. Current practice is to administer alpha-interferon by daily subcutaneous injection with a reduction in dosing frequency to three times a week after 2 or 3 months of treatment in responding patients. The unmaintained response duration in monotherapy trials of alpha-interferon has ranged from 12 to 24 months for complete responders and 8 to 12 months for partial responders. The optimal duration of treatment with alpha-interferon is not known; however, many patients relapse within 6 to 8 months after discontinuation of therapy, and many would advocate continued treatment with alpha-interferon for as long as drug tolerance and tumor responses continue.

The optimal dose of alpha-interferon is also not clearly established. Recent studies using low doses of alpha-interferon (<10 million units) in combination with a nucleoside analog (e.g., zidovudine, didanosine, or zalcitabine) have shown higher response rates than with interferon alone. Responses are also seen in patients with CD4 counts less than 200 cells/mm^3 who ordinarily would not be likely to respond to interferon monotherapy.

CHEMOTHERAPY

For patients with more widely disseminated, rapidly progressive, or symptomatic disease, systemic chemotherapy is generally warranted. Several chemotherapy drugs have been shown to be active against Kaposi's sarcoma. Treatment with combination regimens result in tumor response rates exceeding 70 to 90% with good palliation of symptoms. The effects of these drugs on survival, however, has not been clearly demonstrated. The combination chemotherapy regimens of adriamycin, bleomycin, and vincristine (ABV) or bleomycin and vincristine (BV) are the two most frequently utilized chemotherapy regimens.

Liposomal anthracyclines (doxorubicin, daunomycin) are also effective in reducing tumor regression in advanced, refractory, or relapse Kaposi's sarcoma and are being evaluated in comparison studies with standard combination regimens. Doses up to 20 mg/m^2 biweekly can be tolerated without excess toxicity and 40 mg/m^2 biweekly can be given with granulocyte colony stimulating factor (G-CSF) support. The major toxicities reported have been neutropenia, nausea, and thrombocytopenia. Response in refractory patients may exceed 50%. Other drugs under investigation as salvage therapy for progressive Kaposi's sarcoma include oral etoposide, taxol (paclitaxel), topotecan, and vinorelbine.

RADIATION THERAPY

Radiation therapy is primarily used as palliation for symptomatic disease or for cosmetic improvement of disfiguring lesions. Radiation therapy may be helpful in alleviating pain, bleeding, lessening and edema, and shrinking obstructing lesions.

Radiation should be administered to the targeted lesion and a small area of surrounding normal tissue of no more than 2 cm. For superficial lesions, radiation of limited penetration (approximately 100 KV) works well. For sensitive areas (e.g., cheek, nose, ear lobe), shielding with wrapped thin lead sheet should be used to protect underlying tissue. Relatively low energy electron beam (e.g., 6 MeV) can be used with shielding as an alternative to superficial x-rays. For very large lesions, electron beams are used; however, infiltrating tumors with edema, such as on the legs, are often treated with more penetrating x-ray such as in symptomatic pulmonary disease.

Non-Hodgkin's Lymphoma

EPIDEMIOLOGY

Lymphoma is generally a late manifestation of AIDS and has been increasing in incidence as the survival of patients with AIDS increases. Lymphoma currently comprises approximately 8 to 10% of all initial AIDS-defining conditions, but it accounts for 15 to 20% of all AIDS-related deaths. The estimated risk of developing lymphoma after 3 years of antiretroviral therapy is approximately 20%. The majority of patients present with advanced-stage, high or intermediate grade B cell lymphomas and have a high frequency of extranodal involvement. Primary central nervous system (CNS) lymphoma occurs in 3% of patients with AIDS. Lymphomas occur with approximately equal frequency in all patient groups at risk for HIV infection including intravenous drug users, homosexual and bisexual men, transfusion recipients, and patients with hemophilia. The incidence of lymphoma is 60 times higher in the HIV population than in the general population. Median CD4 counts for patients with systemic lymphoma is 100 to 200 cells/mm^3 while CD4 counts <50 cells/mm^3 are found in the majority of patients with CNS lymphomas.

ETIOLOGY AND RISK FACTORS

AIDS-related lymphoma is believed to arise as a consequence of continued stimulation of B cell proliferation as a result of HIV, Epstein Barr virus (EBV), and cytokines induced by these infections. Genetic errors, including a variety of chromosomal translocations and oncogene activation that occurs in the setting of immune deficiency, can lead to polyclonal and then to monoclonal B cell proliferation.

CLINICAL PRESENTATION

"B" symptoms are seen in approximately 80% of patients with systemic AIDS-related lymphoma and in the majority of those with primary CNS lymphoma. In these patients, it is mandatory to exclude the presence of occult opportunistic infections before ascribing these infections to the lymphoma itself.

Advanced-stage disease is expected in the majority of patients. Extranodal involvement has been reported in 60 to 90% of patients. As the likelihood of dissemination is great, AIDS patients who develop non-Hodgkin's lymphoma must be assumed to have widespread disease at the time of presentation and treated with systemic chemotherapy even if dissemination is not confirmed on routine staging evaluation.

Common sites of extranodal involvement include the CNS in approximately 30%, gastrointestinal track in 25%, and bone marrow in 25%.

SCREENING, DIAGNOSIS, AND PATHOLOGY

Diagnosis of non-Hodgkin's lymphoma requires histologic confirmation by biopsy with immunophenotypic and/or molecular gene rearrangement confirmation of diagnosis. A complete staging evaluation should be done in all patients including computed tomography (CT) or magnetic resonance imaging (MRI) scans of the head, chest, and abdomen, bone marrow aspiration and biopsy, liver function studies, and spinal fluid analyses. The use of polymerase chain reaction (PCR) for EBV in spinal fluid to establish a diagnosis of CNS involvement with immunoblastic or large cell type lymphoma is still under evaluation.

Over 95% of lymphomas are B cell in origin. The majority of AIDS lymphomas are of high grade type (70 to 90%), including the immunoblastic and small non-cleaved types. Diffuse large cell lymphoma constitutes 30% of AIDS-related lymphomas.

Although not considered part of the AIDS epidemic, several cases of T cell lymphomas have been described in HIV-infected individuals. In addition, several case of Ki-1 positive large cell aplastic lymphoma have been reported in HIV-infected patients. The clinical and pathologic characteristics of these lymphomas are similar to those seen in the non-HIV settings.

CNS lymphomas are typically the immunoblastic or large-cell type. The large cell or immunoblastic lymphomas are also more likely to involve the gastrointestinal track and oral cavity than small non-cleaved lymphomas. No major differences have been seen in response to chemotherapy or in survival among the various pathological types of systemic AIDS lymphoma. Patients with primary CNS lymphoma, however, have a particularly poor prognosis with a median survival of only 2 to 3 months.

STAGING AND PROGNOSIS

Staging of AIDS-related lymphoma uses the same Ann Arbor classification system used for staging non-Hodgkin's lymphoma in general. Workup would include imaging studies as well as bone marrow and CSF evaluation.

Four factors have been shown in several retrospective studies to correlate most closely with survival in patients with AIDS-related non-Hodgkin's lymphoma. These include a history of opportunistic infection, CD4 counts <200 cells/mm^3, Karnofsky performance status <70%, and stage IV disease, especially with bone marrow involvement. Patients with one or more of these adverse prognostic factors have a median survival of 4 months compared to a median survival of 11 to 12 months in patients who lack these findings. Patients with polyclonal tumors appear to have better tumor responses to chemotherapy and longer survival. Very intensive high-dose combination chemotherapy regimens have been associated with a statistically shorter survival than moderately intensive regimens.

Patients with primary CNS lymphoma have an extremely poor prognosis with a median survival of only 2 to 3 months despite therapy. These individuals have evidence of profound HIV-related immune deficiency with median CD4 counts (<50 cells/mm^3) and often a prior history of AIDS.

MEDICAL MANAGEMENT

The mainstay of treatment for patients with non-Hodgkin's lymphoma is chemotherapy. Even patients with clinically apparent localized disease should be viewed as having systemic lymphoma and treated with combination chemotherapy. The development of treatment for AIDS lymphoma paralleled that of non-HIV infected patients and used multiagent chemotherapy with non-cross resistant drugs. Multivariate analysis, however, showed that patients who were given greater chemotherapy dose intensity survived for shorter periods of time than did patients who were less intensively treated. Lower dose modification of regimen such as the current mBACOD regimen as evaluated by the ACTG has demonstrated a >50% complete response rate, with long-term lymphoma-free survival in 60% of patients with complete responses. Subsequent studies of mBACOD or CHOP chemotherapy with myeloid hematopoietic growth factors demonstrated better tolerance of these regimens, although no better survival.

A randomized study (ACTG 142) comparing low dose mBACOD with standard dose mBACOD plus GM-CSF to assess the effect of increased dose intensity, did not show any improvement in response rate or survival of patients receiving the more dose-intensive regimen. Similarly, in a study of the CHOP regimen with or without GM-CSF, the complete remission rate was similar in the two groups and there was no difference in overall survival. It is therefore recommended that the majority of patients with AIDS-related lymphoma receive moderately dose-intensive first or second generation chemotherapy regimens (such as CHOP or mBACOD) along with hematopoietic growth factor support and that more dose-intensive regimens should be reserved for selected populations of patients, such as those with small non-cleaved lymphomas. It is also recommended that patients receive effective antiretroviral treatment along with their chemotherapy whenever possible.

RADIATION THERAPY

The role of radiation therapy in systemic lymphoma is limited to the consolidation of chemotherapy effects. For patients with lymphomatous meningitis or radiographically detectable cerebral lymphoma deposits, whole brain radiation is administered along with intrathecal chemotherapy to control microscopic spinal disease. Occasionally, focal radiation therapy can be used to control local lymphoma deposits in specific nodal areas; however, this should not be used as the only modality of treatment.

PRIMARY CNS LYMPHOMA

Patients with primary CNS lymphoma often present with focal neurologic deficits, seizures, or altered mental status. These lesions are usually detectable on MRI or CT scan. Because many of these patients present late in the course of their disease, are often debilitated, and tolerate treatment poorly, the usual standard treatment is whole brain irradiation which can result in complete remission in 20 to 40% of patients, although survival is improved only from a median of 1.4 to 4.5 months with this treatment. Studies to evaluate short courses of combination chemotherapy or drugs that can penetrate the blood-brain barrier followed by whole brain irradiation are currently in progress. Although these approaches appear somewhat efficacious in non-HIV infected patients with primary CNS lymphoma, no data are available yet regarding their effectiveness in AIDS-related lymphomas.

Cervical Carcinoma

EPIDEMIOLOGY

Cervical carcinomas in the setting of HIV infection have been recognized as AIDS-defining malignancies since 1993. Cervical and anal intraepithelial neoplasia (CIN and AIN) are seen in association with HIV infection. These premalignant lesions may count for the high frequency of squamous cell carcinoma of the anus and may foretell a higher incidence of cervical carcinoma among HIV-infected women. These lesions are usually associated with human papilloma virus (HPV), particularly the oncogenic serotypes 16, 18, 3, 33, and 35. HIV seropositive women have up to a ten-fold higher risk of abnormal cervical cytology on routine Pap testing. Several centers have reported abnormal cytology rates of 30 to 60% and Pap smears consistent with cervical dysplasia in 15 to 40%. The prevalence of cervical dysplasia increases with progressively worsening immunodeficiency in HIV-infected women.

ETIOLOGY AND RISK FACTORS

While HIV itself does not appear to cause malignant transformation, the severe cellular immune deficiency associated with HIV infection may allow oncogenic viruses to flourish and compromise the body's natural immunologic defenses that can control the development of neoplasia. There is abundant evidence that HPV infection is related to malignant and premalignant neoplasia in the lower genital track. The prevalence of CIN among HIV-infected women may be as high as 25 to 50%, with many presenting with higher cytologic and histologic grade lesions. Women with a history of STDs, genital condylomatas, and multiple sexual partners are at higher risk for developing these lesions. It is also possible that HIV may function as a promoter that increases the risk of malignant transformation by certain subtypes of HPV.

CLINICAL PRESENTATION AND DIAGNOSIS

Cervical abnormalities are most often detected on routine cytologic evaluation of Pap smears in women with HIV infection. Postcoital bleeding, vaginal discharge, lumbarsocral pain, and urinary obstruction are often symptoms of more advanced invasive disease. Unfortunately, many women with invasive carcinoma present with these late symptoms as their first presenting AIDS symptoms and are otherwise asymptomatic. In a large study of women under the age of 50 with cervical cancer, 19% were HIV seropositive and the majority of these women were asymptomatic with regards to their HIV disease.

Because of this fact, frequent cytologic screening of women at risk for HIV infection must be undertaken. Current screening recommendations are for women with HIV to have pelvic examinations and cytologic screening every 6 months. Pap smears indicating CIN must be take seriously and abnormalities would justify immediate colposcopic evaluation and biopsy. Although abnormalities are sometimes missed by relying solely on cytologic screening, recommendations for the use of routine colposcopy and biopsy have not yet been established. For women who have a history of CIN, more frequent evaluation, cytologic screening, and repeat colposcopy with biopsy would be prudent, as these women are at high risk for developing invasive cancer.

For women with invasive carcinoma, complete staging, including pelvic examination, CT scan of the pelvis and abdomen, chest x-ray, and screening laboratories for hepatic and bone disease should be undertaken. In addition, full evaluation and treatment for HIV and its related complications should be initiated.

STAGING, PROGNOSIS, AND PATHOLOGY

The staging classification for cervical carcinoma as adopted by the International Federation of Gynecology and Obstetrics (FIGO) also applies to AIDS patients. Cervical dysplasias in HIV seropositive women often have higher cytologic and histologic grades. HIV-infected women are more likely to have CIN II-III lesions, tumors at multiple sites, and endocervical lesions. HIV-infected women with invasive cervical carcinoma typically present with high grade tumors with a greater proportion of lymph node and visceral involvement at the time of presentation. The majority of cervical carcinoma is of the squamous cell type, although, rarely, adenocarcinoma and clear cell carcinoma have been diagnosed.

As in preinvasive CIN, women with lower CD4 counts and a history of AIDS typically have more advanced disease and have a worse outcome. Mean time to recurrence after primary treatment is short, and most patients have persistent disease after primary treatment. Median time to death in one series was 10 months in AIDS patients compared to 23 months in HIV seronegative individuals.

MEDICAL TREATMENT

Preinvasive disease is often treated with local therapies including cryotherapy, laser therapy, cone biopsy, and excision. Short-term recurrence rates of 40 to 60% have been reported. Patients with CD4 counts <500 cells/mm^3 are at high risk for developing recurrent disease (>50%), whereas women with CD4 counts >500 cells/mm^3 have recurrence rates only twice that of HIV-negative women. Close surveillance after initial therapy is critical, and repetitive treatment may be necessary to prevent progression to more invasive disease. The use of topical vaginal 5-fluorouracil (5-FU) maintenance therapy as prophylaxis against recurrent CIN in patients with high-grade cervical dysplasia is under investigation.

For patients with invasive cervical carcinoma, the same principles that guide management of the immunocompetent patient should be used. Surgery can be undertaken for the usual indications, and surgical decisions should be based on oncologic appropriateness and not on HIV status. As most AIDS patients with cervical cancer present with advanced disease, radiation therapy is more often indicated. There is no evidence at present to suggest that radiation therapy is less effective in the AIDS patients compared with similarly staged non-HIV-infected individuals. Chemotherapy regimens such as cisplatinum or carboplatinum, bleomycin, and vincristine have been used in patients with advanced or recurrent disease. Vigorous management of side effects and complications of these treatments and of AIDS itself must be provided.

ACKNOWLEDGMENT

Supported in part by grants from the State of California, Universitywide Task Force on AIDS to the UCLA AIDS Clinical Research Center (CC-95-LA-194) and USPHS NIH grants AI-27660, CA-70080, and RR-00865.

SUGGESTED READINGS

KAPOSI'S SARCOMA

Kaplan LD, Northfeld DW. Malignancies associated with AIDS. In: Sande MA, Volberding PA, ed. The Medical Management of AIDS, 4th ed. Philadelphia: WB Saunders, 555–590.

Krown SE, Metroka C, Wernz JC. Kaposi's sarcoma and the acquired immunodeficiency syndrome: a proposal for uniform evaluation, response and staging criteria. J Clin Oncol 7:1201–1207, 1989.

Miles SA, Wang H, Elashoff R, Mitsuyasu RT. Improved survival for patients with AIDS-related Kaposi's sarcoma. J Clin Oncol 12:1910–1916, 1994.

Piedbois P, Frikha H, Martin L, et al. Radiotherapy and the management of epidemic Kaposi's sarcoma. Int J Radat Oncol Biol Phys 30:1207–1211, 1994.

Rabkin CD. Epidemiology of AIDS-related malignancies. Curr Opin Oncol 6:492–496, 1994.

Stelzer KF, Griffin TW. A randomized perspective trial of radiation therapy for AIDS-associated Kaposi's sarcoma. Int J Radiat Oncol Biol Phys 27:1057–1061, 1993.

NON-HODGKIN'S LYMPHOMA

Baumgartner JE, Rachlin JR, Bechstead JH, et al. Primary CNS lymphoma: natural history and response to radiation therapy in 55 patients with AIDS. J Neurosurg 73:206–211, 1990.

Beral V, Peterman T, Berkelman R, Jaffe J. AIDS-associated non-Hodgkin's lymphoma. Lancet 337:805–809, 1991.

Cooper JS. The role of radiation therapy and the management of patients with AIDS. In: Cox JD, ed. Moss' Radiation Oncology: Rationale, Technique, Results, 7th ed. 1994.

Kaplan LD, Kahn JO, Crowe S, et al. Clinical and virologic effects of recombinant human granulocyte-macrophage colony-stimulating factor in patients receiving chemotherapy for HIV-associated non-Hodgkin's lymphoma: results of a randomized trial. J Clin Oncol 9:929–940, 1991.

Levine AM. Acquired immunodeficiency syndrome-related lymphoma. Blood 80:8–20, 1992.

CERVICAL CARCINOMA

Maiman M. Cervical neoplasia in women with HIV infection. Oncology 8:83–88, 1994.

Marte C, Kelly P, Cohen M, et al. Papanicolaou smear abnormalities in ambulatory care sites for women infected with HIV. Am J Obstet Gynecol 163:1232–1237, 1992.

Northfelt DW. Cervical and anal neoplasia and HPV infection in persons with HIV infection. Oncology 8:33–37, 1994.

Neurological Aspects

Human Immunodeficiency Virus (HIV-1) invades the nervous system early in infection and is a common cause of morbidity in advanced HIV-1 disease. In general, health care workers are less familiar with the manifestations and treatment of HIV-1 as associated with neurologic disease (HIV-1 ND) than they are with systemic diseases such as pneumocystis. This lack of knowledge has contributed to a therapeutic nihilism. Many neurologic problems associated with HIV-1 are treatable, and treatment will significantly improve the patients' quality of life.

Epidemiology

In 1988, it was reported that approximately 10% of AIDS patients presented with a central nervous system (CNS) disease as their initial manifestation of AIDS, about forty percent of all AIDS patients developed a neurologic disease during life, and that 70% or more of AIDS patients had one or more neurologic diseases at autopsy (1). These studies did not estimate the incidence or prevalence of neurologic symptoms such as delirium, seizures, or headaches.

Recent studies have redefined the incidence of some neurologic problems in samples of HIV-1 infected persons. About 4–5% of HIV-infected persons will develop dementia as their initial AIDS-defining illness (2). Approximately 7% will develop a full-blown dementia during each year of life after another AIDS-defining illness (2). Overall, HIV-1-associated dementia is estimated to occur in 15–28% of AIDS patients before death. Another report observes that the incidence rates of HIV-1 sensory neuropathy and of primary CNS lymphoma increased from 1985 to 1992 (3). The incidence and prevalence of HIV-1-associated neurologic disease may be expected to grow for the following reasons: first, because more HIV-1-infected people are surviving into the advanced stages of disease when the majority of HIV-1 neurologic diseases occur, and second, because neurologic problems are more common in the very young and in the elderly, and these are growing subgroups of the HIV-1-infected population.

Natural History/Pathogenesis

HIV-1 enters the CNS at the time of primary infection. Evidence for early penetration includes the recovery of HIV-1 from the cerebrospinal fluid (CSF) during primary infection, the detection of antiHIV-1 antibodies synthesized in the brain, the detection of HIV-1 DNA in the CSF of neurologically normal, asymptomatic HIV-seropositive persons (4) and in the brain tissue of an iatrogenically infected patient who died shortly after infection (4). In most cases, HIV-1 infection of the CNS is clinically silent. An unknown number of seroconverters may develop one or more self-limited episodes of an HIV-1 associated aseptic meningitis characterized by headache, stiff neck, and fever, and CSF pleocytosis. Sixty to 90% of neurologically normal, asymptomatic HIV-1 seropositive individuals have CSF abnormalities indicating the presence of HIV-1, such as a mildly elevated CSF white blood cell (WBC) count, elevated CSF total protein level, normal or slightly low CSF glucose, and elevated levels of CSF albumin, IgG, IgG synthesis rate, or the presence of one or more unique CSF oligoclonal bands (4).

Once within the CNS, the bulk of HIV-1 infection is located in non-neural tissues, such as macrophages, monocytes, microglia, and to a lesser extent, astrocytes and capillary endothelial cells (5). Little evidence suggests that HIV-1 infects neurons or oligodendrocytes (the cells that produce myelin). Investigators speculate that when the immune defenses decline, and HIV-1 proliferates, then neurotoxic substances are generated both within the CNS and the periphery, and they damage neural cells. For example, HIV-1-infected macrophages shed fragments of viral proteins, such as gp120 and tat, which are neurotoxic. The HIV-1 coat protein gp120 appears to trigger excessive calcium influx into neurons, which causes dysfunction and eventually, death (6), and tat can disrupt neuronal membrane function, ultimately causing neural cell death (6). Activated immune cells, such as macrophages, can synthesize cytokines such as tumor necrosis factor (TNF) and gamma interferon, which can have harmful effects on the CNS. TNF has been associated with demyelination, headache, and stroke. Elevated levels of gamma interferon induce the enzyme changes which shunt the metabolism of tryptophan into the production of quinolinic acid, which is a neurotoxin and convulsant. Quinolinic acid binds to the N-methyl-D-aspartate receptor found on many neurons, and increases calcium influx into the cell, causing neuronal dysfunction and cell death (7).

Other harmful substances synthesized by infected and/or immunologically activated cells in the CNS include arachidonic acid and prostaglandins. This information about possible indirect mechanisms of HIV-1 CNS disease has led investigators to study drugs which block the effects of these neurotoxins *in vitro,* such as nimodipine and memantine, for the treatment of HIV-1-associated cognitive-motor complex.

In the peripheral nervous system, autoimmune mechanisms play an important role in causing demyelinating neuropathies and HIV-associated myopathy (HIV inflammatory muscle disease). The cause of the most common neuropathy, HIV-1-associated distal sensory neuropathy, remains unknown but is suspected to be an indirect result of viral infection.

HIV-1 Associated Cognitive/Motor Complex

HIV-1-associated cognitive/motor complex (HIV-1 CMC), previously referred to as AIDS Dementia Complex or HIV encephalopathy, is among the most common HIV-1-associated neurologic diseases. HIV-1 CMC is caused solely by HIV-1, and almost always occurs after a significant decline in immunity, such as another AIDS-defining condition, or at CD4 counts which are under 200 cells/mm³. The first patients who were identified as having HIV-1 CMC were in the advanced stages of neurologic and systemic disease. Subsequently, it was appreciated that the cognitive and central motor changes seen in HIV-1-infected patients range in severity from subtle dysfunction that can only be detected on neuropsychological testing, to a disabling dementia and quadriparesis, while other patients may present with CNS motor, spinal cord, or behavioral symptoms which are not properly classified as dementia. The American Academy of Neurology (8) has introduced the term "HIV-1-associated cognitive/motor complex" (HIV-1 CMC) which includes: (a) HIV-1-associated dementia complex for patients with disabling cognitive and central motor impairment who meet the standard criteria for other dementias, (b) HIV-1-associated minor cognitive/motor disorder for patients with nondisabling disease who are still able to function in the home and at work, and (c) HIV-1-associated myelopathy for patients who present with spinal cord disease, but little or no cognitive impairment. The term "dementia" should be reserved for patients with cognitive impairment that causes significant loss of function at home or work. "Dementia" has potential medical-legal implications, e.g., that a patient may be incompetent to manage his/her own affairs, or, in some states, to operate a motor vehicle.

COGNITIVE IMPAIRMENT

There are three key features of HIV-1 CMC, although all three do not need to be present to indicate this diagnosis. The first feature is cognitive impairment, characterized by decline in memory, decreased concentration and attention span, and to a lesser degree, problems with visual-spatial functions. HIV-1 CMC patients report problems with short-term memory but can sometimes respond to cues or "hints." Recall may also be facilitated if they have a longer period of time to respond. These strategies allow patients to compensate, to some degree, for their cognitive impairment. However, compensation can allow slowly progressive deficits to go undetected. Typical complaints include forgetting familiar names or telephone numbers, a need for increased time to complete complex tasks, or increased difficulty maintaining attention while reading, talking or watching television. Patients with HIV-1 CMC often complain about difficulty finding words, slowed speech or dysarthria (slurring). The latter are related to the motor problems described below, and do not represent a true aphasia. In advanced cases, patients develop progressive memory problems, difficulty maintaining a train of thought, severe slowing of thought processes, difficulty producing speech, difficulty following directions, and/or impaired judgment and insight.

CENTRAL MOTOR PROBLEMS

Central motor problems (as opposed to peripheral neuromuscular disorders) are the second component of HIV-1 CMC, and may be the initial feature in some patients. The first signs may be subtle motor slowing, which is detectable by declining performance on timed neuropsychological tests. This slowing may be misinterpreted as depression, generalized weakness, or fatigue. As the disease progresses, patients typically report difficulties with walking, including slowing and/or weakness in one or both legs. This may later involve the arms. Patients may manifest an action tremor, lack of coordination, and loss of balance, resulting in problems such as dropping tools, changes in handwriting, or stumbling. Many patients develop a paucity of spontaneous facial movements such as blinking, reminiscent of Parkinson's disease. In later stages of the disease, patients may have difficulty initiating movement, or develop paraparesis, incontinence, rigidity, spasticity, and severe hyperreflexia with clonus. Some individuals develop movement disorders such as resting tremor, mycolonic jerks, choreoathetosis, or hemiballismus. Clinical features of HIV-1-associated myelopathy include lower extremity weakness and spasticity, leg ataxia, loss of balance in the lower extremities, loss of posterior column functions such as position and vibration sense, and hyperreflexia, despite relatively well-preserved cognitive function. Patients with end-stage disease HIV-1-associated myelopathy may develop total loss of control of the lower extremities and bowel/bladder incontinence.

ORGANIC BEHAVIORAL CHANGES

Organic behavioral changes associated with HIV-1 CMC are the most difficult clinical features to assess. Often, they are reported by the patient's significant other, while the patient is oblivious to the spouse's concerns. The most commonly described pattern is a general loss of interest in usual activities, a loss of drive, apathy, and a general sense of "slowing down." Another common problem is irritability, which can sometimes lead to inappropriate outbursts. A small group of patients with HIV-1 dementia present with a new-onset organic psychosis. Most often, a manic or hypomanic syndrome has been observed, although some patients have a schizophrenic or paranoid picture. These syndromes must be differentiated from delirium, substance abuse or withdrawal, a recurrent episode of a preexisting psychiatric illness, neurosyphilis, brain infections, or tumors, or the adverse effects of prescription medications.

Diagnosis

The diagnosis of HIV-1 CMC is made when an HIV-infected person manifests key clinical features in the absence of another explanation.

There is no single test, or combination of tests, to diagnose this syndrome. Tests are used to exclude other causes of CNS disease. The following pathway can be used as a guide: Neuroimaging (magnetic resonance imaging (MRI) or computed tomography (CT)) is performed to rule out structural diseases of the CNS. Contrast-enhanced MRI, (including T1- and T2-weighted images), is more sensitive for this purpose than contrast-enhanced CT. Many persons with HIV-1 CMC have normal scans; others have cerebral atrophy, ventricular enlargement, or white matter lesions. None of the latter is specific for HIV-1. Cerebrospinal fluid (CSF) exam is performed to rule out treatable infections or malignancies which may escape detection on neuroimaging. Routine tests include cultures for bacteria, acid-fast organisms and fungi, and serology for syphilis, toxoplasmosis, and selected fungal diseases. Opportunistic viral infections such as cytomegalovirus are among the most significant pathogens that can be confused with HIV-1 CMC; however, routine viral cultures of the CSF are rarely productive. If a reliable lab is available, physicians should consider the use of the newer and more sensitive polymerase chain reaction (PCR) tests to detect CNS viral infections such as cytomegalovirus and herpes. Common and treatable causes of altered mental status such as B_{12} deficiency, thyroid disease, syphilis, hypoxia, systemic sepsis, alcohol abuse, drug abuse, and atypical reactions to prescription medications should be routinely evaluated in each patient. Neuropsychologic tests are not necessary to confirm the diagnosis of dementia in persons with advanced disease, but can be exceedingly helpful in detecting early cognitive dysfunction and in distinguishing dementia from psychiatric disease. Additionally, neuropsychological testing can be used as medical-legal documentation of a patient's mental status and as a quantitative baseline to assess the effects of therapy. Selected neuropsychologic tests appear to be the most sensitive indices of response to antiretroviral therapy.

Management

Pharmacotherapy with adequate doses of antiretroviral drugs to achieve therapeutic levels in the CNS is the mainstay of treatment for HIV-1 CMC. Two double-blind, randomized, placebo-controlled studies have evaluated the effects of zidovudine (ZDV) on neuropsychologic impairment. Significant improvement in neuropsychological test scores was demonstrated in previously untreated adult ARC and AIDS patients who received 1000 mg/day of ZDV, versus those who received placebo (9). Sidtis et al. (10) studied previously untreated adults selected by neurologists for HIV-1 CMC. Subjects were treated with placebo versus 1000 mg/day ZDV or 2000 mg/day ZDV. Overall, the neuropsychologic test scores of the treated group improved significantly more than did the scores of the untreated group: however, a dose effect was observed, with the most improvement occurring in the 2000 mg/day group. The presumed mechanism behind this dose effect is the incomplete penetration of ZDV into the CSF/CNS. There are no controlled studies which demonstrate the efficacy of the now-standard 500 mg/day dose, although there are anecdotal reports of patients who improved on low-doze ZDV, as well as reports of patients who failed to improve on 500 mg/day, but improved when their dose was increased to 1000 mg/day. No controlled studies on the treatment of HIV-1 CMC in adults with other antiretroviral drugs are available. As in the treatment of systemic HIV-1 infection, there is a loss of efficacy over time, probably due to the development of drug resistance. Current research is focused on clinical studies of drugs which block the effects of putative neurotoxins in vitro, such as nimodipine, memantine, and pentoxifylline, in addition to antiretroviral therapy. There are also several small studies (11) which report that amphetamines and other stimulants can be used to treat the symptoms of depression and psychomotor slowing in HIV-1 CMC. These drugs do not reverse the underlying disease process or improve judgment, and their effects do not last after the medication is discontinued. Some patients develop labile, irritable, or belligerent behavior, insomnia, or anorexia on stimulant medications.

Patients with HIV-1 CMC may manifest adverse reactions to common medications. Examples include extrapyramidal movement disorders after the administration of low doses of dopamine-blocking drugs, such as neuroleptics or antiemetics, an increased incidence of neuroleptic malignant syndrome, and delirium, sedation, forgetfulness or hypomania with tricyclic antidepressants, antihistamines, anticholinergic agents or benzodiazepines. The elimination of medications which may impair mental status is an important part of the management of HIV-1 CMC.

Nonpharmacologic symptom management in HIV-1 CMC includes structuring the patient's environment, which can significantly improve his/her ability to function, and the use of cognitive techniques such as diaries, posted notes and other reminders. HIV-1 CMC must also be differentiated from common opportunistic infections (OIs) and tumors of the CNS, such as cryptococcal meningitis, toxoplasmosis, progressive multifocal leukoencephalopathy (PML), neurosyphilis, and cytomegalovirus encephalitis.

Differential Diagnosis of HIV-1 CNS Disease

CRYPTOCOCCAL MENINGITIS

Cryptococcal meningitis is the most common CNS OI, affecting approximately 5 to 7% of people with AIDS. The causative organism is *Cryptococcus neoformans,* a fungus which can be spread by the inhalation of spores. The initial nidus of infection is usually the lungs: reactivation may occur when cell-mediated immunity declines and the infection spreads to many sites, including the CNS. Cryptococcal meningitis (12) can present in a fulminant fashion with severe persistent headache, fever, stiff neck, altered mental status, focal neurologic findings, and photophobia; however, it is quite common for the disease to take an indolent course so that the patient presents after several weeks of nonspecific malaise, low-grade temperatures, or mild-to-moderate headache without meningismus, altered mental status, or focal signs. In a few instances, cryptococcus is an "incidental" finding on CSF exams performed as part of a fever workup. Although the CSF profile is typically one of elevated intracranial pressure, CSF pleocytosis, elevated total protein, and low glucose, many cases have been reported of patients with "normal" CSF who had cryptococcus documented by fungal cultures, CSF cryptococcal antigen testing, or India ink stains. Treatment regimens usually include induction in hospital with 1.5 to 2.0 grams of amphotericin B administered intravenously over six weeks, followed by fluconazole 200 to 800 mg po per day as outpatients. Secondary prophylaxis must be continued for life because of the high rate of relapse in AIDS patients.

TOXOPLASMOSIS

Toxoplasmosis is the most common cause of a CNS mass lesion in adults with AIDS, affecting 10 to 30% of patients, depending on the sample studied (13). It is caused by infection with the parasite *Toxoplasmosis gondii,* which is usually acquired by consuming infected food, such as raw meat, fecal oral contamination, or vertically from the mother. The primary infection typically causes few problems, but reactivation may occur when cell-mediated immunity declines. Relatively few infections in adult AIDS patients are acquired de novo, e.g., from handling cat feces. The CNS infection is characterized by an encephalitis which is usually associated with multiple focal brain abscesses, rather than a diffuse infection. The abscesses appear to have a predilection for the basal ganglia and the cortical-white matter junction. At presentation, 97% of patients will have multiple lesions on neuroimaging. These lesions often have a "ring-enhancing" pattern and are surrounded by edema, producing a mass effect which may predispose the patient to increased intracranial pressure, coma, and herniation. There is no MRI or CT pattern which can definitively distinguish toxoplasmosis from lesions such as brain lymphoma, however, without additional diagnostic tests.

Patients with CNS toxoplasmosis often present with focal neurologic signs referable to their lesions, superimposed on a background of headache, malaise, low-grade fever, and/or seizures. Stiff neck is uncommon. Patients may develop delirium, lethargy, stupor, or coma if untreated. CSF exam should be performed only after an MRI or CT demonstrates that the patient is not at risk for herniation. Typical CSF findings are nonspecific, and usually show elevated total protein with a moderate pleocytosis. However, there are instances reported of normal CSF profiles. Toxoplasmosis serology is often unhelpful, because of the high rate of seroprevalence in the population, and because it is uncommon to find rising IgG titers or IgM in time to make these tests useful in diagnosis. CSF titers are often not helpful, as several cases of negative CSF toxoplasmosis titers in the presence of positive serum antibodies and CNS lesions have been reported. However, the absence of serum IgG does make the diagnosis of toxoplasmosis unlikely. Patients with typical multifocal, ring-enhancing lesions are usually treated in hospital for at least two weeks under close observation with pyrimethamine (25 mg po per day) and sulfadiazine (100 mg po per kg per day up to a maximum of 8 gm per day, along with folinic acid to prevent megaloblastic anemia). If the lesions respond (disappearance of clinical symptoms and radiologic improvement), an empirical diagnosis of toxoplasmosis can be made and the patient is given secondary prophylaxis for life. If the patient does not respond, or worsens, a stereotactic brain biopsy is indicated for definitive diagnosis and treatment. The use of steroids should be avoided unless herniation is imminent because they will obscure the neuroradiologic findings, and because many CNS lymphomas, which can have similar presentations, will respond temporarily to steroid treatment.

PROGRESSIVE MULTIFOCAL LEUKOENCEPHALOPATHY (PML)

PML is caused by a papovavirus known as the JC (for John Cunningham, not Jacob-Creuzfeldt) virus (14). This virus is ubiquitous in the human population, with about 60–80% of adults exposed worldwide. Presumably, the virus resides in a latent form in the kidney, and reactivates when immunity declines. About 3–4% of AIDS patients develop PML before death. JC virus infects oligodendrocytes, and to a lesser extent, astrocytes. Patients develop a rapidly progressive demyelinating disease, characterized by focal neurologic deficits referable to the areas of demyelination. Typical presentations include dementia, aphasia, apraxia, visual field cuts, cortical blindness, and cranial neuropathies. Headache, fever, and stiff neck are very uncommon. CSF findings are nonspecific, usually a normal or mildly elevated CSF WBC, total protein, and normal glucose. Recently, PCR technology has been applied to detect the presence of JC virus in CSF and blood. It remains to be seen if CSF PCR is sensitive and specific enough to detect this disease. Otherwise, the neuroradiologic findings of nonenhancing, multifocal, hypodense lesions in the white matter, which show no mass effect, are consistent with the patchy demyelination caused by other viral infections and are not specific for PML. The definitive test is brain biopsy. Most AIDS PML patients die within four months, although a few cases have been reported of prolonged survival, spontaneous remission, and clinical improvement after treatment with zidovudine, cytosine arabinoside, and alpha interferon.

LYMPHOMA

Lymphoma is the second most common CNS mass lesion in adults with AIDS, affecting 2–5% of patients, and lymphoma is the most common cause of CNS mass lesions in children with AIDS. Both primary CNS lymphoma and metastatic disease can involve the CNS. The incidence of AIDS/CNS lymphoma is increasing, possibly due to prolonged survival with severe immunodeficiency. The most common presenting symptoms include confusion, lethargy, memory loss, seizures, headaches and focal neurologic deficits, including multiple cranial nerve palsies.

Primary CNS lymphoma usually shows a homogeneous hyperdense, enhancing lesion, or a ring-enhancing pattern on CT or MRI, typically surrounded by a ring of edema. Lymphoma usually presents as a single lesion, although a substantial minority are multifocal at the time of diagnosis. Unfortunately, there is no neuroimaging pattern which definitively distinguishes brain lymphoma from toxoplasmosis, or other mass lesions in AIDS. Definitive diagnosis is usually made by stereotactic brain biopsy. Lymphoma which metastasizes from a systemic primary can present as a mass, or as lymphomatous meningitis or epidural metastases. If enough malignant cells are shed into the CSF, cytology may confirm the diagnosis. Treatment includes radiation and steroids; clinical trials for various chemotherapy regimens are in progress. Most patients with AIDS/lymphoma die from opportunistic infection and not from tumor.

SYPHILIS

Syphilis is common in the population at risk for HIV-1 infection, and neurosyphilis must be included in the differential diagnosis of any HIV-1 neurologic disease (15). Many patients who have CNS syphilis as diagnosed by a positive CSF VDRL will be neurologically asymptomatic; others will present with meningitis, dementia, strokes, seizures, myelopathy, or psychiatric symptoms. Uncommon manifestations or neurosyphilis that have been reported in HIV-1 positive patients include CNS mass lesions (gummas), optic neuritis, Bell's palsy, sensorineural hearing loss, and peripheral neuropathy. The CSF exam may not be helpful in confirming the diagnosis of neurosyphilis, because nonspecific abnormalities such as elevated CSF WBC and total protein may be present because of HIV-1, and because of the reportedly high rate of false-negative CSF VDRL tests. It has been proposed that HIV-1 infection may alter the natural history of syphilis, accelerating the course of the disease in the CNS and elsewhere. It has also been suggested that syphilis in HIV-1 infected persons may be refractory to the standard doses of penicillin given to seronegatives. It is prudent to perform a CSF exam on all HIV seropositives who present with syphilis. The recommended treatment regimen is intravenous, high-dose aqueous penicillin G, at least 12 million units per day for 10 to 14 days.

CYTOMEGALOVIRUS (CMV) ENCEPHALITIS

CMV encephalitis is a common infection of the CNS in AIDS, which is frequently found at autopsy (16) and infrequently detected during life. CMV may be found incidentally along with other AIDS-related neurologic diseases. However, it may be associated with dementia, seizures, and focal neurologic signs. Some patients progress rapidly from delirium to stupor and coma. The clinical spectrum of CMV neurologic disease in AIDS has not been fully explored, in part because it usually coexists with HIV-1 neurologic disease, which it resembles clinically to some degree, and in part because until the advent of polymerase chain (PCR) technology, CMV was often difficult to detect in the CNS during life. There are few specific neuroradiologic characteristics, except for occasional ventriculitis seen on contrast-enhanced brain MRI. CSF may show polymorphonuclear pleocytosis with elevated total protein and mildly decreased glucose, or may be unremarkable. Although no clinical studies have been performed, anecdotal reports suggest that intravenous ganciclovir and/or foscavir may produce clinical improvement.

HIV-1 Neuromuscular Disorders

HIV-1-associated peripheral neuropathies are of growing importance in the management of HIV/AIDS patients. It is incorrect to lump together all the types of neuropathy which occur in HIV-1 infected patients; in fact, several distinct types of neuropathy occur, and many respond to disease-specific treatment. The most common neuropathies associated with HIV-1 are the inflammatory demyelinating neuropathies (IDPs), mononeuritis multiplex (MM), and predominantly sensory polyneuropathy (PSP): these must be differentiated from secondary neuropathies associated with cytomegalovirus, herpes, varicella, and malignancy, and from neurotoxic neuropathies.

INFLAMMATORY DEMYELINATING NEUROPATHIES (IDPS)

There are two types of IDPs: Acute IDP (AIDP), which resembles Guillain-Barré syndrome in HIV-1 seronegatives, and chronic IDP (CIDP), which resembles CIDP in HIV-1 seronegatives. The mechanism in IDPs is autoimmune demyelination. AIDP tends to occur early in the course of HIV-1 infection, and has been reported to occur during primary infection. Clinically, it is characterized by a rapidly ascending lower motor weakness with decreased or absent deep tendon reflexes, and minimal or no sensory symptoms. Bowel, bladder, and autonomic function are spared. AIDP is a medical emergency requiring hospitalization, so that respiratory function can be monitored and the patient intubated if necessary. The diagnosis can be confirmed by the demonstration of elevated CSF total protein, a CSF White Blood Cell (WBC) count up to $50/mm^3$, normal CSF glucose, negative tests for other pathogens, and the demonstration of slowed nerve conduction velocities and other typical signs of a patchy, demyelinating neuropathy on nerve conduction studies (NCS). No controlled clinical studies have reported on the efficacy of various treatments in HIV-1 AIDP; however, case reports indicate a generally good prognosis with supportive care, as well as response to the treatments used in non-HIV-1-associated Guillain-Barré such as plasmapheresis and IV IgG. Prednisone has also been used in a few cases but has the potential to suppress general immunity. In my experience, some patients will make an incomplete recovery and develop CIDP or a chronic, painful neuropathy with mixed axonal and demyelinating characteristics.

CIDP tends to occur later in the course of HIV-1 disease, often after the patient has developed systemic symptoms. It is characterized by a slowly progressive or relapsing motor weakness usually accompanied by sensory symptoms, and decreased or absent deep tendon reflexes. The bowel and bladder are spared, and there is no sensory level. While HIV-1 CIDP has the potential to involve the bulbar and respiratory muscles, it tends to progress over weeks to months. Therefore, if the patient presents early in the course of CIDP, he/she can be evaluated (promptly) on an outpatient basis. The diagnosis is confirmed by a CSF white cell count which is less than 50 cells/mm³, elevated total protein, normal glucose, and negative tests for other pathogens. Electrodiagnostic studies (17) show predominantly demyelinating disease, (with or without some axonal findings) characterized by slow NCS, partial conduction block, or abnormal temporal dispersion; prolonged distal latencies; and/or absent or prolonged F waves. Nerve biopsies are not essential to the diagnosis, but if performed will show demyelination and remyelination. The latter two studies should be performed by specialists familiar with peripheral nerve diseases. No controlled studies are available regarding the treatment of HIV-1 CIDP; however, case reports indicate good response to treatments used for HIV-negative CIDP, such as plasmapheresis and or IV IgG (18).

HIV-1-ASSOCIATED PREDOMINANTLY SENSORY POLYNEUROPATHY (PSP)

HIV-1-associated predominantly sensory polyneuropathy, also called distal sensory peripheral neuropathy or distal symmetric polyneuropathy, is the most common neuropathy seen in HIV-1-infected patients. It tends to occur in the later stages of infection, and is associated with a decline in immunity. Symptoms tend to occur first in the most distal parts of the extremities, e.g., in the feet, then in the hands. The key features include sensory loss (which may be found on examination before it is reported by the patient), numbness, burning, tingling, or pain, and relatively mild weakness in the distal extremities which creeps proximally over time following the course of the sensory loss. CSF usually shows a normal WBC and minimally elevated or normal protein. Electrodiagnostic studies show a polyneuropathy with an axonal or mixed axonal-demyelinating picture. Nerve biopsies (rarely required for diagnosis) show distal axonal degeneration. Other etiologies (such as syphilis or toxin exposure) should be ruled out by appropriate laboratory tests and/or history. The pathogenesis of HIV-1 PSP is unknown, and there is no specific treatment for the neuropathy itself. Pain and dysesthesias can often be managed with standard therapies such as tricyclic antidepressants, carbamazepine, mexiletene, or topical capsaicin/lidocaine. Patients may require prosthesis or braces for weakness, or to prevent foot drop, and physical therapy to prevent contractures. Patients should be cautioned to protect numb extremities against burns, or penetrating sharp objects.

MONONEURITIS MULTIPLEX (MM)

MM is a relatively less common neuropathy in HIV/AIDS. The most common mononeuritis is a facial nerve (Bell's) palsy, which has been reported to occur at all stages including seroconversion. By definition, MM involves two or more nerves, usually in the form of a rapid loss of motor and sensory function in a mixed nerve or nerve trunk, suggesting a possible ischemia. Electrodiagnostic findings are less well defined than IDP or PSP, but typically are mixed axonal-demyelinating. MM has been reported to occur in association with a vasculitis that sometimes occurs in HIV-1, so a search for other autoimmune illnesses is worthwhile.

HIV-1-ASSOCIATED NEUROPATHIES

HIV-1-associated neuropathies must be distinguished from neuropathies caused by opportunistic infections, such as cytomegalovirus (CMV). CMV polyneuropathy typically occurs in severely immunodeficient patients. Most of these patients will have CMV infections elsewhere; however, CMV can present solely in the nervous system. The clinical picture is that of a rapidly progressing polyneuropathy that usually begins in the legs. It is characterized by progressive weakness, pain, sensory loss, low back pain, and loss of bowel and/or bladder function. I have seen patients present with urinary retention, only to develop the full-blown syndrome within the next two weeks. Untreated, CMV polyneuropathy leads to flaccid paraparesis, double incontinence, and may involve the respiratory, arm, bulbar, and extra-ocular nerves. Patients may develop diffuse CMV neurologic disease, such as encephalitis or myelopathy. The CSF usually shows a pleocytosis with polymorphonuclear leukocytes, elevated protein, and normal or low CSF glucose. Because it may be difficult to culture CMV from the CSF, CMV cultures from other body tissues, and CSF CMV PCR (19) should be sent. The most common electrodiagnostic pattern is that of a radiculopathy. Again, no controlled studies of treatment for neurologic CMV in HIV-1-infected persons have been performed; however, there are numerous case reports of clinical response to intravenous ganciclovir. In my experience, patients usually need to stay at the induction dose for a far longer time than in systemic or ocular CMV disease, and tend to recover more slowly from neurologic than systemic illness. The response to ganciclovir may also to fade over time, possibly due to the development of drug resistance.

Neurotoxic neuropathy can be caused by many drugs, especially antiretrovirals such as dideoxyinosine (ddl), dideoxycytidine (ddC), stavudine (d4T), and antineoplastic drugs such as vincristine. AZT is rarely associated with peripheral neuropathy, but has been associated with a toxic myopathy (see below). Most toxic neuropathies are characterized by pain, burning, or dysesthesias and loss of deep tendon reflexes, with or without motor weakness. Most are length-dependent, starting in the distal lower extremities and proceeding proximally before involving the hands. Recent reports indicate that persons who were treated with neurotoxic drugs in the past are more likely to develop a sensory neuropathy, even when off drug. Some observers have speculated that neurotoxic drugs may "unmask" a subclinical HIV-1-related neuropathy. Toxic neuropathies tend to be dose related, and occur either after a cumulative dose or a certain drug level is reached. In the toxic neuropathies associated with anti-viral drugs, symptoms may take up to six weeks to begin to improve after discontinuing the drug. Most neurotoxic neuropathies from antivirals show an axonal pattern on electrodiagnostic studies. Treatment consists of stopping the drug, and controlling pain. Although some patients can resume the offending drug at a lower dose after the neuropathy remits, most will be susceptible to recurrence if the same drug or another neurotoxic agent is used.

HIV-1-ASSOCIATED MYOPATHY

HIV-1 infected patients can manifest a myopathy which clinically resembles polymyositis in HIV-1 seronegatives (20). HIV-1-associated myopathy can occur at any time in the course of disease, and is characterized clinically by proximal, usually symmetrical muscle weakness, so that patients report difficulty with rising from a chair or climbing stairs. Many patients also report myalgias, muscle tenderness, or cramps. The creatine phosphokinade (CPK) and/or aldolase are elevated. The muscle biopsy shows inflammation. HIV-1-associated myopathy is an autoimmune disease which must be differentiated from toxic myopathy (see below) and wasting syndrome. While no controlled studies have been performed, there are case reports of clinical response to prednisone (which must be administered cautiously due to possible immunosuppressive effects), plasmapheresis, and IV IgG.

A myopathy which is clinically indistinguishable from HIV-1-associated myopathy can be caused by AZT. This myopathy is related to the cumulative dose and duration of treatment and remits when the patient is withdrawn from AZT. Muscle biopsy of persons with AZT myopathy has been reported to have characteristic "ragged red" fibers (which are abnormal mitochondria) on electron microscopic studies (21), as well as cytochrome c oxidase deficiency on histochemistry.

Our ability to understand, identify and treat the neurologic aspects of HIV-1 infection has dramatically improved over the past few years. The current explosion of diagnostic and therapeutic advances in the neurosciences should have an even greater impact on this field in the years to come.

ACKNOWLEDGMENT

Dr. Singer was supported by AIDS Regional Education and Training Center for Southern California, HRSA# 5D35PEOO106, the Neurologic AIDS Research Consortium, and NIMH# MH47281RO1, and the Veterans Health Service and Research Administration, Department of Veterans Affairs.

REFERENCES

1. Rosenblum ML, Levy RM and Bredesen DE, eds. AIDS and the nervous system. New York: Raven Press, Ltd., 1988.
2. McArthur JC, Selnes OA, Glass JD, et al. HIV dementia. Incidence and risk factors. In: HIV, AIS and the brain. Price RW, Perry SW, eds. New York: Raven Press, Ltd., 1994;251–271.
3. Bacellar H, Munoz A, Miller EN, et al. Temporal trends in the incidence of HIV-1-related neurologic diseases: Multicenter AIDS cohort study, 1985-1992. Neurology 1994;44:1892–1900.
4. Marshall DW, Brey RL, Cahill WT, et al. Spectrum of cerebrospinal fluid findings in various stages of HIV infection. Arch Neurol 1988;45:945–958.
5. Wiley CA, Schrier RD, Nelson JA, et al. Cellular localization of human immunodeficiency virus infection within the brains of acquired immune deficiency syndrome patients. Proc Natl Acad Sci USA 1986;83:7089–7093.

6. Dreyer EB, Kaiser PK, Offermann JT, Lipton SA. HIV-1 coat protein neurotoxicity prevented by calcium channel antagonists. Science 1990;248:364–367.
7. Heyes MP, Brew BJ, Martin A, et al. Quinolinic acid in cerebrospinal fluid and serum in HIV-1 infection: relationship to clinical and neurological status. Ann Neurol 1991;29:202–209.
8. American Psychiatric Association. Diagnostic and statistical manual of mental disorders. 4th ed. Washington, D.C.: American Psychiatric Association, 1994.
9. Schmitt FA, Bigley JW, McKinnis R, et al. Neuropsychological outcome of zidovudine (AZT) treatment of patients with AIDS and AIDS-related complex. N Engl J Med 1988;319:1573–1578.
10. Sidtis JJ, Gatsonis C, Price RW, et al. Zidovudine treatment of the AIDS dementia complex: results of a placebo-controlled trial. AIDS Clinical Trials Group. Ann Neurol 1993;33:343–349.
11. Fernandez F, Adams F, Levy JK. Cognitive impairments due to AIDS-related-complex and its response to psychostimulants. Psychosomatics 1988;29:38–46.
12. Kovacs JA, Kovacs AA, Polis M, et al. Cryptococcosis in the acquired immunodeficiency syndrome. Ann Intern Med 1985;103:533–538.
13. Porter S, Sande M. Toxoplasmosis of the central nervous system in the acquired immunodeficiency syndrome. N Engl J Med 1992;327:1643–1648.
14. Bredesen DE, Levy RM, Rosenblum ML. The neurology of human immunodeficiency virus infection. Quart J Med 1988;68:665–677.
15. Berger J, McCarthy M, La Voie L, et al. Neurosyphilis in HIV-seropositive individuals. Neurology 1989;39 (Suppl 1):361.
16. Vinters HV, Kwok MK, Ho HW, Anders KH, Tomiyasu U, Wolfson WL, Robert F. Cytomegalovirus in the nervous system of patients with the acquired immune deficiency syndrome. Brain 1989;112:245–268.
17. Report from an ad hoc subcommittee of the American Academy of Neurology task force. Research criteria for diagnosis of chronic inflammatory demyelinating polyneuropathy (CIDP). Neurology 1991;41:617–618.
18. Miller RG, Parry GJ, Pfaeffl W, et al. The spectrum of peripheral neuropathy associated with ARC and AIDS. Muscle & Nerve 1988;11:857–63.
19. Clifford DB, Buller RS, Mohammed S, et al. Use of polymerase chain reaction to demonstrate cytomegalovirus DNA in CSF of patients with human immunodeficiency virus infection. Neurology 1993;43:75–79.
20. Illa I, Nath A, Dalakas M. Immunocytochemical and virological characteristics of HIV-associated inflammatory myopathies: similarities with seronegative polymyositis. Ann Neurol 1991;29:474–481.
21. Dalakas MC, Illa I, Pezeshkpour GH, Laukaitis JP, Cohen B, Griffin JL. Mitochondrial myopathy caused by long-term zidovudine therapy. N Engl J Med 1990;322:1098–1105.

Ophthalmic Manifestations of HIV Infection

The ophthalmic manifestations of human immunodeficiency virus (HIV) infection can be particularly devastating because of their impact on a patient's quality of life. The majority of patients with acquired immunodeficiency syndrome (AIDS) will develop one or more ophthalmic disorders during the course of their illness, and at least 20% are at risk for severe visual loss from ocular infections. Because even tiny foci of disease in the eye can cause profound visual symptoms, ophthalmic lesions are often an early marker for multifocal disease and disseminated infections.

In most cases of intraocular disease, ophthalmologists depend largely on the clinical appearance and course of lesions in making a diagnosis. However, the immunosuppression associated with HIV infection alters the typical clinical characteristics of many well-known ophthalmic diseases, such as ocular toxoplasmosis. The early and accurate diagnosis of ophthalmic disease is critical. Lesions may be early markers for potentially life-threatening disseminated diseases, and preservation of sight often requires immediate treatment. Retinal tissue that is destroyed cannot be regenerated, and even relatively mild damage to many structures such as the retina, optic nerve, or cornea can cause profound visual loss.

HIV has been recovered from most ocular tissues, but its ability to cause clinically-apparent ocular disease as a direct result of ocular infection remains a subject of debate. HIV has been hypothesized as a cause of nonspecific uveitis, but the occurrence of such cases is probably rare, and HIV-induced uveitis should be a diagnosis of exclusion, after opportunistic infections are ruled out. Secondary disorders make up the bulk of the ophthalmic manifestations of AIDS and fall into four major categories: lesions attributed to microvascular disease of the retina and other tissues; infections; neoplasms; and neuroophthalmic signs of intracranial disease (Table 4.17).

Table 4.17.

Ophthalmic Disorders Associated with HIV Infection

I. Microvasculopathy
  A. Retina
    1. Cotton-wool spots
    2. Retinal hemorrhages
    3. Microaneurysms
    4. Ischemic maculopathy
  B. Conjunctiva
    1. Changes in vessel structure (dilated capillaries, microaneurysms, isolated vascular fragments, vessel segments of irregular caliber)
    2. Altered blood flow ("sludging")
  C. Optic nerve
    1. Ischemic optic neuropathy
II. Opportunistic Infectious Diseases
III. Neoplasms
  A. Kaposi sarcoma
    1. Eyelids
    2. Conjunctiva
    3. Orbit (rare)
  B. Burkitt lymphoma
    1. Orbit
  C. Large cell lymphoma
    1. Intraocular tissues
IV. Neuro-ophthalmic Signs of Intracranial Disease
  A. Cranial nerve palsies
  B. Eye movement abnormalities
  C. Visual field defects
  D. Papilledema
  E. Pupillary abnormalities
  F. Optic atrophy

Table reprinted from Holland GN. Ocular Sequelae. In: Broder S, Merigan TC, Bolognesi D, eds. Textbook of AIDS Medicine. Baltimore: Williams & Wilkins, 1994.

Microvascular Disease of the Eye

The most common ocular lesions in HIV-infected patients are cotton-wool spots (1,2). They are discrete areas of retinal opacification, usually located around the optic nerve head or along the major vascular arcades in the posterior pole. They are the most common manifestations of a diffuse retinal microvasculopathy that probably occurs in all HIV-infected persons. Microvascular abnormalities can also be seen in the bulbar conjunctiva, indicating that vascular damage is widespread in patients with HIV infection (3). Changes are most apparent in the inferior, perilimbal bulbar conjunctiva, and consist of dilated capillaries, isolated vascular fragments, vessel segments of irregular caliber, and sludging of blood flow. Ischemic optic neuropathy may sometimes be seen and results in pale optic nerve heads and visual field loss.

Cotton-wool spots rarely produce gross visual disturbances and are of little clinical significance to the individual patient. Although cotton-wool spots are generally considered to be asymptomatic lesions, some investigators suspect that the underlying retinal microvascular disease may lead to diffuse retinal dysfunction with subtle visual changes.

Infections of the Eye

Infectious agents that have been reported to cause ocular disease in HIV-infected patients are shown in Table 4.18. Infections of the retina and choroid are the most common and most important. Information about these infections that is important for the general care of patients is summarized here.

INFECTIONS OF THE RETINA AND CHOROID

Infections of the retina and choroid vary in prevalence, but all can lead to loss of vision or blindness. CMV retinopathy is the most common; as a group, all other infections probably account for 5% or less of retinal infections seen in HIV-infected patients.

CMV Retinopathy

Although CMV retinopathy is an "index disease" for AIDS, only approximately 2% of patients with AIDS have CMV retinopathy as the first and only manifestation of the syndrome (4). It is estimated that the risk of developing CMV retinopathy as the first manifestation of AIDS is less than 0.5% during the first 7 years after infection with HIV (4). Median survival after diagnosis of CMV retinopathy is currently between 7 and 13 months (5,6). The risk of CMV retinopathy is associated with decreasing levels of CD4 lymphocytes, mostly occurring only after the CD4 count is below 50 mm^3 (7). Little is known of other factors that might increase one's risk of retinal infection. The diagnosis of CMV retinopathy is based on clinical findings. Because of the high prevalence of antiCMV antibodies in the general population, serological tests as well as shedding of virus in urine or other body fluids are of little value in diagnosis.

Table 4.18.
Infectious Agents Associated with Ophthalmic Disease in HIV-Infected Patients

I. Infections of the retina and choroid
    A. *Candida albicans*
    B. *Cryptococcus neoformans*
    C. Cytomegalovirus
    D. Endogenous bacteria
    E. *Fusarium* species
    F. Herpes simplex virus
    G. *Histoplasma capsulatum*
    H. *Mycobacterium avium* complex
    I. *Mycobacterium* tuberculosis
    J. *Nocardia* species
    K. *Pneumocystis carinii*
    L. *Sporotrichum schenckii*
    M. *Toxoplasma gondii*
    N. *Treponema pallidum*
    O. Varicella-zoster virus
II. Infections of the Ocular Surface and Adnexa
    A. Bacteria (most commonly Pseudomonas species and Staphylococcus aureus)
    B. *Candida albicans*
    C. *Chlamydia trachomatis,* serotype L2 (lymphogranuloma venereum).
    D. Herpes simplex virus
    E. Microsporidia
    F. Molluscum contagiosum
    G. Varicella-zoster virus

Table reprinted from Holland GN. Ocular Sequelae. In: Broder S, Merigan TC, Bolognesi D, eds. Textbook of AIDS Medicine. Baltimore: Williams & Wilkins, 1994.

There is a spectrum to the appearance of CMV retinopathy lesions. There can be variable degrees of retinal whitening or opacification and retinal hemorrhage. There may or may not be sheathing of the retinal vessels. All lesions will have an irregular, dry-appearing, granular border, which is the most clinically diagnostic feature of CMV retinopathy. Other clinical features that suggest a diagnosis of CMV retinopathy include relatively slow enlargement of lesions and minimal vitreous and anterior chamber inflammatory reactions.

The location of lesions has important implications for vision. Those in the macula (roughly that area within the major temporal vascular arcades) and around the optic nerve head are considered to be immediately vision threatening, and are considered to be in "zone 1" of the retina (8). Those lesions outside of the major vascular arcades (zones 2 and 3; sometimes referred to as "peripheral retina") are not immediately threatening to central vision. An understanding of the natural history of CMV retinopathy is important in making decisions about treatment. There are usually only one or two foci of infection at presentation, and new lesions develop infrequently, even without treatment. These isolated lesions expand slowly. Lesions tend to spread more rapidly in an anterior direction (toward the ora serrata) than in a posterior direction (toward the optic nerve and macula). CMV retinopathy also tends to be fovea-sparing. New lesions, when they do occur, are rarely located in the fovea, and with progression, the posterior border of lesions tend to spread circumferentially around the fovea, rather than straight toward it. An untreated lesion in the peripheral retina may therefore pose little threat to vision for some time after diagnosis; for that reason, deferral of treatment, especially for small lesions outside the major vascular arcades, for a few days or even a couple of weeks may be acceptable. The short deferral period enables patients to be evaluated medically or even complete business or vacation travel before starting intravenous medical therapy. Although lesions will continue to enlarge during a period of treatment deferral, they will come under control once treatment is started. As yet, there is no evidence that small amounts of lesion enlargement in the peripheral retina affect final visual outcome.

Prolonged deferral of therapy is not advised, however. Extensive retinal involvement, even if it is in the peripheral retina and does not affect central vision, will increase the risk of rhegmatogenous retinal detachments (9-11). Also, treatment will reduce the risk of developing new ocular lesions, and it presumably treats clinically inapparent, nonocular sites of CMV infection that might eventually be life threatening (12). Without treatment, CMV retinopathy lesions continue to enlarge slowly and the entire retina will be destroyed over several months.

Management of CMV

Ganciclovir and foscarnet are two approved drugs currently available for treatment of CMV retinopathy. Both drugs have similar treatment regimens. Patients are given an initial "induction" course of therapy (ganciclovir: 5 mg/kg twice daily for 14 days; foscarnet: 60 mg/kg, three times daily for 14 days), designed to inactivate the virus and prevent further enlargement of lesions. Induction is followed by a lifelong "maintenance" therapy (FDA-approved regimens: ganciclovir: 5 mg/kg daily or 6 mg/kg for five of seven days; foscarnet: 90–120 mg/kg daily) to prevent disease reactivation. Despite maintenance therapy, reactivation and progression of lesions eventually occur in almost all patients. The most easily recognized effect of treatment is a change in retinal opacification, but it is not necessarily a reliable measure of disease control; lesions with very little opacity can continue to enlarge. However, increasing opacification of the lesion border is believed to be a predictor of eventual lesion enlargement (8).

The best management of CMV retinopathy remains a subject of controversy. In recent years, objective methods have been developed for clinical studies (8,9) and trials have been carefully designed to address management issues. A large, prospective, multicenter clinical trial demonstrated no apparent difference between foscarnet and ganciclovir for major clinical endpoints such as final visual acuity and the time to first disease reactivation and progression (6). There was, however, a statistically significant difference between treatment groups for patient survival. Those who received foscarnet had a median survival of approximately 12.6 months, compared to a median survival of approximately 8.5 months for those who received ganciclovir. Although the cause for the differential survival could not be determined, it is possible that survival was prolonged by foscarnet due to its antiretroviral activity. The differential survival might also be attributable, in part, to other factors that were not controlled in the trial. Although analysis did not identify the differential use of other antiretroviral agents as a factor in the survival, patients taking ganciclovir were less able to tolerate zidovudine (13). Compared to ganciclovir, foscarnet therapy was associated with a greater incidence of side effects (primarily renal toxicity) requiring discontinuation of drug administration. Among a subgroup of patients with preexisting renal impairment, survival was actually longer with ganciclovir than with foscarnet. Therefore, the decision to begin treatment with ganciclovir or foscarnet should be based on nonophthalmic factors.

The failure of standard long-term maintenance therapies is the most pressing problem in the management of CMV retinopathy. The cause of late disease reactivations is not entirely clear. Some investigators advocate switching from ganciclovir to foscarnet or vice versa when reactivation occurs. However, in most cases, the first reactivation of CMV retinopathy can be controlled by administering induction-level doses of the same drug that is being used for maintenance therapy, suggesting that the drug levels achieved in standard maintenance therapies are too low to prevent disease reactivation. An inverse relation between ganciclovir dose and CMV viremia in patients receiving maintenance therapy has been shown (14).

The drug doses used for maintenance therapy are limited by their toxicities. Recent experience shows that patients may tolerate prolonged ganciclovir therapy better with the concurrent use of the leukocyte growth factors sargramostim [granulocyte-monocyte colony-stimulating factor (GM-CSF)] and filgrastim [granulocyte colony-stimulating factor (G-CSF)], which increase a patient's neutrophil count (15). The continued administration of induction-level ganciclovir with the concurrent use of leukocyte growth factors has been proposed as a therapy for patients whose lesions reactivate on standard maintenance therapy regimens.

In vitro evidence suggests that ganciclovir and foscarnet act synergistically against CMV (16,17), and combined maintenance therapy using both drugs has been used in some patients with multiple disease reactivations (18). While this therapy may be useful for the most refractory of cases, it may not be practical for routine use. The relative benefits and risks of alternatives for maintenance therapy have never been compared in a large, well-designed, prospective study, and currently, little published data exist to provide a basis for choosing between maintenance therapies. Local administration of drugs is a subject of continuing interest because of the toxicity and inconvenience of intravenous antiviral therapy. Direct injection of ganciclovir into the vitreous has been studied extensively as an alternative to systemic treatment (19,20). These injections are associated with several potential problems, however, including endophthalmitis, a potential increase in the rate of retinal detachment, increased intraocular pressure at the time of injection, scarring of the injection site, and retinal toxicity. It is also impractical to administer injections on a weekly or twice-weekly basis to large numbers of patients. The implantation of devices into the vitreous that slowly release ganciclovir have been advocated as a solution to the latter problem, but these devices remain investigational (21).

On the basis of autopsy studies, CMV retinopathy is believed to be a reliable indicator of tissue-invasive infections in other organs as well (22). In most cases, thse non-ocular sites of infection are not clinically apparent at the time CMV retinopathy is diagnosed, but may eventually be life-threatening. Local therapies do not treat these nonocular sites of disease, nor do they protect the opposite eye if it is not already infected. Patients who are treated with intravenous ganciclovir and/or foscarnet for CMV retinopathy have been found to have significantly fewer nonocular CMV infections at autopsy (12). Most clinicians, therefore, reserve local therapy only for those patients who cannot tolerate any form of systemic treatment. With the availability of oral ganciclovir, interest has developed in the combinatioin of oral drugs (to protect against non-ocular disease) and intraocular implants (to raise the local level of drug for control of retinitis). This combination is being compared to intravenous therapy in clinical trials.

CMV Reactivation

Repeated disease reactivations come at increasingly short intervals even with reinduction therapy, suggesting that the disease becomes harder to control as the patient's immune defenses wane further (6). Long-term survivors may reach a point where their CMV retinopathy can no longer be completely controlled, even with reinduction, and there is continued slow progression of lesions. Even if disease activity cannot be completely eliminated with drug therapy, patients probably receive a therapeutic benefit from continued drug administration by slowing of disease progression (23).

Complications of CMV Retinopathy

Rhegmatogenous retinal detachment occurs in at least 20% of patients with CMV retinopathy. It is generally a late complication of CMV retinopathy, and the risk appears to increase with the duration of infection (11). Detachments can be repaired, but final visual acuity is often poor even if the macula is attached and uninfected. Furthermore the most successful technique (vitrectomy and silicone tamponade) results in several optical problems that make visual rehabilitation difficult, even when visual potential is good. Cataracts are also common in eyes that contain silicone oil.

Differential Diagnosis of CMV

The major disorders in the differential diagnosis of CMV retinopathy include toxoplasmic retinochoroiditis, varicella-zoster and herpes simplex viral retinopathies, and syphilitic retinitis. These disorders can also occur concurrently with CMV retinopathy. In any case of presumed CMV retinopathy with atypical features or with poor response to therapy, concurrent infections should be considered. Intraocular lymphoma with retinal involvement can also be confused with CMV retinopathy (24).

Varicella-zoster Virus (VZV) Retinopathy

Although it is far less common than CMV retinopathy, varicella-zoster virus retinopathy is probably the second most common infection of the retina in HIV-infected patients in the United States. Varicella-zoster virus retinopathy may occur as an isolated infection or concurrently with or after cutaneous zoster in any dermatomal distribution. It is characterized by multifocal deep retinal opaque lesions (believed to be retinal edema) throughout the peripheral retina that quickly coalesce to involve the entire retina (25,26). Perifoveal lesions are also common at presentation. The retina can become completely necrotic over a period of a few days to a couple of weeks. There is little or no vitreous or anterior chamber inflammatory reaction. Vasculitis is not a feature of the syndrome, but patients are left with severe vascular attenuation. The optic nerve may be hyperemic and optic atrophy may result from inflammation and necrosis of the nerve. Most patients develop retinal detachments early in the course of the infection. The extensive distribution of early infection, the rapidity of its progression, and the high rate of retinal detachment make varicella-zoster virus retinopathy by far the most devastating of the retinal infections associated with HIV disease. Most patients with this infection have no light perception in either eye by the time they die.

The results of treatment for varicella-zoster virus retinopathy have generally been disappointing. Even with high-dose intravenous acyclovir disease may progress rapidly (25). Cases have been recently treated with combinations of intravenous acyclovir and foscarnet or ganciclovir and foscarnet (26). However, experience with these therapies is limited, and the best management of this infection is yet to be determined. Even if lesions become inactive with initial therapy, reactivation and progression of disease are common shortly after the termination of antiviral therapy (27), unlike cutaneous zoster lesions. Varicella-zoster virus retinopathy is similar to CMV retinopathy in this respect. Maintenance therapy using intravenous antiviral agents is therefore now used in patients who have retained some useful vision.

Herpes Simplex Virus Retinopathy

Herpes simplex virus infections of the retina in HIV-infected patients have been confirmed histologically, but cases of herpes simplex virus retinopathy in patients with AIDS are so rare that its course, prognosis, and response to therapy have not been established.

Toxoplasma Gondii Infection

Toxoplasma gondii infection of the retina is probably the third most common infection of the retina in patients with AIDS. It is seen only occasionally even by clinicians who care for large numbers of patients with AIDS and retinal disease, and is therefore much less common than intracranial toxoplasmosis. Accurate diagnosis is critical because infection poses a serious threat to vision, but it generally responds well to appropriate treatments. It can have a variety of clinical manifestations in HIV-infected patients, including single lesions, multifocal lesions in one or both eyes, and broad areas of retinal necrosis (28,29). Although the majority of reported cases have been unilateral, bilateral cases are not uncommon. There are several clinical features that appear to be reliable signs of toxoplasmic retinochoroiditis. In cases with full-thickness necrosis, the retina appears to have a thick, wet, and "indurated" appearance with sharply demarcated borders. There is vitreous inflammation and possibly inflammatory vascular sheathing. There is usually little or no hemorrhage.

Patients with suspected ocular toxoplasmosis should also be evaluated for systemic toxoplasmosis. It has been reported that 50% of patients with ocular toxoplasmosis also had CNS involvement, and ocular disease may be recognized before any neurological manifestations of intracranial infection (28,30). Lesions will continue to enlarge without treatment, although progression is generally slow. Spontaneous resolution of toxoplasmic retinochoroiditis in HIV-infected patients has not been reported.

All cases of ocular toxoplasmosis in HIV-infected patients should be treated. Most investigators believe that pyrimethamine in combination with at least one other antiparasitic agent is the most effective of the currently available medications for ocular disease. Lesions generally heal completely within 4 to 6 weeks. Corticosteroids are generally not used in combination with antimicrobial agents for several reasons. Inflammation does not appear to play an important role in tissue destruction; corticosteroids may further impair host defenses; and corticosteroids are generally not necessary for control of vitreous and anterior chamber inflammatory reactions.

Toxoplasmic retinochoroiditis will reactivate if treatment is discontinued. A variety of maintenance therapies have been used successfully, including continued full-dose administration of multiple drugs or single drugs, and intermittent therapy. While some investigators administer pyrimethamine because it is considered to be the most effective treatment, others prefer not to use it because of its potential for bone marrow suppression and interference with zidovudine therapy (28,31). It appears that disease reactivation can be prevented with relatively low-dose therapy that would be inadequate for the initial control of lesions. Single drug therapy with clindamycin or even tetracycline has been reported to be successful anecdotally, but the benefits of one drug compared to another have not been confirmed by a large trial series. Atovaquone has also be used successfully to treat ocular toxoplasmosis in patients with AIDS (32).

Syphilitic Retinal Disease

Syphilitic retinal disease can take a variety of forms in HIV-infected patients. They may have patchy infiltrates, with or without retinal necrosis that can mimic the more indolent-appearing forms of CMV retinopathy. A very characteristic subretinal lesion has also been described in other patients with HIV infection and syphilis (33). It is typically a large, nonelevated, subretinal, plaque-like mass, found in the macular and juxtapapillary area. The borders of the lesion are distinctly yellow, while the central area may be more faded. Retinal disease may be unilateral or bilateral. Vascular sheathing may be present. Syphilitic retinal disease is usually accompanied by marked inflammatory reactions in the vitreous and anterior chamber (33–35). Posterior synechiae are common. Keratic precipitates may be fine white or granulomatous (large, irregular and "greasy") in appearance.

It is generally believed that ocular disease is more common in HIV-infected patients with syphilis than in nonHIV-infected patients with syphilis. Ocular manifestations of syphilis in HIV-infected patients also reported include granulomatous iridocyclitis, vitritis, and optic neuritis. Although ocular disease can occur in patients with secondary or early latent syphilis, most reported patients with HIV infection and syphilitic eye disease have had neurosyphilis (34). It is recommended that all patients with suspected ocular syphilis be evaluated for CNS involvement and treated with antibiotic therapy appropriate for neurosyphilis. Both syphilitic retinitis and subretinal placoid lesions will regress with therapy. Patients may be left with coarse pigmentary stippling of the fundi, but vision is generally good (33–35).

Fungal Infections

Several fungi can infect the retina or choroid in patients with AIDS; however, none are common causes of disease. *Cryptococcus neoformans* is the fungus most commonly reported as a cause of intraocular infection in patients with AIDS. (22,36–40). Intraocular organisms have been found as incidental findings at autopsy (22), where they are seen within retinal and choroidal vessels without associated inflammation. Infection may result in multifocal, discrete, yellow-white choroidal lesions of up to a disc diameter in size with few clinical signs of inflammation (39,40). Lesions have been reported to fade with many weeks of intravenous amphotericin B and oral 5-flucytosine therapy. Lesions predominantly involving the retina have also been reported (36,37). Similar choroidal and retinal lesions have been reported rarely as a result of disseminated *Histoplasma capsulatum* infection (41,42).

Because mucocutaneous candidal infections are very common in HIV-infected patients, some clinicians incorrectly assume that patients are at high risk for candidal chorioretinitis. Candidemia is, in fact, uncommon among HIV-infected patients and intraocular candidal infections are rare. They are probably most common among patients having the same risk factors that are associated with intraocular candidal infections in immunocompetent patients: intravenous drug use, indwelling catheters, and broad-spectrum antibiotic use (22,38).

Mycobacterial Infections

Although tuberculosis occurs frequently in patients with AIDS, ocular involvement is very uncommon, as is true for patients without AIDS who develop pulmonary tuberculosis. Patients with miliary disease are those at highest risk for ocular disease. Multiple choroidal infiltrates, appearing as hypopigmented spots, are the most common finding (43-45). Patients may also have a severe anterior uveitis. Disseminated atypical mycobacterial infections, usually with *M. avium* complex, may also result in choroidal granulomata (22).

Choroidal Pneumocystosis

Choroidal pneumocystosis is one of the few previously unknown ophthalmic diseases that has emerged as a result of the AIDS epidemic. The typical clinical appearance of lesions is a discrete, yellow-white subretinal plaque. Without treatment, choroidal lesions enlarge slowly, and can assume irregular and multilobular shapes (46,47). Large, geographic yellow-white areas can result from lesion coalescence as disease progresses. A vitreous inflammatory reaction does not occur. Patients with choroidal pneumocystosis are frequently asymptomatic. Some may complain of "intermittent blurring" of vision, but objective visual acuity can be as good as 20/25 even if there are subfoveal lesions (48). Choroidal pneumocystosis is clinically important because it can be an early sign of disseminated, life-threatening *P. carinii* infection. Although prophylactic aerosolized pentamidine may be effective in preventing pneumonia, it does not protect against extrapulmonary *P. carinii* infections. Choroidal pneumocystosis has always been an uncommon problem, but is seen even less frequently now, since many patients receive oral prophylaxis in lieu of inhaled aerosolized pentamidine.

Choroidal pneumocystosis lesions respond to either intravenous pentamidine or trimethoprim-sulfamethaxazole (49). Oral trimethoprim and dapsone have also been used successfully (48). Lesions may resolve within 3 weeks of initiating treatment (49), but regression usually takes many weeks or months (48). Some lesions will fade, but not resolve completely. Without continuous or frequent intermittent suppressive therapy, lesions will recur. Average survival after diagnosis of choroidal pneumocystosis is reported to be 4 months (47). Among choroidal infections, pneumocystosis has received the most attention, but a variety of choroidal infections, including cryptococcosis and mycobacterial granulomata, can present in a similar manner.

Infections of the Ocular Surface and Adnexa

Severe infections of the ocular surface also occur in HIV-infected patients, although they are less prevalent than CMV retinopathy. The most common problem is zoster ophthalmicus, characterized by cutaneous lesions in the distribution of the first division of the trigeminal nerve. If the nasociliary branch is involved, patients can develop keratitis and anterior uveitis. Zoster ophthalmicus can be seen relatively early in the course of a patient's HIV disease, and is believed to be a harbinger of further deterioration in the patient's immune status.

Oral acyclovir (800 mg five times a day), used at the onset of skin lesions, has been shown to reduce the severity and incidence of ocular involvement in immunocompetent hosts. Acyclovir presumably has a similar beneficial effect in patients with HIV infection, although this issue has not been studied specifically. Because of the risk of disseminated varicella-zoster infection, many clinicians now treat patients having newly diagnosed zoster ophthalmicus with intravenous acyclovir.

In immunocompetent patients, zoster keratitis is an immunological reaction, and virus cannot be recovered from the cornea. In contrast, patients with HIV infection can develop a productive varicella-zoster virus infection of the corneal epithelium, as described below. Noninfectious zoster keratitis and zoster anterior uveitis may persist long after cutaneous lesions have resolved. The use of topical corticosteroids may be necessary to control the inflammation associated with zoster uveitis.

Patients with HIV disease can develop a chronic, productive varicella-zoster virus infection of the corneal epithelium, which resembles herpes simplex virus epithelial keratitis (50). This keratitis occasionally follows zoster ophthalmicus, with isolation varicella-zoster virus from corneal lesions many weeks after the resolution of cutaneous vesicles. In other patients there is no history of cutaneous zoster. In many cases, varicella-zoster virus epithelial keratitis in HIV-infected patients responds to topical acyclovir ointment (which is not commercially available in the United States); it does not respond to trifluridine solution (the most commonly used topical antiviral agent). Some patients with varicella-zoster virus keratitis have responded only to intravenous foscarnet.

Herpes simplex virus epithelial keratitis has been reported in patients with HIV infection, although there is no indication that it is more prevalent among patients with AIDS than in the general population. When it does occur, however, it tends to be more prolonged and severe; it is more likely to be adjacent to the corneal limbus; and there is a higher subsequent recurrence rate than in healthy individuals (51). Episodes appear to respond to conventional antiviral therapies, such as topical trifluridine.

Molluscum contagiosum lesions are difficult to eliminate from the eyelid margins. Very large lesions can be excised surgically. Cryotherapy is successful in reducing the size of lesions, and is well tolerated. Recurrences are common with both treatment modalities.

Neoplasms of the Eye

KAPOSI'S SARCOMA

Kaposi's sarcoma (KS) is the most common tumor to involve the eye in HIV-infected patients. Ocular involvement has been reported to occur in 20% of patients with AIDS-related Kaposi's sarcoma, and in fact Kaposi's sarcoma may make its first appearance on or around the eye (52). The eyelids are the most common sites of ophthalmic involvement. Conjunctival tumors are also seen frequently, whereas orbital involvement is rare. Conjunctival tumors are also seen frequently, whereas orbital involvement is rare. Conjunctival tumors can occur anywhere on the surface of the eye or lining of the eyelids, but are most common in the inferior fornix. Bilateral disease is frequent. Lesions can be missed if the lower eyelids are not pulled down on examination. They will be bright to deep red or violaceous, and may initially be mistaken for chronic subconjunctival hemorrhages. Conjunctival lesions spread slowly throughout the fornix, but do not invade the eye, nor do they involve the cornea. Intraocular Kaposi sarcoma has not been reported. Kaposi's sarcoma, therefore, presents little or no threat to a patient's vision.

Ophthalmic Kaposi sarcoma lesions may respond well to systemic chemotherapy. They can also be treated locally with radiation therapy, cryotherapy, or surgical excision. There is as yet no evidence that either radiation therapy or cryotherapy is safer or more effective than the other for local therapy of Kaposi sarcoma.

LYMPHOMAS

A growing problem in ophthalmology is the occurrence of intraocular lymphomas among patients with AIDS. Manifestations can include a cellular reaction in the vitreous fluid or an ill-defined subretinal mass. If the retina is involved, the lymphoma can be mistaken for CMV retinopathy or other necrotizing viral infections. Intraocular lymphoma may respond to systemic chemotherapy or local radiation, although there is little long-term experience in treating this problem because of the high mortality among these patients. Patients may also develop orbital lymphomas, with proptosis typically being the first manifestations (53). Treatment consists of radiation therapy and/or systemic chemotherapy, but the prognosis for the such patients is guarded.

Neuro-ophthalmic Disorders

Patients with intracranial infections and neoplasms may develop a variety of neuro-ophthalmic abnormalities, including cranial nerve palsies, abnormal eye movements, visual field defects, papilledema, pupillary abnormalities, and optic atrophy (54-56). The associated visual symptoms or ophthalmic signs may bring patients to the attention of an ophthalmologist before other neurological problems develop. A mass lesion on one side of the brain may produce a profound homonymous hemianopsia on the opposite side. Losing half of the visual field may be misinterpreted by patients as a problem with the eye on that side. Cryptococcal meningitis is the most common cause of papilledema in patients with AIDS. Patients with cryptococcosis occasionally also develop an unusual syndrome of very sudden, severe, bilateral visual loss, with or without papilledema. Its pathogenesis is not fully understood. It occurs in the absence of intraocular *Cryptococcus neoformans* infection, and is believed to be the result of a retrobulbar or intracranial process.

Conclusion

With continued spread of the AIDS epidemic, greater attention is being focused on its ophthalmic manifestations. Patients and their primary care providers should learn the signs and symptoms of intraocular disease, such as floaters, blind spots, and blurring of vision; patients who develop these problems should seek help from an ophthalmologist immediately. Because of the blood-retina barrier and the lack of blood vessels in some ocular tissues, many drugs reach sites of infection with difficulty. These factors, in addition to the severe immunosuppression associated with the later stages of AIDS, mean that immediate, aggressive, and prolonged therapy will usually be required to control HIV-related opportunistic infections of the eye. Because intraocular infections are usually a manifestation of disseminated disease, systemic therapy should be the mainstay of treatment. For most intraocular infections, chronic low-dose antimicrobial therapy will be necessary to prevent reactivation of disease. Prophylaxis against ophthalmic infections is not currently given in most cases. With regard to ocular surface infections, topical antiviral drugs are too toxic to corneal epithelium for prolonged prophylactic use, and topical antibacterials may select for resistant organisms. Until risk factors for CMV retinopathy are better understood, and more convenient and less toxic anti-CMV drugs become available, prophylaxis against this infection in all patients is not practical. Previously rare ocular infections and neoplasms have emerged as frequent manifestations of AIDS and it is likely that additional rare disorders will emerge as the epidemic continues. As the availability of new drugs and information about these diseases emerge, concepts about their diagnosis and management will undoubtedly change.

This chapter was adapted from Holland G. Ocular Sequelae. In: Broder S, Merigan TC, Bolognesi D, eds. Textbook of AIDS Medicine. Baltimore: Williams & Wilkins, 1994.

REFERENCES

1. Holland GN, Pepose JS, Pettit TH, Gottlieb MS, Yee RD, Foos RY. Acquired immune deficiency syndrome: ocular manifestations. Ophthalmology 1983;90:859–873.
2. Jabs DA, Green WR, Fox R, Polk BF, Bartlett JB. Ocular manifestations of acquired immune deficiency syndrome. Ophthalmology 1989;96:1092–1099.
3. Engstrom RE, Holland GN, Hardy WD, Meiselman HJ. Hemorheologic abnormalities in patients with human immunodeficiency virus infection and ophthalmic microvasculopathy. Am J Ophthalmol 1990;109:153–161.
4. Sison RF, Holland GN, MacArthur LJ, Wheeler NC, Gottlieb MS. Cytomegalovirus retinopathy as the initial manifestation of the acquired immunodeficiency syndrome. Am J Ophthalmol 1991;112:243–249.
5. Holland GN, Sison RF, Jatulis DE, et al. Survival of patients with the acquired immunodeficiency syndrome after development of cytomegalovirus retinopathy. Ophthalmology 1990;97:204–211.
6. Studies of Ocular Complications of AIDS (SOCA) research group in collaboration with the AIDS Clinical Trials Group (ACTG). Foscarnet-ganciclovir retinitis trial: 3. Morbidity and toxic effects associated with ganciclovir or foscarnet therapy in a randomized cytomegalovirus retinitis trial. Arch Intern Med 1995;155:65–74.
7. Kuppermann BD, Petty JG, Richman DD, Mathews WC, Fullerton SC, Rickman LS, Freeman WR. Correlation between CD4+ counts and prevalence of cytomegalovirus retinitis and human immunodeficiency virus-related noninfectious retinal vasculopathy in patients with acquired immunodeficiency syndrome. Am J Ophthalmol 1993;115:575–582.
8. Holland GN, Buhles WC, Mastre B, Kaplan HJ. CMV retinopathy study group. A controlled retrospective study of ganciclovir treatment for cytomegalovirus retinopathy: Use of standardized system for the assessment of disease outcome. Arch Ophthalmol 1989;107:1759–1766.
9. Freeman WR, Henderly DE, Wan WL, et al. Prevalence, pathophysiology, and treatment of rhegmatogenous retinal detachment in treated cytomegalovirus retinitis. Am J Ophthalmol 1987;103:527–536.
10. Holland GN, Sidikaro Y, Kreiger AE, et al. Treatment of cytomegalovirus retinopathy with ganciclovir. Ophthalmology 1987;94:815–823.
11. Jabs DA, Enger C, Haller J, de Bustros S. Retinal detachments in patients with cytomegalovirus retinitis. Arch Ophthalmol 1991;109:794–799.
12. Morinelli EN, Dugel PU, Lee M, Klatt EC, Rao N. Opportunistic intraocular infections in AIDS. Trans Am Ophthalmol Soc 1992;90:97–108.
13. Hochster H, Dieterich D, Bozzette S, et al. Toxicity of combined ganciclovir and zidovudine for cytomegalovirus disease associated with AIDS. An AIDS clinical trials group study. Ann Intern Med 1990;113:111–117.
14. Jennens ID, Lucas CR, Sandland AM, Maclean H, Hayes K. Cytomegalovirus cultures during maintenance DHPG therapy for cytomegalovirus (CMV) retinitis in acquired immunodeficiency syndrome (AIDS). J Med Virology 1990;30:42–44.
15. Hardy WD. Combined ganciclovir and granulocyte-macrophage colony-stimulating fac-

tor in the treatment of cytomegalovirus retinitis in AIDS patients. Rationale for and preliminary results from a phase II randomized trial (ACTG 073). In: Spector SA, ed. Ganciclovir therapy for cytomegalovirus infection. New York: Marcel Dekker, Inc., 1991.

16. Freitas VR, Fraser-Smith EB, Matthews TR. Increased efficacy of ganciclovir in combination with foscarnet against cytomegalovirus and herpes simplex virus type 2 in vitro and in vivo. Antiviral Res 1989;12:205–212.

17. Manischewitz JF, Quinnan GV, Jr., Lane HC, Wittek AE. Synergistic effect of ganciclovir and foscarnet on cytomegalovirus replication in vitro. Antimicrob Agents Chemother 1990;34:373–375.

18. Nelson MR, Barter G, Hawkins D, Gazzard BG. Simultaneous treatment of cytomegalovirus retinitis with ganciclovir and foscarnet [letter]. Lancet 1991;338:250.

19. Cochereau-Massin I, LeHoang P, Lautier-Frau M, et al. Efficacy and tolerance of intravitreal ganciclovir in cytomegalovirus retinitis in acquired immune deficiency syndrome. Ophthalmology 1991;98:1348–1355.

20. Heinemann MH. Long-term intravitreal ganciclovir therapy for cytomegalovirus retinopathy. Arch Ophthalmol 1989;107:1767–1772.

21. Martin DF, Parks DJ, Mellow SD, Ferris FL, Walton RC, Remaley NA, et al. Treatment of cytomegalovirus retinitis with an intraocular sustained-release ganciclovir implant. A randomized controlled clinical trial. Arch Ophthalmol 1994;112:1531–1539.

22. Pepose JS, Holland GN, Nestor MS, Cochran AJ, Foos RY. Acquired immune deficiency syndrome: pathogenic mechanisms of ocular disease. Ophthalmology 1985;92:472–84.

23. Holland GN, Shuler JD. Progression rates of cytomegalovirus retinopathy in ganciclovir-treated and untreated patients. Arch Ophthalmol 1992;110:1435–1442.

24. Schanzer MC, Font RL, O'Malley RE. Primary ocular malignant lymphoma associated with the acquired immune deficiency syndrome. Ophthalmology 1991;98:88–91.

25. Margolis TP, Lowder CY, Holland GN, et al. Varicella-zoster virus retinitis in patients with the acquired immunodeficiency syndrome. Am J Ophthalmol 1991;112:119–131.

26. Engstrom RE, Holland GN, Margolis TP, Muccioli C, Lindley JI, Belfort R, et al. The progressive outer retinal necrosis syndrome: A variant of necrotizing herpetic retinopathy in patients with AIDS. Ophthalmology 1994;101:1488–1502.

27. Johnston WH, Holland GN, Engstrom RE, Rimmer SO. Recurrence of presumed varicella-zoster virus retinopathy in patients with acquired immunodeficiency syndrome. Am J Ophthalmol 1993;116:42–50.

28. Holland GN, Engstrom RE, Glasgow BJ, et al. Ocular toxoplasmosis in patients with the acquired immunodeficiency syndrome. Am J Ophthalmol 1988;106:653–667.

29. Holland GN. Ocular toxoplasmosis in the immunocompromised host. Int Ophthalmol 1989;13:399–402.

30. Gagliuso DJ, Teich SA, Friedman AH, Orellana J. Ocular toxoplasmosis in AIDS patients. Trans Am Ophthalmol Soc 1990;88:63–86.

31. Engstrom RE, Holland GN, Nussenblatt RB, Jabs DA. Current practices in the management of ocular toxoplasmosis. Am J Ophthalmol 1991;111:601–610.

32. Lopez JS, de Smet MD, Masur H, Mueller BU, Pizzo PA, Nussenblatt RB. Orally administered 566C80 for treatment of ocular toxoplasmosis in a patient with the acquired immunodeficiency syndrome. Am J Ophthalmol 1992;113:331–333.

33. Gass JDM, Braunstein RA, Chenoweth RG. Acute syphilitic posterior placoid chorioretinitis. Ophthalmology 1990;97:1288–1297.

34. McLeish WM, Pulido JS, Holland S, Culbertson WW, Winward K. The ocular manifestations of syphilis in the human immunodeficiency virus type 1-infected host. Ophthalmology 1990;97:196–203.

35. Stoumbos VD, Klein ML. Syphilitic retinitis in a patient with acquired immunodeficiency syndrome-related complex. Am J Ophthalmol 1987;103:103–104.

36. Schuman JS, Orellana J, Friedman AH, Teich SA. Acquired immunodeficiency syndrome (AIDS). Surv Ophthalmol 1987;31:384–410.

37. Denning DW, Armstrong RW, Fishman M, Stevens DA. Endophthalmitis in a patient with disseminated cryptococcosis and AIDS who was treated with itraconazole. Rev Infect Dis 1991;13:1126–1130.

38. Schuman JS, Friedman AH. Retinal manifestations of the acquired immune deficiency syndrome (AIDS): cytomegalovirus, *Candida albicans, Cryptococcus,* toxoplasmosis, and *Pneumocystis carinii.* Trans Ophthalmol Soc UK 1983;103:177–190.

39. Winward KE, Hamed LM, Glaser JS. The spectrum of optic nerve disease in human immunodeficiency virus infection. Am J Ophthalmol 1989;107:373–380.

40. Carney MD, Combs JL, Waschler W. Cryptococcal choroiditis. Retina 1990;10:27–32.

41. Macher A, Rodrigues MM, Kaplan W, et al. Disseminated bilateral chorioretinitis due to *Histoplasma capsulatum* in a patient with the acquired immunodeficiency syndrome. Ophthalmology 1985;92:1159–1164.

42. Specht CS, Mitchell KT, Bauman AE, Gupta M. Ocular histoplasmosis with retinitis in a patient with acquired immune deficiency syndrome. Ophthalmology 1991;98:1356–1359.
43. Blodi BA, Johnson MW, McLeish WM, Gass JD. Presumed choroidal tuberculosis in a human immunodeficiency virus infected host. Am J Ophthalmol 1989;108:605–607.
44. Croxatto JO, Mestre C, Puente S, Gonzalez G. Nonreactive tuberculosis in a patient with acquired immune deficiency syndrome. Am J Ophthalmol 1986;102:659–660.
45. Menezo JL, Martinez-Costa R, Marin F, Vilanova E, Cortes-Vizcaino V. Tuberculous panophthalmitis associated with drug abuse. Intl Ophthalmol 1987;10:235–240.
46. Holland GN, MacArthur LJ, Foos RY. Choroidal pneumocystosis. Arch Ophthalmol 1991;109:1454–1455.
47 Shami MJ, Freeman W, Friedberg D, Siderides E, Listhaus A, Ai E. A multicenter center study of Pneumocystis choroidopathy. Am J Ophthalmol 1991;112:15–22.
48. Koser MW, Jampol LM, MacDonell K. Treatment of *Pneumocystis carinii* choroidopathy. Arch Ophthalmol 1990;108:1214–1215.
49. Dugel PU, Rao NA, Forster DJ, Chong LP, Frangieh GT, Sattler F. *Pneumocystis carinii* choroiditis after long-term aerosolized pentamidine therapy. Am J Ophthalmol 1990; 110:113–117.
50. Engstrom RE, Holland GN. Chronic herpes zoster virus keratitis associated with the acquired immunodeficiency syndrome. Am J Ophthalmol 1988;105:556–558.
51. Young TL, Robin JB, Holland GN, et al. Herpes simplex keratitis in patients with acquired immune deficiency syndrome. Ophthalmology 1989;96:1476–1479.
52. Shuler JD, Holland GN, Miles SA, Miller BJ, Grossman I. Kaposi sarcoma of the conjunctiva and eyelids associated with the acquired immunodeficiency syndrome. Arch Ophthalmol 1989;107:858–862.
53. Antle CM, White VA, Horsman DE, Rootman J. Large cell orbital lymphoma in a patient with acquired immune deficiency syndrome: case report and review. Ophthalmology 1990;97:1494–1498.
54. Friedman DI. Neuro-ophthalmic manifestations of human immunodeficiency virus infection. Neurologic Clin 1991;9:55–72.
55. Keane JR. Neuro-ophthalmologic signs of AIDS: 50 patients. Neurology 1991;41: 841–845.
56. Mansour AM. Neuro-ophthalmic findings in acquired immunodeficiency syndrome. J Clin Neuro Ophthalmol 1990;10:167–174.

Oral Manifestations

Most of the oral diseases occurring in persons with HIV infection, can also be encountered in persons who are not infected. Importantly, in the HIV-positive patient, the oral lesions are more widespread, manifest atypical clinical features and persist longer than in seronegative individuals (1,2). In most cases, soft tissue biopsy will be needed to confirm any clinical suspicions. Oral manifestations common in persons with HIV infection are summarized below.

Candidiasis

Candidiasis is a superficial fungus infection caused by *Candida albicans* or, occasionally, other species of Candida (3,4). Often, this is encountered among patients with a recent history of antibiotic therapy or among immunocompromised patients. The oral lesions are clinically characteristic, assuming three forms: (a) pseudomembranous, (b) erythematous, and (c) angular cheilitis. Multiple curdled mild-appearing papules characterize the pseudomembranous type and are distributed throughout the oral cavity. They may be associated with an erythematous base. These white plaques and papules may be generally dislodged with a firm scraping of a tongue blade. A cytologic smear should be procured and submitted to the oral pathology laboratory for a statin to demonstrate fungal mycelia. The erythematous form may show a concomitant white component or may appear exclusively as diffuse red macules. In angular cheilitis, the oral commissures are ulcerated and red.

Hairy Leukoplakia

Hairy leukoplakia is a viral infection of the tongue that appears to be specific to HIV-positive patients (5–7). This white plaque is found primarily along the lateral border of the tongue with occasional localization on the ventral surface. These lesions cannot be rubbed away. Vertical white stria are aligned about a white plaque and resemble a radiating fringe of hairy-like configurations. Microscopic features of this lesion resemble flat genital warts. The surface parakeratin layer may be colonized by candida hyphae and has a thickened appearance. The upper spinous epithelial cells show a hollow appearance and are termed koilocytes. These cells are infected by Epstein-Barr virus. Progression to AIDS has been observed in over 20% of patients with hairy leukoplakia who were followed 16 to 24 months. Unlike other forms of oral leukoplakia, this HIV/EBV-associated lesion is not precancerous.

Condyloma Acuminatum

Condylomas or genital warts are benign papillomatous lesions caused by the human papilloma virus (HPV) (8). Oral mucosal condylomas are occasionally present in persons without HIV infection, however they are more common among homosexuals, particularly those with concurrent HIV infection. Condylomas can be sexually transmitted and therefore can be passed to oral mucosa as a consequence of genital-oral contact. These oral lesions are most commonly seen on the lips, gingiva and tongue, appearing as cauliflower-shaped papillary masses with a tendency for multiplicity, although they can appear as multiple papules resembling focal epithelial hyperplasia (Heck's disease).

Herpetic Gingivostomatitis

Herpes simplex viruses (HSV) cause primary and recurrent infections in the oral cavity (HSV type 1) (9–11). Although HSV type 2 is generally sexually transmitted and associated with penile, vulvar or vaginal infections; genital-oral transmission of HSV 2 occurs commonly among both homosexuals and heterosexuals. Most persons have been exposed to HSV and possess circulating antiherpes antibodies by age 21, and the vast majority of the population experience subclinical infection. Immunity to HSV 1 does not always confer immunity to HSV 2. Clinical features are the same for both types 1 and 2. Vesicles appear on the mucosa of the lips, tongue and buccal mucosa as well as on the gingiva. The primary infection resembles acute necrotizing ulcerative gingivitis, yet it is associated with fever. Secondary herpes infections are localized to the lips and focal areas of the oral cavity. The lesions are usually more severe and widespread among persons with HIV infection than those seen in persons who are HIV negative.

Shingles

Shingles (zoster) is a unilateral cutaneous vesicular eruption, caused by a latent infection of varicella-zoster virus (2,9). Shingles usually occurs on the skin of the trunk and in people over 50 years of age. Persons with HIV infection are prone to develop zoster with a more severe clinical course; the lesions can be orofacial and involve the trigeminal nerve pathways. Zoster or shingles is uncommon in healthy young adults.

Atypical Tuberculosis

This is caused by *Mycobacterium avium intracellular*, a bacterium that is localized to tissue sites other than the pulmonary tract, as seen in the usual form of tuberculosis. There have been cases of *Mycobacterium avium intracellular* that involve the oral mucosa. The oral lesions appear as a moveable tumefactions or nodules, and biopsy is required to obtain a definitive diagnosis. Similarly, granulomatous fungi, particularly histoplasmosis, may present in the oral cavity as nonhealing tumefactive ulcerations (12).

Pigmented Macules

Melanotic pigmentation is reported to occur in the mouth among HIV-infected patients and is not associated with Addison's disease. The oral pigmentations are macular and usually multifocal involving the buccal mucosa and palate (13).

Oral Ulcers

Aphthous-like ulcerations are common in HIV-infected tissues and may be solitary or multiple in nature. These ulcers can be deep, over one centimeter in diameter and are very painful. They may persist for many weeks and may not heal without steroid therapy. Biopsy must be performed to rule out a specific viral etiology since some of these ulcers can be caused by cytomegalovirus (2,3,14)

Kaposi's Sarcoma

Kaposi's sarcoma (KS) is a malignant vascular neoplasm with multicentric distribution located primarily in cutaneous tissues and lymph nodes. Most cases of KS in patients with HIV infection appear in an nonaggressive form and KS lesions will appear on the trunk, limbs, head and neck, tip of the nose and oral mucosa. The lesions may begin as pink, red or violet macules, papules or nodules that often coalesce into large plaques. Internal organs are commonly involved, particularly the lungs, gastrointestinal tract and lymphatic system. Oral KS lesions most commonly occur on the palate, but may also be present on the gingiva or lip (15,16). Oral lesions may be asymptomatic or go unnoticed until swelling or bleeding from trauma. Intralesional injection of sclerosing agents (3% sodium tetradecyl sulfate) can eliminate mucosal lesions (17).

Lymphoma

Lymphoma is the second leading malignancy in persons with HIV infection. Lymphomas in these persons have been marked by poor response to treatment, rapid progression and death. The clinical appearance of intraoral lymphomas may be nonspecific intraoral swelling, nodule or mass (18,19). Cervical and/or submandibular lymphadenopathy may or may not be present. The intraoral lesions may appear to be fibrous growth, a granular type of reactive tissue surrounding a tooth or a nonspecific nodular ulceration. Lesions of these types should be submitted for histologic diagnosis.

REFERENCES

1. Silverman S Jr, Migliorati DA Lozada-Nur F, et al. Oral findings in people with or at high risk for AIDS: a study of 375 homosexual males. J Am Dent Assoc 1986; 112:187–192.
2. Reichart P, Gelderblom HR, Becker J, Kuntz A. AIDS and the oral cavity: the HIV-infection—virology, etiology, origin, immunology, precautions and clinical observations in 110 patients. Int J Oral Maxillofac Surg, 1987;16:129–153.
3. Lynch DP. Oral Candidiasis. Oral Surg Oral Med Oral Pathol, 1994;78:189–193.
4. Challacombe, SJ. Immunologic aspects of oral candidiasis. Oral Surg Oral Med Oral Path 1994;78:202–210.
5. Greenspan D, Greenspan JS, Conant M, Petersen V, Silverman S Jr, DeSouza Y. Oral 'hairy' leucoplakia in male homosexuals: evidence of association with both papillomavirus and a herpes-group virus. Lancet 1984;2:831–832.
6. Eversole LR, Stone CE, Beckman AM. Detection of EBV and HPV DNA sequences in oral hairy leukoplakia by in-situ hybridization. J Med Virol 1988;26:271–277.
7. Ficarra G, Barone R, Gaglioti D, et al. Oral hairy leukoplakia among intravenous drug abusers: a clinicopathologic and ultrastructural study. Oral Surg Oral Med Oral Pathol 1988;65:421–426.
8. De Villiers E-M. Prevalence of HPV-7 papillomas in the oral mucosa and facial skin of patients with human immunodeficiency virus. Arch Dermatol 1989;125:1590.
9. Eversole LR. Viral Infections of the head and neck among HIV-seropositive patients. Oral Surg Oral Med Oral Pathol 1992;73:155–163.
10. Glick M, Muzyka BC, Lurie D, Salkin LM. Oral manifestations associated with HIV-related disease as markers for immune suppression and AIDS. Oral Surg Oral Med Oral Pathol 1994;77:344–349.
11. Greenspan D, Greenspan J, Pindborg JJ, Schiødt M. AIDS and the dental team. Copenhagen: Munksgaard, 1986.
12. Samaranayake L. Oral mycoses in HIV infection. Oral Surg Oral Med Oral Pathol 1992;73:171–180.
13. Ficarra G, Shillitoe EJ, Adler-Storthz K, et al. Oral melanotic macules in patients infected with HIV. Oral Surg Oral Med Oral Pathol 1990;70:748–755.
14. Scully C. McCarthy G. Management of oral health in persons with HIV infection. Oral Surg Oral Med Oral Pathol 1992;73:215–225.
15. Ficarra G, Berson AM, Silverman S Jr, et al. Kaposi's sarcoma of the oral cavity: a study of 134 patients with a review of the pathogenesis, epidemiology, clinical aspects and treatment. Oral Surg Oral Med Oral Pathol 1988;66:543–550.
16. Epstein JB, Lozada-Nur F, McLeod WA, Spinelli J, Oral Kaposi's sarcoma in acquired immunodeficiency syndrome: review of management and report of the efficacy of intralesional vinblastine. Cancer 1989;64:2424–2430.
17. Lucatorto FM, Sapp JP. Treatment of oral Kaposi's sarcoma with a sclerosing agent in AIDS patients. Oral Surg Oral Med Oral Pathol 1993;75:192–198.

18. Green TL, Eversole LR. Oral lymphomas in HIV-infected patients: association with Epstein-Barr virus DNA. Oral Surg Oral Med Oral Pathol 1989;67:437–442.
19. Ficarra G, Eversole LR. HIV related tumors of the oral cavity. Crit Rev Oral Biol Med 1994;5:159–185.

Tuberculosis and HIV Infection

Epidemiology

After three decades of declining rates of tuberculosis (TB), the number of reported TB cases increased in 1986. Between 1985 to 1993, the Centers for Disease Control (CDC) reported a 20% increase in the cases of tuberculosis (1). Several observations suggest that the HIV epidemic has played a major role in the resurgence of tuberculosis: a) the largest numbers of TB cases have been reported from large urban areas with high HIV seroprevalence rates; b) African-Americans and Hispanics between the ages of 25-44 years have the highest cumulative incidence of AIDS and the greatest reported increases in tuberculosis incidence; c) estimates of HIV seroprevalence rates in TB clinics have ranged between 0–46%, and high rates of HIV co-infection in TB patients have been found in the homeless, intravenous drug users, prison inmates, and patients seen in county hospital TB clinics; and d) individuals infected with *M. tuberculosis,* have a 100-fold greater risk of developing active TB if they are also HIV infected (1–6). In 1993, the case definition for acquired immunodeficiency syndrome (AIDS), which already included extrapulmonary TB, was expanded to include pulmonary TB as an AIDS-defining illness (7). Most cases of tuberculosis in HIV-infected patients are due to reactivation of previous infection. However, the presence of HIV infection also greatly increases the risk of clinical tuberculosis in those recently exposed to a TB contact. Tuberculosis usually occurs at an earlier stage than other opportunistic illnesses in HIV-infected patients. Since tuberculosis may be the first recognized manifestation of HIV infection, HIV testing is recommended for all newly diagnosed cases of TB, which will allow early identification of HIV infection and initiation of appropriate antiretroviral and prophylactic therapy (1,3–6,8).

MULTIDRUG-RESISTANT TUBERCULOSIS

The emergence of multidrug-resistant (MDR) TB has become a serious public health problem. In 1991, 33% of all isolates of TB in New York City were resistant to at least one drug and 19% were resistant to isoniazid and rifampin (9). Outbreaks of MDR-TB have occurred in institutional settings such as hospitals and correctional facilities. In most institutional outbreaks, a high prevalence of HIV infection has been found in MDR-TB cases; HIV-infected cases with tuberculosis also experienced a short interval from diagnosis to death (4 to 16 weeks), with a mortality rate of 72 to 89%. Delays in appropriate anti-tuberculosis therapy for MDR-TB patients contributed to the high mortality rate and prolonged infectiousness observed during these outbreaks (6,9–12).

Transmission and Pathogenesis

Tuberculosis is a bacterial disease caused by *Mycobacterium tuberculosis*. TB is spread to a susceptible person (contact) primarily through airborne droplets produced by coughing or sneezing in patients with pulmonary or laryngeal disease. Tubercle bacilli enter the alveoli, multiply and establish infection. Later, these organisms spread through lymphatic channels to regional lymph nodes and then to distant organs via the blood stream. The tuberculin skin test is used to identify individuals infected with *M. tuberculosis*. A significant test reaction usually occurs within 3 months following initial infection (10, 13).

Close contacts of untreated cases of pulmonary tuberculosis are at high risk of becoming infected with the tubercle bacilli. Approximately 30% of close contacts (e.g., household members) will develop latent infection with *M. tuberculosis* (2). The highest rates or tuberculous infection are seen in contacts of cases with cavitary lung disease and positive acid-fast bacilli (AFB) sputum smears. About 10% of individuals with positive tuberculin skin tests will develop active disease over their lifetime, the risk being greatest within the first 2 years after infection, unless they receive preventive therapy. However, the risk of tuberculosis is much higher in HIV-infected individuals. HIV-infected individuals with positive tuberculin skin tests have an 8–10% chance per year of developing active tuberculosis. In one study, clinical disease occurred in 37% of HIV-infected contacts of TB cases within five months of exposure (4,8,14).

Clinical Features of Tuberculosis in HIV Infection

Tuberculosis may occur at any time during HIV infection. Although active TB most commonly affects the lungs, any organ may be involved, and disseminated (miliary) disease may be the initial presentation. The clinical presentation of TB is dependent on the degree of immune suppression. Patients with relatively preserved immune function, with CD4+ cell counts above 200/mm^3, are more likely to have classic upper lobe disease and cavitary changes characteristic of reactivation disease. Although tuberculosis should be suspected in any HIV-infected patient with pulmonary systems, clinical symptomatology, such as fevers, sweats, cough and weight loss, are not helpful in distinguishing TB from other opportunistic illnesses. Extrapulmonary TB frequently occurs with HIV infection, and is seen in close to 70% of patients with CD4+ cell counts less than 100/mm^3. Patients with miliary tuberculosis may have involvement of any organ including the gastrointestinal tract, central nervous system, bone marrow and skin. Since extrapulmonary disease is common in HIV-infected individuals, and classic pulmonary symptoms may be absent, any patient with a persistent, unexplained fever should be evaluated for TB (4, 5, 14,15).

DIAGNOSIS

Initial evaluation of patients should include a physical examination, a tuberculin skin test, chest radiography and microscopic examination and culture of sputum and other appropriate clinical specimens (e.g., blood, urine). Three serial sputa for AFB stains and cultures should be obtained, preferably morning specimens which have the highest yield of acid-fast bacilli. Chest radiographic features suggestive of tuberculosis include cavitation and upper lobe infiltrates in patients with CD4+ counts above 200/mm^3. Radiographs from patients more severely immunosuppressed may show a miliary pattern and hilar lymphadenopathy. Apical or subapical abnormalities obscured by bony structures can be further evaluated by obtaining lordotic views. Other HIV infected processes, such as pneumocystic pneumonia (PCP), fungal diseases, cytomegalovirus (CMV) infection, and neoplasms may present with similar findings suggestive of tuberculosis. In addition, TB may occur simultaneously with other opportunistic illnesses such as PCP (4). The lack of positive acid-fast smears should not rule out presumptive TB and delay therapy, as smears may be negative in over 50% of HIV-infected patients, especially in patients without cavitary disease. Cavitation on chest radiograph is strongly associated with positive acid-fast smears. Bronchoscopy with lavage and transbronchial biopsy will aid in the diagnosis of TB in patients when the diagnosis remains uncertain (5,16).

Clinical specimens from nonpulmonary sites (e.g., blood, urine, cerebrospinal fluid, stool, bone marrow) should be submitted if extrapulmonary disease is suspected. Additional imaging modalities may be used such as computerized tomography and magnetic resonance imaging, to evaluate extrathoracic disease. Lymphadenitis and bacteremia are the most frequently reported extrapulmonary sites of disease. Tuberculous lymphadenitis may be diagnosed by lymph node aspiration, which yields acid-fast organisms in over 65% of patients with lymphadenitis. Distinguishing *M. tuberculosis* infection from that due to atypical mycobacteria, which may also cause enlarged lymph nodes with positive AFB smears, depends on culture results, although the presence of tender lymphadenopathy with abnormal chest radiographic findings is more typical of infection with *M. tuberculosis*. Histologic examination of lymph node or other biopsy specimens may not show the characteristic caseating granulomas. Fluorochrome staining of tissue may be useful in identifying mycobacteria pending culture results. Blood cultures are positive in 26–42% of HIV-infected patients with tuberculosis using the lysis-centrifugation method. Positive blood cultures are more likely to be found in patients with less than 100/mm^3 CD4+ cell counts (4,5,14,16)

Tuberculous meningitis occurs five times more frequently in HIV-infected patients compared to other populations. Patients typically present with headache, fevers and altered mental status. Cranial nerve deficits may be presented on exam. Computerized tomography is used to define the presence and extent of hydrocephalus, basilar meningitis and cerebral infarction. Tuberculous may be seen as mass lesions and are usually ring-enhancing. Examination of spinal fluid typically demonstrates a pleocytosis with a lymphocytic predominance, low glucose, and high protein. One-third or less of CSF specimens will have positive acid-fast smears, although serial lumbar punctures with larger volumes of CSF will increase this yield. Patients presenting with persistent abdominal pain or fever should be evaluated for intraabdominal disease, which is characterized most frequently by regional lymphadenopathy. Hepatic and splenic abscesses can be evaluated using ultrasonography or computerized tomography. Genitourinary involvement is diagnosed through microscopic examination of first-morning voided urine specimens or specimens of cervical discharge and endometrial (4,5,14–16).

Mycobacterial cultures are necessary to confirm the diagnosis of tuberculosis and to evaluate drug susceptibilities. It normally takes up to 6 weeks for culture results to be obtained, although radiometric testing using BACTEC shortens this interval to 2 weeks. Diagnostic tests are available to rapidly identify *M. tuberculosis* from sputum and other specimens. Rapid direct tests on smears include fluorochrome stains, ELISA, and agglutination tests. Highly sensitive assays, such as gas chromatography for tuberculostearic acid, and nucleic acid detection by polymerase chain reaction (PCR) may be useful tools in the future when TB is clinically suspected and specimens are acid-fast smear negative. The use of the BACTEC radiometric system with DNA probes reduces the time in differentiating *M. tuberculosis* from other mycobacterial species to 10–14 days. At the present, serologic assays for antimycobacterial antibodies do not appear to be useful in the diagnosis of tuberculosis. Research tools to rapidly identify drug resistance are under development and appear promising (e.g., luciferase reporter assay) (5,14,16).

Treatment of Tuberculosis

PULMONARY TUBERCULOSIS

Delays in the diagnosis and treatment of pulmonary TB contribute to increased morbidity, and mortality, and nosocomial spread of tuberculosis. Empiric treatment for tuberculosis should be considered in patients with respiratory symptoms and compatible chest radiographs, regardless of sputum AFB smear results. Standard antituberculosis drug regimens are extremely effective in treating most HIV-infected patients with TB. Because the frequency of drug-resistant TB is rising in many parts of the United States, initial treatment requires administration of three or four drugs until drug susceptibilities are available. Drug susceptibility testing should be done initially on all *M. tuberculosis* isolates. Drug susceptibilities should also be obtained on patients who have persistently positive mycobacterial cultures after 2 months of appropriate therapy or if there is clinical evidence of failure to respond to therapy (17,18).

Effective therapy for TB is divided into 2 phases: an initial 2-month bactericidal phase and a sterilizing phase which is 4 months or longer. The recommended treatment options are outlined in Table 4.19. A four-drug regimen which includes isoniazid (INH), rifampin (RIF), pyrazinamide (PZA), and ethambutol (EMB) is preferred for the initial, empiric treatment of pulmonary tuberculosis. Streptomycin (SM) may be substituted for ethambutol in patients who cannot take that drug. Sputum conversion is accomplished more rapidly with a four-drug regimen,

Table 4.19.

Regimen Options for the Initial Treatment of TB in HIV-infected Patients[1]

Option 1	Option 2
Administer daily isoniazid, rifampin, and pyrazinamide for 8 weeks, followed by 16 weeks of isoniazid and rifampin. Ethambutol (or streptomycin) should be added to the initial regimen until isoniazid and rifampin sensitivities are established.[1] An expert in the treatment of tuberculosis should be consulted if the patient continues to be symptomatic or if the smear/culture is positive after 3 months of therapy.	Administer daily isoniazid, rifampin, pyrazinamide, and ethambutol (or streptomycin)[1] for 2 weeks followed by 2 times/weekly administration of the same drugs for 6 weeks (by DOT).[2,3] Thereafter, continue isoniazid and rifampin twice weekly for 16 weeks (by DOT).[4] An expert in the treatment of tuberculosis should be consulted if the patient continues to be symptomatic or if the patient continues to be symptomatic or if the smear/culture is positive after 3 months of therapy.

Adapted from American Thoracic Society. Treatment of tuberculosis and tuberculosis infection in adults and children. Am J Respir Crit Care Med 1994;149:1365.
[1]Unless local INH resistance documented to be <4%.
[2]Directly-observed therapy
[3]DOT may be given 3 times/weekly; some authors recommend DOT 3 times/weekly immediately after the diagnosis of TB.
[4]Unless susceptibility studies indicate isoniazid or rifampin in resistance.

and most patients will receive an adequate regimen even if they are found to have isolated INH or RIF resistance. In patients with a low risk of infection with drug-resistant TB (i.e., no prior history of TB treatment, no known exposure to drug-resistant cases, community drug resistance <4%, and not from a country with an increased level of drug resistance), therapy may be initiated with INH, RIF, and PZA. When drug susceptibility data are available, the regimen should be altered as appropriate. In patients with drug-susceptible TB, a 6-month regimen of INH, RIF and PZA given for 8 weeks, followed by INH and RIF for 16 weeks is recommended. Ethambutol (or streptomycin), which should be included in the *initial* regimen unless there is little possibility of drug resistance, may be discontinued once drug susceptibilities demonstrate pansensitivity (18). In patients who cannot tolerate PZA, a 9-month regimen of INH and RIF is also acceptable. Although 6-month regimens have been proven to be effective in HIV-infected patients, it is important to periodically evaluate the clinical and bacteriologic response to therapy. Patients may need a longer duration of therapy if response to treatment is suboptimal (17,18).

Drug susceptibility tests may be unavailable because they were not initially performed or cultures were negative. In this situation, regimens should be based on the probability of drug resistance locally. If the prevalence of INH resistance is ≥ 4%, EMB or SM should be continued along with INH and RIF for the entire course of therapy (17). Table 4.20 summarizes the dosage recommendations for drugs used in the initial treatment of tuberculosis.

Table 4.20.

Recommended Drugs for the Initial Treatment of Tuberculosis in Children and Adults

Drug	Daily Dose (mg/kg)		Maximum Daily Dose in Children & Adults	Twice Weekly Dose (mg/kg)	
	Children	Adults		Children	Adults
Isoniazid[a,b]	10–20	5	300 mg	20–40 Max. 900 mg	15 Max. 900 mg
Rifampin[a]	10–20	10	600 mg	10–20 Max. 600 mg	10 Max. 600 mg
Pyrazinamide	15–30	15–30	2 gm	50–70 Max. 4 gm	50–70 Max. 4 gm.
Ethambutol[c]	15–25	15–25	2.5 gm	50 Max. 2.5 gm	50 Max. 2.5 gm
Streptomycin[d,e,f]	20–40	15	1 gm	25–30 Max. 1.5 gm	25–30 Max. 1.5 gm

Adapted from CDC. Initial therapy for tuberculosis & tuberculosis infection in adults and children. MMWR 1993;42 (No. RR-7)
[a]Isoniazid and rifampin available as a combination capsule (Rifamate) containing 150 mg of isoniazid and 300 mg of rifampin. A combination of isoniazid, rifampin and pyrazinamide in a single tablet (Rifater) is being introduced.
[b]Pyridoxine should be given in patients who may be malnourished (e.g., AIDS, alcoholism), pregnant or diabetic.
[c]Daily dose 25 mg/kg for the first 4–8 weeks or if isolate is INH-resistant.
[d]Available from Pfizer (800-254-4445).
[e]In persons 60 years or older, the daily dose should be limited to 10 mg/kg daily with a maximum dose of 750 mg; decrease dose in renal insufficiency.
[f]Given intramuscularly.

TREATMENT OF PATIENTS WITH DRUG RESISTANCE

For patients initially started on the recommended 4-drug regimen and found to have isolated INH resistance, INH should be discontinued and PZA continued along with RIF and EMB for the entire 6 months. Alternatively, patients may be treated with RIF and EMB for a minimum of 12 months. For patients initially started on INH and RIF and found to have isolated INH resistance, repeat susceptibilities should be obtained, INH should be discontinued, and 2 new drugs (e.g., PZA, EMB) added to PIF until results of the repeat susceptibilities are available. Solitary rifampin resistance may be treated with INH and EMB, with or without PZA. In HIV-infected patients with drug-resistance TB, a longer duration of therapy may be necessary if the clinical and bacteriological response to therapy is suboptimal. Some experts recommend that INH or PIF resistance be treated for a minimum of 18 months, or 1 year past sputum conversion (whichever is longer) (17,19). HIV-infected patients with drug-resistant TB should receive directly-observed therapy to assure compliance with antituberculosis regimens (see below).

The presence of INH and RIF resistance is associated with treatment failure rates up to 70% and a high mortality rate in HIV-infected patients. Consequently, at least three effective agents should be used to treat multiple-drug resistant (MDR) TB, based on drug susceptibilities, and four or five agents may be preferable (18–20). In cases of tuberculosis occurring after exposure to drug-resistant TB cases, the initial regimen is based upon drug susceptibilities from the contact case (17,18). Table 4.21 lists some of the second-line agents used for drug-resistant cases. The drug regimen and duration of therapy for patients with drug-resistant tuberculosis should be determined with the assistance of physicians experienced in the treatment of tuberculosis.

EXTRAPULMONARY TUBERCULOSIS

Regimens which are adequate for the treatment of pulmonary TB are generally effective in treating extrapulmonary disease (13). Although a 6–9 month duration of treatment appears to be sufficient to treat many sites of extrapulmonary disease, a longer duration of therapy (12 months) is recommended for some sites including miliary TB, bone or joint disease, and tuberculosis meningitis in infants and children. In addition, higher doses of isoniazid (10 mg/kg) is recommended for tuberculosis meningitis. Adjunctive therapy, such as surgery or corticosteroids, may also be necessary in the prevention or treatment of complications of extrapulmonary TB (e.g., constrictive pericarditis, tuberculosis meningitis) (17,18).

TREATMENT OF INFANTS AND CHILDREN

The same drug regimens used in adults may be used in infants and children; however, the dosage will vary (Table 4.20). In children whose visual acuity cannot be monitored, the use of EMB is generally not rec-

Table 4.21.

Second-line Drugs Used in the Treatment of Multidrug-resistant Tuberculosis

Drug	Dosage in Adults (Daily)	Dosage in Children (Daily)
Capreomycin[a]	15 mg/kg IM	15–30 mg/kg
Kanamycin[a]	15 mg/kg IM, IV	15–30 mg/kg
Amikacin[a]	15 mg/kg IM, IV	15–30 mg/kg
Ethionamide[a]	250–500 mg bid PO	15–20 mg/kg[d]
Para-amino salicylic acid (PAS)[b,c]	4–6 gm bid[e] PO	150 mg/kg[d]
Cycloserine[a,f]	250–500 mg bid PO	10–20 mg/kg
Ciprofloxacin	500–750 mg bid[e] PO	Not recommended
Ofloxacin	300–400 mg bid[e] PO	Not recommended
Clofazamine[g]	100–200 mg PO	1 mg/kg

Adapted from The Medical Letter 1993;35(908):101.
[a]Dosage not to exceed 1 gm
[b]Available from the CDC (404-639-8123)
[c]Dosage not to exceed 12 gm
[d]In divided doses
[e]Some authorities recommend that this drug be given in one single dose.
[f]Some authors recommend pyridoxine 50 mg for every 250 mg of cycloserine to decrease the incidence of psychiatric effects.
[g]Efficacy unproven

ommended except in cases with drug-resistance. Infants are at particular risk for dissemination of tuberculosis, regardless of HIV status, therefore evaluation and treatment need to be initiated immediately if TB is suspected. Clinical isolates for susceptibility studies may be difficult to obtain from young children, therefore the choice of drugs will depend on the drug susceptibility pattern of the adult source case. Extrapulmonary TB, including lymphadenitis, can be treated with the same 6- or 9-month regimen as with pulmonary TB. A 12-month regimen is recommended for miliary TB, bone or joint disease, and tuberculosis meningitis (17,18,21).

TREATMENT DURING PREGNANCY AND LACTATION

Effective therapy for tuberculosis should not be delayed because of pregnancy. Initial therapy usually includes INH and RIF, with EMB if INH resistance is suspected. Pyrazinamide is not routinely used because of limited teratogenicity data. The use of streptomycin is contraindicated because of its association with ototoxicity in the fetus. Pyridoxine should be given during treatment with isoniazid. In the setting of multiple drug resistance, the risks and benefits of PZA and other second-line agents will need to be considered. The small concentrations of antituberculosis drugs excreted in breast milk should not discourage breast feeding in mothers receiving treatment for tuberculosis. Some authors recommend that mothers take their medications after breast feeding with the substitution of a bottle at the next feeding (17,18)

DIRECTLY-OBSERVED THERAPY

Noncompliance with antituberculosis therapy is a major factor in the development of drug-resistant TB and treatment failure. The use of directly-observed therapy (DOT) allows for the supervised administration of medications two or three times a week by a health worker. There is no evidence that intermittent therapy is less effective in those who are HIV-infected. DOT therapy should be considered for all new HIV-infected patients diagnosed with pulmonary TB and is necessary for any patients with drug resistance (9,18). In addition, DOT should be used for patients who are at high risk for non-compliance (e.g., intravenous drug users), who have not converted sputum cultures after 2 months of therapy or who are documented treatment failures/relapses (17). The dosage recommendations for initial drug therapy for both daily and intermittent treatment are shown in Table 4.20.

EVALUATION OF RESPONSE TO TREATMENT

The effectiveness of an anti-tuberculosis regimen may be assessed by several measures. The most effective means of assessing therapeutic response in patients with pulmonary TB is through monthly sputums for acid-fast smears and cultures. More than 85% of patients will convert their sputum from positive to negative after 2 months of therapy which includes isoniazid and rifampin. Patients with negative sputum cultures after 2 months of therapy should have at least one additional AFB smear and culture by completion of therapy (18). Persistently positive sputum cultures after 2–3 months of therapy suggests the possibility of disease due to drug-resistant organisms or non-compliance with therapy. Additionally, patients with AIDS are at increased risk of malabsorption of antituberculosis drugs resulting in lower serum drug levels. In the treatment of MDR-TB, these decreased serum levels may contribute to treatment failure. Therapeutic drug monitoring of serum levels in HIV-infected patients who fail to respond to appropriate therapy may optimize management.

A follow-up chest radiograph should be obtained at completion of treatment. Patients with significant residual radiographic findings should have another chest radiograph in 6 months. In patients who were treated presumptively for TB, because of inability to obtain a microbiologic diagnosis or negative cultures, response to therapy should be guided by clinical examinations and a follow-up chest radiograph at 3 months. Failure of radiographic abnormalities to improve after 3 months of therapy should lead to reexamination of the diagnosis.

Evaluation of response to treatment of extrapulmonary TB should be individualized according to the site and extent of disease. For example, clinical examination, radiographic modalities (e.g., computerized tomography), and bacteriologic examination of urine specimens are used to evaluate response to therapy in patients with TB lymphadenitis, intraabdominal TB, and genitourinary TB respectively.

DRUG TOXICITY AND MONITORING

Adverse events are more frequently reported with anti-tuberculosis agents in HIV-infected patients (5,21). However, the frequency of reactions due to these agents may be overestimated because of the multiple medications these patients may be taking. Major adverse drug reactions to antituberculous drugs are listed in Table 4.22. Only serious or life-threatening side effects warrant the discontinuation of therapy.

Patients begun on antituberculosis treatment need baseline measurements of hepatic enzymes, bilirubin, serum creatinine, blood urea nitrogen, and a complete blood count with platelets. Serum uric acid measurements are obtained if PZA will be given since this agent may cause hyperuricemia, although asymptomatic increases do not warrant discontinuation of this drug. Baseline and periodic monitoring of visual acuity and color vision is necessary with ethambutol therapy. Vestibular testing, audiometry and monitoring of renal function is recommended when using streptomycin and other aminoglycosides. Patients should be followed monthly to assess response to therapy, and to monitor possible drug toxicity by clinical exam with periodic laboratory testing. Patients may need to be seen more frequently or hospitalized if their clinical condition deteriorates. Instructions regarding possible toxicities of drug regimens should be given to each patient, including the symptoms suggestive of hepatitis, which may be due to isomazid or rifampin, and less frequently pyrazinamide. Common symptoms of hepatitis include

Table 4.22.
Major Adverse Reactions to Antituberculosis Drugs

Drug	Adverse Reactions
Isoniazid	Hepatitis, peripheral neuropathy, skin rashes, neurologic disturbances
Rifampin	Hepatitis, skin rashes, flu-like syndrome, renal failure, thrombocytopenia, hemolytic anemia
Pyrazinamide	Hepatitis, skin rashes, hyperuricemia
Ethambutol	Optic neuritis
Ethionamide	Gastrointestinal disturbance, hepatitis, skin rashes, photosensitivity, peripheral neuropathy, arthralgia
Cycloserine	Psychiatric symptoms, seizures
Para-aminosalicylic acid	Anorexia, nausea, vomiting, diarrhea, hepatitis, high sodium load, skin rashes
Streptomycin, kanamycin, capreomycin	Vestibular and auditory toxicity, nephrotoxicity, skin rashes
Ciprofloxacin	Nausea, vomiting, diarrhea, abdominal pain
Ofloxacin	Skin rashes, nausea, abdominal pain
Clofazimine	Brownish pigmentation of skin, gastrointestinal disturbance

anorexia, nausea, vomiting, malaise, abdominal pain, dark urine or yellowing discoloration of skin. Mild abnormalities in liver chemistries may be seen without symptoms, but elevations threefold or greater above baseline are more likely to be associated with drug toxicity. Therapy with INH is infrequently associated with peripheral neuropathy in patients who are malnourished or have chronic debilitating diseases (e.g., diabetes, AIDS, alcoholism) and is preventable by administration of pyridoxine (10–50 mg/day).

Many HIV-infected patients receive other medications that may interact with antituberculosis therapy or are associated with similar toxicities. INH or RIF may decrease serum levels of antifungal agents, such as ketoconazole or fluconazole, and intraconazole, and limit their efficacy. Ketoconazole may cause decreased RIF levels by decreasing absorption if they are taken together. Rifampin may accelerate the clearance of many drugs metabolized by the liver including coumadin, estrogen derivatives, dapsone, anticonvulsants and glucocorticoids (4,18). The frequency of neuropathy associated with the use of certain antiretroviral agents (zalcitabine, didanosine) may potentially be increased by the concomitant use of isoniazid. One study found the combination of zidovudine and antituberculosis treatment well tolerated (22).

Screening and Preventive Therapy for Tuberculosis Infection

Screening for tuberculosis infection is important to identify individuals at high risk for disease who would benefit from preventive therapy with isoniazid. All HIV-infected persons should have tuberculin skin testing at the initial visit. The intradermal Mantoux method is recommended using 5 tuberculin units (TU) of purified protein derivative (PPD). In those HIV-infected, a skin induration of 5 mm or greater is considered significant whether or not persons have received a BCG vaccine. The absence of a reaction to tuberculin testing does not rule out tuberculous infection, since many patients with AIDS and TB may have negative skin tests secondary to decline in immune function (anergy) (3). Also, patients recently exposed to TB contacts may not develop a significant reaction. HIV-related anergy to skin testing appears to correlate with the degree of immune suppression. One study found that over 60% of HIV-infected patients with tuberculosis and a CD4+ cell count exceeding $100/min^3$ reacted to tuberculin skin testing with greater than 5 mm induration. Patients with CD4+ cell counts less than $100/mm^3$ were unlikely to react (4). The use of mumps, *Candida,* or tetanus toxoid antigens as controls to test for cutaneous anergy is helpful in interpreting a negative PPD response in HIV-infected patients (see Table 4.23). Preventive therapy should be offered to anergic patients who have a history of positive PDD, radiographic evidence of old, healed tuberculosis, or recent exposure to an infectious TB case. In addition, preventive therapy should be considered in those populations at high risk for TB infection (prevalence >10%). Preventive therapy should never be initiated until clinical and radiographic examinations exclude active disease. If abnormalities are present on the chest radiograph, further evaluation, including a clinical examination and acid-fast smears and cultures of sputum, should be performed.

Isoniazid is used for preventive therapy of tuberculosis infection. Twelve months of INH in a single dose of 300 mg per day for adults and 10 mg/kg per day (not to exceed 300 mg) for children is recommended as preventive therapy. Although 6 months of isoniazid preventive therapy has been shown to offer nearly comparable benefit, 12 months of treatment is currently recommended for those HIV-infected (18). INH may also be given twice-weekly under directly-observed therapy (DOT) in a

---

Table 4.23.
CDC Guidelines for Anergy Testing

- All persons with HIV infection should receive a purified protein derivative (PPD)-tuberculin skin test (5TU, PPD by Mantoux method).
- Persons with HIV infection should also be evaluated for DTH anergy at the time of PPD testing. Companion testing with 2 DTH skin-test antigens (i.e., *Candida,* mumps, or tetanus toxoid) administered by the Mantoux method is recommended. However, a multipuncture device which administers a battery of DTH antigens may be used.
- Any induration to a DTH antigen measured at 48 hours to 72 hours is considered evidence of DTH responsiveness; failure to elicit a response is considered evidence of anergy.
- Persons with a positive (induration of 5 mm or larger) PPD are considered infected with *M. tuberculosis* and should be considered for 1 year of isoniazid preventive therapy, after active tuberculosis has been excluded.
- Persons who demonstrate a DTH response but have a negative PPD reaction are, in general, considered to be uninfected with M. tuberculosis.
- Anergic, tuberculin-negative persons whose risk of tuberculous infection is estimated to be greater than 10% should also be considered for INH preventive therapy after excluding active tuberculosis.
- CD4 counts are not a substitute for anergy evaluation.

Adapted from CDC. Purified protein derivative (PPD)-tuberculin anergy and HIV infection: Guidelines for anergy testing and management of anergic persons at risk of tuberculosis. MMWR 1991;40 (No. RR-5):27–32

dose of 15 mg/kg (not to exceed 900 mg). Preventive regimens are being studied using rifampin and pyrazinamide for shorter courses. Close contacts of INH-resistant cases may receive preventive therapy with rifampin (600 mg/day for 6 months). Preventive regimens for close contacts of MDR-TB cases should be tailored to the susceptibility pattern of the resistant isolate. Close contacts of MDR-TB cases with both INH and RIF resistance may be treated with a combination of pyrazinamide (PZA) with ethambutol (EMB) or a quinolone (ciprofloxacin or ofloxacin). The efficacy of alternative preventive regimens is uncertain since long-term studies have not been performed with preventive regimens other than INH (3,9,18).

REFERENCES

1. Centers for Disease Control and Prevention. Expanded tuberculosis surveillance and tuberculosis morbidity—United States, 1993. MMWR 1994;43(20):361–363.
2. Centers for Disease Control and Prevention. Screening for tuberculosis and tuberculosis infection in high risk populations, and The use of preventive therapy for tuberculosis infection in the United States: Recommendations of the Advisory Committee for Elimination of Tuberculosis. MMWR 1990;39(No.RR-8).
3. Centers for Disease Control and Prevention. Purified protein derivative (PPD)-tuberculin anergy and HIV infection. Guidelines for anergy testing and management of anergic persons at risk of tuberculosis. MMWR 1991;40(No.RR-5):27–32.
4. Barnes PF, Bloch AB, Davidson PT, et al. Tuberculosis and human immunodeficiency virus infection. NEJM 1991;324(23):1644–1650.
5. Castro KG. Tuberculosis as an opportunistic disease in persons infected with human immunodeficiency virus. Clin Infect Dis 1995;21(Suppl 1):S66–71.
6. McGowan JE. Nosocomial tuberculosis: new progress in control and prevention. Clin Infect Dis 1995;21:489–505.
7. Castro KG, Ward JW, Slutsker L, et al. 1993 revised classification systems for HIV infection and expanded surveillance case definition for AIDS among adolescents and adults. Clin Infect Dis 1993;17:802–10.
8. Selwyn PA, Hartel D, Lewis VA, et al. A prospective study of the risk of tuberculosis among intravenous drug users with human immunodeficiency virus infection. N Engl J Med 1989;320:546–550.
9. Centers for Disease Control and Prevention. National action plan to combat multidrug-resistant tuberculosis. Meeting the challenge of multidrug-resistant tuberculosis: management of persons exposed to multidrug-resistant tuberculosis. MMWR 1992;41(No.RR-11).
10. Centers for Disease Control and Prevention. Guidelines for preventing transmission of tuberculosis in health-care settings, with special focus on HIV-related issues. MMWR 1990;39(No.RR-17).
11. Centers for Disease Control and Prevention. Nosocomial transmission of multidrug-resistant TB to health-care workers and HIV-infected patients in an urban hospital—Florida. MMWR 1990;39:718–722.
12. Centers for Disease Control and Prevention. Nosocomial transmission of multidrug-resistant tuberculosis among HIV-infected persons—Florida and New York, 1988–1991. MMWR 1991;40(34):585–591.
13. American Thoracic Society. Diagnostic standards and classification of tuberculosis. Am Rev Respir Dis 1990;142:725–735.
14. Chaisson RE and Slutkin G. Tuberculosis and human immunodeficiency virus infection. J Infect Dis 1989;159(1):96–100.
15. Chaisson RE, Schecter GF, Theuer CP, et al. Tuberculosis in patients with the acquired immune deficiency syndrome. Am Rev Respir Dis 1987;136:570–574.
16. Wolinsky E. Conventional diagnostic methods for tuberculosis. Clin Infect Dis 1994;19:396–401.
17. Centers for Disease Control and Prevention. Initial therapy for tuberculosis in the era of multidrug resistance: Recommendations of the Advisory Council for the Elimination of Tuberculosis. MMWR 1993;42(No.RR-7).

18. American Thoracic Society. Treatment of tuberculosis and tuberculosis infection in adults and children. Am J Respir Crit Care Med 1994;149:1359–74.
19. Goble M. Drug-resistant tuberculosis. Sem Respir Inf 1986;4:220–229.
20. Goble M, Horsburgh R, Waite D, Madsen L, et al. Treatment of isoniazid and rifampin-resistant tuberculosis. Am Rev Respir Dis 1988;137(Suppl):24A.
21. Small PM, Schecter GF, Goodman PC, et al. Treatment of tuberculosis in patients with advanced human immunodeficiency virus infection. N Engl J Med 1991;324:289–294.
22. Kavesh NG, Holzman RS, Seidlin M. The combined toxicity of azidothymidine and antimycobacterial agents: a retrospective study. Am Rev Respir Dis 1989;139:1094–1097.

Guidelines for Nutritional Management

HIV and Nutrition

Weight loss, multiple nutrient deficiencies, and malnutrition, particularly protein calorie malnutrition (PCM) are common among persons living with AIDS (PLWA). As HIV disease progresses, there is a decrease in lean body tissue, and an increase of both intracellular and extracellular water. Malabsorption, diarrhea, oral/esophageal complications, nausea/vomiting, and fever can compromise nutritional status (1–3). The severe malnutrition that frequently accompanies AIDS increases morbidity and compromises the quality of life.

Persons living with AIDS (PLWAs) have also demonstrated disturbances in lipid metabolism, which may contribute to alterations in immune function. Cholesterol is important in maintaining cell structure, lymphocyte proliferation, and specific immune processes. Despite higher cholesterol and saturated fat intake, HIV-positive persons have lower levels of cholesterol (total, low- and high-density lipoprotein cholesterol) and elevated levels of $\beta2$ microglobulin during early stages of HIV-1 infection compared to seronegative individuals (4). Malnutrition in HIV infection also included reports of micronutrient and vitamin deficiencies such as zinc, iron, selenium, vitamin A, vitamin B_{12}, and folate (1,5–7), however, study results have been variable (1). Deficiencies of zinc and selenium have been hypothesized to contribute to immune and organ dysfunction (8) and evidence has suggested that zinc and selenium deficiency is associated with HIV disease progression (1,6,7). Among HIV-infected patients, low levels of vitamins B_6 and A have been reported; vitamin B_{12} deficiency has been associated with cognitive dysfunction in patients (1).

Etiology of Malnutrition

Malnutrition, itself, has been shown to cause significantly reduced immune response, and shortened survival (7,8). Cellular immune defects, abnormal macrophage function, wasting, recurrent fevers, gastrointestinal dysfunction, and increased susceptibility to opportunistic infections all have been described in patients with protein calorie malnutrition and other nutritional deficiencies (9,10). Evidence of protein calorie malnutrition among PLWAs includes the loss of lean body mass, and decreases in circulating levels of export proteins (e.g., serum albumin, prealbumin, retinol binding protein) in the presence of progressive weight loss (1). Loss in body mass and weight is associated with HIV disease progression, and a greater decrease in body mass associated with opportunistic infections (11). A fall in serum albumin levels among PLWAs has been associated with decreased survival time (3). Malnutrition in HIV patients may be caused by a number of reasons: decreased dietary intake, malabsorption, diarrhea, metabolic changes secondary to infections and fever (1–3). Decreased food intake may be caused by depression, or a systemic response to infection, side effects of medication, altered taste sensations, oral lesions (e.g., thrush), and fatigue. It can also be difficult for persons living with HIV to carry out daily chores (e.g., shopping and preparing food), which would limit their access to good nutrition (3). Malabsorption can be caused by secondary infections which involve the gastrointestinal tract (e.g., Cryptosporidium, Isospora, Campylobacter, Salmonella). In severe malnutrition, the integrity of the gastrointestinal mucosa becomes compromised, exacerbating malabsorption. Metabolic changes occur during HIV disease, resulting in loss of lean tissue and increased energy needs. Metabolic rates have been shown to be elevated in asymptomatic HIV patients and to be increased with the occurrence of secondary infections (7). The decreased dietary intake that usually accompanies these infections results in more weight loss, which in turn predisposes an individual to further infection.

Benefits of Nutrition

Nutritional intervention can ameliorate immune dysfunction that is caused by malnutrition, improve quality of life, restore lean tissue, and prolong survival. Enteral tube feedings or parenteral intravenous feedings have been shown to partially restore body weight, body fat, and lean body mass. However, the benefits of parenteral feeding appears to be greater for patients with gastrointestinal infections than for patients with systemic opportunistic infections (1,7). Dietary intake may also affect AIDS progression. A six-year longitudinal study of an HIV-positive cohort revealed that higher intake of micronutrients (i.e., iron, vitamin E, riboflavin) was associated with higher CD4 counts at baseline measurements, daily multivitamin use was associated with a reduced hazard of AIDS and a reduced risk for low CD4 counts at baseline (12). Nutritional intervention can have a therapeutic benefit in nutritional status despite a progressive drop in CD4 counts, although it does not appear to decrease disease progression (3).

Goal of Nutritional Therapy

The major aims of nutritional therapy are to preserve lean body mass; to provide adequate levels of nutrients; and to minimize symptoms of malabsorption (1,13). Optimizing the nutritional status of people with AIDS is essential in overall medical management. Early nutritional assessment, initiating corrective measures, and follow-up may result in slower weight loss and avoidance of nutritional complications seen in later stages of the disease (13,14).

Oral food intake is the first choice for providing good nutrition. When not possible, enteral nutrition, using various routes, must be considered; total parenteral nutrition (TPN) is considered as the last option (13).

Nutritional Assessment and Counseling

At the time of HIV diagnosis, individuals should have their baseline nutritional status assessed and receive nutritional counseling. The nutritional assessment, routine follow-up, and nutritional counseling should be provided in consultation with a registered dietician or nutrition support team. Recommended components of a nutritional assessment (13) are shown in Table 4.24.

Nutrition histories should include a detailed weight evaluation (e.g., current, usual, and desirable weight). Any weight changes should be noted, to determine percentage of weight loss. In HIV-infected persons, weight loss of 10% or more accompanied by fever or diarrhea is clinically significant (15). Symptoms which can interfere with nutrition (e.g., diarrhea, vomiting) should also be noted. Nutritional counseling should stress the importance of a balanced diet, and include information about nutritional management of symptoms, nutritional support and food safety (1,12,13) (See Chapter 10, *Self Care for Persons Living with HIV*). Counseling should be oriented towards making the fewest changes in lifestyle and dietary habits to encourage adherence to the recommendations. Suggested measures should be prioritized, explained in simple terms, and patients assisted in their implementation. In addition to the patient, persons who may be willing to share the tasks should be included in the counseling session (1). The topics of megadosing and alternative diets should be discussed, as high doses of some minerals and fat soluble vitamins may impair immunity and organ functions (16).

Table 4.24.

Nutritional Assessment for Persons Living with HIV

Diet and nutrition history (past and present)
Calculation of nutrient intake
Anthropometric measurements (e.g., weight, height, skinfold thickness, and midarm circumference to measure somatic protein stores)
Laboratory tests for anemia (blood count), long-term PCM[a] (serum albumin)
Investigation for specific micronutrient deficiencies (e.g., selenium and zinc)
Functional measurements of muscle power (e.g., handgrip strength)
When PCM suspected, measurement of short-term visceral protein deficits (serum retinol-binding protein and prealbumin)

Adapted from Task Force on Nutrition Support in AIDS. Guidelines for Nutrition Support in AIDS. Nutrition 1989;5(1):39–46.
[a]PCM = protein calorie malnutrition

Nutritional Requirements

The Harris Benedict equation can be used to calculate calorie requirements with modification to fit the goal of nutrition therapy (3) (e.g.,
weight gain = basal energy expenditure (BEE) × 1.5; weight maintenance = BEE × 1.3). Protein requirements have been recommended to
be similarly calculated (e.g., 1.0 to 1.2 g protein per kg of body weight
daily for repletion; 0.8 to 1.0 g for maintenance). In the presence of malabsorption, protein requirement may need to be modified (3). A vitamin
and mineral supplement may be beneficial but megadoses beyond the
recommended daily allowance are not recommended. Folic acid supplements may be indicated when antifolate drugs (e.g., TMP-SMX) are being used to treat opportunistic infections (17).

Supplementing Calories and Nutritional Support

Because there may be an increased need for protein and calories
among PLWAs, the patient should be given suggestions regarding the
addition of calories and protein to the daily diet (See also *Self Care for
Persons with HIV*). Appetite stimulants are available and appear to be
helpful. Megestrol acetate is an FDA-approved appetite stimulant which
has been shown to increase appetite, dietary intake, and weight in patients with AIDS (3,18). However, side effects include venous thrombo-
sis, edema, and impotence. Dronabinol, a substance derived from
cannabis has also been shown to increase appetite and body weight in
AIDS patients (3,19). Nutritional support should be introduced when dietary needs cannot be met by a regular, well-balanced diet, and given before the patient becomes malnourished.

Studies have suggested that aggressive alimentation of PLWAs can
lead to increase or maintenance of body cell mass if the primary cause of
wasting is decreased food intake. Studies on the effects of hyperalimentation on nutritional status of malnourished PLWAs with reduced dietary intake have reported improvement in body composition indicators
(e.g., body cell mass, fat, serum albumin) (20). An increase in total lymphocyte counts was also reported, although there was no change in the
CD4+ cell number (20). The use for home TPN for patients with severe
eating disorders or significant malabsorption but without infection resulted in weight gain and improvement in indices of body cell mass and
fat content (21). Using home TPN for patients with systemic infection
(e.g., CMV or MAI), resulted in weight gain and increase in body fat, but
no improvement in lean body mass (21).

ENTERAL AND PARENTERAL FEEDING

When nutrient intake is inadequate or significant weight loss recorded,
enteral formulas should be used to supplement or replace the regular oral
diet. If oral nutrient support provides inadequate calories and protein,
and malabsorption is not a significant factor, enteral feeding by tube
should be considered. Depending on the patient's condition and preference
either a nasal feeding tube or a surgically placed gastrostomy tube may be

used. The enteral route is preferable as it is simpler, and maintains the physiologic functions of the gastrointestinal mucosa (1). Intestinal mucosa can become significantly atrophied if the patient receives no food by mouth for an extended period of time (3). The enteral formula should be lactose free and may have to be restricted in fat content (7), to maximize absorption in a compromised GI tract, the formula should be delivered over 8 to 10 hours at night (3). Enteral feedings are effective as adjuncts to regular oral intake, which should be continued as tolerated. If enteral feeding was required due to a secondary opportunistic infection and consequent acute weight loss, once the secondary infection is controlled, tube feeding may be discontinued (3). Continuous infusion of nutrients with nasogastric, nasoduodenal, or nasojejunal feeding tubes are preferred to provide all or most of the individual's nutrition (13). The nasogastric route allows for intermittent or nocturnal use for ambulatory individuals. When long-term feeding is indicated, or when oral/esophageal complications preclude the nasal route, percutaneous endoscopic gastrostomy (PEG) and small-bore feeding tubes placed into the small intestine are appropriate (13).

Only if enteral routes are not feasible or effective should parenteral nutrition be used as the sole source of nutrition. (13,22). Peripheral parenteral nutrition (PPN) is delivered via a peripheral vein and is appropriate for a short-term (7–10 days) in the hospital to preserve lean body mass (13). Central parenteral nutrition (CPN), which is delivered via a central vein, should be reserved for patients with totally nonfunctional gastrointestinal tracts. CPN can also be used together with enteral feeding to meet high caloric requirements (13). Total parenteral nutrition (TPN) is used to avoid aspiration when recurrent vomiting or obstruction occurs. It may be the only effective means of alimentation in the presence of severe diarrhea or significant malabsorption (22). TPN is also associated with an increased risk of infection of PLWAs (22). Although TPN is potentially valuable for persons with HIV infection, it is still experimental. Consequently, patients should be given an informed consent for TPN (23).

Diarrhea, often considered an inevitable consequence of tube feedings, is more often the result of underlying problems. Bacterial contamination of a nutritional formula, improper rate and strength of administration, and formula temperature are also potential causes of diarrhea. Before discontinuing therapy, all other possible causes of diarrhea should be ruled out (3).

Management of HIV-related Symptoms

Persons living with HIV will commonly have symptoms, signs and adverse effects which affect their nutritional intake. Symptoms as well as recommendations for their management by the AIDS Task Force on Nutrition in AIDS and others (1–3,13) are summarized below; dietary modifications to manage complications can be found in Chapter 10, *Self Care for Persons with HIV*.

ANOREXIA/WEIGHT LOSS

Anorexia is a loss or change in appetite with a relative decrease in food intake which may occur as a direct consequence of AIDS symptoms (e.g., malabsorption, diarrhea, systemic infections, fever, altered endogenous metabolism) or in response to drug therapy. Appetite may be depressed as the result of oral and esophageal ulcers, dysphagia, fever, malaise, dysgeusia, and specific nutritional deficiencies as well as psychological factors (e.g., anxiety, depression). Dietary modifications such as catering to personal tastes, eating in a pleasant atmosphere, and having frequent, small meals or nutritionally dense food items may be helpful in stimulating food intake. A more aggressive approach (e.g. enteral formulas to supplement or replace the regular oral diet) may be indicated if nutritional intake is insufficient or if weight loss is significant.

ORAL/ESOPHAGEAL COMPLICATIONS

Oral and esophageal complications are common among PLWAs and may result in obstruction, difficulty in swallowing, and aspiration, possibly interfering with the ability to eat. Most lesions are responsive to therapy and short-term dietary modification may enable the person with AIDS to maintain oral food intake. Maximum oral intake through diet modification as well as good oral and dental hygiene should be encouraged. Diet can be modified to stimulate tastes via food temperature and texture adjustments and use of agents to increase saliva production. If aspiration is a potential problem, a specialist (ENT, speech pathologist) trained in this area should be consulted.

NAUSEA AND VOMITING

A loss of body cell mass, resulting in electrolyte imbalances and dehydration may be caused by protracted nausea and vomiting. Nausea and vomiting are often temporary and intermittent, occurring as a consequence of drug therapy. The use of nutritional support depends on the etiology and duration of the nausea and vomiting, and the anticipated outcome of drug therapy. If the problem is persistent and unrelated to drug therapy, organic causes, (e.g., infectious, gastrointestinal, or malignant) may be present which require appropriate treatment. If medication is responsible for causing nausea and vomiting the following options can be considered:

- Discontinuation of medication
- Modification of dosing schedule
- Provision of antiemetics
- Nutritional support, if treatment is expected to be longer than 2 weeks, if prognosis is good, and/or if there is unintentional weight loss of 10% or greater.

INFECTION AND SEPSIS

Infection and sepsis are frequent events in PLWAs. Metabolic and physiological consequences of infection, such as hypermetabolism, urinary losses, negative nitrogen balance and catabolism can affect nutritional status (24). The synergistic effect of nutritional deficiencies and recurrence of infection may impair the immune response.

In patients with fever, the Basal Energy Expenditure (BEE) increases 7% for every degree Fahrenheit of body temperature over normal, requiring that caloric needs be adjusted for the febrile individuals. Although this calorie recommendation may not be attainable, attempt to meet these needs as closely as possible. Parenteral feedings may be associated with catheter-related septic complications and therefore should be used only when aggressive nutrient repletion is desired for longer than seven to 10 days during which the GI tract is unavailable. In the presence of sepsis, it may not be advisable to give iron parenterally. Because septic patients may be glucose intolerant, formulas should be diluted so that they are iso-osmolar. Blood glucose should be monitored and insulin use encouraged to maintain a blood sugar of less than 200 mg/dl (13).

NEUROLOGICAL DISEASES

Central nervous system (CNS) manifestations of AIDS can significantly affect the individual's ability to maintain adequate nutritional intake. Reduced appetite, impaired ability to self-feed, and altered metabolic activity may result. When the swallowing reflex is depressed, there is a risk of aspiration. If may be difficult to separate the effects of AIDS complications from the effects of protein calorie malnutrition and specific nutrient deficiencies on the CNS. Some malnourished patients may be showing neurological and behavioral abnormalities which are induced by malnutrition; these are reversible.

Appropriate diagnostic procedures should be conducted to determine the cause of central nervous system impairment. If malnourishment is suspected, a short-term trial of moderate doses (5 to 10 times the RDA) of micronutrients should be introduced to ascertain whether nutritional deficiencies are responsible for the observed dementia (13). For patients who are unable to feed themselves because of neurological difficulties, assistance from the family and friends should be encouraged. For people with severe dementia and a poor prognosis, the decision whether to provide nonvolitional nutrition support should involve the family or friends, the primary care giver, and should consider the patient's prior wishes.

BOWEL DISEASE/DIARRHEA

Diarrhea may be associated with malabsorption due to villus abnormalities, producing a defective mucosal barrier. When mucosal damage occurs, the chance of sepsis increases (13). Hypoalbuminemia, antibiotic therapy, and consequences of nutritional support via tube feedings are also potential causes of diarrhea. The causes of AIDS enteropathies can be divided into four categories: total small bowel disease, partial small bowel disease, large bowel disease, and nonspecific enteropathy. Recommendations for their management by the Task Force on Nutrition Support in AIDS (13) are summarized below and in Table 4.25.

Table 4.25.
Recommendations for Bowel Disease/Diarrhea

	Clinical Diagnosis	Diet Modification	Enteral Formula Administration	Parenteral Administration
Small bowel disease	Biopsy or absorption tests	Fat less than 20 % Low fiber Low residue Lactose-free Avoid caffeine	(Only with partial or total reversal) Low residue Low lactose Fat less than 5% (e.g., elemental)	Primary feeding route
Partial small bowel disease	Exclusion or x-ray	Fat less than 20% Low residue Low lactose Avoid caffeine	Low residue Low lactose Fat less than 5% (e.g., elemental) Low fiber	Rarely indicated
Large bowel disease	Endoscopy and/or biopsy	Low fat or MCT[a] Low fiber Low residue Low lactose Avoid caffeine	Low residue Low lactose Low fat, as tolerated Low fiber	Rarely indicated
Nonspecific enteropathy	No identifiable pathogen Volume and frequency of stool	Include bulking agent (pectin) Low lactose Low fat, as tolerated	Low lactose Low fat, as tolerated	Rarely indicated

Adapted from Task Force on Nutrition Support in AIDS. Guidelines for Nutrition Support in AIDS. Nutrition 1989;5(1):39–46.
[a]MCT = medium chain triglyceride

Total Small Bowel Disease

Because malabsorption is so severe in this enteropathy, it is the only instance that parenteral delivery of calories is considered as the treatment of choice. If the condition is partially or totally reversed, a minimal fat (less than 5%), lactose-free diet should be provided to stimulate gut function (e.g., elemental enteral diet). Hypoalbuminemia with increased interstitial edema is a manifestation of malnutrition and may also contribute to diarrhea. Therefore, serum albumin should be monitored and nitrogen intake adjusted to promote its repletion.

Partial Small Bowel Disease

For partial small bowel disease, small, frequent feedings consisting of low fat, low-lactose and caffeine-free foods are recommended with maximum caloric intake taken early in the day. A low-fat formula to decrease bile salt flow is recommended. If ileal function becomes severely limited and bile salts entering the colon result in steatorrhea with fatty acid diarrhea, an elemental diet (defined formula with less than 5% fat) is recommended.

Large Bowel Disease

Small, frequent feedings that are low in fiber, residue, lactose, fat, and caffeine should be encouraged to minimize the number of bowel movements.

Nonspecific Mild Enteropathy

A bulking agent, such as bran or pectin, should be provided to solidify stool consistency. When nutritional support is indicated, an enteral formula should be provided. If condition worsens, or persists beyond 2 to 3 days, the formula should be changed to a less complex formula.

A growing amount of evidence suggests that immune dysfunction can be ameliorated by nutritional intervention, improving the quality of life by slowing weight loss and maintaining/restoring lean tissue. Optimizing the nutritional status for persons with HIV through aggressive nutritional therapy and providing nutritional intervention and education is an important component of overall medical management.

REFERENCES

1. GT Keusch and DM Thea. Guidelines for nutrition support in AIDS. Med Clin North Am 1993;77(4):795–814.
2. Bunce LV. Practical approaches to nutrition in AIDS Patients. AIDS Clinical Care 1993;5(11):88–89.
3. Mascioli EA. Nutrition and HIV infection. AIDS Clinical Care 1993;5(11):85–87.
4. Shor-Posner G, Basit A, Lu Y, et al. Hypocholesterolemia is associated with immune dysfunction in early human immunodeficiency virus-1 infection. Am J Med 1993; 94:515–519.
5. Corman LC. Effects of specific nutrients on the immune response. Med Clin North Am 1985;69:759–791.
6. Cirelli A, Ciardi M, de Simone C, et al. Serum selenium concentration and disease progress in patients with HIV infection. Clin Biochem 1991;24:211–214.

7. Kotler DP. Malnutrition in HIV infection and AIDS. AIDS 1989;3(Supple 1) S175–S180.
8. Keithley JK, Zeller JM, Szeluga DJ, Urbanski PA. Nutritional alterations in persons with HIV infection. IMAGE: Journal of Nursing Schools 1992;24:183–189.
9. Harakch S, Jariwalla RJ, Pauling L. Suppression of human immunodeficiency virus replication by ascorbate in chronically and acutely infected cells. Proc Natl Acad Sci USA 1990;87:7245–7249.
10. Nicholas SW, Leung J, Fennoy I. Guidelines for nutritional support of HIV-infected children. J Pediatr 1991;119:S59–S62.
11. Castro M, Pereiro C, Pedreira JD, et al. Alterations in body mass index (BMI) and weight in progressive HIV disease. IX international Conference on AIDS, Berlin June 1993;PO–B36–2362:529.
12. Abrams B, Duncan D, Hertz-Picciotto. A prospective study of dietary intake and acquired immune deficiency syndrome in HIV-seropositive homosexual men. J Acquir Immune Defic Syndr 1993;6:949–958.
13. Task Force on Nutrition Support in AIDS. Guidelines for nutrition support in AIDS. Nutrition 1989;5:39–46.
14. McKinley MJ, Goodman-Brock J, Salbe AD. Improved nutritional status as a result of nutrition intervention in adult HIV+ outpatients. (abstract) IX international Conference on AIDS. Berlin June 1993; POB36–2365:529.
15. Fernandez L. Assessing nutrition in HIV-infected patients. AIDS Clinical Care 1989;1:52–53.
16. Fenton M. Diet, immunity and nutritional therapies. Focus 1990;5:1–2.
17. Glatt AE, Chirgwin K, Landesman S. Treatment of infectious associated with human immunodeficiency virus. N Engl J Med 1988;318:1439.
18. Oster M, Enders S, Samuels S, et al. Randomized double-blind study comparing high-dose megestrol acetate and placebo in cachectic patients with acquired immunodeficiency syndrome (AIDS). (abstract) IX International Conference on AIDS. Berlin, June 1993;PO–B36–2360:528.
19. Beal J, Olson R, Shepard KV. Effect of dronabinol on appetite and weight in AIDS: Long-term follow-up. (abstract) IX international Conference on AIDS. Berlin, June 1993;PO–B36–2354:527.
20. Kotler D, Tierney A, Ferraro R, et al. Effect of enteral hyperalimentation upon body cell mass in patients with acquired immunodeficiency syndrome. Am J Clin Nutr 1991;53:149–154.
21. Kotler DP, Tierney AR, Culpepper-Morgan JA, et al. Effect of home total parenteral nutrition upon body composition in patients with AIDS. JPEN 1990;14:454–458.
22. Grunfeld C, Kotler DP. Wasting in the acquired immunodeficiency syndrome. Seminars in Liver Dis 1992;12:97–109.
23. Lo B. Total parenteral nutrition: ethical issues. AIDS Clinical Care 1989;1:53.
24. Scrimshaw NS. Effect of infection on nutrient requirements. Am J Clin Nutr 1977;30:1536–1544.

CHAPTER 5

Women and HIV Infection

Counseling and Testing Considerations for Women

There are additional considerations for women regarding HIV testing and counseling (See HIV Counseling and Testing). Women will have concerns regarding their future or current pregnancy and their unborn child. HIV education, counseling and testing programs should aim to prevent HIV infection among seronegative women and to present all HIV-infected women with choices concerning their health care and reproduction.

HIV Testing and Women

In 1985, the Centers for Disease Control (CDC) recommends HIV antibody testing for women at high risk (1). However, targeting women at risk for screening programs may be problematic. Women with substance abuse problems may be suspicious or unconnected to the health care system; a documented history of substance abuse also be threatening to women who are concerned about losing their children (2). In addition, many women are often unaware of their or their partner's risk and may not identify with a risk category (2,3). Therefore, it has therefore been recommended that testing and counseling programs be offered to all women of childbearing age, irrespective of acknowledgment of risk, (2–4). It has also been suggested that women who receive their routine health care in the emergency room, all prenatal patients, and postpartum patients who have received no prenatal care should be educated about HIV disease and offered testing and counseling (2,5). In areas where providing these services is not feasible, an alternative approach is to provide general HIV education and allow self-selection for testing. Because of the availability of intervention strategies which significantly reduce the rate of HIV transmission from mother to child, a universal approach should be taken—all pregnant women should be given HIV counseling and offered voluntary testing, regardless of their risk for infection or the prevalence of HIV infection in their community (5). A nondirective approach to

HIV testing (i.e., patients are told that the test is available, but testing is neither encouraged nor discouraged) may be helpful (5).

Contraception Counseling

HIV prevention should be discussed with all methods of contraception and family planning issues. If nonbarrier contraception methods are selected (e.g., oral contraceptive, diaphragm, surgical sterilization), the importance of also using latex condoms and nonoxynol-9 as protection against HIV transmission should be emphasized. Intrauterine device (IUD) use should be discouraged because of the possibility that ascending infection could be enhanced in HIV-positive women and that the efficacy of the IUD may be immune mediated.

Counseling Women Who Are Pregnant or Planning Pregnancy

In addition to general counseling information, perinatal transmission and the effect of HIV infection on a woman's reproductive choice should be discussed (e.g., contraceptives, pregnancy) (2,6). The availability of therapy which reduces the risk for perinatal transmission, emphasizes the importance of offering HIV testing and counseling to women before or early in pregnancy so that informed and timely reproductive decisions can be made. Women who consider HIV testing are concerned about the impact of HIV on their pregnancies, its role in causing pediatric disease, and their own health. Women may not choose to be tested unless counseling is individualized (7,8). Decisions regarding pregnancy options may be less complex if reproductive counseling is done prior to pregnancy. Since heterosexually acquired AIDS is a common mode of HIV exposure for women, risk reduction to prevent sexual transmission should be emphasized for women. If one child is diagnosed as vertically infected with HIV, the siblings, the mother, and the mother's partner are frequently infected with HIV. In instances when a child is first diagnosed as HIV positive, it has been suggested to approach parental pretest counseling as soon as the child's diagnosis is confirmed (5). Counseling and testing the entire family (parents and the child who may be HIV positive) at the same time have been recommended (5). Linking the family to follow-up care and social and psychological support is important.

REPRODUCTIVE COUNSELING

Reproductive counseling is preferable when the patient is not pregnant. Counseling about pregnancy options should be informative, client oriented, and nondirective. In one counseling model, the patient is assisted to develop her own risk-benefit analysis in order to make an informed reproductive choice, focusing on several scenarios (9). The patient is helped to develop strategies which support her decision-making process (9). To assist HIV-infected women make a decision regarding childbearing, all factual information of HIV disease, including all available data and options should be given. This includes current estimates of perinatal disease transmission, knowledge about factors influencing risk of perinatal transmission, the diagnosis of infants, and therapeutic options for infected infants (2,4,6). In addition, transmission to sex partners, contraception, and contingency plans for the future care of children should also be discussed. Reproductive options, including termination of pregnancy should be addressed. Factors which may play a role in decision making concerning pregnancy and contraception choices should also be discussed (e.g. age, attitudes and beliefs, general health status, pregnancy history, maternal stage of HIV infection, social support) (6).

Although the Centers for Disease Control recommends HIV-positive women avoid pregnancy until more is known about perinatal transmission (1), many women will choose to continue their pregnancy or become pregnant. Reproductive counseling should be nondirective. The woman should make her own informed reproductive decision and her decision supported (3,4,6,10).

HIV-negative Pregnant Women

Uninfected pregnant women who continue practicing high-risk behaviors (e.g. IDU, unprotected sex with a partner at high risk) should be counseled to avoid further exposure to HIV and be retested for HIV in the third trimester of pregnancy (4). Risk-reduction counseling should be given.

HIV-positive Pregnant Women

COUNSELING (1–6,9–12)

Counseling a woman who is HIV infected is often complex, since the existence of children is frequently involved. Besides her own infection and illness, HIV-infected women must often cope simultaneously with the illness and death of a spouse or life partner, and possibly of her children. The immediate needs of the woman will be support and counseling. If the woman has other children, it has been suggested to first address the issues for the pregnant patient, and delay the testing and counseling of the other children (5). HIV-infected women should be encouraged to obtain HIV testing for any of their children born after they became infected. If women are unaware when they became infected, children born after 1977 should be tested (4). Children older than 12 years of age should be tested with informed consent of the parent and agreement of the child (4). The absence of signs and symptoms suggestive of HIV in older children does not necessarily indicate that the child is uninfected; some perinatally infected children remain asymptomatic for several years (4). If the child is first diagnosed with HIV, discuss the implications of the child's diagnosis for the woman's health and assist the mother in obtaining care for herself. Health care needs and options specific to the woman's own health and pregnancy should be outlined, access to current and planned clinical trials discussed, as well as the importance for follow-up care for the woman and her children (if indicated). Specific topics for discussion include: the current health status of the woman; the interaction between pregnancy on HIV; the risk of perinatal HIV transmission; the prognosis of HIV infection in infants; child care issues; reproductive choices; treatment options; HIV prevention; and risk reduction. Medical and social service referrals that focus on the needs of the entire family should be ensured. Topics to discuss during counseling may include the following:

THE EFFECT OF HIV-RELATED TREATMENT TO THE WOMAN AND FETUS DURING PREGNANCY

Immediate and long-term health concerns should be discussed, and health care needs specific to pregnancy outlined. Current prophylactic treatment of HIV disease and possible impact on pregnancy should be discussed. Recent studies (ACTG 076) have shown that *the risk of fetal-maternal transmission can be decreased approximately two-thirds by timely administration of zidovudine (ZDV)* during pregnancy, labor, delivery, as well as to the newborn during the first six weeks of life (13). The effect of zidovudine on the fetus is not clearly known but recent studies (ACTG 076) have thus far shown no or minimal side effects for mothers and infants. Further follow-up of mothers and infants is being conducted to determine any late adverse effects from zidovudine administration. Based on these findings, the Public Health Service (PHS) issued recommendations regarding ZDV therapy to reduce perinatal transmission (14). The long-term risk of zidovudine therapy is still unknown as is the effectiveness of ZDV therapy in women who have different clinical characteristics (e.g., CD4+ T-lymphocyte count and previous ZDV use) as those who participated in the trial (4). Both the benefits and potential risks should be reviewed with the woman before therapy is initiated. The final decision to accept or reject ZDV treatment is the woman's responsibility.

THE RISK OF TRANSMISSION FROM MOTHER TO FETUS

Rates of transmission from mother to fetus have been variable, ranging from 13% in Europe, to 45% in Kenya (15–18). In the United States, HIV is transmitted to approximately 20% to 30% of babies born to HIV-infected pregnant women (19). Factors which influence transmission rates include clinical status of the mother, viral load, seroconversion during pregnancy and maternal coinfections. There is evidence that cesarean section does not prevent infection in the child (20).

THE EFFECTS OF PREGNANCY ON THE PROGRESSION OF HIV INFECTION

Preliminary data suggest pregnancy in HIV-infected women has little effect on disease progression (17). Pregnancy, itself, alters cellular immunity so that and other viral diseases can be more serious in pregnancy (11). Because HIV disease leaves a host susceptible to a variety of opportunistic infections, concern is centered on whether pregnancy could aggravate the immune insult caused by HIV infection. At present, there is no evidence that pregnancy and childbirth have a direct adverse effect on HIV disease progression (6,12,17,20,21).

THE EFFECT OF HIV ON PREGNANCY OUTCOMES

Early studies showed an association with maternal HIV infection and low birth weight, stillbirth, prematurity, and premature death (5,22). However, more recent studies, controlled for substance abuse, socioeconomic status, smoking, etc. have showed no difference between HIV-infected asymptomatic and noninfected women. Women with AIDS or low CD4 counts have a poorer perinatal outcome secondary to intervening maternal disease.

THE IMPACT OF PREGNANCY DECISIONS ON THE FAMILY

The potential impact of pregnancy decisions and its consequences on the family should be discussed. This includes the basic course of pediatric HIV disease, including both the possibility of asymptomatic infection and of early development of symptoms, AIDS, and potential death of the child (2). In addition, the potential loss of a parent or parents and the impact within the family should be discussed (e.g., issues related to caring for children who have lost their parents: foster care, emotional well-being of both HIV-infected and uninfected children). Women should be encouraged to discuss these issues with their partners or other who play a supportive role (6).

HIV-infected Women Continuing Pregnancy

If the woman chooses to continue with the pregnancy, the woman's decision should be supported and antepartum care tailored to her individual needs (17). She should be given information regarding the meaning of a positive HIV test in the infant and diagnosis of HIV infection, and counseled on how to care for the potentially infected newborn (11).

ZDV THERAPY

ZDV has been approved by the FDA for therapy to reduce perinatal HIV transmission (14). Treatment recommendations are based on the available data from ACTG Protocol 076 and current information regarding factors associated with transmission (14). HIV-infected women should be informed about the substantial benefit and short term safety of ZDV administered during pregnancy and the neonatal period observed in ACTG Protocol 076. However, women should also be informed that the long term risks of ZDV to themselves and their children are unknown. The benefits of potential risks of ZDV therapy to the HIV-infected woman and her child should be weighed. Discussion of treatment options should be noncoercive, linguistically and culturally appropriate and tailored to an individual's educational level.

BREAST FEEDING

Breast milk has been implicated as a means of transmission from mother to infant. Breast feeding is not recommended for HIV-infected mothers in the United States (1,4,6). Only in developing countries where breast milk is the principal source of calories and protein for newborns, is breast feeding recommended.

The importance of medical follow-up for HIV-infected women and their children after pregnancy should be discussed. HIV-infected women should receive ongoing HIV-related medical care, and their children follow-up care to determine their infection status, to initiate prophylactic therapy to prevent PCP, and if infected, to determine the need for anti-retroviral and other prophylactic therapy to monitor disorders in growth and development. Recommended vaccinations should be given to HIV-infected children and other children in households with HIV-infected persons. Social and medical service referrals which focus on the family needs should be given.

REFERENCES

1. CDC. Recommendations for assisting in the prevention of perinatal transmission of human T lymphotropic virus type III/lymphadenopathy-associated virus and the acquired immunodeficiency syndrome. MMWR 1985;34:721–32.
2. Tuomala R. Human Immunodeficiency Virus Education and Screening of Prenatal Patients. Obstet and Gyn Clinics of North America 1990;17:571–583.
3. Holman S. HIV counselling for women of reproductive age. Baillere's Clin Obstetrics and Gyn 1992;6:53–68.
4. CDC. U.S. Public Health Service Recommendations for Human Immunodeficiency virus counseling and voluntary testing for pregnant woman. MMWR; 1995;44 (RR-7).
5. Fox HE. Obstetric issues and counseling women and parents. In: Pizzo PA, Wilfert CM, eds. Pediatric AIDS: the challenge of HIV infection in infants, children and adolescents. Baltimore: Williams and Wilkins, 1991;669–683.
6. El-Sadr W, Oleske JM, Agins BD, et al. Evaluation and management of early HIV infection. AHCPR Publication No. 94-0572. Rockville, MD: Agency for Health Care Policy and Research, Public Health Service, US Department of Health and Human Services, January 1994.
7. Sachs BP, Tuomala RE, Frigoletto FD. Acquired immunodeficiency syndrome: suggested protocol for counseling and screening in pregnancy. Obstet Gynecol 1987; 70:408–411.
8. Selwyn PA, Carter RJ, Schoenbaum EE, et al. Knowledge of HIV antibody status and decisions to continue or terminate pregnancy among intravenous drug users. JAMA 1989;261:3567–3671.
9. Bermon N. Reproductive counseling. AIDS Clinical Care June 1993;5:45–47.
10. Holman S. Berthaud M, Sunderland A, Moroso, et al. Women infected with human immunodeficiency virus: counselng and testing during pregnancy. Seminars in Perinatology 1989;13:7–15.
11. Hauer LB, Dattel BJ. Management of the pregnant woman infected with human immunodeficiency virus. J of Perinatology 1988;8:258–262.
12. Nanda D, Minkoff HL. Pregnancy and women at risk for HIV infection. Prim Care 1992;19:157–169.
13. Connor EM, Sperling RS, Gelber R, et al. Reduction of maternal-infant transmission of human immunodeficiency virus type 1 with zidovudine treatment. N Engl J Med 1994;331:1173–1180.
14. CDC. Recommendations of U.S. Public Health Service Task Force on the use of zidovudine to reduce perinatal transmission of HIV. MMWR 1994;43 (No. RR-11).
15. European Collaborative Study. Children born to women with HIV-infection: natural history and risk of transmission. Lancet 1991;337:253–260.
16. Blanche S, Rouzioux C, Guihard Moscato ML, et al. A prospective study of infants born to women seropositive for human immunodeficiency virus type 1. N Eng J Med 1989; 320:1643–1648.
17. ACOG Technical Bulletin. Human immunodeficiency virus infection. Int J Gynecol Obstet 1993;41:307–319.
18. Ryder RW, Nsa W, Hassig SE, et al. Perinatal transmission of the human immunodeficiency virus type 1 to infants of seropositive women in Zaire. N Eng J Med 1989; 320:1637–1642.

19. Von Seidlein L, Bryson YJ. Maternal-fetal transmission of the human immunodeficiency virus type 1. Seminars in Pediatric Infectious Diseases 1994;5:78–86.
20. Newell ML, Peckham CS. HIV-1 infection in pregnancy: implications for women and children. AIDS 1990;4(Suppl 1):S111–S117.
21. Nanda D, Minkoff HL. HIV in pregnancy—transmission and immune effects. Clin OB GYN 1989;32:456–466.
22. Temmerman M, Plummer FA, Mirza NB, et al. Infection with HIV as a risk factor for adverse obstetrical outcome. AIDS 1990;4:1087–1093.

Clinical Management of HIV-infected Women

Relatively little is known about the gender-specific course of HIV disease progression among women and the gender appropriate clinical care of HIV-infected women. Information about HIV has been primarily derived from gay white males, while studies in women have been principally of pregnant women focusing on perinatal issues. Candida vaginitis, genital herpes, syphilis, pelvic inflammatory disease and human papilloma virus disease (condyloma acuminatum, cervical dysplasia, and cervical carcinoma) have been reported to occur with greater frequency and severity among women with HIV disease. HIV infection appears to modify the course of several gynecological diseases. Among HIV-infected women, pelvic inflammatory disease (PID), cervical intraepithelial neoplasia (CIN), and cervical cancer are often more aggressive, with frequent recurrence and decreased response to standard therapies.

Gender Differences

The AIDS surveillance case definition is similar for male and female adults and many nongynecological HIV manifestations do not differ between men and women. However, it has been suggested that gender differences may have possible effects on the course of HIV disease progression (1,2). Studies have demonstrated a higher rate of candida esophagitis (versus *Pneumocystis carinii* pneumonia) reported as the AIDS-defining diagnosis in women and a higher rate of mycobacterium recovery by blood culture in women compared to men (3,4). Although the clinical features of HIV-related *Pneumocystis carinii* pneumonia are similar in both men and women, respiratory failure occurs more often in women and is more likely to be fatal (5). Gender may also affect the pharmacokinetics of drugs or the interaction with commonly used drugs (e.g. methadone, oral contraceptives), possibly resulting in different responses to drug therapies (2,6). Shorter survival time from AIDS diagnosis to death in women compared to men has been reported (7), while other studies have showed no difference. This may be due to a number of external factors, including delayed medical diagnosis, poor access to gynecologic or general health care, and research trials (2,5).

Evaluation of HIV-infected Women

Given the strong association between HIV infection and the occurrence of abnormal gynecologic conditions, the evaluation and appropri-

Table 5.1.

Targeted Evaluation for the HIV-infected Woman

Gynecologic history	Menstrual history Obstetrical history Contraceptive use history History of previous STDs, vaginal and pelvic infections Review of previous Pap smear results History of sexual practices
Physical examination	Clinical breast exam Inspection of the external genitalia, vaginal canal, cervix, and perianal area Rectal and bimanual examination Special attention should be given to genital ulcerative lesions and nonulcerative genital lesions (e.g., genital warts, molluscum contagiosum) Monitor Candida infections for frequency and response to antifungal treatment
Laboratory evaluation	Pap smear Wet mount, KOH prep Culture for Chlamydia organisms, gonorrhea Serologic test for syphilis Pregnancy test (if indicated)
Other	Mammogram for women between 35 and 39 years of age, then every other year through age 49. An annual mammogram for women 50 years and older

ate gynecologic care of HIV-infected women are important. Once diagnosed with HIV infection, a woman should have a targeted evaluation, in addition to the standard evaluation for HIV-infected individuals. Recommended elements of this targeted evaluation (2,5) are summarized in Table 5.1. Counseling regarding risk reduction, family planning, and information regarding access to clinical trials should also be given. Referrals for psychological counseling and social support should be made as indicated.

Follow-Up

Follow-up intervals are not yet clear, although some have suggested that the pelvic examination, Pap smear, and serologic studies and cultures for sexually transmitted diseases (i.e., syphilis, gonorrhea, chlamydia) should be done every six months (8,9).

Another recommendation is that Pap smears be done twice in the first year (10) and annually thereafter when the initial Pap smears are normal and interpretable (2,10,11). If no endocervical cells are seen, the Pap smear should be repeated immediately (10). Pap smears should be repeated every six months when the following occurs (10).

- There is a history of HPV infection
- Previous Pap smear shows squamous intraepithelial lesions (SIL)
- Woman with symptomatic HIV infection
- Following treatment of any cervical lesion or underlying cause of an inflammation.

The use of colposcopy as an initial screening test for detection of cervical cytologic abnormalities in HIV-infected women is not recommended (2,10). Referral for colposcopy is indicated when the Pap smear indicates an abnormality such as: atypical cells of undetermined significance; low-grade or high-grade SILs; cellular changes of HPV; or carcinoma; or if there is a history of untreated SILs (5,10). Evaluation should include a visual examination of the vulva, vagina, and cervix; endocervical curettage; and biopsy of any visible lesions (5,10). Cervical intraepithelial neoplasias or SILs should be colposcoped as soon as possible; treatment of overt cervical disease should be managed aggressively and should not be altered because of HIV status (2,5,12).

Treatment of HIV-related Gynecologic Conditions

VAGINAL CANDIDIASIS

Recurrent vaginal candidiasis is common among HIV-infected women. The initial therapeutic approach is the use of a standard topical antifungal medication. Oral therapy (e.g., ketoconazole) should be initiated for patients with recurrent candidiasis or candidiasis unresponsive to therapy in the absence of correctable causes (e.g. antibiotics, oral contraceptives) (2,5,12). The concomitant use of antacids should be avoided to optimize gastric absorption. The use of ketoconazole (400 mg/day for 14 days followed by a five-day course each month for six months) is recommended (2,6,13). Liver function tests should be monitored closely during treatment and ketoconazole therapy discontinued if transaminases are three times the normal value (5). Oral fluconazole is another treatment alternative, starting with a dose of 200 mg/day and a maintenance dose of 100 mg/day for five days per month with monitoring of liver function tests (5).

CERVICAL INTRAEPITHELIAL NEOPLASIA (CIN)

Evidence suggests a more fulminant course of cervical disease and more false-negative cytologic findings in HIV-infected women. Pap smears should be done regularly (e.g., annually or biannually) with colposcopy performed as indicated. Overt cervical disease in HIV-infected women should be managed aggressively; HIV disease is not contraindication for a surgical approach (2,12).

HERPES SIMPLEX

Following confirmation of diagnosis by viral culture, oral acyclovir therapy is recommended (200 mg four or five times a day) and may be supplemented with acyclovir 5% ointment, applied at three-hour intervals (5,6). Oral acyclovir may be continued indefinitely at a lower dosage (200 mg two times daily); however, renal functioning should be monitored and dosing intervals extended in the event of renal insufficiency (5). Intravenous foscarnet has been reported to be effective in treating acyclovir resistant stains of herpes simplex (0.6 mg/kg at eight-hour intervals, reducing dosage in patients with renal impairment) (5).

PELVIC INFLAMMATORY DISEASE (PID)

HIV-infected women with pelvic inflammatory disease (PID) appears to have different manifestations, being less likely to have a leukocytosis and more likely to have abscesses and require surgical intervention (13). It has also been suggested that PID in women with HIV infection may be more severe. Given that immunocompromise is sufficient justification for inpatient management of PID, it has been recommended that HIV-infected women be treated for PID on an inpatient basis (2,12,13). Initial treatment regimens do not differ from that of HIV-negative women (12).

GENITAL ULCERS

Most patients with genital ulcers in the U.S. have genital herpes, syphilis, or chancroid. Evaluation of all persons with genital ulcers should include a serologic test for syphilis and possibly other tests. Specific tests for the evaluation of genital ulcers include: darkfield examination or direct immunofluorescence test for *Treponema pallidum;* culture or antigen test for HSV; and culture for *Hemophilus ducreyi* (14). Since treatment often begins prior to the availability of test results, treatment should be for the most likely diagnosis. If the diagnosis is unclear or if the patient resides in a community where chancroid morbidity is notable, treating for both chancroid and syphilis has been recommended by many experts (14).

SYPHILIS

Syphilis appears to have a more aggressive course in women with HIV infection (15). When clinical findings suggest the presence of syphilis, but serologic tests are nonreactive or confusing, alternative tests (e.g. biopsy of a lesion, darkfield examination, or direct fluorescent antibody staining of lesion material) may be helpful. Neurosyphilis should be considered in the differential diagnosis of neurologic disease among HIV-infected persons. It has been suggested that persons with early syphilis are at increased risk for neurologic complications and have higher rates of treatment failure with current recommended regimens (16).

Treatment of HIV-infected patients with primary or secondary syphilis is the same as for those without HIV infection (i.e. benzathine penicillin G 2.4 million units IM) with careful follow-up (14,16). Others recommend additional treatments (e.g., multiple doses of benzathine penicillin G, or supplemental antibiotics); higher antibiotic dose has also been suggested to prevent progression of neurosyphilis (14,17). Although CSF abnormalities are common among HIV-infected individuals, the prognostic significance is unknown. It has been suggested that CSF of all HIV-infected patients who have any form of syphilis should be examined routinely (16,17). HIV-infected patients diagnosed with neurosyphilis should be treated with parenteral penicillin, as opposed to oral erythromycin or tetracycline (16).

Syphilis Screening and Treatment in Pregnant Women

Given the recent resurgence of congenital syphilis reported in selected urban centers in the U.S. (18), early diagnosis and treatment of syphilis in pregnant women is indicated. HIV-infected pregnant women should be evaluated for syphilis with a nontreponemal test (RPR or VDRL) at entry into prenatal care, during the third trimester, at delivery, and if the patient is exposed to or presents with symptoms or signs of an STD (10). Evaluation during the third trimester is important if treatment is to be completed in time to reliably prevent congenital syphilis. Treatment and follow-up of syphilis is the same for pregnant women as for nonpregnant adults (10). The therapy for syphilis during pregnancy is designed to effectively treat the mother, while preventing congenital infection of the fetus (18). Penicillin is the only therapy known to be effective for both mother and fetus. Although oral therapies such as erythromycin, tetracycline, and its derivatives are effective treatment for the mother, they do not effectively treat the fetus (19). Tetracyclines are not indicated during pregnancy due to their adverse effects on the bones and teeth of the fetus (20). Penicillin therapy must be completed at least 4 weeks before delivery to reliably prevent the sequelae of congenital syphilis (10). All infants born to women with syphilis should be assessed for congenital syphilis and appropriately managed.

Drug Therapy

Initiation of anti-retroviral therapy for women is similar to men. Asymptomatic HIV-infected women should be offered antiretroviral therapy when CD4 cell count falls below 500 cells/μL (10). PCP prophylaxis should be started when the CD4 count falls below 200 cells/μL when there has been a prior episode of PCP, or in the presence of other specific signs or symptoms (10). Treatment guidelines for tuberculosis do not differ by gender.

ZDV Therapy for Pregnant Women with HIV Infection

Recently, it has been shown that the risk of perinatal transmission can be reduced by approximately two-thirds with the timely administration of ZDV (21–23). In this clinical trial (ACTG 076), ZDV was administered to HIV-infected women during pregnancy and delivery, as well as to the newborn during the first 6 weeks of life. Both women and infants in the study tolerated ZDV therapy well and there were no associated serious short-term effects. However, the long-term risks of ZDV therapy to women and their children are unknown. There are also other limitations of the study which should be considered: a) Although, ZDV administration reduced perinatal transmission, it did not eliminate perinatal transmission; b) the therapy efficacy is unknown for HIV-infected pregnant women who have advanced disease, who have received prior antiretroviral therapy or who have ZDV-resistant virus strains; and c) It is not known whether the use of ZDV during pregnancy will affect the

Table 5.2.

Eligibility Criteria for HIV-infected Pregnant Women Participating in AIDS Clinical Trials Group Protocol 076

- Pregnancy at 14–34 weeks of gestation.
- No antiretroviral therapy during the current pregnancy.
- No clinical indications for antenatal antiretroviral therapy.
- CD4+ T-lymphocyte count ≥200 cells/μL at the time of entry into the study.

Source: CDC Recommendations of the U.S. Public Health Service Task Force on the use of zidovudine to reduce perinatal transmission of the human immunodeficiency virus. MMWR 1994;43:RR-11.

Table 5.3.

Zidovudine Regimen from AIDS Clinical Trials Group Protocol 076

- Oral administration of 100 mg of zidovudine (ZDV) five times daily, initiated at 14–34 weeks of gestation and continued throughout the pregnancy.
- During labor, intravenous administration of ZDV in a 1-hour loading dose of 2 mg per kg of body weight, followed by a continuous infusion of 1 mg per kg of body weight per hour until delivery.
- Oral administration of ZDV to the newborn (ZDV syrup at 2 mg per kg of body weight per dose every 6 hours) for the first 6 weeks of life, beginning 8–12 hours after birth.

Source: CDC Recommendations of the U.S. Public Health Service Task Force on the use of zidovudine to reduce perinatal transmission of the human immunodeficiency virus. MMWR 1994;43:RR-11.

drug's efficacy for the woman when it becomes clinically indicated for her own health. The results of the ACTG 076 are directly applicable to women who meet the entry criteria for the study (Study-eligibility criteria and regimen are shown in Tables 5.2 and 5.3). Based on the available data from ACTG 076 and current information regarding factors associated with transmission, treatment recommendations for various circumstances that commonly occur in the clinical practice have been published by the U.S. Public Health Service (Summary in Table 5.4) (23). Recommendations regarding the use of ZDV regimen for women whose clinical conditions differ from ACTG 076 eligibility criteria were derived from consensus interpretation of available scientific data (23). It should be noted that not all potential clinical circumstances can be described and in many cases, definitive evidence on which to base recommendations may not be available. A woman's decision to use ZDV to reduce the risk of HIV transmission to her infant should be balanced between the benefits, the potential risks of the regimen to herself and to her child, and the gaps in knowledge relating to her clinical situation.

MONITORING FOR MOTHERS AND INFANT DURING THE ZDV REGIMEN (23)

Monitoring the ZDV regimen during pregnancy should include monthly assessment for ZDV-associated hematologic and liver chemistry abnormalities. Indications of toxicity which might require interrupting or stopping the dose of ZDV include:

Table 5.4.

Clinical Situations and U.S. P. H.S. Recommendations for Use of Zidovudine* to Reduce Perinatal HIV Transmission

1. Pregnant HIV-infected women with CD4+ T-lymphocyte counts ≥200 cells/μL who are at least 14–34 weeks of gestation and who have no clinical indications for ZDV and no history of extensive (>6 months) prior antiretroviral therapy.
   Recommendation: The health-care provider (HCP) should recommend the full ACTG 076 regimen to all HIV-infected pregnant women in this category. This recommendation should be presented to the pregnant woman in the context of a risk-benefit discussion: a reduced risk of transmission can be expected but the long-term adverse consequences of the regimen are not known. The decision about this regimen should be made by the women following a discussion with her health-care provider.
2. Pregnant HIV-infected women who are at >34 weeks of gestation, who have no history of extensive (>6 months) prior antiretroviral therapy, and who do not require ZDV for their own health.
   *Recommendation*s: The HCP should recommend the full ACTG 076 regimen in the context of a risk-benefit discussion with the pregnant woman. The woman should be informed that ZDV therapy may be less effective than that observed in ACTG 076, because the regimen is being initiated late in the third trimester.
3. Pregnant HIV-infected women with CD4+ T-lymphocyte counts <200 cells/μL who are at 14–34 weeks of gestation, who have no other clinical indications for ZDV, and who have no history of extensive (>6 months) prior antiretroviral therapy.
   Recommendation: The HCP should recommend initiation of antenatal ZDV therapy to the woman for her own health benefit. The intrapartum and neonatal components of the ACTG 076 regimen should be recommended until further information becomes available. This recommendation should be presented in the context of a risk-benefit discussion with the pregnant woman.
4. Pregnant HIV-infected women who have a history of extensive (>6 months) ZDV therapy and/or other antiretroviral therapy before pregnancy.
   Recommendation: Because data are insufficient to extrapolate the potential efficacy of the ACTG 076 regimen for this population of women, the HCP should consider recommending the ACTG 076 regimen on a case-by-case basis after a discussion of the risks and benefits with the pregnant woman. Issues to be discussed include her clinical and immunologic stability on ZDV therapy, the likelihood she is infected with a ZDV-resistant HIV strain, and, if relevant, the reasons for her current use of an alternative antiretroviral agent (e.g., lack of response to or intolerance of ZDV therapy). Consultation with experts in HIV infection may be warranted. The HCP should make the ACTG 076 regimen available to the woman, although its effectiveness may vary depending on her clinical status.
5. Pregnant HIV-infected women who have not received antepartum antiretroviral therapy and who are in labor.
   Recommendation: For women with HIV infection who are in labor and who have not received the antepartum component of the ACTG 076 regimen (either because of lack of prenatal care or because they did not wish to receive antepartum therapy), the HCP should discuss the benefits and potential risk of the intrapartum and neonatal components of the ACTG 076 regimen and offer ZDV therapy when the clinical situation permits.
6. Infants who are born to HIV-infected women who have received no intrapartum ZDV therapy.
   Recommendation: If the clinical situation permits and if ZDV therapy can be initiated within 24 hours of birth, the HCP should offer the ACTG 076 postpartum component of 6 weeks of ZDV therapy for the infant in the context of a risk-benefit discussion with the mother. Data from animal prophylaxis studies indicate that if ZDV is administered, therapy should be initiated as soon as possible (within hours) after delivery. If therapy cannot begin until the infant is >24 hours of age and the mother did not receive therapy during labor, no data support offering therapy to the infant.

*These recommendations do not represent approval by the Food and Drug Administration (FDA) or approved labeling for the particular product or indications in question.
Adapted from CDC. Recommendations of the U.S. Public Health Service Task Force on the use of zidovudine to reduce perinatal transmission of the human immunodeficiency virus. MMWR 1994;43:RR-11.

Table 5.5.
PCP Prophylaxis for Pregnant HIV-Infected Women

CD4+ T Lymphocyte Counts (cells/μL)	PCP Prophylaxis
<200	Woman should receive PCP prophylaxis
<600	Evaluate CD4+ T lymphocyte counts each trimester
Postpartum	Measure CD4+ T lymphocyte counts at 6 weeks and 6 months postpartum to evaluate whether antiretroviral therapy is indicated

Source: CDC Recommendations of the U.S. Public Health Service Task Force on the use of zidovudine to reduce perinatal transmission of the human immunodeficiency virus. MMWR 1994;43:RR-11

- hemoglobulin < 8 gm/dL
- absolute neutrophil count <750 cells/μL
- AST (SGOT) or ALT (SPGT) greater than five times the upper limit of normal

To determine if prophylaxis for opportunistic infections (e.g. PCP) should be initiated, CD4+ T-lymphocytes counts should be monitored. The recommended therapy regarding PCP prophylaxis (23), is shown in Table 5.5. Antepartum testing (sonographic and nonstress testing, intrapartum fetal monitoring) should be performed only when clinically indicated, and not specifically because the patient is receiving ZDV therapy during pregnancy.

INFANT MONITORING

A complete blood count and differential should be taken at birth (i.e., baseline measures). Repeat measurements of hemoglobin at 6 and 12 weeks of age are recommended. Infants born with severe anemia (hemoglobulin <8 gm/dL) should be administered ZDV with caution; if ZDV is administered the anemia should be treated and the infant intensively monitored. Guidelines concerning diagnosing HIV infection in infants and initiating PCP prophylaxis and antiretroviral therapy for HIV-infected children are addressed elsewhere (*See Pediatric AIDS*). The potential efficacy of ZDV for HIV-infected children who require antiretroviral therapy and who received ZDV in utero and during infancy has not been determined. A specialist in pediatric HIV infection should be consulted if therapy is necessary for HIV-infected infants whose mother received ZDV during pregnancy.

FOLLOW-UP AND SURVEILLANCE

There are concerns regarding the use of ZDV during pregnancy and the long-term effects among women. These concerns include the development of ZDV-resistant virus and the potential effect that such resistance could have on disease progression for the woman. Among women who receive ZDV during pregnancy solely to reduce the risk of perinatal transmission, viral resistance and disease progression should be addressed. Monitoring should include Pap smears and gynecologic examinations (14,23) and if appropriate referral to family planning consultation and services. Long term follow-up of both infected and uninfected infants born to mothers receiving ZDV is important, with an emphasis on assessing organ system toxicities, neurodevelopment, pubertal development, reproductive capacity, and development of neoplasms.

An Antiretroviral Pregnancy Registry has been established to collect observational data concerning pregnancy outcomes of women who receive ZDV during pregnancy. The registry will provide surveillance for possible teratogenicity among infants born to women who received ZDV during pregnancy. To register patients, health-care providers can register patients at the following numbers:

(800) 722-9292, extension 8465—in the United States
(919) 315-8465 for calls outside the United States

Written reports can be obtained from the Antiretroviral Pregnancy Registry, P.O. Box 12700, Research Triangle Park, NC 27709, USA.

PCP Prophylaxis for Pregnant Women with HIV Infection

PCP prophylaxis for HIV-infected pregnant women are similar to those for the nonpregnant adult (10). The effects of specific PCP prophylaxis mediations on the fetus should be considered. TMP-SMX is the recommended drug of choice for PCP prophylaxis during pregnancy, with the recommended dosage similar to that recommended for nonpregnant adults (10). Trimethoprim crosses the placenta and reaches similar levels in the mother and fetus (24). There is a theoretical risk of teratogenicity, although no known cases of fetal anomalies can be attributed to its use during pregnancy. Similarly, sulfamethoxazole presents a theoretical risk for kernicterus during pregnancy but no cases have been reported in the current literature. Aerosolized pentamidine has also been used during pregnancy for PCP prophylaxis. The negligible serum levels of pentamidine achieved following aerosol administration are unlikely to pose a threat to the fetus (25). For pregnant women who are intolerant of or experience side effects with TMP-SMX or pentamidine, dapsone is an alternative. Dapsone has been shown to be used safely in pregnant women with leprosy (26).

Evaluation and Management of Tuberculosis in Pregnant Women

If appropriate precautions are taken, PPD testing and chest x-rays are both reliable and safe for use with pregnant women (27–29). In asymptomatic women, chest x-rays should be performed only after the first trimester, and a lead apron should be used to shield the abdomen (10,30,31). Women who have symptoms suspicious for TB should be x-rayed with a lead apron shield irrespective of stage of pregnancy, and even if the tuberculin skin test is negative (10,30–32). Preventive INH therapy is not contraindicated in pregnant women and should be initiated as recommended for nonpregnant HIV-infected adults and adolescents (*See also Tuberculosis and HIV Infection*). Treatment of tuberculosis in the pregnant women has been modified for pregnant women because of potential teratogenic effects of specific medications (e.g., streptomycin and pyrazinamide) (30,31,33). Pregnant women with drug-susceptible organisms can be safely treated with INH, rifampin (RIF), and ethambutol (EMB), but treatment must be continued for 9 months (30,31,33). The coadministration of pyridoxine with INH is recommended in pregnant women to provide supplementation to the mother and prevent neurotoxicity in the fetus (34,35).

REFERENCES

1. Kline MW, Shearer WT. Impact of human immunodeficiency virus infection on women and infants. Infectious Disease Clinics of North America 1992;6:1–17.
2. Minkoff HL, DeHovitz JA. Care of women infected with the human immunodeficiency virus. JAMA 1991;266:2253–2258.
3. Carpenter CC, Mayer KH, Fisher A, Desai MD. Natural history of acquired immunodeficiency syndrome in Rhode Island. Am J Med 1989;86:771–775.
4. Moty MR, Saltzman B, Levi MH, McKitrick JC, et al. The recovery of *Mycobacterium avium complex* and *Mycobacterium tuberculosis* from blood specimens of AIDS patients using the nonradiometric BACTEC NR 660 medium. Am J Clin Pathol 1990; 94:84–86.
5. Allen MH, Marte C. HIV infection in women: presentations and protocols. Hosp Pract 1992;27:155–162.
6. Wofsy CB, Padian NS, Cohen JB et al. Management of HIV disease in women. In: Volberding P, Jacobson MA, eds. AIDS Clinical Review, New York: Marcel Dekker, Inc. 1992;301–328.
7. Brettle RP, Lee CLS. The natural history of HIV and AIDS in women. AIDS 1991;5:1283–1292.
8. Minkoff H, DeHovitz JA. HIV infection in women. AIDS Clin Care 1991;3:33–35.
9. New York State Department of Health AIDS Institute. HIV medical evaluation and primary care: gynecologic services. Albany, NY: New York State Department of Health; January 1991.
10. El-Sadr W, Oleske JM, Agins BD, et al. Evaluation and management of early HIV infection. AHCPR Publication 94-0572. Rockville, MD: Agency for Health Care Policy and Research, Public Health Service, US Department of Health and Human Services, January 1994.
11. CDC. Risk for cervical disease in HIV-infected women—New York City. MMWR 1990;39:846–849.
12. Anonymous. ACOG Issues report on HIV infection in women. Am Fam Physician 1992;46:579–585.
13. DeHovitz JA, Sadovsky R. Initial clinical assessment and management of HIV infection. Primary Care 1992;19:35–56.
14. CDC. 1993 sexually transmitted diseases treatment guidelines. MMWR 1993;42 (RR-1).
15. Tramont EC. Syphilis in the AIDS era. N Engl J Med 1987;316:1600–1601.
16. CDC. Recommendations for diagnosing and treating syphilis in HIV-infected patients. MMWR 1988;37:600–607.
17. Musher DM, Hamil RJ, Baughn RE. Effect of human immunodeficiency virus on the course of syphilis and on the response to treatment. Ann Intern Med 1990;113: 872–888.
18. New York City Dept. of Health. Congenital syphilis: its prevention and control. City Health Information 1989;8:1–4.
19. CDC. Guidelines for preventing the transmission of tuberculosis in health care settings, with special focus on HIV-related issues. MMWR 1990;39 (RR-17)

20. Kline AH, Blatter RJ, Lunin M. Transplacental effect of tetracycline on teeth. JAMA 1964;188:178–180.
21. CDC. Zidovudine for the prevention of HIV transmission from mother to infant. MMWR 1994;43:285–287.
22. National Institute of Allergy and Infectious Diseases. Clinical alert: important therapeutic information on the benefit of zidovudine for the prevention of the transmission of HIV from mother to infant. Bethesda, MD: National Institutes of Health, National Institute of Allergy and Infectious Diseases, February 20, 1994.
23. CDC. Recommendations of the U.S. Public Health Service Task Force on the use of zidovudine to reduce perinatal transmission of the human immunodeficiency virus. MMWR 1994;43:RR-11.
24. Briggs GG, Bodendorfer TW, Freeman RK, Yagge SJ. Drugs in pregnancy and lactation. A reference guide to fetal and neonatal risk. Baltimore: Williams & Wilkins, 1983.
25. Conte JE, Chernoff D, Feigal DW et al. Intravenous or inhaled pentamidine for treating Pneumocystis carinii pneumonia in AIDS. Ann Intern Med 1990;113:203–209.
26. Kahn JO. Dapsone is safe during pregnancy. J Am Acad Dermatol 1985;13:838–839.
27. Bonebrake CR, Noller KL, Loehnen CP et al. Routine chest roentgenography in pregnancy. JAMA 1978;240:2747–2748.
28. Montgomery WP, Young RC, Allen MP, Harden KA. The tuberculin test in pregnancy. Am J Obstet Gynecol 1968;100:829–831.
29. Swartz HM, Reichling BA. Hazards of radiation exposure for pregnant women. JAMA 1978;239:1907–1908.
30. CDC. Tuberculosis among pregnant women—New York City, 1985-1992. MMWR 1993;42:605, 611–612.
31. Vallejo J, Starke J. Tuberculosis and pregnancy. Clin Chest Med 1992;13:693–707.
32. Hamadeh MA, Glassroth J. Tuberculosis and pregnancy. Chest 1992;4:1114–1120.
33. CDC. Initial therapy for tuberculosis in the era of multidrug resistance: recommendations of the Advisory Council for the Elimination of Tuberculosis. MMWR 1993;42:RR-7.
34. Atkins JN. Maternal plasma concentration of pyridoxal phosphate during pregnancy: adequacy of vitamin B6 supplementation during isoniazid therapy. Am Rev Resp Dis 1982;126:714–716.
35. Snider DE, Layde PM, Johnson MW, Lyle MA. Treatment of tuberculosis during pregnancy. Am Rev Resp Dis 1980;122:65–79.

Prevention Considerations for Women

Women currently comprise the fastest growing category of people diagnosed with the Acquired Immunodeficiency Syndrome (AIDS) (1), with AIDS being the fourth leading cause of death among U.S. women, aged 25 to 44 (2). The primary modes of AIDS transmission among women are injecting drug use and heterosexual contact with an at-risk partner (3). Heterosexual contact is the most rapidly increasing transmission category for women (4) and accounts for 36% of the AIDS cases among women in the United States through mid-1995 (3). Given that the early epidemiologic characteristics of HIV infection affected primarily male communities (i.e. homosexual/bisexual and injection drug users [IDUs]), there is a greater probability for a heterosexual woman to encounter an HIV-infected male partner (5,6). In addition, the efficiency of HIV transmission appears to be greater from male to female than from female to male (5,6). Injection drug use (IDU) also plays a major role in direct and indirect HIV transmission among women. Among women with AIDS, IDU accounts for 47% of cases and heterosexual contact with an IDU for 18% (3). Although female IDUs typically have sexual relationships with male IDUs, 80% of male IDUs are involved with women who are not using injecting drugs (7). HIV infection in women is clustered geographically, ethnically and economically, is associated with the demographics of injection drug use (8), and is more common among women of color and low social and economic status. Furthermore, AIDS continues to disproportionately affect racial/ethnic minorities; 75% of women with AIDS in the United States are among African-American and Latina women (3). The social aspects, gender differences, and reproductive choices are special issues which concern women with HIV and should be considered in HIV-prevention efforts.

Barriers to Prevention

Women and children with AIDS represent a greater diversity of a racial and socioeconomic mix than do adult males with AIDS. This diversity creates a sense of social isolation which can make it more difficult for women to organize socially or politically in the same way gay men successfully have (9). Women as a group lack a common denominator to receive education, prevention, and support. Women frequently perceive AIDS agencies to be gay-oriented and therefore inappropriate for them (10). Women may also be hesitant to undergo HIV testing because of the possible discovery of drug use or the likelihood of losing their children (11,12). Social and cultural pressures may affect a woman's ability to protect themselves from HIV infection, compromising her ability to negotiate safer sex behaviors. In general, women have less direct control of sexual behavior change. Women may participate in unsafe sex from fear of a partner's response (e.g. anger, violence, rejection, or abandonment) (13,14) or may be unable to protect themselves if they are in a violent, manipulative, or coercive relationship (14). Furthermore, impoverished women engaging in HIV-risk behaviors are more likely to experience life stresses, low self-esteem, emotion-focused coping style and greater depression as compared with impoverished women who are not practicing such risky behaviors (15,16).

Women at greatest risk for HIV are poor, persons of color, and live in urban areas (6,17). HIV-infected women are usually poorer than infected men, limiting their access to adequate shelter, food, social and medical services (10,18). Access to routine health care may be complicated by limited finances, lack of insurance and transportation, child care needs, fear of discrimination and language and cultural barriers (19). The immediate daily realities for many women may outweigh the risk of acquiring HIV infection (20). Avoiding exposure to HIV may have relatively low priority when food, shelter, and employment are immediate concerns (21). Women who engage in survival sex, i.e., sex used to obtain sustenance, are unlikely to utilize condoms (22).

PERCEPTION OF HIV RISK

Many women may perceive themselves to be at low risk of HIV infection, which may explain why they continue to engage in high-risk behavior. Women may fail to see their partner's behavior as risky to themselves or their children (22). In a survey of women who were identified as infected while donating blood, 44% could not identify a factor that placed them at risk (23). Similarly, 58% and 42% of HIV-positive women in prenatal programs in the Bronx and Brooklyn, respectively, had no identified risk factor (24,25). Women surveyed at a sexual transmitted disease (STD) clinic revealed that 84% of women with multiple partners perceived their risk for HIV infection to be somewhat low, very low, or none (26). Women are more likely than men to be initially reported without a risk for HIV; a woman's or her partners' risk behaviors may not be recognized or reported by the woman or her health care provider (4).

PARTNER SELECTION

Partner selection, or knowing one's partner well before having sex is considered an important component of preventing HIV transmission. Although women are encouraged to identify high-risk behaviors in potential sexual partners, this has been shown to be uncommon. Studies have shown a majority of women to be unaware of their partner's drug or sexual history, and few women question partners about prior sexual behaviors (27). Among college students in California, only 38% of women questioned their partners about prior sexual behaviors (28).

UNEQUAL POWER RELATIONSHIP

Many heterosexual relationships are characterized by an imbalance of power since a woman may depend on her spouse or partner for housing, and financial support. In addition, cultural factors may defer most decisions, including sexual ones, to the man. Consequently, women may be unable to effectively assert the need for safe sexual practices, including the use of condoms. Unlike the certain contraceptives that are under a woman's control (e.g. oral contraceptives, IUD), HIV prevention requires a partner's cooperation and safer sex involves the behavior of men as well as women (6).

SAFER SEX AND CONDOM USE

Overall reported condom use by women is low. Of women surveyed in an STD clinic, only 30% reported using a condom at their last sexual encounter (29). National surveys of high school students have also shown that condom use is lower among females than males (30,31). In relationships which allow self protection, women may not use a condom for a number of reasons: they do not perceive themselves as being at risk; they are unaware that condom use reduces risk of transmission; they lack knowledge of proper condom use and sexual negotiation skills; other birth control methods are used; their partner does not appear to practice at-risk behaviors, or they perceive that using a condom destroys the spontaneity of sex (32–35). A woman may also desire to have a child or fear abuse from her partner (35). Partner anger, less self-efficacy, negative attitudes toward condoms, and having fewer friends who use condoms have also been reported as barriers to condom use (33,36). In a survey of women attending an STD clinic, only 30% reported using a condom during their last sexual encounter (29). Variables associated with low condom use included a decrease in sexual pleasure, feeling in love with a partner, and the partner's unwillingness to use condoms (29). Factors associated with irregular or no condom use among Canadian university students included embarrassment about buying condoms, difficulty discussing condom use with a prospective partner, use of oral contraceptives, the belief that condoms interfere with sexual pleasure, and having insufficient knowledge of HIV (37).

The perception that a partner is unwilling to use condoms has been associated with noncondom use among women. However, women may falsely believe that men are less willing to use condoms. In a survey of STD clients having multiple sex partners or crack-using partners, 56% of women (compared to 30% of the men) thought that condom use was a turn-off for their partners (38). Women were also more likely than men to report difficulty in finding a sex partner who wanted to use a condom (71% versus 53%, respectively) (38). Most men surveyed (91%) reported using condoms was a sign of respect for their partners (38). In other surveys of residents in high AIDS incidence areas, men were more likely than women to report condom use (39,40).

CONTRACEPTION

Women may choose nonbarrier contraceptive methods which prevent pregnancy but do not protect against HIV or other sexually transmitted diseases (STDs). Condoms, although effective in protecting against HIV transmission, are less effective as a contraceptive as well as outside a woman's control. Women must use one form of contraception to protect against pregnancy, and another to prevent HIV transmission. The use of birth control methods other than a condom has been reported to be associated with noncondom use (33,37). In the United States, surgical sterilization is the most common contraceptive method for women older than 30 years of age and is used by 28% of women age 15–44 years old (41). It is also more common among women of color, and women who reside in low socioeconomic, inner city communities (42). Compared to nonsterilized women, more women who had been surgically sterilized reported never using condoms (78% versus 46%) (41). Similar findings have been reported among sterilized women in drug treatment programs. Women who are using nonbarrier contraceptive methods may wrongly perceive themselves to be at no risk for HIV infection and should be counseled regarding the use of condoms, safer sexual practices, and the risk for HIV (43).

REPRODUCTIVE CHOICES

Despite being HIV-infected, many women will continue their pregnancy or become pregnant (44,45). The profound meaning of childbearing may be more important to women of many cultures than external factors like illness or economics (12). Women often find childbearing and raising children as their most fulfilling role. Having children may be the only means to obtain a sense of identity and status (6,21). For women whose opportunities are limited by poverty and racism, having children may be considered an important contribution to her community. In the black community, the ability to reproduce has been seen as a powerful tool to fight for liberation and against racism (46). Other reasons for continuing pregnancy may be religious or ethical beliefs; denial of HIV infection; varying perception of risk; barriers to abortion services; drug use; and psychiatric and/or emotional problems (12).

Chemically Dependent Women

For the female injection drug user, there is not only potential HIV transmission through sharing of needles, but also from unprotected sexual intercourse. The dependence on drugs decreases a woman's ability to negotiate safer sex, and safer sex guidelines may also be difficult to adhere to when drug or alcohol use is uncontrollable (12). Female IDUs are often involved in prostitution to support their partners, their children and their addiction (7). Because women IDUs are more likely to have drug-using sex partners (47,48), negotiating safer sex behaviors within a relationship can be difficult, particularly if it is complicated by gender, cultural and financial issues. Female IDUs are often in a high-risk environment where they have little control (e.g., emotional and physical abuse) (17,19,47) and may be dependent on the partner for the supply of drugs, financial support and housing. In addition, women IDUs often have health problems related to their drug use (e.g., poor nutrition, STDs) and do not seek early medical care (7,9). Reported risks associated with injection drug use alone among women IDUs have been needle sharing and lack of disinfection of injecting equipment (35). Perceived barriers to needle disinfection among women IDUs have included: not having their own needles, being high, lack of disinfectant, a need to hide their needles, and unfamiliar surroundings (35).

Being pregnant or having children can also be a motivating factor for women to seek treatment (49). However, drug treatment programs often have excluded pregnant women and women with children; if admitted, the woman must either bring children, which causes interruptions, or leave them with inadequate child care (50). Drug treatment programs may not consider women's special relationship needs (e.g. care of children, family, sex partners, and friends) and confrontational methods used in treatment programs may be damaging for women, particularly for individuals with low self-esteem (49,51). For women in recovery, feelings of guilt and self-blame need to be reduced (51). It has been suggested that programs use nonconfrontational and nonabusive methods and help women establish a love relationship based on choice rather than dependency (49). Many women in recovery have a history of physical, sexual, or emotional abuse, and relationships which are imbalanced in power. For women in treatment, there is a need for positive role models as well as relationships with other women based on trust and support (49). In addition, not all women will have heterosexual relationships; homosexuality is reported more frequently among women substance abusers than among male substance abusers (50). Treatment programs should consider a woman, her circumstances, and the ways which she can alter her lifestyle (e.g. child care, employment training and parenting skills). Job skills training may not be offered to women in the manner it is offered to men (50). This should be considered as unemployment rates have been reported to be high among female IDUs, and remain high following treatment (49).

Lesbian and Bisexual Women

Women who are lesbian or engage in bisexual behavior should also be considered in prevention programs for women. It has been estimated that 3% to 4% of all women may be homosexual or bisexual (52–54). Female-to-female sex is not currently designated as an exposure category by the Centers for Disease Control for women with AIDS. Consequently, the lack of attention given to female-female transmission may lead to the misperception that lesbian sexual practices are relatively safe (55,56). Sexual practices among women having same-sex contact may include cunnilingus, tribadism (genital to genital stimulation) and sadomasochism (56,57). There may be vaginal- and/or anal-digital intercourse, vaginal and/or anal fisting, rimming (mouth to anus), and full body rubbing. Dildos and other sex toys may also be used and shared (56). Only anecdotal reports of possible female-to-female sexual transmission have been reported (58,59). Lesbian and bisexual women may acquire HIV infection via injection drug use, sexual contact with men, sexual contact with IDUs, receipt of infected blood and blood products, or artificial insemination (56). Women having same-sex contact may be at risk for HIV-infection if their partner is HIV-infected or engages in high-risk behaviors (60–62).

Women who have sex with women may engage in multiple risk behaviors other than exposure to their female partner. Injection drug use and heterosexual contact have been linked to HIV serpositivity in lesbian and bisexual women (52,53) with injection drug use reported as a risk behavior among lesbian and bisexual women with AIDS in national surveillance data (62,63). The practice of high-risk sexual behavior, such as having sex with multiple partners, high-risk male partners, and the exchange of sex for money, have also been described among women with same-sex contact (52,56,64–66).

To help women better assess their personal risks for HIV, health providers should be aware of current information regarding lesbians and HIV and feel comfortable in discussing lesbian sexuality (56). Prevention efforts should focus on the specific educational needs of lesbian and bisexual women, as well as women who have sexual contact with other women, but who do not self-identify as lesbian.

Implications for Prevention

Prevention of HIV infection among women remains a primary goal, and counseling and education must be provided to enable women to protect themselves from infection, as well as make reproductive choices for themselves and their families (27). Known strategies to prevent HIV infection in women include increasing the level of perceived risk, identifying and assessing women engaging in at-risk behaviors, and assisting in risk reduction (e.g. safer sex, partner selection, reduction in the number of partners, and the elimination of risky sexual practices). However, standard prevention messages for sex transmission may be ineffective for women because they seem irrelevant and suggest that women can control a man's sexual behavior (67). Messages of abstinence, monogamy, or condom use may equate to a woman losing her partner and may disregard her need for love and support (67). Although women are counseled to know the sexual and drug history of their partners, they may want to initiate or continue a relationship with a man, despite the risk, for many reasons, including love, companionship, status, or support for herself and children. Further, women may not wish to jeopardize the relationship by questioning their partner about their past sexual or drug use history, or by insisting on the use of condoms (6). Interventions which rely on women to introduce condoms into a sexual situation may require women to assume new roles in an intensely emotional and private situation and upset the existing balance of power in the relationship. In many cultural contexts, negative connotations of condom use include presumptions of infidelity, distrust, disease, or trying to control a man's sexuality (6,20,40). Male partners may react with sexual rejection, domestic violence, and termination of the relationship.

To be effective, education and prevention efforts must consider the diversity of women. Programs must be individualized, culturally and ethnically relevant, linguistically appropriate, and delivered in a sensitive and understandable manner. Women, preferably peers who share the same group identity, should be included in interventions. To reach women, prevention efforts can take place at locations that are part of women's daily lives. Places women visit frequently regardless of HIV or risk status, such as hospitals, churches, beauty shops, supermarkets, and shopping centers might be important opportunities to present and/or disseminate HIV information (46,68). Community-based peer programs have been shown to be helpful for women at high risk in increasing condom use and intention to use condoms (69).

Obstacles to changing sexual behavior include lack of knowledge, denial of risk (by a woman or her partner), embarrassment about discussing sex and AIDS, difficulty in being assertive, lack of control in relationships with men, and lack of partner cooperation (70). Information alone is insufficient to change behavior. Because most women do not personalize being at risk for HIV, education should be aimed at increasing women's levels of perception of risk and enabling participants to assess their risk accurately. Interventions must be personalized, relevant, and sensitive to the realities of each woman's life (20,27) and counseling supportive of decisions made by women and their partners to reduce risk behaviors (71).

Training should be based on social cognitive (72) theories emphasizing specific behavioral skills necessary to implement risk reduction behaviors (e.g., communicative skills), and enhancing women's motivation to act on perceived risk with appropriate behavioral skills (27). The use of individual or group settings can be used for focused skill training. A benefit of a small group setting would be the sense of peer support that develops as women seek solutions together (73). Role playing can assist the woman to anticipate and plan how she might integrate safe sex behavior into her unique circumstances. Risk reduction should also assist in communication skills, risk reduction problem solving, sexual assertiveness; behavioral self-management including how safer sex and condoms can be a part of an enjoyable sexual experience may facilitate compliance with guidelines and enjoyment (74–76). In a study of discordant heterosexual partners (i.e., one partner HIV seropositive, the other seronegative) who received risk reduction, couples having a history of frank sexual communication and varied sexual behavior found it easier and more fulfilling to comply with risk reduction guidelines than couples who lacked that history (74). For women who choose nonbarrier methods of contraception, educational efforts should emphasize the need for continued barrier protection (i.e., condom use) and its importance in preventing HIV and STDs. Because men control or influence the majority of women's decisions about sexual behavior, it may be necessary to include men in prevention efforts (e.g., couple counseling) (20). Since many women may believe that a male partner may be unwilling to use condoms, consequently inhibiting condom use, men should be encouraged to verbalize their feelings about condom use to women (38). For relationships where the partner is unwilling to use condoms, non-penetrative sex or alternatives that offer some protection (e.g., use of spermicidal agent with a diaphragm) should be explored (77). In addition, women should be informed how to access available local, state, and national resources. Referrals to social, mental health, financial, legal, and medical sources of support are important to help decrease the sense of isolation women at risk and infected women may feel. As approximately half of AIDS cases among women are attributed to injecting drug use, prevention must also address drug addiction in women and their partners, providing risk reduction counseling regarding safer injection practices.

Prevention efforts must consider the diverse population of social, cultural, and economic mix that women at risk for HIV infection represent. Understanding the issues relevant to women and the complexity of behavior change for women is important in developing strategies which are effective in assisting women prevent HIV infection.

REFERENCES

1. Chu S, Buehler J, Berkelman R. Impact of the human immunodeficiency virus epidemic on mortality of women of reproductive age, United States. JAMA 1990;264: 225–229.
2. National Institute of Allergy and Infectious Disease (NIAID). Women and HIV Infection. April 1994. NIAID.
3. CDC. HIV/AIDS Surveillance Record. Whole booklet (pg 1–34) publisher—CDC Atlanta Georgia. Mid-year edition 1995; 7(1).

4. CDC. Heterosexually acquired AIDS—United States 1993. MMWR 1994;43:155–160.
5. Guinan, ME Hardy A. Epidemiology of AIDS in women in the United States. JAMA 1987;257:2039–2042.
6. Anastos K and Palleja SM. Caring for women at risk of HIV infection. J Gen Int Med 1991;6(Jan/Feb Suppl):S40–S46.
7. Cohen JB, Hauer LB, Wofsy CB. Women and IV drugs: parenteral and heterosexual transmission of human immunodeficiency virus. Journal Drug Issues 1989;19:39–56.
8. Landesman SH. Human immunodeficiency virus infection in women: an overview. Seminars in Perinatology 1989;13:2–6.
9. Stuntzner-Gibson D. Women and HIV disease: an emerging social crisis. Social Work 1991;36:22–27.
10. Buckingham SL, Rehm SJ. AIDS and women at risk. Health and Social Work 1987;12:5–11.
11. Tuomala R. Human immunodeficiency virus education and screening of prenatal patients. Obstet and Gyn Clinics of North America 1990;17:571–583.
12. Holman S. Berthaud M, Sunderland A, Moroso, et al. Women infected with human immunodeficiency virus: counseling and testing during pregnancy. Seminars in Perinatology 1989;13:7–15.
13. Macks J. Women and AIDS: countertransference issues. Social Casework 1988;69:340–347.
14. Shernoff M, Palacios-Jimenez L. AIDS: prevention is the only vaccine available: an AIDS prevention educational program. J Social Work & Human Sexuality 1988;6:135–150.
15. Nyamathi A, Stein J, Brecht ML. Psychosocial predictors of AIDS risk behavior and drug use behavior in homeless and drug addicted women of color. Health Psychology 1995;14:1–9.
16. Nyamathi A, Wayment H, Dunkel-Schetter C. Psychosocial correlates of emotional distress and risk behavior in African-American women at risk for HIV infection. Anxiety, Stress and Coping 1993;6:133–48.
17. Worth D and Rodriguez R. Latina women and AIDS. Siecus Rep 1987;Jan-Feb:5–7.
18. Andriote J. For women at risk, prevention begins with self-esteem. The NAN Monitor 1988;3:12–14.
19. Public Health Reports. Report of the second public health service AIDS prevention and control conference. J U.S. Public Health Serv 1988;13(Suppl 1):66–71, 88–98.
20. Wofsy CB, Padian, Cohen JB, et al. Management of HIV disease in women In: Volberding P, Jacobson MA, eds. AIDS Clinical Review. New York: Marcel Dekker, Inc, 1992:301–328.
21. Nyamathi A, Shin D. Designing a culturally sensitive AIDS educational program for black and hispanic women of childbearing age. NACOOG's Clinical Issues in Perinatal and Woman's Health Nursing 1990;1(1):86–98.
22. Stuber ML. Children, adolescents and AIDS. Psychiatric Medicine 1991;9:441–454.
23. Ward J, Kleinman S, Douglas D. Epidemiologic characteristics of blood donors with antibody to human immunodeficiency virus. Transfusion. 1988;28:298–301.
24. Checola R, Hand I, Wiznia A, et al. Maternal drug abuse and perinatal HIV seropositivity (Abs). In: Proceedings of the Fifth International Conference on AIDS. Ottawa, Ontario: International Development Research Centre, 1989:313.
25. Landesman S, Minkoff H, Holman S, et al. Serosurvey of human immunodeficiency virus infection in parturients. JAMA 1987;258:2701–2703.
26. Wettrich M, Dillon B. Perception of risk for HIV/AIDS, self-efficacy for behavior change and sexual behaviors among STD clinic clients. U.S. 1991. (Abs). Presented at IXth International Conference on AIDS. June 1993. PO–D23–4121. Berlin.
27. Nolte S, Sohn MA, and Koons B. Prevention of HIV infection in women. Journal of Obstet Gynecol Neonatal Nursing 1993;2:128–134.
28. Cochran SD, Leidan J, Kalechstein A. Sexually transmitted diseases and acquired immunodeficiency syndrome (AIDS). Sexually Transmitted Diseases 1990;17:80–86.
29. CDC. Heterosexual behaviors and factors that influence condom use among patients attending a sexually transmitted disease clinic—San Francisco. MMWR 1990;39:685–688.
30. Collins J, Holtzman D, Kann L, Kolbe L. Predictors of condom use among U.S. high school students. (Abs) Presented at the IXth International Conference on AIDS, Berlin, June 1993 (WS-C13-4).
31. CDC. Premarital sexual experience among adolescent women—United States, 1970, 1988. MMWR 1991;39:929–932.
32. Njeri N. A new sexuality? Essence. 1989;January:114–118.

33. Gomez C. Can women demand condom use?: gender and power in safe sex. (Abs). Presented at IXth International Conference on AIDS, Berlin, June 1993 (PO–D03–3502).
34. Catania JA, Coates TH, Kegeles S, Fullilove MT, Peterson J, Marin B, et al. Condom use in the multiethnic neighborhoods of San Francisco: The population-based AMEN (AIDS in multiethnic neighborhoods) study. Am J Public Health 1992;82:284–287.
35. Nyamathi AM, Lewis C, Leake B, Flaskerud J, Bennett C. Barriers to condom use and needle cleaning among impoverished minority female injection drug users and partners of injection drug users. Public Health Rep 1995;110:166–172.
36. Jemmott JB, Jemmott LS, Fong GT. Reductions in HIV risk-associated sexual behaviors among black male adolescents: effects of an AIDS prevention intervention. Am J Public Health 1992;82:372–377.
37. MacDonald NE, Wells GA, Fisher WA, Warren WK, et al. High risk STD/HIV behavior among college students. JAMA 1990;263:3155–3159.
38. Walsh C, Wettrich M, Campbell C. Perceptions of cond use among STD clinic clients by gender, U.S., 1991. (Abs) Presented at IXth International Conference on AIDS, Berlin, June 1993(PO–D37–4403).
39. CDC. Sexual behavior and condom use—District of Columbia, January-February, 1992. MMWR 1993;42:390–391,398.
40. Choi KH, Rickman R, Catania J. What do US heterosexual adults believe about condoms. (Abs) Presented at IXth International Conference on AIDS, Berlin, June 1993(PO–C22–3146).
41. CDC. Surgical sterilization among women and use of condoms—Baltimore, 1989-1990. MMWR 1992;41:568–569,575.
42. Mosher WE. Contraceptive practice in the United States, 1982–1988. Fam Plann Perspect 1990;22:198–205.
43. CDC. 1993 Sexually Transmitted Diseases Treatment Guidelines. MMWR. 1993;42 (RR-1).
44. Selwyn PA, Carter CJ, Schoenbaum EE, et al. Knowledge of HIV antibody status and decisions to continue or terminate pregnancy among intravenous drug users. JAMA 1989;261:3567–3571.
45. Johnstone FD, MacCullum L, Brethle R, et al. Does infection with HIV affect the outcome of pregnancy? Br Med J 1988; 196:467.
46. Mays V, Cochran S. Issues in the perception of AIDS risk and risk reduction activity by black and Hispanic/Latina women. Am Psychol 1988;43:949–957.
47. Mondanaro J. Chemically dependent women: assessment and treatment. Lexington, Massachusetts: Lexington Books, 1989.
48. Turner CF, Miller HG, Moses LE. AIDS, sexual behavior and intravenous drug use. Washington D.C.: National Academy Press, 1989.
49. Wells DVB, Jackson JF. HIV and chemically dependent women: recommendations for appropriate health care and drug treatment services. Int J Addict 1992;27:571–585.
50. Peluso E, Peluso LS. Women and drugs: getting hooked, getting clean. Minneapolis: Compcare Publishers, 1988.
51. Reed BG. Drug misuse and dependency in women: the meaning and implications of being considered a special population or minority group. Int J Addict 1985;20:13–61.
52. McCombs SB, McCray E, Wendell DA, Sweeney PA, Onorato IM. Epidemiology of HIV-1 infection in bisexual women. J Acquir Immune Defic Syndr. 1992;5:850–852.
53. Petersen LR, Doll L, White, Chus S, and the HIV Blood Donor Study Group. No evidence for female-to-female HIV transmission among 960,000 female blood donors. J Acquir Immune Defic Syndr. 1992;5:853–855.
54. Wellings K, Field J, Wadsworth J, Johnson AM, Anderson RM, Bradshaw SA. Sexual lifestyles under scrutiny. Nature. 1990;348:276–278.
55. Einhorn L. New data on lesbians and AIDS. Off Our Backs 1989;19:10.
56. Cole R, Cooper S. Lesbian exclusion from HIV/AIDS education: ten years of low-risk identity and high-risk behavior. SIECUS Report, December 1990/January 1991: 18–23.
57. Califia P. Lesbian sexuality. J of Homosexuality, 1979;4:255–266.
58. Marmor M, Weiss LR, Lyden M, et al. Possible female-to-female transmission of human immunodeficiency virus. Ann Intern Med 1986;105:969.
59. Monzon OT, Capellan JM. Female-to-female transmission of HIV. Lancet 1987;1: 40–41.
60. Perry S, Jacobsberg L, Fogel K. Orogenital transmission of the human immunodeficiency virus. Annals of Internal Medicine. 1989;11:951–952.
61. Spitzer PT, Weiner NJ. Transmission of HIV infection from a woman to a man by oral sex. N Engl J Med 1989;320:251.

62. Chu SY, Hammett TA, Buehler JW. Update: epidemiology of reported cases of AIDS in women who report sex only with other women, 1980–1991. AIDS 1992;6:518–519.
63. Chu SY, Buehler JW, Fleming PL, Berkelman RL. Epidmeiology of reported cases of AIDS in lesbians, United States 1980–89. Am J Public Health. 1990;80:1360–1381.
64. Cohen H, Marmor M, Wolfe H, Ribble D. Risk assessment of HIV transmission among lesbians. J Acquir Immune Defic Syndr. 1993;6:1173–1174.
65. Young RM, Weissman G, Cohen JB. Assessing risk in the absence of information: HIV risk among women injection drug users who have sex with women. AIDS Public Policy J. 1992;7:175–183.
66. Bevier PJ, Chiasson MA, Hefferman RT, Castro KG. Women at a sexually transmitted disease clinic who reported same-sex contact: their HIV seroprevalence and risk behaviors. Am J Public Health. 1995;85:1366–1371.
67. Cohen JB. Why woman partners of drug users will continue to be at high risk for HIV infection. J Addic Res 1991;10:99–110.
68. Berman S, Lindsay M, Hadgu A. Reaching minority women at risk for HIV: the potential for pre-gestational access by churches and inner-city hospitals. (Abstr) Presented at IXth International Conference on AIDS. Berlin, June 1993 (PO-D13-3746).
69. Tross S, Abdul-Quader AS, Simons PS, et al. Evaluation of a peer outreach HIV prevention program for female sexual partners (FSPs) of injecting drug users (IDUs) in New York City (NYC). (abstr) Presented at IXth International Conference on AIDS. Berlin, June 1993. (PO-D13-3737)
70. Ehrhardt AA. Preventing and treating AIDS: the expertise of the behavior sciences. Bull NY Acad Med 1988;64:513–519.
71. CDC. Update: AIDS Among Women—United States, 1994. MMWR. 1995;44:81–84.
72. Bandura A. Perceived self-efficacy in the exercise of control over HIV infection. In S.J. Blumenthal, A. Eichler, G. Weissman, eds. Women and AIDS. Washington DC: American Psychiatric Press, 1994.
73. Raisler J. Safer Sex for Women. NACOOG's Clinical Issues in Perinatal and Woman's Health Nursing 1990;1:28–32.
74. Moore L, Padian NS. The social context of sexual risk taking in a cohort of heterosexuals. (abstr) Presented at IXth International Conference on AIDS. Berlin, June 1993 (PO-D15-3873).
75. Malow RM, Corrigan SA, Cunningham SC, et al. Psychosocial factors associated with condom use among African-American drug abusers in treatment. AIDS Educ Prev 1993;5:244–253.
76. Washington CD, Kelly JA, Murphy DA et al. Effects of group behavior change intervention for high risk women seen in urban primary health care clinics. (Abstr) Presented at IXth International Conference on AIDS. Berlin, June 1993 (PO-C22-3143).
77. Moroso G, Holman S. Counseling and Testing Women for HIV. NACOOG's Clinical Issues in Perinatal and Woman's Health Nursing 1990;1:10–19.

CHAPTER 6

Pediatric AIDS

Diagnosis and Evaluation of HIV-infected Children

Vertical transmission of HIV from mother to child accounts for the majority of children infected with HIV. With larger numbers of women of childbearing age contracting HIV infection, the epidemic is growing in children born to these mothers. However, there is recent evidence that early identification and therapy of the mother-infant pair with zidovudine significantly reduces vertical transmission. Advances have also been made to improve the quality and duration of life of infected children. Guidelines have become available which help the practitioner with the diagnosis, management, and therapy of HIV-infected children. (For purposes of this section, newborns are defined from birth to 30 days of age, infants are from 30 days to two years of age and children are up to 12 years old.)

Maternal-fetal transmission is the primary mode of HIV transmission for children in the United States, accounting for 90% of pediatric HIV infections. Infection through blood products has been virtually eliminated through improved screening practices. Of vertically infected children, 60% had mothers who were injecting drug users (IDU) or had sex with an IDU (1). Recent data from the CDC suggest an increasing number of mothers have no identifiable risk factor other than heterosexual intercourse. This suggests that the epidemic is no longer confined to identified high-risk groups and therefore neither practitioner nor patient will know either are at risk. In large prospective studies the rate of transmission of HIV infection from mother to child is between 13% and 39% with an average of 20–25% in U.S. studies (2). It is estimated that approximately 1,800 newly infected infants are born each year in the United States (3). The mechanism and timing of vertical transmission is still uncertain, however HIV can be transmitted from mother to infant in utero, intrapartum, or postpartum by breast feeding.

Morbidity and Mortality

HIV-infected children progress more rapidly than do adults, with distinct patterns of disease presentation, which makes early and aggressive intervention a priority. Recently a bimodal pattern of disease presentation in children has been recognized (4). One group of children presents within the first three to six months of life, while another group remains asymptomatic for the first year of life. Children who present early may be at risk of rapid loss of CD4 cells and also for *Pneumocystis carinii* pneumonia (PCP), wasting syndrome, cytomegalovirus (CMV) coinfection, or encephalopathy. Children who become symptomatic, after the first year of life frequently have a more indolent course. These children may present with lymphoid interstitial pneumonitis (LIP) or other lymphoproliferative disorders (5). The authors feel that the most convincing explanation for this phenomenon lies in the biologic characteristics of the virus and the timing of infection of the fetus. In utero-infected infants can be expected to show earlier signs of disease than children who are infected during the birth process. Only a minority of children infected vertically have been found to survive beyond eight years; however as the epidemic progresses and new therapies are introduced, older HIV-infected children are expected to be seen more frequently.

Importance of Testing and Counseling

To provide appropriate counseling and prenatal care to HIV-infected women, they must first be identified. Indications for HIV testing and counseling are described elsewhere in the book. Given that heterosexual transmission is the primary mode of HIV exposure among women, *all* pregnant women should be offered HIV testing and counseling, even in areas of low seroprevalence. Considering the recent findings from the AIDS Clinical Trials Group (ACTG) 076 study, which shows that the rate of HIV transmission from mothers to infants has been reduced from 25.5% to 8.3% by treatment with zidovudine (ZDV), (6,7) it is crucial to diagnose and treat HIV-infected women during pregnancy.

Management for the HIV-infected Pregnant Woman

ANTEPARTUM AND INTRAPARTUM CARE (8,9)

Management and care for women who are HIV-infected should include the following:

- A thorough history and physical examination.
- Nondirective counseling with the focus on the woman and her needs, rather than on the beliefs held by the provider. It is also important to determine whether the women is able to access care for a pregnancy termination if that is her decision.

- Due to the resurgence of syphilis in urban centers, HIV-infected women should be screened for syphilis with a nontreponemal test (RPR or VDRL) at entry into prenatal care, during the third trimester, at delivery and if the patient becomes exposed to or presents with symptoms of syphilis.

- The woman should be screened for other infectious diseases including: gonorrhea, herpes simplex, tuberculosis, hepatitis B, chlamydia, cytomegalovirus (CMV), and candidiasis.

- A Pap smear should be obtained at least once during prenatal care, any cytologic abnormality should be investigated by colposcopy. Any abnormality should be followed up with consultation from a gynecologist. A Pap smear should be repeated following delivery.

- Whenever possible the following procedures should be avoided: amniocentesis, chorionic villus sampling, percutaneous umbilical blood sampling, and fetal scalp electrodes and fetal scalp sampling during labor.

- CD4 counts should be followed monthly and PCP prophylaxis should be initiated as recommended by the guidelines from the Centers of Disease Control (CDC).

- The risks and benefits of the initiation of antiretroviral therapy should be discussed with all patients, independent of their lymphocyte (CD4) counts.

ZIDOVUDINE REGIMEN FOR HIV-INFECTED PREGNANT WOMEN AND THEIR INFANTS

- Oral administration of 100 mg zidovudine (ZDV) five times daily, initiated at 14–36 weeks' gestation and continued for the remainder of pregnancy.

- During labor intravenous administration of ZDV in a loading dose of two mg per kg body weight given over one hour, followed by continuous infusion of one mg per kg body weight per hour until delivery.

- Oral administration of ZDV to the newborn (ZDV syrup at two mg per kg body weight per dose given every six hours) given for the first six weeks of life, beginning 8–12 hours after birth.

Diagnosis of the HIV-Infected Infant

The diagnosis of infants born to HIV-infected mothers is complicated by the presence of passively transferred maternal antibodies (Ab) which may persist for up to 18 months. HIV infection is diagnosed in infants/children over 18 months by a positive ELISA and confirmation of Western blot analysis or another federally approved assay as are adults. Alternatively HIV infection can be diagnosed clinically in children by onset of HIV-related symptoms as defined by the CDC. Diagnosis by these methods may delay the benefits of intervention of infants and children who develop complications before one year of age.

Tests that detect the HIV-1 independent of Ab, for example, virus culture, proviral DNA by polymerase chain reaction, and immune complex dissociation (ICD) by p24 can be used to diagnose HIV infection in the majority of at-risk infants by three to six months. If the infant is infected during the birthing process (intrapartum), the minuscule viral load may escape detection at birth, but can be detected as early as two weeks or rarely as late as six months after birth. Using these techniques, 30–50% of infected infants have been diagnosed at birth and the remainder before six months of age. *The infant born to a HIV infected mother should be tested as soon as possible after birth with an HIV specific test that does not depend on antibody. If tests are negative the child should be retested at three and six months of age. Infants with a negative test at six months of age should have an Ab-dependent HIV test performed at 15 and 18 months of age to document their HIV status and loss of passively transferred maternal antibody (9).*

WHERE TO TEST PEDIATRIC PATIENTS FOR HIV-1

At present, since these tests may not be widely available to the clinician in the community, consultation with a specialist in pediatric HIV care should be considered. Collaborative management between primary health care provider and specialist may significantly improve survival and quality of health of the infected child as well as the family. Information for referral can be found in the Resources chapter, "Resources."

Evaluation of a Child with HIV

A detailed timetable for clinical, laboratory and additional testing is shown in Table 6.1. This table contains information on how frequently history and physical examination, laboratory evaluation, diagnostic imaging and additional testing like developmental, audiology and ophthalmology are recommended.

IMMUNOLOGIC TESTING

Whenever a child is found to be HIV seropositive, an initial CD4+ cell count should be measured to rapidly evaluate the child's need for PCP prophylaxis. *Expert opinion recommends obtaining CD4 counts and percentages in all infants born to HIV-infected mothers at one, three and six months of age and then at three-month intervals until the HIV status of the child is known. Thereafter, CD4 counts and percentages should be monitored at three- to six-month intervals in children proven to be HIV infected (9).*

If the CD4+ cell count is approaching the age-adjusted threshold level for initiation of prophylaxis, the CD4+ lymphocyte count should be assessed more frequently (at one-month intervals) to evaluate the rate of decline and the need to initiate prophylaxis. PCP prophylaxis for infants and children is described elsewhere in this section. In young infants between 6 weeks and 3 months of age, PCP prophylaxis may be started prior to a definitive diagnosis of HIV and stopped if the child is found to be negative.

Table 6.1.

Guidelines for Clinical and Laboratory Evaluation for Infants or Children Younger than 2 Years Born to HIV-Infected Women

Evaluation	Birth	1–2 wk	1 mo	2 mo	3 mo	4 mo	6 mo	9 mo	12 mo	15 mo	18 mo	21 mo	24 mo
History, physical exam	◆	◆	◆	◆		◆	◆	◆	◆	◆	◆	◆	◆
Developmental assessment	◆		◆			◆	◆	◆	◆	◆	◆	◆	◆
Ht, wt, head circumference	◆	◆	◆	◆		◆	◆	◆	◆	◆	◆	◆	◆
Complete blood count & platelets	◆		◆			◆	◆	◆	◆	◆	◆	◆	◆
Chemistry panel	◆		◆			◆	◆	◆	◆	◆	◆	◆	◆
Urinalysis	◆		◆			◆	◆	◆	◆	◆	◆	◆	◆
Immunoglobulins	d							◆	◆	◆	◆	◆	◆
ELISA/Western blot													
Lymphocyte subsets					◆		◆	c	c	c	c	c	c
p24 antigen	◆		◆		◆		◆						
HIV culture	◆				◆		◆						
PCR	◆				◆		◆		◆				
CMV urine	◆			◆		◆							
PPD control													
Neurologic evaluation	Every 3 to 6 months												
Ophthalmology evaluation	At 1–2 years												
Dental exam	At 1–2 years												
Audiology	a												
If mother positive or unknown													
Hepatitis B serology	◆		◆		◆		◆		◆				
Syphilis serology	◆	c			◆		◆		◆				
Toxoplasmosis (IgG, IgM)	◆	b		◆		◆							
For HIV-infected child, or if clinically indicated													
Chest x-ray	Baseline, then if clinically indicated												
CT/MRI	Only if clinically indicated												
Echocardiogram	Only if clinically indicated												
Electrocardiogram	Baseline, then if clinically indicated												

Modified from Kovacs A, Oleske J. Antiretroviral Treatment for Children with HIV Infection. In: Pizzo PA, Wilfert CM. Pediatric AIDS. Baltimore: Williams & Wilkins, 1994:734.

a = routinely at 2 years or if indicated; b = every 3 months after age 6 months; c = if positive; d = see text; CT = computed tomography; MRI = magnetic resonance imaging.

For children more than two years of age, CD4+ cell counts should be monitored at least every six months, as recommended for HIV-infected adults. Every attempt should be made to diagnose HIV infection definitively as soon as possible so that children may receive appropriate treatment if indicated. In addition, depending on clinical findings, other diagnostic evaluation or treatment may be needed. PCP prophylaxis should be considered for a young infant who is thought to be at risk of PCP because of the presence of a constellation of HIV-related symptoms, even if a CD4+ cell count is not yet available.

NEUROLOGIC TESTING

CNS dysfunction occurs in as many as 20% of all HIV-infected infants and children and may be twice as high in symptomatic patients (10). The most frequent manifestations are impaired brain growth, motor dysfunction, loss or plateau of milestones, and cognitive impairment (9). Abnormal CNS findings may be caused by HIV encephalopathy, opportunistic infections (OIs), intercerebral hemorrhage or CNS neoplasms. OIs in adults are frequently secondary to reactivation of previously acquired organisms and are less frequently seen in infants and children.

A neurologic examination and developmental assessment should be performed on all HIV-infected infants and children. A follow-up neurologic examination should be part of each clinic visit. Full developmental assessment should be performed every three months during the first two years of life and in children above 2 years every 6 months. CT scan and MRI should be reserved to diagnose the cause of neurologic deterioration, although some specialists feel that baseline neuroimaging is justified in the absence of neurologic deficits.

HIV encephalopathy is diagnosed by exclusion and should be treated with antiretroviral agents, preferably by a neurologist with experience in HIV disease. Studies are presently undertaken in certain centers using continuous intravenous infusion of ZDV for HIV encephalopathy unresponsive to oral therapy. Other combined antiretroviral regimens are also under study. Intervention has to be a team effort involving physical, occupational, and speech therapy. Nutritional supplements may be required in patients with advanced neurologic disease.

REFERENCES

1. CDC. HIV/AIDS surveillance report. Mid-Year Edition Atlanta, GA: Center for Disease Control, 1995;7:1.
2. Von Seidlein L BY. Maternal-fetal transmission of HIV-1. Seminars in Pediatric Infectious Diseases 1994;5:78–86.
3. Chin J. Current and future dimensions of the HIV/AIDS pandemic in women and children. Lancet 1990;336:221–224.
4. Blanche S, Tardieu M, Duliege A, et al. Longitudinal study of 94 symptomatic infants with perinatally acquired human immunodeficiency virus infection. Evidence for a bimodal expression of clinical and biological symptoms. Am J Dis Child 1990;144:1210–1215.
5. Oxtoby M. Vertically acquired HIV infection in the USA. In: Pizzo PA WC, ed. Pediatric AIDS. The challenge of HIV infection in infants, children, and adolescents. 2nd ed. Baltimore: Williams & Wilkins, 1994: 3–20.

6. Cotton P. Trial halted after drug cuts maternal HIV transmission rate by two thirds [news]. Jama 1994;271:807.
7. CDC. Zidovudine for the prevention of HIV transmission from mother to infant. MMWR 1994;43:285–287.
8. Boyer PJ. HIV infection in pregnancy. Pediatr Ann 1993;22:406–408, 411–412.
9. US Dept Health and Human Service. Evaluation and management of early HIV infection. In: Clinical practice guideline. US Department of Health and Human Services, 1994: vol 7. Rockville, MD
10. Butler KM, Husson RN, Balis FM, et al. Dideoxyinosine in children with symptomatic human immunodeficiency virus infection. N Engl J Med 1991;324:137–144.

RECOMMENDED READING

Pizzo PA, Wilfert CM. Pediatric AIDS. The challenge of HIV infection in infants, children, and adolescents. 2nd ed. Baltimore: Williams & Wilkins. 1994

Antiretroviral Therapy in Children with HIV

Initiating Antiretroviral Therapy

All children with established diagnosis of HIV infection should be considered for antiretroviral therapy. The decision of when to start should be made by a practitioner who is expert in the management of pediatric HIV infection. Whenever possible, we try to enroll our patients in clinical trials so that they may have access to new retroviral therapies, which may benefit the individual patient as well as other HIV-infected infants and children. Current trials are focusing on aggressive, early therapy of newly diagnosed infants using triple therapy in an effort to block high level viremia during primary infection at <6 months of age. Information about trials can be found in the resource section. All children with evidence of significant immune deficiency or HIV-associated symptoms should be considered for antiretroviral drug therapy. In addition, administration of zidovudine (ZDV) to the newborn of an HIV-infected mother should be strongly considered. (For dosages see: Zidovudine regimen for HIV-infected pregnant women and their infants).

CD4 Criteria for Initiation of Antiretroviral Therapy

Current recommended CD4 criteria for initiation of antiretroviral therapy (1) are listed in Table 6.2. Children who are infected with HIV and those with indeterminate HIV infection status should have their CD4 parameters (absolute, relative, and percentage) measured every three months. Abnormal CD4 parameters have to be repeated to validate the result as well as to establish a baseline value.

Clinical Criteria for Initiation of Antiretroviral Therapy

Clinical criteria used for initiation of antiretroviral therapy regardless of the CD4 lymphocyte count have been recommended (1) and are listed in Table 6.3.

Table 6.2.
CD4 Lymphocyte Values for Initiating Antiretroviral Therapy

Age	CD4(%)	CD4 (cells/mm^3)
Younger than 1 year	<30	<1750
1 to 2 years	<25	<1000
2 to 6 years	<20	<750
Older than 6 years	<20	<500

Modified and reprinted with permission from the Working Group on Antiretroviral Therapy. Antiretroviral therapy & medical management of the human immunodeficiency virus-infected child. Working Group on Antiretroviral Therapy: National Pediatric HIV Resource Center. Pediatr Infect Dis J 1993;12:513–522.

Table 6.3.
Clinical Criteria for Initiating Antiretroviral Therapy

s   AIDS-defining opportunistic infection
s   Wasting syndrome or failure to thrive[a]
s   Thrombocytopenia (platelet count <75,000 cells/mm^3 on at least 2 occasions)
s   Hypogammaglobulinemia (total IgG/IgM/IgA <250/mm^3)
–   Lymphoid interstitial pneumonitis (LIP)
–   Parotitis
–   Splenomegaly
–   Oral candidiasis persisting >1 month
–   Unexplained, persistent, or recurrent diarrhea (≥3 loose stools per day for ≥2 weeks)
–   Symptomatic cardiomyopathy
–   Nephrotic syndrome
–   Severe hepatic transaminitis (>5-fold normal)
–   Chronic bacterial infections
–   ≥2 episodes of herpes simplex/varicella zoster (VZV) infection within a 1-year period
–   Neutropenia (<750/mm^3)
–   Age-corrected anemia on at least 2 occasions over 1 week.

s Clinical conditions which warrant institution of antiretroviral treatment independent of CD4 lymphocyte count.
– Clinical conditions which may warrant initiation of antiretroviral therapy depending on the overall clinical profile of the child and judgment of health care providers regarding the risk/benefit.
[a] Defined as crossing two percentiles for weight over time or being below the 5th percentile for age and falling from the growth curve.

DRUG AND REGIMEN OF CHOICE

ZDV, ddI, and 3TC are the only antiretroviral drugs approved by the FDA for treatment of HIV infection in children under 13 years of age at the time of this writing. A recent study (ACTG 152) showed that ZDV monotherapy, although effective, was not the ideal treatment when compared to either ddI monotherapy or ZDV/ddI in combination. Therefore, primary therapy outside of the newborn period of ZDV prophylaxis should consist of ZDV plus ddI or ddI alone. Efficacy trials of combined ZDV and 3TC in children are underway which may also become an option. In addition, stavudine (D4T) has also been evaluated in phase I/II trials. Recommended dosages for administration of ZDV, ddI, ddc, and 3TC are listed in Table 6.4.

Table 6.4.
Recommended Dosages of ZDV, ddl, ddC and 3TC for Children

	Dosage	Side Effects
ZDV		
0 to 2 weeks old	2 mg/kg per dose every 6 hours	Anemia, neutropenia, increased transaminase, nausea, and vomiting
2 to 4 weeks old	3 mg/kg per dose every 6 hours	
4 wks to 13 yrs	180 mg/m^2 per dose every 6 hours	↓
13 years and older	600 mg/day	
ddl	100 mg/m^2 per BID	Pancreatitis, peripheral neuropathy
ddC	0.01 mg/kg TID	Peripheral neuropathy, oral ulcers
3TC	4 mg/kg/dose BID	Rash, insomnia/headache, peripheral neuropathy, pancreatitis

The minimum acceptable dosage is 75 mg/m^2 every 6 hours po, but should not be used in patients with progressive neurologic involvement.

Monitoring ZDV Treatment

The primary adverse effects of ZDV treatment are anemia and neutropenia, which are more common among children receiving high dosage of ZDV or children with advanced HIV disease (2). Monthly monitoring of blood counts (CBC and platelets) is necessary. Liver function and creatine phosphokinase should be monitored regularly. Up to a quarter of children using ZDV require dose reduction secondary to anemia or neutropenia; however discontinuation of ZDV is only rarely required (3). The use of erythropoietin and granulocyte colony-stimulating factor (GCSF) is described below. Other adverse effects like vomiting, headaches, insomnia, neuropathy are rarely seen in children. A suggested management plan and monitoring schedule for children receiving ZDV is shown in Table 6.5.

ADVERSE EFFECTS OF ZDV

Anemia

If the hemoglobin drops below 8 gm/dl, ZDV should be reduced by 30%. Blood transfusion with 10–15 ml per kg of packed red blood cells are recommended in symptomatic children. In case of recurrent transfusion requirement (greater than two per month), treatment with erythropoietin 150–600 units/kg s.c. three days per week is indicated.

Neutropenia

If the absolute neutrophil count (ANC) drops below 500, ZDV therapy should be reduced and if it remains low it should be stopped. If recovery to above 500 does not occur within one month, granulocyte colony-stimulating factor (GCSF) should be administered: 1–20 mg/kg per day s.c. An alternative explanation for neutropenia could be the use of TMP-SMX

Table 6.5.

Management and Monitoring Plan for Children Receiving ZDV

		Weeks of Treatment														
	Pre	0	2	4	8	12	16	20	24	28	32	36	40	44	48	52
History & P.E.	◆	◆		◆	◆	◆	◆	◆	◆	◆	◆	◆	◆	◆	◆	◆
CBC, differential, retics	◆	◆	◆	◆	◆	◆	◆	◆	◆	◆	◆	◆	◆	◆	◆	◆
Electrolytes, liver function tests				◆		◆			◆			◆			◆	
Urinalysis									◆			◆				
IgG, IgA, IgM				◆		◆			◆			◆			◆	
Lymphocyte subsets				◆		◆			◆			◆			◆	
p24 antigen									◆			◆			◆	
Chest x-ray																
EKG[a]																
CT or MRI[b]																

Modified & used with permission from the Working Group on Antiretroviral Therapy. Antiretroviral therapy & medical management of the human immunodeficiency virus-infected child. Working Group on Antiretroviral Therapy: National Pediatric HIV Resource Center, Pediatric Infect. Dis J 1993;12:513–522.

[a]Repeat as needed to monitor cardiac symptoms
[b]Repeat as needed to monitor CNS disease

PE = physical exam   CBC = complete blood count   retics = reticulocytes
CT = computerized tomography   MRI = magnetic resonance imaging   EKG = electrocardiogram

and is discussed under PCP prophylaxis. *In the opinion of the authors all efforts should be aimed at maintaining zidovudine at least at a minimum of 90 mg/m²/dose Q6hrs.*

Monitoring DDI Therapy

The most common side effects of ddI are nausea and a dislike of the oral formulation, leading to non-compliance. The most severe side effects of ddI include pancreatitis and peripheral neuropathy. Careful monitoring of pancreatic amylase and lipase should be done. Routine questioning of symptoms of peripheral neuropathy should occur every 3 to 6 months. Transaminases should also be monitored for liver toxicity.

Antiretroviral Therapy and Follow-Up of Disease Status

The most common reason to change antiretroviral therapy is intolerance or disease progression of children. For this reason, it is necessary to follow the HIV disease status closely using the following parameters:

- Physical examination (including anthropomorphic measurements)
- Laboratory assessment (electrolytes, liver and renal function, ECG, etc.)
- Opportunistic infections (e.g., pneumonias, recurrent bacterial infections)
- Immune function (CD4 parameters)
- Virologic assessment (viral load/phenotype)
- CNS evaluation (neurologic exam, neurodevelopmental assessment and neuroimaging)
- In some centers tests for in vitro drug sensitivity may be available (for ZDV)

Table 6.6.
Symptoms Suggesting the Failure of Antiretroviral Therapy

Growth failure (dropping greater than 2 percentile lines from the established curve or a sustained deviation from a parallel curve for children who are below the 5th percentile for weight)
Neuropsychologic behavioral deterioration: decline in brain growth, cognitive function, and clinical neurologic function
Symptomatic cardiomyopathy
Opportunistic infections
Drop in CD4 parameters
Increase in p24 antigen values
Increase in RNA PCR levels

Failure of therapy may be suggested by the presence of symptoms shown in Table 6.6. Alternative or combination of therapies should be considered when these symptoms are evident.

Alternative Therapy

Other antiretroviral drugs currently used are: zalcitabine (ddC) or 3TC, but only 3TC is FDA approved for children. Other drugs (d4t, Nevirapine, and protease inhibitors) are presently being studied in clinical trials, before FDA approval can be considered. This points again to the necessity to enroll infants and children into drug trials. Recently published trials have shown that ddC is at least as efficacious as ddI in delaying disease progression and death in adult patients. (4) Since not all toxicities are overlapping, sequential or simultaneous combination of antiretroviral therapy can be considered. 3TC was recently approved for use in children who can't tolerate ZDV/ddI or in whom the HIV disease is progressing. 3TC should be used in combination with ZDV for a prolonged effect.

REFERENCES

1. Working Group on Antiretroviral Therapy. Antiretroviral therapy and medical management of the human immunodeficiency virus-infected child. Working Group on Antiretroviral Therapy: National Pediatric HIV Resource Center. Pediatr Infect Dis J 1993;12: 513–522.
2. McKinney RJ, Maha MA, Connor EM, et al. A multicenter trial of oral zidovudine in children with advanced human immunodeficiency virus disease. N Engl J Med 1991; 324:1018–1025.
3. US Dept Health and Human Services. Evaluation and management of early HIV infection. In: Clinical practice guideline. United States Department of Health and Human Services, 1994:7. Rockville, MD
4. Abrams DI, Goldman AI, Launer C, et al. A comparative trial of didanosine or zalcitabine after treatment with zidovudine in patients with human immunodeficiency virus infection. N Engl J Med 1994;330:657–662.

Opportunistic Infections (OIs)—Prevention and Prophylaxis

The six most commonly reported opportunistic infections (OIs) in children reported from 1982–1992 were: *Pneumocystis carinii* pneumonia (PCP), recurrent bacterial infections, *Candida* esophagitis, Cytomegalovirus disease, Pulmonary candidiasis, and *Mycobacterium avium* infection (MAI). With increasing number of children on prophylaxis against PCP, it is expected that a much smaller number of children will become infected with PCP. Other infections like MAI will become among the most commonly reported AIDS-indicator diseases. Further prophylactic strategies will be recommended in the future.

Intravenous Immunoglobulins (IVIG) for Recurrent Bacterial Infections

Infants and children with evidence of humoral immune defects, including hypogammaglobulinemia, poor functional antibody development or significant recurrent infections despite therapy with appropriate antimicrobials, are appropriate candidates for routine IVIG prophylaxis. The recommended dosage is 400 mg/kg/dose every 28 days. A recent study (ACTG 051) concluded that IVIG decreases serious bacterial infections in children with advanced HIV disease receiving zidovudine who are not receiving TMP-SMX prophylaxis, but appears to provide no additional protection from serious bacterial infections in children receiving zidovudine and TMP-SMX prophylaxis. Survival is unaffected by intravenous gamma globulin usage (1).

IVIG is also used for thrombocytopenia (<20,000 platelets). Treatment consists of high dose IVIG (0.5 to 1 g/kg/dose) for 3 to 5 days. Unresponsive children should be considered for alternative therapies, such as steroids, rhogam or danazole.

Immunizations for Children with HIV

In general, immune compromised patients including children with HIV infection should not be given live vaccines, with the exceptions noted.

POLIO (2)

Polio immunization for a child with HIV, their household members, or other close contacts should be given IPV, rather than OPV. Although a protective immune response cannot be assured in the immunocompromised patient, some protection may be provided. The use of IPV eliminates any theoretical risk to the vaccine and prevents the possibility of prolonged shedding of vaccine virus in feces resulting in spread to immune compromised close contacts. Because of the possibility of immunodeficiency in the child's other family/household members, no family members should receive OPV unless the immune status of the intended recipient and all other children in the family is known.

DTP AND HIB (2)

Inactivated childhood vaccines (e.g., DTP or Hib) should be given to HIV-infected children regardless of whether HIV symptoms are present. Immunizations may be less effective than it would be for immunocompetent children.

MEASLES, MUMPS, AND RUBELLA (2,3)

The Advisory Committee on Immunization Practices (ACIP) recommends measles, mumps, and rubella (MMR) vaccine, a live virus vaccine for asymptomatic HIV-infected children. MMR should also be considered for all symptomatic HIV-infected children since measles disease can be severe in symptomatic HIV-infected children. Limited studies of MMR immunization in both asymptomatic and symptomatic HIV-infected patients have not documented serious or unusual adverse events.

If vaccinations are given, symptomatic HIV-infected children should receive MMR vaccine at 15 months, the age currently recommended for vaccination of children without HIV infection and for those with asymptomatic HIV infection. When there is an increased risk of exposure to measles, such as during an outbreak, these children should receive vaccine at younger ages. At such times, infants six to 11 months of age should receive monovalent measles vaccine and should be revaccinated with MMR at 12 months of age or older. Children 12–14 months of age should receive MMR and do not need revaccination. Presently, studies are underway to compare a combination of Attenuvax© and MMR, and MMR by itself.

An MMR vaccine may be ineffective if administered to a child who has received intravenous immune globulin (IVIG) during the preceding three months (3,4). The AAP recommends deferring measles vaccine for 8 months after the last dose of immune globulin. Physicians should consider administering MMR vaccine at least 14 days before initiating non-emergency therapy with IVIG to allow sufficient time for an active response to the vaccine without interference (4).

CHILDREN EXPOSED TO MEASLES (3)

Immune globulin (IG) (16.5 gm% protein) can be used to prevent or modify measles infection in HIV-infected children if administered within 6 days of exposure. IG is indicated for measles-susceptible household contacts of children with asymptomatic HIV infection, particularly for those under 1 year of age and for measles-susceptible pregnant women. The recommended dose is 0.25 mL/kg intramuscularly (maximum dose, 15 mL). (Note: a person is measles-susceptible if s/he is unvaccinated or does not have laboratory evidence or physician documentation of previous measles disease).

Exposed symptomatic HIV-infected patients should receive IG prophylaxis regardless of vaccination status. The standard postexposure measles prophylaxis regimen for such patients is 0.5 mL/kg of IG intramuscularly (maximum dose, 15 mL). This regimen corresponds to a dose of protein of approximately 82.5 mg/kg (maximum dose, 2,475 mg). Intramuscular IG may not be necessary if a patient with HIV infection is receiving 100–400 mg/kg IVIG at regular intervals and received the last dose within three weeks of exposure to measles. Based on the amount of protein that can be administered, high-dose IVIG may be as effective as IG given intramuscularly. However, no data exist on the efficacy of IVIG administered postexposure in preventing measles. The time interval to administration of measles vaccine should be increased to six months (4).

PNEUMOCOCCUS

Pneumococcal vaccine is recommended for any child over two years of age infected with HIV.

INFLUENZA (2,5)

An annual immunization with inactivated influenza vaccine is recommended for children with symptoms of HIV infection over 6 months of age.

HBV (1)

Because of similar risks of HBV and HIV among adults and potential transmission to infants and children, prevention of hepatitis B should be considered a high priority and the newly recommended schedule should be applied to populations at high risk even if they are presently known to be free of hepatitis B.

Summary of ACIP recommendations for children infected with HIV are in Table 6.7. These are applicable to adolescents and adults in addition to children (3).

Prophylactic Therapies

PNEUMOCYSTIS CARINII PNEUMONIA (PCP)

Initiation of PCP Prophylaxis

PCP is the most frequent OI in nonprophylaxed infants under one year of age. This high morbidity and the high mortality associated with PCP even if treated appropriately make prophylaxis a top priority in the management of HIV-infected children (6,7). An optimal prophylaxis program will involve identification of HIV-exposed infants as soon as possible so that prophylaxis can be initiated when indicated. Currently, CD4

Table 6.7.
Recommendations for Routine Immunization of HIV-infected Children

Vaccine	HIV Infection	
	Known Asymptomatic	Symptomatic
DTP	Yes	Yes
OPV	No	No
IPV	Yes	Yes
MMR	Yes	Yes[a]
Hib	Yes	Yes
Pneumococcal	Yes (at 2 years of age)	Yes
Influenza	No[b]	Yes
HBV	Yes[c]	Yes[c]

DTP = Diphtheria and tetanus toxoids and pertussis vaccine
OPV = Oral, attenuated poliovirus vaccine; contains poliovirus types 1, 2 and 3
IPV = Inactivated poliovirus vaccine; contains poliovirus types 1, 2 and 3
MMR = Live measles, mumps, and rubella viruses in a combined vaccine
Hib = Conjugate *Haemophilus influenza* b vaccine
[a]Should be considered
[b]Not contraindicated
[c]Recommended by the Working Group on Antiretroviral Therapy: National Pediatric HIV Resource Center
Adapted from CDC. General recommendations on immunization. MMWR 1989;38:205–227.

Table 6.8.
Criteria for Initiation of PCP Prophylaxis in HIV-infected and Exposed Children

Age	Absolute Criteria CD4 cells/mm^3
1 to 12 months	<1500
12 to 23 months	<750
24 months through 5 years	<500
6 years and older	<200

counts provide the most practical way to distinguish HIV-infected children at risk of early PCP disease. The age-adjusted CD4 cell count indicator levels for initiation of prophylaxis have been recommended by CDC (6) and are found in Table 6.8. If a child has a CD4 percentage less than 15%, prophylaxis should be initiated regardless of the absolute count.

Primary PCP prophylaxis should begin in all infants born to HIV-positive mothers within the first 4 to 6 weeks of life until they are determined not to be infected (8). Children who cannot have their HIV-infection status determined should remain on PCP prophylaxis for the first year of life. Once a child is determined to be HIV infected, the previous guidelines should be followed.

Recommended PCP Chemoprophylaxis Regimen

The drug of choice for PCP prophylaxis of HIV-infected or -exposed children is trimethoprim-sulfamethoxazole (TMP-SMX, Bactrim®). Recommended drug regimens are shown in Table 6.9. Doses should not exceed 320 mg TMP with 1600 mg SMX. Any child who has had a prior episode of PCP *should be started on daily PCP prophylaxis* regardless of age or CD4+ count.

When starting TMP-SMX prophylaxis:

- A baseline CBC, differential count, and platelet count should be obtained.

- CBC, differential count, and platelet count should be monitored monthly during the first three months and after that only during routine blood draws.

- CD4 counts should be monitored at least every three months.

If life-threatening toxicity (anaphylaxis, Stevens-Johnson syndrome, or hypotension) occurs, the drug should be permanently discontinued. If other potentially drug-related reactions are noted (i.e., rash, neutropenia), the drug should be temporarily discontinued, and tried again within two weeks. Some patients with documented adverse reactions to TMP-SMX have been successfully desensitized. If desensitization is attempted, administration of TMP-SMX should then be given daily be-

Table 6.9.

Recommended Drug Regimens for PCP Prophylaxis in Children with HIV Infection

I. Recommended regimen for children ≥1 month of age
150 mg TMP/m^2/day with 750 mg SMX/m^2/day given orally in divided doses twice a day (BID) 3 times per week on consecutive days (e.g., Monday-Tuesday-Wednesday)
Any child who has had an episode of PCP should be started on daily PCP prophylaxis regardless of age or CD4+ count.

Alternative TMP-SMX dosage schedules:

A. 150 mg TMP/m^2/day with 750 mg SMX/m^2/day given orally as a single daily dose 3 times per week on consecutive days (e.g., M-T-W)	B. 150 mg TMP/m^2 with 750 mg SMX/m^2/day orally divided BID and given 7 days/week	C. 150 mg TMP/m^2/day with 750 mg SMX/m^2/day given orally divided BID and given 3 times per week on alternate days (e.g., M-W-F)

II. Alternative regimens, if TMP-SMX is not tolerated

A. Aerosolized pentamidine (≥5 years of age) 300 mg given via Respirgard II inhaler monthly.	B. Dapsone (≥1 month of age) 1 mg/kg (not to exceed 100 mg) given orally once daily.	C. If neither aerosolized pentamidine nor dapsone is tolerated, some clinicians use intravenous pentamidine (4 mg/kg) given every 2 or 4 weeks.

cause of the potential for serious adverse reaction upon reintroduction of the drug after any interruption of dosing.

Discontinuation of PCP Prophylaxis

Some children initially placed on prophylaxis will not subsequently warrant continuation of prophylaxis based on HIV-infection status or CD4+ lymphocyte count. Discontinuation of prophylaxis is recommended for infants who were initially seropositive (as a result of transplacentally acquired antibody) but who are later shown not to be infected with HIV. Also, prophylaxis can be discontinued for HIV-infected or seropositive children who have CD4+ cell counts above indicated prophylaxis thresholds on two sequential measurements at least 1 month apart, unless there are special clinical circumstances—for instance if children are receiving medications that could alter the CD4+ cell count (corticosteroids, cytotoxic agents or antiretroviral therapy). Regardless of symptoms or CD4+ cell counts, children with a previous episode of PCP should continue on life-long prophylaxis to prevent recurrence.

PCP Prophylaxis Other Than TMP-SMX

The CDC has suggested alternative regimens for TMP-SMX-intolerant individuals (Table 6.9). Aerosolized pentamidine is recommended for HIV-infected children 5 years of age or older via the Respirgard II jet nebulizer. The dose is 300 mg diluted in 6 ml of sterile water and delivered at 6 L/min from a 50 pounds per square inch (PSI) compressed air source until the reservoir is dry. If cough or bronchospasm occurs, interrupt therapy and administer a bronchodilator; for mild coughing, lowering the flow rate of the nebulizer has helped in some instances. Although routine pulmonary function tests are not recommended, clinical awareness of the potential for pulmonary compromise is warranted.

Dapsone can be considered for patients who cannot tolerate TMP-SMX. (7) The dose is 2 mg/kg/day, but the total daily dose should not exceed 100 mg per day. Although dapsone is not available as a liquid preparation, the tablets (25 mg or 100 mg) can be crushed to administer the appropriate dose and to give the drug with or in food. Weekly complete blood counts with differential and platelet count should be performed for the first month, and then monthly for those children receiving dapsone prophylaxis to assess hematologic toxicity. Intravenous pentamidine can also be administered. The dose is 4mg/kg every 2–4 weeks. Other alternate treatments such as atovaquone are currently being evaluated in children.

TUBERCULOSIS PROPHYLAXIS (1)

HIV-infected children frequently fail to mount a response to *Mycobacterium tuberculosis* and remain PPD negative. Tuberculosis prophylaxis should be given to children with a significant reaction to PPD ($\geq$5 mm), a prior positive test result without treatment, or in children who have had contact with a person with active tuberculosis. INH alone is the drug of choice for INH-susceptible *Mycobacterium tuberculosis* for a duration of 9–12 months. The dosage is: 10 to 15 mg/kg/dose/po every 24 hours (maximum dose 300 mg) or 20 mg/kg/dose/po twice weekly (maximum dose 900 mg) (after 1 month of daily therapy).

If the contact person has INH-resistant tuberculosis, the drug regimen is rifampin 10–20 mg/kg (max 600 mg) po or IV QD × 12 mo (8).

VARICELLA ZOSTER VIRUS (VZV) PROPHYLAXIS

Like all immune suppressed children who come in contact with a VZV-infected person, HIV-infected children should receive passive immunization with varicella zoster immune globulin (VZIG). Dosage: 125 units/10 kg IM (125 units to maximum dosage of 625 units) given $\leq$96 hours after exposure, ideally within 48 hours. Children who receive routine IVIG should receive VZIG if exposure is <14 days after last IVIG treatment.

MYCOBACTERIUM AVIUM COMPLEX (MAC)

With the use of routine prophylaxis for pneumocystis infection, the most common illness in HIV-infected patients is now *Mycobacterium avium* complex disease. Prophylaxis may be indicated in selected high-risk children with less than 75 CD4 lymphocytes/mm^3 in children 6–12 years old (1). Oral rifabutin (300 mg/day) may delay and prevent MAC bacteremia. In children <6 years of age, the dose is 5 mg/kg po QD. Alternatives include azithromycin 7.5 mg/kg/day divided into two doses or clarithromycin 5–12 mg/kg each day.

TOXOPLASMOSIS

In children with severe immunosuppression (CD4 <100/ml) a dose of TMP-SMX 150/750 mg/m^2/d divided into two doses can be given 3 days each week (preferably consecutive days). It can be given daily if this improves compliance. Alternative for TMP/SMX intolerant children include dapsone 2 mg/kg (max 25 mg) each day plus pyrimethamine 1 mg/kg/day plus leukovorin 5 mg po every 3 days (8).

Multidisciplinary Approach

Children with HIV infection have a chronic, presently incurable disease. In vertically infected children the management is additionally complicated by disease of the mother and frequently other family members. Successful management of the multilayered challenges which this disease invariably generates requires a multidisciplinary approach. Such a team can include a primary care giver (either a physician or a nurse practitioner), a case manager or a social worker, a multitude of medical subspecialists including developmental specialists. Mental health support of child and family may require guidance of a social worker, psychiatrist or psychologist. Home health care and respite workers, pharmacists, nutritionists and eventually home hospice care may become highly valuable during the course of the disease.

Close coordination of the patient's outpatient care and care during hospitalization can be easily overlooked. Close communication between the team responsible for in- and out-patient care may prove crucial for the patient's health and her family's trust in her health care providers. At present there is no single structure which can respond to the requirements of all patients equally well. There is agreement that successful management should be individualized for the individual patient, depending on the patient's medical, cultural and social characteristics, the community where the patient lives, and the support available to the patient.

REFERENCES

1. Working Group on Antiretroviral Therapy. Antiretroviral therapy and medical management of the human immunodeficiency virus-infected child. Working Group on Antiretroviral Therapy: National Pediatric HIV Resource Center. Pediatr Infect Dis J 1993;12:513–522.
2. CDC. General recommendations on immunization. MMWR 1989;38:205–227.
3. CDC. Immunization of children infected with human immunodeficiency virus—supplementary ACIP statement. MMWR 1988;37:181–183.
4. Mueller BU, Karina M, Butler MB, et al. Clinical and pharmakinetic evaluation of long-term therapy with didanosine in children with HIV infection, Pediatrics 1994; 94:724–731
5. CDC. Immunization of children infected with HTLV-III/LAV. MMWR 1986;35:595–606.
6. CDC. Guidelines for prophylaxis against *Pneumocystis carinii* pneumonia for children infected with human immunodeficiency virus. MMWR 1991;40(RR40).
7. Barnett ED, Mirochnik M, Cooper ER. Dapsone for prevention of pneumocystis pneumonia in children with acquired immunodeficiency syndrome. Pediatric Infectious Disease Journal 1994;13:72–4.

8. CDC. US PHS/IDSA guidelines for the prevention of opportunistic infections in persons infected with human immunodeficiency virus: A summary. MMWR 1995;44(RR-8): 1–32.

Nutritional Guidelines for Children With HIV

Failure to thrive and multiple nutritional deficiencies, particularly protein calorie malnutrition are seen in children with HIV (1–3). Intrauterine exposure to drugs and associated poor prenatal care, suboptimal maternal weight gain, and premature birth can be cofactors affecting nutritional status in HIV-positive infants. Malnutrition, growth failure and weight loss may be secondary to other nutritional complications (e.g., anorexia, fatigue, persistent diarrhea, chronic infections). Caloric needs may be increased by infections and recurrent fevers, and inadequate caloric intake and increased malabsorption may further exacerbate malnutrition. Maintaining optimal nutrition is crucial for children with AIDS to help gain weight, facilitate growth, prevent nutritional deficiencies. Early nutritional intervention may prevent severe malnutrition, decrease the incidence and severity of infection, and provide some protection of the immune system, enabling a better quality of life for children infected with HIV children (1,4–6). Recommended guidelines concerning the nutritional management of children infected with HIV children are summarized below (1,4,7).

Patient Assessment

Frequent assessment of children infected with HIV increases the likelihood of detecting growth failure as early as possible. During routine pediatric visit, the following should be included (1):

- Measurements of height or length, weight, head circumference, and weight for length; these should be plotted on a growth chart to show longitudinal changes. More information regarding fat stores and lean body mass includes measurements of skin fold thickness and midarm circumference.

- An interval history inquiring about diet, intermittent fevers, diarrhea, vomiting, or other problems

- Hemoglobin and hematrocrit readings with red blood cell indices every three months.

A wide variety of etiologies may lead to weight loss or failure to gain weight (see Table 6.10). Frequent fevers and infection in a children infected with HIV can cause an increase in basal metabolic rate and poor appetite; nutrient metabolism may also be altered in acute and chronic phases of infection. The presence of oral and/or esophageal lesions may make feeding difficult as can a lack of or regression of feeding skills caused by neurodevelopmental delays and HIV encephalopathy. Gas-

Table 6.10.
Mechanisms of Weight Loss or Failure to Gain Weight

Poor intake
- Dysgeusia (loss of smell), dysphagia, odynophagia (pain when swallowing), esophagitis, abdominal pain, early satiety, malaise, depression, central swallowing problems (CNS), vomiting, inadequate diet.

Malabsorption
- Infections (treatable): entamoeba, giardia, salmonella, campylobacter, shigella.
- Infections (untreatable): rotavirus, adenovirus, astrovirus, cryptosporidium, microsporidium.
- HIV enteropathy, small bowel overgrowth, lactose intolerance, biliary obstruction, pancreatic insufficiency, mucosal atrophy.

Metabolic alterations
- Hypermetabolic state, increased resting energy expenditure, protein wasting, cytokine dysregulation.

Neuroendocrine dysfunction

Micronutrient deficiency

Table 6.11.
Evaluation and Management of Growth Failure in Children with HIV

Assess health status, including medical history, medication profile, physical exam and measurements, laboratory profile of nutritional and related parameters (e.g., serum albumin and protein serum iron, total iron-binding capacity
Investigate treatable causes of growth failure or weight loss
Take a 72-hour recall history of food intake, if possible (otherwise a 24-hour recall is sufficient)
Calculate the approximate daily intake of calories and protein and analyze nutrient consumption, particularly calcium, vitamins D, E, and B complex, iron, zinc, and selenium
Measure visceral and somatic protein stores (e.g., albumin, prealbumin, serum retinol-binding protein); vitamin and mineral status (e.g., iron, iron-binding capacity, ferritin)
Estimate catch-up caloric requirements
Develop an altered diet, and plan for follow-up if indicated

trointestinal dysfunction is common among children with HIV, causing diarrhea and malabsorption. When growth is inadequate, a nutritionist or registered dietitian should be consulted. An evaluation of a malnourished child and recommendations to manage growth failure (1,7) are shown in Table 6.11.

Nutritional Management for the Asymptomatic Child

Breastfeeding has been implicated in the transmission of HIV infection. Therefore it is prudent to discourage children infected with HIV mothers from breast feeding, at least when alternatives are available. No standardized recommendations are available for pediatric HIV infection. Unless frequent infections, diarrhea, malabsorption, or other complications occur, growth can be achieved with the caloric intake level recommended by the RDA (required daily allowance). A high calorie/high protein diet is generally recommended, although the diet should be individualized for each child. Vitamin and mineral supplementation should not be greater than two times the RDA for the age and sex. Whenever possible, oral food intake should be encouraged. Caloric requirements should be increased for catch-up growth, or under conditions of stress to accommodate the metabolic response to injury and illness (e.g., fever, acute diarrhea, sepsis). Diet modification as well as commercial nutritional supplements are available for additional calories and protein.

Children infected with HIV are at risk for micronutrient deficiencies. Serum levels of iron, selenium, zinc, thiamine, vitamin B_{12} and vitamin B_6 are frequently decreased and may be associated with immune dysfunction and other pathologies. For children with chronic diarrhea, monitoring of serum zinc levels should be considered. Measurement and targeted supplements of these micronutrients may enhance a nutritional rehabilitation program. However, micronutrient supplementation should be carefully approached, since the potential for immune function impairment exists (1). Children with AIDS are more susceptible to foodborne illness than are healthy children and necessary precautions should be used. (*See Precautions for Persons Living with HIV*). Nutritional problems seen in children infected with HIV and recommended intervention strategies (4) are shown in Table 6.12.

Nutritional Reasons for Weight Loss or Failure to Gain Weight

As mentioned, there are a variety of etiologic reasons why a child infected with HIV may experience weight loss or a failure to gain weight. When growth begins to slow or weight begins to decrease, an immediate assessment and aggressive, proactive intervention are important. Exclusion of treatable causes has absolute priority (diet, stool culture, ova and parasites, endoscopy). After treatable causes have been excluded, absorptive function tests (D-Xylose) and pancreatic function (Bentiromide) may help optimize strategies.

Simple interventions should first be considered: using bottle nipples that decrease the work of sucking; having smaller and more frequent feedings; identifying and correcting maternal behaviors that interfere with feeding; and modifying diets to give foods appropriate for a particular child's level of development (1). For children experiencing inadequate growth, calorie and protein requirements can be calculated using the following formula (1,7):

$$kcal/kg = (RDA \times ideal\ weight\ for\ height)/actual\ weight$$
$$protein\ (in\ grams)/kg = (RDA \times ideal\ weight\ for\ height)$$

The optimal nutritional management in children infected with HIV with inadequate weight gains is unknown. General recommendations for oral feedings include small, frequent meals, using nutritionally dense foods (i.e., diet high in caloric density and protein). High calorie formulas, with the addition of carbohydrates or fat (e.g., polyglycose, medium chain triglyeride oil) should be given as needed. For children two to four

Table 6.12.

Strategies for Nutritional Problems in HIV-infected Children

Weight loss/poor weight gain/growth failure
- Give a high calorie-high protein diet, including foods from all food groups
- Give frequent snacks, i.e., fruits, juices, vegetables, soup, cheese, peanut butter, ice cream, pudding, bread, cereal, crackers, cookies
- Increase calories, protein, and fat (if tolerated)

Loss of appetite/fatigue

- Build meals around favorite foods. Variety is not as essential as calorie intake
- Give small frequent meals and snacks. Children should be encouraged to eat slowly. Drink fluids after meals, because fluids may cause a full stomach
- If appetite is better in morning, serve a large breakfast or have dinner foods early in the day
- Increase protein and calories to food without adding volume (e.g., add dry milk powder to milk, soups, eggs).
- If meat is not well liked, give fish, poultry, beans, eggs or cheese
- Present food attractively. Vary shape, color, texture, and arrangement of food. Garnish dishes with fresh fruit or vegetable slices
- When possible involve the child in meal preparation, food shopping, and setting the table
- Give finger foods, and bite-size pieces such as crackers, fruit, or vegetable slices (if tolerated)
- Position the child to sit comfortably (i.e., high chair with feet supported)
- Encourage self-feeding skills as much as possible
- Create a relaxed pleasant environment for eating. Eat with the child. Tell a story. Be supportive
- Adequate rest, fresh air, and moderate exercise may stimulate appetite

Feeding problems (neurological impairment)

- Bottle or spoon feed, as needed.
- Use special feeding utensils, if needed.
- Modify consistency of foods, i.e., puree, fork-mashed.
- Consult with appropriate therapist to evaluate child's feeding position

Diarrhea/malabsorption

- Give fruit or vegetable juice, diluted fruit nectars, broth, gelatin, ices or popsicles to replace fluid losses

- Give salty foods (e.g., crackers or soup) to replace sodium losses
- Replace potassium losses with bananas, apricots, oranges, potatoes, meats, fish, and other fruits and vegetables
- Encourage children to eat small portions of food slowly
- Use foods low in dietary fiber (e.g., canned or cooked fuits and vegetables). Certain types of "soluble" fiber (pectin and gums) may help. Eat oatmeal, beans, apples, pears, or potatoes. Avoid bran and "whole grain" breads and cereals that may exacerbate diarrhea
- Use foods low in lactose (milk sugar). Use soy-based milk (flavor with cinnamon or vanilla), lactose-reduced milk, or nondairy creamer[b] instead of high lactose milk, cheese, yogurt, ice cream, sherbet, pudding, custard, cream, malted milk, instant cocoa, and cream soups
- Avoid giving fried and high fat foods such as cold cuts, frankfurters, pastry, chips, nuts, mayonnaise, margarine/butter, oils, cream, sauces, gravies, and high fat cheese (i.e., cheddar)

Difficulty chewing and swallowing

- Give foods at room temperature or cold foods; avoid very hot foods
- Give foods that are soft, mildly flavored, and nonirritating (e.g., cooked eggs, cream soups, pudding, pastry, potatoes, cereals, ground meats, baked fish, soft cheese, ice cream, gelatin dessert)
- Mash or puree foods in a blender (fruits and vegetables)
- Moisten foods with sauce, gravy or broth
- Serve high calorie/high protein nonacidic beverages (e.g., milkshakes)
- Give non-acidic juices (e.g., vitamin C fortified apple or grape juice) or fruit nectars (dilute with water, if needed)
- Give canned fruits or fruits without skin or seeds.
- Popsicles eaten before a meal can help numb the mouth making eating easier
- Drink liquids through a straw

Infection/fever

- Treat treatable causes
- Give a high calorie/high protein diet.
- Increase fluids

Modified from Cowell C, Rubin KW. Children with AIDS living at home: A challenge for a community support team. Nutrition Focus 1989 4(5):1–5. Univ of Washington, Seattle WA.
NOTE: DO NOT GIVE raw honey; DO NOT GIVE honey to infants under one year of age.
[b]Use appropriate vitamin supplements

years of age, a high-calorie formula for children can be used; adult formulas may be used for children older than four years of age. High-calorie formulas (24 or 27 kcal/oz) may be used in children younger than two years of age. The most reliable indicator of adequate intake is steady weight gain. However, during actively catabolic states, only weight maintenance may be realistic. If inadequate growth continues, a possible diagnosis to consider is nonorganic failure to thrive. Hospitalization may be warranted to determine whether sufficient growth occurs when adequate caloric intake is provided.

After treatable causes have been excluded and an adequate diet has been assured, consultation with a gastroenterologist, pediatric nutritionist, and a home nutrition service should be considered. If it is impossible to give the child adequate calories by mouth, placement of a nasogastric (NG) tube should be discussed with the caregivers. Supplementing daytime oral intake with evening parenteral feedings may be an option. If after one or two months, the need for nutritional support continues and NG feedings have improved growth, placement of a gastrostomy tube should be considered. If calorie absorption through the intestines is impossible secondary to intractable diarrhea or pancreatitis, parenteral nutrition as an option should be discussed with the caregiver and practitioners experienced in home TPN care. Home TPN care will require close monitoring.

Several pharmacological agents are under investigation for their potential benefit for weight gain. Megesterol acetate has been shown to increase appetite but most of the weight gain is fat and not the desired lean body mass (8). Other agents like cannabinol, growth hormone and anabolic steroids are presently studied in adults, but there is currently only little experience in children.

REFERENCES

1. Nicholas SW, Leung J, Fennoy I. Guidelines for nutritional support of HIV-infected children. J Pediatr 1991;119:S59–S62.
2. Miller TL, Orav EJ, McIntosh, Lipschultz SE. Is selenium deficiency clinically significant in pediatric HIV infection? IXth International Conference on AIDS. 1993 (abstr PO-B05-1023).
3. Chadwick EG, Freeman I, Yogev R, Brown RR. Tryptophan (TRP) depletion associated with failure to thrive (FTT) in pediatric AIDS. IXth International Conference on AIDS. 1993 (abstr PO-BO2-0918).
4. Cowell C, Rubin KW. Children with AIDS living at home: a challenge for a community support team. Nutrition Focus 1989;4(5):1–5
5. Henderson RA, Saavedra JM. Nutritional considerations and management of the child with human immunodeficiency virus infection. Nutrition 1995;11:121–128.
6. Henderson RA, Saavedra JM, Perman JA, Hutton N, Livingston RA, Volken RH. Effects of internal tube feedings on growth of children with symptomatic human immunodeficiency virus infection. J Peds Gastr Nutr 1994;18:429–434.
7. Newman CF, Capitelli S. Nutrition in pediatric AIDS. PAAC Notes. 1992;(December):401–403
8. Brady MT, Koranyi KI, Hunkler JA. Megestrol acetate for treatment of anorexia associated with human immunodeficiency virus infection in children. Pediatric Infectious Disease Journal 1994;13:754–756.

CHAPTER 7

Adolescents and HIV Infection

Recent statistics have indicated that the age at the time of HIV infection is significantly declining as the epidemic progresses (1). In the early 1980s, the estimated median age of HIV infection was greater than 30 years; from the period 1987–1991, the median age decreased to 25 years

(1). Moreover, from 1987 to 1991, approximately 25% of newly HIV-infected persons in the U.S. were younger than 22 (1). As more effective treatment of HIV develops, there will be an increase in the number of children infected perinatally or through blood or blood products that will reach adolescence. The temporal trend toward a younger age at the time of HIV infection points to the importance of HIV prevention efforts for adolescents and the provision of services which consider the unique attributes of this age group.

Adolescence is a period marked by great psychosocial and physiologic changes which potentially place adolescents at risk for acquiring HIV infection. Psychosocial changes occurring during adolescence include the process of separation from the family, development of independent thought and action, and the emergence of sexual identity (2). The development and expression of ideas, social relationships, sexuality, independence, and experimentation with alcohol and other drugs have a direct effect on an adolescent's behavioral risk for HIV infection. For example, sexual identity is often explored during adolescence and same-sex experiences may occur. Anal sex may be practiced as a part of sexual experimentation, as a part of the sexual repertoire of gay/bisexual men or as a method to avoid pregnancy or maintain virginity (3,4). Adolescents may also have involuntary sex experiences. Half of all rape victims and 17% to 30% of reported sexual abuse cases are adolescents (5). Victims of sexual abuse often initiate voluntary sexual activity at an earlier age, and have higher rates of alcohol and drug use than their non-abused peers (6). Needle-sharing practices among adolescents include injecting drug use, tattooing, body piercing, or injecting steroids. Adolescents explore and experiment with various behaviors and lifestyles, and are vulnerable to peer pressure.

A shift from concrete to abstract reasoning also takes place during adolescence. Since physical and cognitive development can be asynchronous, it is important to assess the adolescent's cognitive level rather than rely on the adolescent's physical appearance. The ability to understand the future consequences of behavior is limited in adolescents who are concrete thinkers (2,7). However, even for those who can think abstractly, peer pressure may override abstract and distant risks (7). Physiological and anatomical changes also occur during adolescence. One physiologic factor which may place females at greater risk is the increased amount of ectopy of the uterine cervix that exists during adolescence (2,8). Adolescents having sexual intercourse at an early age have a high rate of abnormal Pap smears and a high prevalence of human papilloma virus (HPV) infection (9,10). A similar mechanism could be postulated for cervical ectopy causing an increased risk for HIV.

The provision of HIV prevention and treatment services for adolescents is complicated by limited data on HIV disease progression during adolescence, limited standards for routine management of HIV-infected youth, and unique issues regarding confidentiality and HIV testing and treatment. Consideration of the unique attributes of this age group is required in providing adolescents with focused and effective HIV prevention, testing and counseling, and health care services.

REFERENCES

1. Rosenberg PS, Biggar RJ, Goedert JJ. Declining age at HIV infection in the United States. N Engl J Med 1994;330:789–790.
2. Friedman LS, Goodman E. Adolescents at risk for HIV infection. Primary Care 1992: 19;171–190.
3. Jaffe LR, Seehaus M, Wagner C, Leadbeater BJ. Anal intercourse and knowledge of acquired immunodeficiency syndrome among minority-group female adolescents. J Pediatr 1988;112:1005–1007.
4. Moscicki A-B, Millstein SG, Broering J, Irwin CE. Risks of human immunodeficiency virus infection among adolescents attending three diverse clinics. J Pediatr 1993: 122;813–820.
5. Hamptom RL, Newberger EH. Child abuse incidence and reporting by hospitals: significance of severity, class and race. Am J Public Health 1987;8:188–197.
6. Harrison PA, Hoffman NG, Edwall GE. Differential drug use patterns among sexually abused adolescent girls in treatment for chemical dependency. Int J Addict 1989; 24:499–514.
7. Hein K. AIDS in adolescence. J of Adolescent Health Care 1989;10:10S–35S.
8. Futterman D, Hein K. Medical management of adolescents. In: Pizzo PA, Wilfert CM. eds Pediatric AIDS: the challenge of HIV infection in infants, children and adolescents. Baltimore: Williams & Wilkins, 1991:546–550.
9. Hein K, Schreiber K, Cohen MI, et al. Cervical cytology: the need for routine screening in the sexually active adolescent. J Pediatr 1977;91:123–126.
10. Rosenfeld W, Vermund S, Saed S, et al. HPV infections of the cervix in adolescents. Pediatr Res 1987;21:177A.

Risk Assessment

Although hemophilia/coagulation disorders account for approximately 30% of AIDS cases among adolescents age 13–19 years (1), current donor screening procedures and practices of heat treatment have virtually eliminated the risk of HIV infection. Therefore, almost all new cases of HIV infection among adolescents are related to sexual activity or injection drug use. For this reason, a comprehensive health care for adolescents must include the assessment of risk factors for HIV infection. This assessment should include questions concerning sexual activity, pregnancy history, contraceptive use, history of sexually transmitted infections, alcohol and other drug use, as well as injuries or accidents caused by their use (2–5). The goal is to identify youth at risk for HIV, and recommend testing and counseling as appropriate. Preventive and risk reduction measures should be individualized for each adolescent.

Interviewing Considerations

The interviewer should be empathetic, nonthreatening and nonjudgmental (6). Sexual behavior, alcohol and other drug use should not be discussed in the presence of a parent or other adult, unless specifically requested by the teenager (7). The presence of a parent was demonstrated to be the most common reason that substance-abusing adolescents reported for not honestly answering questions about drug use posed during a medical interview with a physician (8). Adolescents should be interviewed separately and privately (9). Procedures regarding confidentiality should be explained at the beginning of the session. Adolescents must be assured that every conversation is confidential and will not be shared with parents or authorities without specific patient consent (unless rape, child/sexual abuse, threatened suicide or homicide are disclosed). The adolescent should be informed that some of the questions may be very personal but are important to his/her health care.

Generally, the adolescent should be told that the provider has an interest in him/her as a person, and that knowledge of his/her lifestyle will enable the provider to give better medical care (9). By being informed of the reasons for disclosure, the adolescent may feel more comfortable in sharing his/her feelings. Vocabulary, methods of questioning, terminology, and explanations should be appropriate and understandable to the adolescent. The provider can use cues taken from the adolescent's language and vocabulary to appropriately modify their interview (5). Wording of questions should be clear and unambiguous. "Have you ever had sex?" may be better than "Are you sexually active?" which is often misinterpreted by adolescents (2). Questions that are concrete and specific, e.g., "Have you ever had sex to obtain drugs or money?" versus "Have you ever been a prostitute?" should be used as much as possible. A combination of specific closed-ended and open-ended questions should be used, depending on the adolescent's response (5). Open-ended questions (i.e., questions that facilitate an explanation) may sometimes be more effective than questions that require a yes/no answer (i.e., closed-end questions). Using closed-end questions may be more effective when open-ended questions are presumptive in nature and may offend the younger patient (e.g., "Have you ever had anal sex?" may be less offensive than "How often do you have anal sex?") (5). Because the adolescent's cognitive and the psychological development may vary and abstract thinking may be limited, open-ended questions may not always be productive during early adolescence (11–13 years old for females, 12–14 for males) to middle adolescence (13–16 females, 14–17 for males) (2). The difficulty of the subject content should be acknowledged and questions from the adolescent encouraged (2). One method of interviewing to consider is directing the interview as a conversation, exchanging information rather than as a question-and-answer session (9).

School and Social Environment

Information regarding the living situation, education level, literacy and family support should be ascertained (4,9,10). Specific points of inquiry include has the teen ever run away from home, are there conflicts between the adolescent and their parents (e.g., violation of curfew, arguments about friends), and how much time is spent alone or away from home. In the adolescent who is attending school, address the areas of academic performance, attendance, relationships with school personnel and how is the time between leaving school and arriving home spent. Young adolescents should be asked how satisfied they are with their academic performance and what goals do they have for the near and distant future (9). Older adolescents should be asked about their career aspirations and plans for further education or training. A sudden decrease in performance or poor attendance may indicate substance abuse (9). Adolescents who do not attend school regularly should be asked how they spend their time while not in school. Youths who are not in school (e.g., homeless, runaways, juvenile offenders, migrant youth) may be at higher risk for HIV exposure due to an increased likelihood of exposure to the virus and need accessible prevention services. Homeless and runaway youth are more likely to have experienced survival sex (sex for housing, food, clothes, or money) and have higher rates of injecting drug use and sexually transmitted diseases (STDs) (11). Compared to adolescents (aged 14 to 19 years) attending school, out-of-school adolescents were significantly more likely to engage in at-risk behaviors for HIV, including sexual intercourse, having four or more sexual partners, and alcohol, marijuana or cocaine use (12).

Inquiries about leisure activities and friends can assist in understanding the adolescent's social network. Having friends who are involved with drug or alcohol use has been found to be closely associated with an adolescent's own use (13). If the adolescent has a job, how much is he/she working? Is the work enjoyable? Does it interfere with school? Adolescents under stress may be at greater risk for alcohol or marijuana use as a coping mechanism (7). Adolescents with low self-esteem or who are depressed are also at increased risk for substance abuse (9). To explore self-esteem, ask the adolescent how he/she feels about him/herself, what his/her strengths are and what attributes would he/she change (9). A history of psychological functioning, suicidal thoughts or attempts, depression, anxiety, psychiatric medications and hospitalizations should be solicited (4,10).

Sexual Activity

A sexual history should be obtained from all adolescents. An increasing proportion of adolescents are having sexual intercourse, and are initiating sex at a younger age (14). In a 1990 national school-based U.S. survey, approximately half of females and 61% of male high school students reported ever having sex (15). In a 1991 national survey, 33% of males and 20% of females initiated sexual activity before the age of 15 (16). Sexual intercourse at an early age has been associated with greater numbers of both recent and lifetime sex partners (14), and an increased number of cumulative sex partners is associated with a greater risk of acquiring viral infections such as human papilloma virus, genital herpes, hepatitis B, HPV, and HIV (17). Moreover, unprotected sexual intercourse among U.S. adolescents appears to be prevalent, as evidenced by the high rates of teenage pregnancy and STDs. Approximately 1 million adolescent females become pregnant each year (18), and 86% of all STDs occur among persons aged 15–29 years (19). Adolescents have higher rates of gonorrheal and chlamydial infection than do older age groups (20). Adolescent fe-males have the highest age-specific rates of pelvic inflammatory disease (PID), when adjusted for sexual activity (21). STDs not only reflect the types of risk-taking behavior that are associated with HIV transmission (e.g., unprotected sex, multiple partners) but STD-associated genital ul-cers may increase susceptibility to HIV infection. Adolescent females may also be more susceptible to HIV and other STDs because of the larger area of cervical ectropion that occurs during adolescence (22). High rates of unprotected anal, vaginal, and oral sex, as well as sex with multiple partners were reported among adolescents attending three diverse clinic sites in San Francisco (23). Condom use during the last sexual intercourse was reported by only 49% of male and 40% of female sexually active high school students (15). Receptive anal intercourse, a sexual practice with a higher risk for HIV transmission, may be practiced frequently among some adolescents as a part of sexual experimentation, as a method of birth control, or to maintain virginity (23,24).

Heterosexual orientation should not be presumed when inquiring about sexual activity. Questions asked should encourage gay, lesbian, or bisexual youth to share their experiences, feelings, and concerns (e.g., "Have you had any sexual partners who were male, female or both?" ver-sus "How many boyfriends have you had?"). Some adolescent males, re-gardless of eventual sexual orientation, may have had at least one sex-ual experience with another male. Surveys of young men in America have reported a 17% to 32% incidence of homosexual activity (25,26). Same gender sexual experimentation may be prevalent among adoles-cents who do not self-identify with being gay, lesbian, or bisexual (27). Same-sex sexual experimentation is common in early adolescence and does not necessarily predict future sexual orientation (2).

Specific questions should include age of first intercourse; age and sex of first and subsequent partners; number of partners; type (e.g., vaginal, anal, oral) and frequency of sex; and if any of the sexual partners had other risk behaviors (3,5,10). The ages of current and past sex partners should be asked, since having older friends and sex partners may expose the adolescent to developmentally inappropriate experiences. An adoles-cent with a much older partner is at greater risk for HIV exposure than if the partner were a peer, because of higher rates of HIV infection in older persons (2). In general, male sexual partners of adolescent females tend to be two to three years older (28), and male sexual partners of ho-mosexual adolescent males are an average of seven years older (25).

Questions regarding prior infection with STDs should be asked. Ado-lescents may not know if they have had an STD, or a clinical diagnosis may not have been established. Naming each STD and its symptoms, asking if medication was received for a problem on or in their penis or vagina, and the types of treatments/names of medications received may be necessary (3). Questions about contraception should include the types of contraception used, as well as the frequency and consistency of use for each method used. In recent research, the strongest predictor of condom use among high school students was whether students relied on birth control pills as their primary form of contraception; fewer students using birth control pills reported condom use (18%) compared to other sexually active students (54%) (29). The characteristics of condom use should be assessed: what type of condoms (latex or natural) is used; is the condom being used correctly; and when and with whom are condoms more (or less) likely to be used (3). Was the condom used the last time during sex? Why or why not? What makes it hard to use condoms? Females should be asked if they have ever been pregnant, had a baby, an abortion, or miscarriage. Questions should also include whether the adolescent has ever: a) used alcohol or drugs before sex, b) experienced survival sex (Have you ever had sex in exchange for food, money, drugs or a place to stay?) or c) been sexually abused (Has anything ever happened to you during sex that hurt or scared you? Were you ever forced to do something that you didn't want to?) Adolescents should be asked if they have any questions or concerns about current sexual experiences, their knowledge about safer sex, and what they are doing to protect themselves from HIV.

Substance Use

Injection drug use among adolescents has been reported to be increasing (30), and may be more common in certain subpopulations such as inner city and street youth (24,31). Multiple sex partners and noncondom use are more likely to be reported by students who inject drugs and share needles (32). Users of crack/cocaine may exchange sex for drugs or money, and consequently be at higher risk for STDs. The use of alcohol and other drugs may indirectly contribute to HIV exposure by impairing judgment, increasing the likelihood of participation in unsafe sexual behaviors such as noncondom use (33). Adolescents frequently use illicit substances or alcohol in conjunction with sex (23) and first-time use of injectable drugs frequently occurs under the influence of alcohol and other drugs (2). As substance use progresses from alcohol and cigarettes to marijuana, cocaine and other illicit drugs, the likelihood increases that adolescents report sexual risk behaviors (e.g., multiple sex partners, noncondom use at last intercourse) (34). Common behavioral characteristics and beliefs have been found among adolescents who are problem drinkers or use marijuana regularly. For example, adolescents involved with alcohol and other drug use have reported lower academic expectations, and value independence more than academic achievement (35). Needle-sharing should also be discussed with persons involved in both building (secondary to the potential use of steroids), body piercing, or tattooing (4).

Many teens who abuse alcohol and other drugs do not consider themselves to have a drug problem and will often not relate such questions to their own health consequences. In addition, these behaviors may not be considered dangerous or abnormal among the adolescent's peers (2). Questions about drugs and alcohol should be presented as an essential part of determining the patient's physical well-being, and not an arbitrary prying into personal behavior. One strategy may be to first ask about peer group behavior surrounding drugs and alcohol, and later lead into the patient's own drug use (6). Another strategy might be to start by asking less threatening questions and moving on towards more sensitive or potential threatening questions (9,36). The progression might start with questions about dietary patterns, proceeding to prescribed medica-

Table 7.1.

HEADSS Assessment

H	Home	Where do you live? Whom do you live with? How much time do you spend at home? What do you and your family argue about? Can you go to your parents with problems? Have you ever run away from home?
E	Education	What grade are you in? What grades are you getting? Have they changed? Do you work after school or on weekends? Have you ever failed any classes or a grade? Do you ever cut classes?
A	Activities	What do you do for fun? What activities do you do during and after school? Are you active in sports? Do you exercise? Whom do you do fun things with? Who are your friends? Whom do you go to with problems? What do you do on weekends? Evenings?
D	Drugs	Do you drink coffee or tea? Do you smoke cigarettes? Have you ever smoked one? Have you ever tried alcohol? When? What kind and how often? Do any of your friends drink or use drugs? What drugs have you tried? Have you ever injected steroids or drugs? When? How often do you use them?
S	Sexual Activity/Identity	Have you ever had sex with men? Women? Both? Have you ever had sex unwillingly? How many sexual partners have you had? How old were you when you first had sex? Have you ever been pregnant? Have you ever had an infection as the result from sex? Do you use condoms and/or another form of contraception/ STD prevention? (Use specific names for STDs) Have you ever traded sex for money, drugs, clothes, or a place to stay? Have you ever been tested for HIV? Do you think it would be a good idea to be tested?
S	Suicide/Depression	How do you feel today on a scale of 0–10 (0 = very sad, 10 = very happy)? Have you ever felt less than a 5? What made you feel that way? Did you ever think about hurting yourself, that life wasn't worth living, or hope that when you went to sleep you wouldn't wake up again?

Adapted from Anderson MM. Principles of care for the ill adolescent. Adolescent Medicine: State of the Art Reviews 1991;2(3):441–458.

tions, over-the-counter medications tobacco products, alcohol use, marijuana, and finally to other illicit drugs. If drugs are being used, then the age at which they were first used, periods of highest use, current use pattern, and history of needle use should be determined. Other questions may include: how he/she gets money to obtain drugs, if sex has ever been exchanged for drugs, has he/she ever had problems (with the law, school, job) because of drug use, does he/she think he/she has a problem with drugs; and what treatment programs or methods (if any) have they used to cut down or discontinue drug use (5)? Certain behavioral characteristics and beliefs have been found to be common among adolescents who are problem drinkers or frequent marijuana users. Adolescents significantly involved with alcohol or other drug use are more likely to report lower academic expectations, and value independence more than academic achievement (35).

Adolescents Reporting At-risk Behaviors

The HEADSS (Home, Education, Activities, Drugs, Sexuality, Suicide/depression) psychosocial assessment tool (37) may be useful in assessing an adolescent's risk and evaluating his/her social support system; examples of HEADSS questions are found in Table 7.1. An adolescent's report of behaviors which place him or her at high risk for HIV infection should invariably prompt the practitioner to engage them in a discussion about HIV (including an option for testing). In addition, providers should be prepared to provide the adolescent with appropriate resources and referrals to local community agencies (e.g., HIV testing and counseling, drug and alcohol treatment programs, support groups for gay and lesbian youth) (2,5).

REFERENCES

1. CDC. HIV/AIDS surveillance report. 1995 Mid-year edition. Atlanta, GA: Centers for Disease Control, 1995;7(1).
2. Friedman LS, Goodman E. Adolescents at risk for HIV infection. Primary Care 1992; 19:171–190.
3. Kipke MD, Futterman D, Hein K. HIV infection and AIDS during adolescence. Medical Clin North Am 1990;74:1149–1167.
4. Anderson MM, Morris RE. HIV and adolescents. Pediatric Annals 1993;22:436–446.
5. Kunins H, Hein K, Futterman D, et al. Module three: HIV/AIDS medical management. J Adolescent Health 1993;14:36S–52S.
6. Marks A, Fisher M. Health assessment and screening during adolescence. Pediatrics 80:135–158,1987.
7. MacKenzie RG. Approach to the adolescent in the clinical setting. Med Clin North Am 1990;74(5):1085–1095.
8. Friedman LS, Johnson B, Brett AS. Evaluation of substance-abusing adolescents by primary care physicians. J Adolesc Health Care 1990;11:227–230.
9. Anglin TM. Interviewing guidelines for the clinical evaluation of adolescent substance abuse. Pediatric Clin North Am 1987;34:381–398.
10. Futterman D, Hein K. Medical care of HIV-infected adolescents. AIDS Clinical Care 1992;4:95–98.
11. Yates GL, Mackenzie RG, Pennbridge J, Swofford A. A risk profile comparison of homeless youth involved in prostitution and homeless youth not involved. J Adoles Health 1991;12:545–548.

12. CDC. Health risk behaviors among adolescents who do and do not attend school—United States, 1992. MMWR 1994;43:129–132.
13. Bachman JG, Johston LD, O'Malley PM. Smoking, drinking and drug use among American high school students: correlates and trends, 1975–1979. Am J Public Health 1981;71:59–69.
14. CDC. Premarital sexual experience among adolescent women—United States, 1970–1988. MMWR 1991;39:929–932.
15. CDC. Sexual behavior among high school students—United States, 1990. MMWR 1992;40;885–889.
16. CDC. Selected behaviors that increase risk for HIV infection and other sexually transmitted diseases, and unintended pregnancy among high school students—United States, 1991. MMWR 1992;41:944–951.
17. Aral SO, Holmes KK. Epidemiology of sexual behavior and sexually transmitted diseases. In: Holmes KK, Mardh PA, Sparling FP, et al. eds. Sexually transmitted diseases. New York: McGraw-Hill, 1990.
18. Hayes CD, ed. Risking the future: adolescent sexuality, pregnancy and childbearing. Vol 1. Washington DC: National Academy Press. 1987.
19. CDC. Division of STD/HIV prevention annual report, 1990. Atlanta: US Department of Health and Human Services, Public Health Service, 1991.
20. Shafer M-A, Sweet RL. Pelvic inflammatory disease in adolescent females: epidemiology, pathogenesis, diagnosis, treatment, and sequelae. Pediatr Clin North Am 1989; 36:513–532.
21. Bell TA, Holmes KK. Age-specific risks of syphilis, gonorrhea, and hospitalized pelvic inflammatory disease in sexually experienced U.S. women. Sex Transm Dis 1984;11:291–295.
22. Cates W. Teenagers and sexual risk taking: the best of times and the worst of times. J Adolesc Health 1991;12:84–94.
23. Moscicki AB, Millstein MS, Broering J, Irwin Jr. CE. Risks of human immunodeficiency virus infection among adolescents attending three diverse clinics. J Pediatr 1993:122: 813–820.
24. Gayle HD, D'Angelo LJ. Epidemiology of AIDS and HIV infection in adolescents. In: Pizzo PA, Wilfert CM. eds. Pediatric AIDS. Baltimore: Williams & Wilkins, 1991: 38–50.
25. Remafedi GJ. Preventing the sexual transmission of AIDS during adolescence. J Adolesc Health Care 1988;9:139–143.
26. Fay RE, Turner CF, Klassen AD, Gagnon JH. Prevalence and patterns of same-gender sexual contact among men. Science 1989;243:338–348.
27. Remafedi G. Adolescent homosexuality: psychosocial and medical implications. Pediatrics 1987;79:331–337.
28. Hein K. AIDS in adolescence. J of Adolescent Health Care 1989:10:10S–35S.
29. Collins J, Holtzman D, Kann L, Kolbe L. Predictors of condom use among U.S. high school students. IXth International Conference on AIDS. Berlin 1993;(abstr WS-C13-4).
30. Lindegren ML, Hanson C, Miller K, et al. Epidemiology of human immunodeficiency virus infection in adolescents, United States. Pediatr Infect Dis J 1994;13:525–535.
31. Strunin L, Hingson R. Acquired immunodeficiency syndrome and adolescents: knowledge, attitudes, beliefs and behaviors. Pediatrics 1987;79:825–828.
32. Holtzman D, Anderson JE, Kann L, et al. HIV instruction, HIV knowledge, and drug injection among high school students in the United States. Am J Public Health 1991;81:1596–1601.
33. Hingson RW, Strunin L, Berlin B, et al. Beliefs about AIDS, use of alcohol and drugs, and unprotected sex among Massachusetts adolescents. Am J Public Health 1990; 80:1–5.
34. Lowry R, Holtzman D, Truman BI et al. Substance use and HIV-related sexual behaviors among US high school students: are they related. Am J Public Health. 1994:84:1116–1120.
35. Jessor R, Chase JA, Donovan JE. Psychosocial correlates of marijuana use and problem drinking in a national sample of adolescents. Am J Public Health 70:604–613, 1980.
36. Chychula NM. Screening for substance abuse in the primary care setting. Nurse Pract 1984;9:15–24.
37. Cohen E, Mackenzie RG, Yates GL. HEADSS, a psychosocial risk assessment instrument: implications for designing effective intervention programs for runaway youth. J Adolesc Health 1991;12:539–544.

Counseling and Testing Considerations for Adolescents

The developmental characteristics of an adolescent are important in determining when and how HIV testing should be discussed. Issues to consider include an adolescent's limited perspective of the future; their egocentrism; concrete thinking and sense of invulnerability. They have a significant capacity for denial, they may have fears of isolation, or loss of control, helplessness, or hopelessness. They are impulsive, and subject to potential extremes of acting out (1). These traits may influence how the clinician will approach an at-risk youth and whether the adolescent chooses to be tested and/or how he/she might respond upon receiving the test results (1). The benefits of treatment in prolonging and improving quality of life should be stressed to adolescents who might only have incorporated fearful images of those infected with HIV. The psychological impact of testing and the difficulties that accompany a positive result should be considered. A discussion of HIV and voluntary testing should be considered when an adolescent presents behaviors or circumstances which may have exposed him or her to HIV. Because it can be difficult to elicit a history of risky behaviors, HIV counseling should be more routinely incorporated into primary care of youth. These are similar to indications for HIV testing in adults (*See Indications for HIV Counseling & Testing*).

Although there may be adverse psychological effects of being identified as HIV positive, it is important for the clinician to help the adolescent understand that the test has not given them the infection but rather is a first step in coping with a reality in their lives and getting important health care. Adverse effects for an adolescent may include depression, suicidal ideation or attempts, acting out behaviors, or increased risk-taking behaviors (2,3). In a survey of teens and young adults attending an alcohol and drug rehabilitation program, 83% believed they would leave treatment; 64% would return to drugs, and 62% would to alcohol if found to be HIV positive (2). Over half indicated they would increase other risk-taking behavior (driving fast or while intoxicated), or would not continue with school (2). In another survey of adolescents, 21% of the respondents spontaneously wrote they would commit suicide if HIV positive (4). Although many youths express these types of fears, no studies have documented an increase in suicides or risky behaviors in HIV-positive youth. HIV testing is frequently associated with issues of high stress and anxiety and the availability of support services to assist youths in coping with testing is particularly important.

Consent

A written informed consent should be obtained from all adolescents, before any HIV testing is done, even if not required by state laws (2). Informed consent should be obtained in writing, to help verify that the adolescent both understands and has consented to testing. Preferably this would be obtained during the pretest counseling session. The consent process should include the following (3):

- A comprehensive explanation of the risks and benefits of HIV testing which is age-appropriate and culturally relevant

- Specification of which information will be disclosed in the medical record as well as the persons who will have access to the information (including the test result)

- Identification of a significant supportive adult by the adolescent

For adolescents judged to be incapable of giving an informed consent (e.g., mental retardation), consent should be obtained for testing from a parent, legal guardian, or the court, but only if there is demonstrated risk of HIV exposure for the adolescent (3). Adolescents have the right to refuse testing and test results should not be released without their permission.

Considerations for Counseling and Support

Adequate pre and posttest counseling and support must be provided to any adolescent being tested for HIV. Counseling information should be specific to the adolescent's needs, and consider special subpopulations (e.g., immigrants, homeless and runaway youth, residents of institutions, youth involved in survival sex, youth in foster care, youth in detention facilities). Counseling should be sensitive, as well as developmentally-, age-, and culturally-appropriate (2,3,5). Ideally, an adolescent should be tested where comprehensive services (medical, psychiatric, and social) are available and the counselor is trained, experienced and flexible (2,6). Rapport between the adolescent and counselor is essential, although it may be difficult since the counselor may be viewed as an authority figure (7). Test results should always be given in person, and if possible, pre and posttest counseling performed by the same individual. A minimum of one pre and one posttest counseling session should be given, although some adolescents will require additional pre and posttest counseling sessions (5). The option of anonymous testing and its benefits and disadvantages compared to confidential testing should be also explained, and a referral given if desired by the adolescent.

The benefits of confidential testing include enhanced ability to follow up on linkages to care. General counseling information is described in *HIV Counseling and Testing*.

PRETEST COUNSELING (2,3,5,8)

Adequate counseling and support should be provided before the adolescent is tested for HIV. If counseling is conducted in several sessions, the adolescent's risk for HIV should be assessed, a psychosocial assessment performed, the adolescent's support system identified, and information on HIV testing provided during the initial session. If the adolescent is asymptomatic, any problems that emerge (e.g., homelessness, psychological state, including risk for suicide) may need to be addressed first before proceeding with testing. The adolescent should be assisted in assessing the risks and benefits of being tested. Potential benefits include: improved quality and duration of life with medical intervention in HIV-positive individuals; motivating behavior change; and decreasing anxiety for both high- and low-risk youth who are HIV negative. Potential risks include: social ostracism, loss of friends or family, discrimination, depression, and providing a false sense of security for those high-risk individuals who test negative. The family support, coping mechanisms in previous crises, and anticipated coping mechanisms if results are HIV positive should be explored and discussed. Adolescents who have reservations should be encouraged to take a few days to consider and review the given information before taking the test. However, testing should not be delayed if the individual strongly desires it and is psychologically stable, or if medical indications warrant testing.

Counseling should provide adolescents with information about AIDS and the HIV antibody test to help them make an active, informed choice about testing. This includes basic HIV information (e.g., modes of transmission), the meaning of a positive and negative test result; interventions for prevention and risk reduction, as well as limitations of confidentiality. Adolescents should be encouraged to identify an adult (family member, guardian, case worker/social worker, or other significant adult) who will provide social and emotional support and be available for the adolescent during and after the testing process.

POSTTEST COUNSELING

Counseling HIV-negative Individuals (2,3,5,7–9)

Posttest counseling is a continuation of the pretest counseling, discussing the social, psychological, medical and the preventive implications of the test result. For adolescents who test negative, the time lag between exposure and the development of detectable antibodies (a few weeks to six months or more) should be explained. The adolescent should be encouraged to return for testing in six months or one year if at high risk. For adolescents practicing high-risk behavior, it should be explained that a negative test result does not provide immunity from HIV and continuing risk behaviors may result in HIV infection. Risk-reduction strategies should be discussed with the individual.

Counseling HIV-infected Individuals (5,7,8,10–12)

An adolescent's reactions to receiving an HIV-positive result may depend upon the stage of illness, life history, social and family support, levels of cognitive and moral development, emotional maturity, and self-acceptance (7). The adolescent should be given time to react to the results. The distinction between HIV infection and AIDS should be clarified. HIV infection should be conveyed as a chronic disease rather than an acute illness (10,11); a sense of hope should be conveyed and all treatment possibilities presented. Adolescents may have difficulty under-standing they are infected, particularly if no overt signs of infection are present. Until adolescents are capable of thinking abstractly, youths are predominantly egocentric, view the world in very concrete terms, and may perceive themselves as immortal. Information which may appear to be basic may be relatively unknown to adolescents, especially if they are members of disenfranchised populations (e.g., homeless/runaway, gay/lesbian, ethnic minorities, incarcerated youth) (7). The adolescent's un-derstanding of the meaning of the test result should be verified, and the biology of the disease explained. Information about HIV transmission, prevention and plans for risk reduction should also be reviewed, and the available medical interventions described. Avoiding further exposure to HIV and the benefits of health maintenance, such as eating a good diet and getting enough sleep, should be discussed. The adolescent's risk for self-harm should be assessed. In addition, financial counseling, including assistance in obtaining Medicaid or other benefits may be necessary. Linkages should be made for follow-up care and referral for additional supportive services (e.g., city, county or state public health services, com-munity agencies, gay and lesbian services, drug rehabilitation services, or local hospital and psychosocial services).

Disclosure Issues (7,13)

Disclosure issues should be discussed and the adolescent assisted in deciding with whom and how to share test results. The importance of in-forming the support person identified in the pretest counseling should be discussed; the supportive adult may not necessarily be a parent. Po-tential consequences of disclosure should be discussed: "Would the par-ent support or reject the adolescent? Would they provide emotional and financial support? Does the adolescent want to tell his or her parents, or does he/she feel compelled (7)?" Role playing with the adolescent, or be-ing present with the adolescent and adult during the disclosure may be helpful.

LEGAL ISSUES

Special aspects of HIV testing and counseling are unique to adoles-cents. These include legal issues regarding consent, confidentiality and disclosure. Every physician who provides care to adolescents should be familiar with the legal statutes in his/her particular state.

Adolescents in many states have the right to seek and receive treat-ment for certain specific medical conditions without the consent of a par-ent or guardian. In almost all states, parental consent is not necessary for adolescents to seek and receive treatment for a sexually transmitted disease (STD) or substance-abuse problems (2). In some states, there are provisions for minors to consent to diagnosis and treatment of STDs (in-cluding HIV testing), and specific HIV statutes have been created for adolescents in others (3,14). Currently, all states give "legal authority" to perform HIV antibody testing on "mature and competent" adolescents (14). Confidentiality of diagnoses and treatment varies from state to state. The limitations to confidentiality should be established prior to testing. To establish informed consent, the health provider must clearly document and record that the teenager fully understands the condition and the treatment under question.

Adolescents' involvement in research or drug treatment protocols is also an issue. Proposed federal guidelines posit that the legal ability of an adolescent to receive medical treatment without parental permission under state law is an indicator of an adolescent's capacity to consent to minimal risk research protocols. However, stricter standards of consent apply in research involving new medications. Because state laws vary widely, the adolescent's ability to seek independent diagnosis and treatment may be limited (15).

REFERENCES

1. Hein K. AIDS in adolescence. J of Adolescent Health Care 1989:10:10S–35S.
2. Friedman LS and Goodman E. Adolescents at risk for HIV infection. Primary Care 1992;19:171–190.
3. English, A. AIDS Testing and Epidemiology for Youth: Recommendations of the Working Group. J of Adolescent Health Care 1989;10:52S–57S.
4. Goodman E and Cohall AT. Acquired immunodeficiency syndrome and adolescents: knowledge, attitudes, beliefs, and behaviors in an NYC adolescent minority population. Pediatrics 1989;84:36–42.
5. Kipke MD, D. Futterman, K Hein. HIV infection and AIDS during adolescence. Med Clin North Am 1990;74:1149–1167.
6. Massachusetts Department of Public Health, Comprehensive guidelines for adolescent HIV antibody counseling and testing, Boston: Massachusetts Department of Public Health 1990.
7. Eliot AS. Counseling for HIV-infected adolescents. Focus. 1993;8(9):1–4.
8. Anderson MM, Morris RE. HIV and adolescents. Pediatric Annals 1993;22:436–446.
9. Hein K, Futterman D. Medical management in HIV-infected adolescents. J Pediatr 1991;119:S18–S20.
10. Spiegel L, Mayero A. Psychosocial aspects of AIDS in children and adolescents. Pediatric Clinics of North America 1991;38:153–167.
11. Kunins H, Hein K, Futterman D, et al. Module three: HIV/AIDS medical management J Adolescent Health 1993;14:36S–52S.
12. Futterman D, Hein K. Medical management of adolescents. In: Pizzo PA, Wilfert CM, eds. Pediatric AIDS: the challenge of HIV infection in infants, children and adolescents. Baltimore, MD: Williams and Wilkins, 1991;546–560.
13. El-Sadr W, Oleske JM, Agins BD, et al. Evaluation and management of early HIV infection. AHCPR Publication No. 94-0572. Rockville, MD: Agency for Health Care Policy and Research, Public Health Service, US Department of Health and Human Services, January 1994.
14. North RL. Legal authority for HIV testing of adolescents. J Adolesc Health Care 1990; 11:176–186.
15. Rogers AS, D'Angelo L, Futterman D. Guidelines for adolescent participation in research: current realities and possible resolutions. NRB 1994;16:1–5.

Prevention Considerations for Adolescents

Adolescent characteristics such as feelings of invulnerability, incomplete development of abstract thought processes, conformity to peer pressure, and risk-taking behavior (1,2) make educational and prevention efforts challenging. Prevention messages delivered by adults may not be acceptable because of adolescents' distrust of authority figures (3). Risk-taking behavior has been identified as a normal part of psychological development and a necessary experience for adolescents to transform into well-adjusted adults (4). Experimentation, in itself, may not be psychologically destructive. The task for prevention programs is to assist adolescents and young adults in distinguishing between appropriate and inappropriate risks, rather than to attempt to eliminate all risky behaviors from life (4). Adolescents have been shown to engage in sex for reasons other than pleasure, such as peer approval, rebellion, expression of hostility, and escape (5). Because peer friendship is an important aspect of psychological well-being and should not be eliminated, prevention programs which focus on reducing "peer pressure" as an influence on sexual, alcohol and drug behaviors should not devalue its worth (4). Prevention strategies should include not only information about HIV infection but also assist in the development of the skills which enable adolescents to reduce their risk for HIV. Prevention efforts for adolescents must be individualized, flexible, consider the developmental changes that take place, and focus on characteristics that may influence behavioral change.

Enhancing Perception of Risk

An individual's perceived susceptibility to HIV is considered an important determinant of taking preventive action (6,7). Among inner city adolescents, knowing someone with HIV, perceiving oneself to be at risk, and having knowledge of HIV, were protective factors associated with negative serostatus (8). Unless adolescents perceive themselves at risk, they will probably not change their behavior. Condom use among adolescents has been associated cross-sectionally with beliefs about the susceptibility to getting AIDS and the benefits and barriers of condom use (9). Suggestions to enhance perception of risk include: encouraging adolescents to examine their own sexual and drug use behaviors and estimating their own risk, interactive games illustrating how random encounters can lead to transmission; talking to a person with HIV from a similar background, age and risk behaviors (10,11). It may be difficult for adolescents to consider the future consequences of their behaviors if the risk of HIV infection does not appear immediate. Even if the risks are known, including death, adolescents may not personalize this knowledge (12). Because studies have shown that perceived risk does not always affect condom use, interventions should focus on specific preventive actions individualized to the adolescent's own risk-taking behavior (13). Socio-environmental influences on preventive behaviors should also be addressed; these include beliefs about norms, values, and self-efficacy, individual/cognitive interventions (14). Adolescents should be helped to clarify their personal values relating to preventive actions, and to understand the effects of outside influences (e.g., peer pressure) on those values (14).

Decision Making, Skill Provision, and Communicative Skills

Adolescents should be assisted in developing decision making, problem-solving, communicative and negotiating skills to reduce their risk, and promote self-protective behavior regarding sex, contraception, and drug use (11,15,16). Values such as the responsibility for one's own body should be taught and supported (17). Adolescents should be encouraged to discuss their thoughts, feelings, and to ask questions; the adolescents' sexual behaviors and sexuality should be discussed positively to promote a healthy sexual identity (11). Special attention and support should be given to gay youth, who may feel isolated or be struggling with their sense of worth (11,18). Adolescents should be supported in their decision to delay or abstain from sexual intercourse and if sexually active, encouraged to take the appropriate precautions to reduce risk.

It is important that adolescents develop communication and assertiveness skills to negotiate condom use with a sexual partner and resist peer pressure in participating in at-risk behaviors (11). The adolescent should be assisted in setting risk reduction objectives (e.g., avoiding casual sex, using condoms regularly) and in deciding on ways to carry these out. Providing the skills necessary for risk reduction can enhance self-efficacy (14); this may involve teaching adolescents how to clarify a partner's request or intention; avoid/refuse to practice risk-related behaviors; discuss risk reduction with a partner, and propose alternative low-risk activities (11). Interventions which specifically promote thinking and talking about condoms may be more effective at increasing condom use than interventions aimed at promoting general communication between partners regarding HIV exposure (19). Asking a partner to use a condom was the strongest predictor of condom use at last intercourse in one study (13). Interventions can include using peer group discussion, peer counseling, role playing, and modeling (e.g., watching a videotape depicting how to persuade a partner to use condoms) (20,21). Role-playing in emotionally charged situations may help adolescents confront their feelings, practice skills, and prepare for future situations. Peer counseling and group discussion can provide a setting where condom use is clearly communicated as being acceptable to peers, and therefore also for the individual.

Facilitating communication between adolescents and parents has also been associated with reduced risk behaviors (22,23). Adolescents receiving HIV instruction have been shown to be more likely to communicate with adult family members about HIV, and adolescents who talked to family members were less likely to have multiple sex partners and inject drugs (22). Among black adolescents, consistent condom use was significantly associated with insisting on condom use, talking about HIV with parents, younger age (12–15 years old), perceiving that peer norms support condom use, and never having an STD (23). Prevention efforts might be focused on younger adolescents, improving their communication skills, promoting discussions about sex among adolescents and parents, and developing community interventions which promote new behavioral standards and social norms (23).

Safer Sex

Regardless of previous sexual experience, the topic of condom use should be discussed with all adolescents. Adolescents who carried condoms and discussed AIDS with a physician were 2.7 and 1.7 times more likely to use them (24). Discussing AIDS with a physician predicted increased condom use by adolescents in another study (25). Since adolescents have reported concern over condom breakage (26), instruction concerning how to correctly use condoms is especially important. Both females and males should practice how to put condoms on and take them off correctly. Females should not assume men have condoms or know how to use them properly. Condoms must be used not only correctly but also consistently to be effective in preventing the transmission of HIV and other STDs. The importance of consistent condom use when having sex should be emphasized and the maintenance of this behavior reinforced. Because female adolescents who use oral contraceptives as a method of birth control may be less likely to use condoms, the importance of barrier methods in preventing STDs and HIV infection should be emphasized. Information should also include where to buy condoms and what types (latex) to buy. The availability of condoms in the office might decrease barriers to their use and emphasize the importance of protected sex (27). It should be reiterated that condoms are the only contraceptive which also reduces the risk of HIV transmission. Among adolescents, condom use has been associated with the desire to prevent pregnancy rather than AIDS (28). To link the importance of preventing pregnancy and AIDS prevention, HIV interventions are best structured within the context of family planning/preventing pregnancy (28).

Obstacles to safer sex for the adolescent should be discussed. Adolescents may fear that insisting on condom use would reveal HIV status or result in a loss of relationship. Youth having same-sex relationships may not be ready to acknowledge that they are gay or bisexual. For urban youths, the risk of violence and crime may be more immediate than the consequences of not using a condom. Moreover, for safer sex to be effective, it must be satisfying. Adolescents have reported discomfort and a reduction of sexual pleasure associated with condom use (25). Effective condom use most likely requires not only technical skills and the social skills to negotiate their use, but the perception that condoms can be a part of a pleasurable sexual relationship (9). To address this, instruction can be obtained concerning the use of appropriate lubricants, methods of partner arousal, and how condoms can be used during foreplay to increase pleasure (25). Although the practitioner or counselor can assist the adolescent in determining what practices are safe and which have some risk, if the adolescent makes his/her decisions regarding safer sex, adherence is more likely.

There has been controversy whether sex and AIDS education (including condom use) encourages sexual activity in young people. Because premature initiation of sexual activity is associated with risk, young people should be encouraged to postpone sexual activity. Adolescents who do not have sex should be supported and a health-oriented social norm regarding sexuality among youth encouraged (29). However, it is also essential that messages regarding safer sex and condom use are given because many adolescents will engage in sexual activity. A review of 19 studies regarding the effects of sex education in school revealed no evidence that sex education led to earlier or increased sexual activity (30). Of these, six studies showed sex education led either to delaying the onset of sexual activity or decreasing overall sexual activity. Moreover, ten studies demonstrated that sexually active youth who were exposed to sex education increased their adoption of safer sex practices. School programs promoting both postponement of sex and protected sex when sexually active were found to be more effective than those promoting abstinence alone. Among school-based sex education programs, those provided before youth became sexually active, and which emphasized skills and social norms rather than knowledge, were found to be more effective (30).

REFERENCES

1. English, A. AIDS testing and epidemiology for youth: recommendations of the working group. J of Adolescent Health Care 1989;10:52S–57S.
2. Hein K. AIDS in adolescence. J of Adolescent Health Care 1989:10:10S–35S.
3. Elkin D. All grown up and no place to go. Reading. Mass: Addison-Wesley, 1985.
4. Hochhauser M. Moral development and HIV prevention among adolescents. Focus 1991;6:1–4.
5. Cohen MW, Friedman, SB. Nonsexual motivation of adolescent sexual behavior. Medical Aspects of Human Sexuality 1975;9:9–31.
6. Janz NK. Becker MH. The health belief model: a decade later: Health Education Quarterly 1984;11:1
7. Becker MH, Joseph JG. AIDS and behavioral change to reduce risk: a review. Am J Public Health, 1988;78:394.
8. Futterman D, Elliot A, Hein K, et al. HIV+ adolescents: factors linked to transmission and prevention. IXth International Conference on AIDS. Berlin 1993; (abstr P0-C19-3049).
9. Hingson RW, Strunin L, Berlin BM, Heeren T. Beliefs about AIDS, use of alcohol and drugs, and unprotected sex among Massachusetts adolescents. Am J Public Health 1990;80:295–299.
10. Goodman E. Cohall AT. Acquired immunodeficiency syndrome and adolescents: knowledge, attitudes, beliefs, and behaviors in an NYC adolescent minority population. Pediatrics 1989;84:36–42.
11. Kipke MD, Futterman D, Hein K. HIV infection and AIDS during adolescence. Med Clin North Am 1990;74:1149–1167.
12. Price JH, Desmond S, Kukula G. High school students' perceptions and misperceptions of AIDS. J School Health 1985;55:107–109.
13. Weisman CS, Nathanson CA, Ensminger M, et al. AIDS knowledge, perceived risk and prevention among adolescent clients of a family planning clinic. Family Planning Perspec 1989;21:213–217.
14. Walter HJ, Vaughan RD, Gladis MM, et al. Factors associated with AIDS risk behaviors among high school students in an AIDS epicenter. Am J Public Health 1992;82:528–532.
15. Lindegren ML, Hanson C, Miller K, et al. Epidemiology of human immunodeficiency virus infection in adolescents, United States. Pediatr Infect Dis J 1994;13:525–535.
16. Cates W. Priorities for sexually transmitted diseases in the 1980s and beyond. Sexually Transmitted Diseases 1986;13:114–117.
17. Prothrow-Stith D. Excerpts from address. J of Adolesc Health Care 1989;10:5S–7S.
18. Friedman LS, Goodman E. Adolescents at risk for HIV infection. Primary Care 1992;19:171–190.
19. Norris AE. Condom use by urban, minority youth. IXth International Conference on AIDS. Berlin 1993;(abstract PO-D02-3429).

20. Flora JA, Thoresen CE. Reducing the risk of AIDS in adolescents. American Psychologist 1988;43:965.
21. Solomon MZ, DeJong W. Preventing AIDS and other STDs through condom promotion: a patient education intervention. Am J Public Health 1989:79:453.
22. Holtzman D, Kann L, Collins J, Kolbe L. HIV instruction, knowledge, communication with parents and peers, and risk behaviors among high school students in the United States, 1989. IXth International Conference on AIDS. Berlin 1993;(abstr PO-D02-3447).
23. DiClemente R, Lodico, Evans P, et al. Some African-American adolescents in a high-risk urban environment use condoms consistently. IXth International Conference on AIDS. Berlin 1993;(abstr PO-D02-3439).
24. Hingson R, Strunin L. Monitoring adolescents' response to the AIDS epidemic: changes in knowledge, attitudes, beliefs, and behaviors. In: DiClemente RJ, ed. Adolescents and AIDS: a generation in jeopardy. Newbury Park, Calif: Sage Publications;1992:17–33
25. DiClemente RJ. Psychosocial determinants of condom use among adolescents. In: DiClemente RJ, ed. Adolescents and AIDS: a generation in jeopardy. Newbury Park, Calif: Sage Publications;1992:34–51.
26. Ford K, Norris A. Urban African-Americans and Hispanic adolescents and young adults: who do they talk to about AIDS and condoms? What are they learning? AIDS Education and Prevention 1991;3:197–206.
27. Anderson MM, Morris RE. HIV and adolescents. Pediatric Annals 1993;22:436–446.
28. Langer LM, Zimmerman RS, Katz JA. Which is more important to high school students: preventing pregnancy or preventing AIDS? Family Planning Perspectives 1994;26:154–159.
29. Roper WL, Peterson HB, Curran JW. Commentary: condoms and HIV/STD prevention-clarifying the message. Am J Public Health 1993;501–503.
30. Baldo M, Aggleton P, Slutkin G. Does sex education lead to earlier or increased sexual activity in youth? IX International Conference on AIDS. Berlin 1993;(abstr PO-D02-3444).

Medical Management of HIV-infected Adolescents

The natural history of HIV and its predominant clinical manifestations are not yet fully defined for the adolescent age group (1). Because HIV infection in adolescents occurs after the immune system is developed, it is thought that HIV infection in adolescents is more similar to adults than to children. Although it has been shown that, compared to young children and adults with hemophilia, HIV disease progression among adolescents is slower (2–4), anecdotal clinical experience has suggested that once adolescents are infected, their immune function deteriorates at the same rate as adults (5). Therapies which have been evaluated in national clinical trials have not been adequately studied in pubertal adolescents. Consequently, it is unclear in what ways, if any, therapies should be altered for adolescents.

Initial Medical Evaluation of an HIV-infected Adolescent

There are limited standards for routine management of HIV-infected youth, but guidelines have been suggested (1–3,6–9). It has been recommended that an initial evaluation of an adolescent should be conducted over several visits (6–8). During this time, the adolescent's ability to cope can also be assessed and support given (7–8). Elements of an initial evaluation include a complete medical history, psychosocial history (e.g., sexuality/sexual activity, substance abuse, coping support systems), review of systems, physical exam, neurologic assessment, and laboratory testing (1,2,6,7). Other elements include psychosocial assessments and

Table 7.2.
Primary Care Focus of Treatment for HIV-Infected Adolescents

Risk assessment and risk reduction
HIV testing and counseling
Staging of HIV infection
Appropriate immunizations
Routine gynecologic care
Treatment of HIV
Prophylaxis against and early diagnosis of opportunistic infections
Education and emotional support
Coordination of care (e.g., psychosocial, specialists)
Referrals for legal, psychological, and other services as needed

Adapted with permission of Elsevier Science, Inc. from Kunins H, Hein K, Futterman D, et al. Module three: HIV/AIDS medical management. J Adolescent Health 1993;14:36S–52S.

counseling, HIV education, information, counseling about the HIV test, financial planning, and entitlements (6). As the provider, it is important to establish a trusting rapport with the youth (10). It may also be helpful to encourage the adolescent to view HIV as a chronic disease which requires ongoing management (6,11). Recommended elements of primary care for the HIV-infected adolescent are summarized in Table 7.2.

MEDICAL HISTORY AND REVIEW OF SYSTEMS

The medical history should include questions about social, psychological, sexual, drug use, and family histories. A complete medical history should include the following (1,2,6–9):

Why does the adolescent want to take or has already taken an HIV test? If testing was performed, when was it done? If positive, determine how the adolescent is coping, and who knows his/her serostatus. Confirm HIV positive serostatus with written records. If not available, retest.

Evidence of seroconversion illness to help date the acquisition of HIV. Symptoms may include a mononucleosis-like syndrome of fever, malaise, lymphadenopathy, variable multiple system involvement (12).

History of conditions that may represent HIV infection. These include opportunistic infections, weight loss, recurrent infections, and failure to grow or gain weight during pubertal growth spurt.

History of prior illness. (For example: tuberculosis, sinusitis, pneumonia, STDs).

History of childhood diseases.

History of sources of care. Inquire about hospitalizations and chronic medication use.

History of blood transfusions or receipt of blood products.

Immunization history.

Alcohol and other drug use history. This includes alcohol, tobacco, marijuana, cocaine, and steroids. Further questions include route, amount, frequency, and injection history.

Sexual history. Inquire about age at first intercourse, types of sex activity (vaginal, oral, anal), number and sex of partners, sexual orientation, and sexual abuse.

A history of sexual transmitted diseases (STDs) and their sites. Each STD and their symptoms should be named, since adolescents may not realize they have had one. Include: gonorrhea, chlamydia, syphilis, genital herpes, warts. Inquire if females have ever had a pelvic exam and if Pap smear results are known or are available from other providers.

Menstrual and pregnancy history. Include contraceptive history and current sexual practices, condom use, number of pregnancies (including abortions, miscarriages, live births) and intention to have children.

Psychosocial history. Include living situation, education level, literacy, employment, school and work status, social support, peer relationships, legal problems. Determine if anyone knows about the adolescent's HIV infection. Assess psychological functioning including past/present depression, anxiety, suicidal thoughts and/or attempts, psychoses, hospitalizations, treatment.

Review of systems

Aspects of the sexual, substance use, and psychosocial history are discussed in detail in the Risk Assessment for the Adolescent. Elements of an HIV-oriented review of systems are shown in Table 7.3 (1,2,6,7,9).

PHYSICAL EXAM

The changes in body size, composition, organ and cognitive function that accompany adolescence should be considered when doing a physical exam and staging of HIV infection. Physical or psychological regression as well as failure to progress should be noted. During the age of 10 to 20 years, weight normally doubles and height increases by 15% to 20% (2). Failure to gain weight or height at the expected rate should be further

---

Table 7.3.
Review of Systems

	Symptoms
General	• Fever, fatigue, night sweats, malaise, weight loss or failure to gain weight during growth spurt, anorexia, rash, skin changes, nail changes, changes in, or low school and workplace performance.
HEENT (Head, eyes, ears, nose, throat)	• Enlarged lymph nodes, visual changes, recurrent sinusitis/otitis, oral lesions or masses, thrush, painful swallowing, recurrent ulcers, gum disease, tooth decay.
Respiratory	• Cough, dry or productive, dyspnea with exertion, wheezing, shortness of breath.
Gastrointestinal	• Abdominal pain, diarrhea, vomiting.
Genitourinary/ gynecologic	• Genital/rectal pain and growths, rectal bleeding, urethral discharge, penile ulcers or growths, previous pelvic inflammatory disease, previous abnormal Pap smears, chronic vaginal infections, pelvic pain.
Neuromuscular	• Peripheral paraesthesias, weakness, myalgia, abnormal pain or sensations.
Neuropsychiatric	• Personality changes, headaches, depression, anxiety, difficulty concentrating, short-term memory loss. Some of these complaints may be indistinguishable from chronic drug use.

Table 7.4.
Physical Exam of an HIV-infected Adolescent

- General exam: include vital signs, growth assessment, nutritional status, skin assessment, and height and weight (including changes over time)
- Lymph nodes examination (if lymphadenopathy is present, describe the location, number, size, consistency, and persistency)
- Head, eyes, ears, nose throat (HEENT) exam: include assessment of visual acuity, a fundoscopic examination (looking for evidence of CMV or toxoplasma retinitis), assess sinuses, and oral examination (oral lesions, gum or dental diseases)
- Lung and heart examination
- Abdominal examination (noting the presence of masses or hepatosplenomegaly)
- Genitalia exam (including Tanner staging of sexual maturity)
- Pelvic exam and PAP smear for sexually active females, or those over 18 years old
- Rectal exam for all adolescents (inspection—digital exam/anoscopy if symptoms)
- Neurological assessment: assess cranial nerves, reflexes, strength, sensation, cerebellar function; baseline mental health status; ability of the adolescent to generalize or think abstractly; perform neuropsychological testing performed if neurological involvement suspected)

investigated. HIV wasting, defined as weight loss in adults, is additionally defined as failure to gain weight during puberty because this is a period when height and weight should be increasing significantly (2,6). The pulse rate and blood pressure ranges also increase during adolescence. Although common skin problems such as acne, dermatophyte infections and eczema may develop during adolescence, HIV-related dermatologic disorders that signal disease progression may also occur. The Tanner and Whitehouse Sexual Maturity Rating Scale (13) is a more reliable indicator of pubertal development than is chronological age and should be used when assessing development during adolescence (3,6). This scale describes the development of pubic hair, breasts and male genitalia during puberty. Yearly or twice yearly pelvic exams with appropriate laboratory tests and inspection for vaginal candida should be performed for women who have had sexual intercourse, have unexplained pelvic pain, or, as some have recommended, patients who are over 18 (2). A rectal exam (inspection) should be done of all males and females (even those who deny anal intercourse) (2,6). Elements of a thorough physical exam are listed in Table 7.4 (1,2,6,9).

LABORATORY ASSESSMENT

Laboratory assessment of HIV-infected adolescents parallels that done in adults. Normal values which are adolescent-specific should be considered where available and different from other age groups (2,6). For example, there are adolescent-specific norms for complete blood count based on Tanner staging. During puberty, hemoglobin dramatically increases in males, (due to increased androgens) compared to females (4). Alkaline phosphatase levels are elevated during the adolescent growth spurt, but elevation may also be associated with disseminated MAC (2,6). The best marker of disease progression is the use of CD4 cell counts. Available studies have demonstrated CD4 counts in

Table 7.5.
Laboratory Assessment

Serum/blood
  CBC and platelets
  Liver/kidney/nutritional chemistries
  Rubella titer (after second MMR)
  Screening test for syphilis
  Hepatitis B, C serologies
Immunologic assessment
  CD4+, total number and percentage of total lymphocyte count and CD4:CD8 ratio; initially
    and every 6 months; if CD4 count approaches 500, repeat every 3 months
  HIV antibody testing (ELISA and Western blot)
  Optional: p24 antigen, beta-2 microglobulin levels, neopterin, quantitative immunoglobulins
Opportunistic infection screening
  Epstein-Barr virus serology
  Serum cryptococcal antigen titer
  Toxoplasmosis titers
  Blood culture: bacteria, MAC, fungal dependent on symptoms
Other
  Urinalysis and urine culture as needed
  Skin test for tuberculosis (PPD) with anergy panel (Merieux multitest or Candida, mumps
    and tetanus antigen)
  Baseline chest x-ray for patients who are PPD positive and/or anergic
Sexually active adolescents
  Pap smear for females and colposcopy when indicated
  Culture for gonorrhea (oral, anal, and genital)
  Chlamydia test (immunofluorescent, DNA probe, or culture)
  Herpes culture, if indicated
  Gram stain to detect inflammation, Candida or gonorrhea (in males)
  KOH preparation for Candida
  Wet prep for trichomonads, WBC, or clue cells
  Pregnancy test as indicated
  Typing of condyloma if indicated

adolescents are similar to adult values (14); however normal values during puberty have not been established. In postpubertal adolescents, adult values apply (2). Baseline laboratory assessments should be performed in all HIV-positive adolescents and follow-up values obtained at regular intervals to monitor changes in immunologic and other markers. Elements of the laboratory evaluation are listed in Table 7.5 (2,6,8).

Staging Classification

Based on clinical and laboratory parameters, the stage of HIV infection is evaluated to assess immune function, risk of disease progression and the appropriate course of treatment (1,2,6,7). Knowing the stage of infection allows the provider to assess the need for early intervention as well as to plan for prevention, care, and treatment. Classification systems include those developed by the CDC for adults and adolescents (15). The criteria for this classification system were not developed specifically for adolescents and may need to be modified (1,2,6).

Immunizations

Immunizations for HIV-infected adolescents should include standard adolescent immunizations [e.g., diphtheria tetanus immunization (at age 15), and measles-mumps-rubella (MMR)] (6,7). In addition, HIV-infected adolescents should be given a pneumococcal vaccine and yearly influenza immunization (16,17). For females, immunity to rubella should be assessed and those without prior immunity should be immunized (6). Hepatitis B vaccine should be given to those who are sexually active and/or inject drugs (unless patient is immune, or hepatitis B surface antigen positive) (18). Currently, the American Academy of Pediatrics recommends that all teens receive hepatitis B vaccine. Although oral polio vaccine is contraindicated for HIV-positive patients and their household members, inactivated polio vaccine is recommended if not previously given (19).

Follow-up Visits

The HIV antibody test should be confirmed or documented. Follow-up of baseline measurements of CD4 cell counts and percentages (optional—p24 antigen, neopterin, β2 microglobulin) should be taken at three- to six-month intervals (6,9). For HIV-infected, sexually active females, PAP smears should be taken every six months (6,9). Follow-up visits for asymptomatic adolescents with CD4 >500 should be scheduled at three- to six-month intervals with routine blood-work (CBC and chemistry panels), and a PPD and anergy panel every six to twelve months (1,6). Adolescents with CD4 counts of 500 or less should have follow-up visits for physical exam and repeat laboratory assessment every three months (1,6). Adolescents on drug protocols will require frequent visits (e.g., monitoring the effect of zidovudine on complete blood count and blood chemistry) (1,6). Patients who are symptomatic and/or with CD4 cell counts of 200 or less may be seen from once every three months to monthly, as immune dysfunction progresses. Guidelines for follow-up of the HIV-infected adolescent (3,6) are shown in Table 7.6 but should be modified to meet individual needs (6). Colposcopy should be performed for females with abnormal Pap results.

Treatment and Dose Adjustment for Therapies

Antiretroviral treatments available include zidovudine (ZDV), ddI (didanosine), d4T (stavudine), 3TC (Lamivudine) and ddC (Zalcitabine), and protease inhibitors should be used in combination treatment due to rapid development of resistance. ddI may be used alone or in conjunction with ZDV, and ddC is generally used in conjunction with ZDV. Treatment for HIV infection and prophylaxis of opportunistic infection (OIs) are currently similar to those in adults and shown in Table 7.7 and Table 7.8. Information regarding protease inhibitors are addressed separately (*See Protease Inhibitors–A New Approach to HIV Therapy*). How-

Table 7.6.

Follow-up Guidelines for HIV-Infected Adolescents

Procedure	Frequency
Update medical history	Every visit
Review of systems	Every 3 months or if symptomatic
Physical examination	Every 3–6 months
Complete blood count	Every 3–6 months
Patients with CD4 >600	Every 6 months
Chemistry panels	
For patients with CD4 >600	Every 6 months
For patients taking potentially toxic medications	Every 3–6 months
Immune function monitoring	
Patients with CD4 >600	Every 6 months
Patients with CD4 <500	Every 3 months
Pap smear	Every 6 months
Screening for STDs	Every 6–12 months
PPD/anergy panel	Every 6–12 months
Toxoplasmosis assessment in unexposed patients	Yearly
Immunizations	As recommended

Adapted with permission of Elsevier Science, Inc. from Kunins H, Hein K, Futterman D, et al. Module three: HIV/AIDS medical management. J Adolescent Health 1993;14:36S–52S.

Table 7.7.

Recommendations for Antiretroviral Medications and Prophylaxis for Opportunistic Infections

CD4 Counts	Antiretrovirals and OI prophylaxis
>500	No routine administration
200–500	Consider antiretrovirals:
	• ZDV 200 mg tid (Initial treatment. If intolerant or CD4 decreases, use ddI, ddC alone or in combination)
	• ddI 200 mg bid or
	• ddC 0.75 mg tid
	OI prophylaxis
	• None
100–200	Antiretrovirals: recommended as above
	OI prophylaxis
	• PCP: TMP/SMX, 1 DS 3 times per week or daily
<100	Antiretrovirals: as above
	OI prophylaxis
	• PCP: As above
	• MAC: Rifabutin, 200 mg qd
	• Fungal: Fluconazole, 100 mg qd
	Candida (if recurrent oral thrush, candida esophageal or vaginitis)
	Cryptococcus—consider

ever, adolescent-specific normal values should be used when evaluating the efficacy and toxicity of medications. Three forms of prophylaxis for *Pneumocystis Carinii* pneumonia are currently recommended: trimethoprimsulfamethoxazole (TMP-SMX), aerosolized pentamidine, and, dapsone.

Currently, pediatric dose schedules are recommended for adolescents who are Tanner stage I and adult doses given to those in Tanner stage V

Table 7.8.
Commonly Used Medicines in HIV/AIDS

Antiretroviral Medications*	Dosage
Zidovudine (ZDV)	200 mg every 8 hours.
Didanosine (ddI)	125 or 200 mg every 12 hours.
Zalcitabine (ddC)	0.375 or 0.75 mg every 8 hours.
Stavudine (d4T)	20 or 40 mg every 12 hours.
Lamivudine (3TC)	150 or 300 mg every 12 hours.
Saquinavir	600 mg every 8 hours.
Ritonavir	600 mg every 12 hours.
Inidinavir	800 mg every 8 hours.

Opportunistic Infections	Prophylactic Medications
Pneumocystis carnii pneumonia (initiate when CD4 cells$<$200/mm^3)	Trimethoprimsulfamethoxazole (TMP/SMX); dapsone, atovaquone or pentamidine
Toxoplasmosis gondii (initiate when CD4$<$100 mm^3)	TMP/SMX or dapsone plus pyrimethamine
Mycobacterium avium complex (when CD4$<$75 mm^3)	Rifabutin or clarithromycin
Mycobacterium tuberculosis (if PPD positive or anergic)	Isoniazid or rifampin
Cytomegalovirus (if antibody positive and CD4$<$50/mm^3	Ganciclovir

*Licensed by the FDA, often used in combination; demonstrate the ability to prolong and/or improve the quality of life.

(3,6,7). Appropriate dosages recommendations for adolescents in Tanner stages II, III, and IV have not been clarified (6,7,15). Adolescents in such stages should be monitored closely for toxicity and efficacy (6). It has been suggested that pediatric doses be given to adolescents in Tanner stage II, and adult doses to those in Tanner stage IV (3). Changes in body composition and organ function characteristic during puberty may affect drug distribution and metabolism; changes in drug dose and interval of drug administration may be necessary (2,3). Because the use of tobacco, alcohol, or drugs may alter drug efficacy and toxicity, an accurate drug history is essential.

Adherence to Treatment Plans (6,7,12,20)

Adherence to treatment by adolescents may be challenging. The characteristics of adolescence (e.g., feeling of immortality, denial) and the developmental level of an adolescent will affect his/her ability to comply to treatment regimen. In addition, other problems may exist which have higher priority (e.g., seeking shelter and food) and must be first addressed to promote adherence. Adolescents may be unfamiliar with the basic knowledge concerning HIV and may need a review of medical terminology and repetition of basic facts of their illness. Adolescents who understand the implications of an HIV test may still be in denial about their health. Characteristics of adolescence, such as concrete thought processes and self-perception of immortality may intensify denial (e.g.,

"If I look and feel good, how can I be sick?") (9). For asymptomatic adolescents, visiting the provider and taking antiviral medication may be a reminder that they are "sick" and may impede compliance (6,9). This may translate to missed clinic appointments, inconsistent compliance with medication, and avoidance of others who are HIV infected. Providers may need to reorient adolescents to the realities of HIV disease and help them integrate their seropositivity with other aspects of their sense of self (20). Providing adolescents with a more mature perspective and necessary structure may be needed; this may require helping adolescents to verbalize feelings and discuss the consequences of actions planned (20). This may discourage acting out in potentially self-destructive ways (e.g., suicide gestures, refusal to keep appointments, noncompliance)—behaviors which may camouflage other feelings such as fear, anger, or despair. Because a patient's adverse response to therapy may impact his/her compliance, these issues should be explored (e.g., for a former crack addict, aerosolized pentamidine may arouse fears of returning to addiction) (9).

Since adolescents tend to think in concrete terms, clinical values such as CD4 cell counts should always be discussed in the context of medical status and level of functioning; otherwise, for the teen, a fixed CD4 value may equate to a specific serious illness or to death. The spectrum of illness versus specific cutoff levels for disease diagnosis and progression should be explained, as well as the usefulness of CD4 counts as a guideline for medication and prophylaxis. Assisting the adolescent to integrate medications into the daily schedule, tailoring it to the individual's lifestyle, and anticipating obstacles and problem solving together may be helpful. Instructions should be simple, and confirmed by having the adolescent repeat the directions. Adherence should be encouraged and demonstrated adherence should be praised. While many adolescents may be unresponsive to abstract concepts such as good health or longevity, they will respond to strategies that enhance their self-esteem, and that assist them in constructing and achieving concrete short-term goals (7,9).

Modified from Module Three: HIV/AIDS Medical Management by Kunins H, Hein K, Futterman D, et al. Journal of Adolescent Health Vol 14;36S–52S. Copyright 1993 by the Society of Adolescent Medicine.

REFERENCES

1. Kipke MD, D. Futterman, K Hein. HIV infection and AIDS during adolescence. Med Clin North Am 1990;74:1149–1167.
2. Futterman D, Hein K. Medical care of HIV-infected adolescents. AIDS Clinical Care 1992;4:95–98.
3. El-Sadr W, Oleske JM, Agins BD, et al. Evaluation and management of early HIV infection. AHCPR Publication 94-0572. Rockville, MD: Agency for Health Care Policy and Research, Public Health Service, US Department of Health and Human Services, January 1994.
4. Goedert JJ, Kessler CM, Aledort LM, et al. A prospective study of human immunodeficiency virus type 1 infection and the development of AIDS in subjects with hemophilia. N Engl J Med 1987;321:1142–1148.

5. Futterman D, Hein K, Reuben N, et al. Human immunodeficiency virus-infected adolescents: the first 50 patients in a New York City program. Pediatrics 1993;91: 730–735.
6. Kunins H, Hein K, Futterman D, et al. Module three: HIV/AIDS medical management. J Adolescent Health 1993;14:36S–52S.
7. Anderson MM, Morris RE. HIV and adolescents. Pediatric Annals 1993;22:436–446.
8. Hein K, Futterman D. Medical management in HIV-infected adolescents. J Pediatr 1991;119:S18–S20.
9. Futterman D, Hein K. Medical management of adolescents. In: Pizzo PA, Wilfert CM, eds. Pediatric AIDS: the challenge of HIV infection in infants, children and adolescents. Baltimore, MD: Williams and Wilkins, 1991;546–560.
10. Hooht FM, Soloway B. HIV infection: a primary care approach. Massachusetts Medical Society, 1992. Waltham: Mass.
11. Spiegel L, Mayers A. Psychosocial aspects of AIDS in children and adolescents. Pediatric Clin North Amer 1991;38:153–167.
12. Tindall B, Cooper DA, Donovan B, Penny R. Primary HIV infection: clinical and serological aspect. Infect Disease Clin North America 1988;2:329.
13. Tanner JM. Growth at adolescence with a general consideration of the effects of hereditary and environmental factors upon growth and maturation from birth to maturity. 2nd ed. Oxford: Blackwell Scientific Publications, 1962.
14. Tollerud DJ, Ildstad ST, Brown LM et al. T-cell subsets in healthy teenagers: transition to the adult phenotype. Clin Immunol Immunopathol 1990;56:88–96.
15. CDC. 1993 revised classification system for HIV infection and expanded surveillance case definition for AIDS among adolescents and adults MMWR 1992; 41(17):1–17.
16. CDC. Pneumococcal polysaccharide vaccine. MMWR 1990;39:5–22.
17. CDC. Prevention and control of influenza. MMWR 1992;41:1–17.
18. CDC. Protecting against viral hepatitis: recommendations of the Immunizations Practices Advisory Committee. MMWR 1990;39:5–22.
19. CDC. ACIP: General recommendations on immunization. MMWR 1989;38(13): 205–227.
20. Eliot AS. Counseling for HIV-infected adolescents. Focus. 1993;8(9):1–4.

SUGGESTED READINGS

Guide to adolescent HIV/AIDS program development. J Adolescent Health 1993:14: 36S–52S.
El-Sadr W, Oleske JM, Agins BD, et al. Evaluation and management of early HIV infection. Clinical Practice Guideline No.7. AHCPR Publication 94–0572. Rockville, MD: Agency for Health Care Policy and Research, Public Health Service, U.S. Department of Health and Human Services, January 1994.
Futterman D, Hein K. Medical care of IIIV infected adolescents. AIDS Clin Care 1992:4; 95–98.
Futterman D, Hein K. AIDS and HIV infection. In: Friedman S, Fisher M, Schonberg SK, eds. Comprehensive adolescent health care. Minneapolis: Quality Medical, 1992: 521–531.
Futterman D, Hein K. Medical management of HIV-infected adolescents. In: Pizzo P, Wilfert C, eds. Pediatric AIDS: the challenge of HIV infection in infants, children and adolescents. Baltimore: Williams and Wilkins, 1990:546–560.

CHAPTER 8

Precautions for the Health Care Worker

Universal Precautions

Universal precautions were developed to minimize the risk of exposure of health care workers (HCWs) to blood and body fluids of all patients. These recommendations emphasize the need for HCWs to treat all blood and other body fluids from all patients as potentially infective and to take the necessary precautions.

Infection control programs should incorporate universal precautions (i.e., appropriate use of handwashing, protective barriers, and care in the use and disposal of needles and other sharp instruments) (1–3). These precautions should be maintained in all health care settings, and proper application should assist in minimizing the risk of transmission of HIV, HBV, or HBC from patient to HCW, HCW to patient, HCW to HCW, patient to environment, environment to patient, or patient to patient. Universal blood and body-fluid precautions or universal precautions should be used in the care of all patients, especially including those in emergency care settings in which the risk of blood exposure is increased and the infection status of the patient is usually unknown. The following precautions have been recommended by the Centers for Disease Control (CDC) (1,2).

- All HCWs should routinely use appropriate barrier precautions to prevent skin and mucous membrane exposure when in contact with blood, body fluids containing visible blood, and other body fluids to which universal precautions apply. The type of protective barrier(s) should be appropriate for the procedure being performed and the type of exposure anticipated. Gloves should be worn for touching blood and body fluids, mucous membranes, or nonintact skin of all patients, for handling items or surfaces soiled with blood or body fluids, and for performing venipuncture and other vascular access procedures. Gloves should be changed after contact with each patient. Masks and protective eyewear or face shields should be worn during procedures that are likely to generate droplets of blood or other body fluids to prevent exposure of mucous membranes of the mouth, nose and eyes. Gowns or aprons should be worn during procedures that are likely to generate splashes of blood or other body fluids.

- Hands and other skin surfaces should be washed immediately and thoroughly if contaminated with blood, body fluids containing visible blood, and other body fluids to which universal precautions apply. Hands should be washed immediately after gloves are removed.

- All HCWs should take precautions to prevent injuries caused by needles, scalpels, and other sharp instruments or devices during procedures, when cleaning used instruments, during disposal of used needles, and when handling sharp instruments after procedures. To prevent needlestick injuries, needles should not be recapped, not purposely bent or broken by hand, not removed from disposable syringes, nor otherwise manipulated by hand. After use, disposable syringes and needles, scalpel blades, and other sharp items should be placed in puncture-resistant containers to be used for disposal; the puncture-resistant containers should be located as close as is practical to the use area, preferably in each patient room. Large-bore reusable needles should be placed in a puncture-resistant container for transport to the reprocessing area.

- There has been one possible case in which saliva has been implicated in HIV transmission; therefore, the need for emergency mouth-to-mouth resuscitation should be minimized. Mouthpieces, resuscitation bags, or other ventilation devices should be available for use in areas in which the need for resuscitation is predictable. Disposable airway equipment and devices should be used. Use once and dispose.

- HCWs who have exudative lesions or weeping dermatitis should refrain from all direct patient care and from handling patient care equipment until the condition resolves.

- Pregnant HCWs are not known to be at greater risk of contracting HIV infection than nonpregnant HCW; however, if a HCW develops HIV infection during or prior to pregnancy, the infant is at risk of infection resulting from perinatal transmission. Because of this risk, pregnant HCW should be especially familiar with and strictly adhere to precautions to minimize the risk of HIV transmission.

- Isolation precautions (e.g., enteric, "AFB") should be used as necessary if associated conditions, such as infectious diarrhea or tuberculosis, are diagnosed or suspected.

Body Fluids to Which Universal Precautions Apply

Universal precautions apply to the following fluids: blood and other body fluids containing visible blood, semen, vaginal secretions, cerebrospinal fluid (CSF), synovial fluid, pleural fluid, peritoneal fluid, pericardial fluid, and amniotic fluid (2,4).

Semen and vaginal secretions are strongly implicated as sources of transmission during sex. The risk of transmission in other circumstances is unknown, although HIV has been isolated from CSF, synovial, saliva, and amniotic fluid. The other fluids listed above have not been implicated in any cases of HIV infection but are included because of a theoretical possibility of transmission and a lack of data to disprove the contention (2).

Body Fluids to Which Universal Precautions Do Not Apply

There are fluids and excretions to which universal precautions do not apply, based upon epidemiological studies that have shown the risk of HIV transmission to be extremely low or negligible. These include feces, nasal secretions, sputum, sweat, tears, urine, and vomitus, unless they contain visible blood (2). However, prudent infection control procedures apply to these fluids and excretions and should be practiced where indicated.

Precautions for Other Body Fluids (2,4)

Although HIV has been isolated from breast milk, and this fluid has been implicated in perinatal transmission of HIV, there have been no cases of occupational exposure. In settings where exposure to breast milk is frequent, e.g., in breast milk banking, gloves should be worn by HCWs. Protective eye goggles should also be worn if there is the possibility of conjunctival exposure.

Universal precautions do not apply to saliva. General infection control practices that currently exist, i.e., wearing gloves for digital examination of mucous membranes and for endotracheal suctioning, and hands washed after exposure to saliva should minimize the minute risk, if any, for salivary transmission of HIV and HBV (4). Gloves do not need to be worn when feeding patients and when wiping saliva from the skin. Special precautions do exist for dentistry and are described elsewhere. During dental procedures, contamination of saliva with blood, trauma to HCWs' hands, and spattering of blood may be common.

Use of Protective Barriers (2,4)

Protective barriers reduce the risk of exposure of the health care worker's skin or mucous membranes to potentially infective materials. Examples of barriers include gloves, gowns, masks, and protective eyewear. Gloves can reduce the incidence of contamination of the hands, although they cannot prevent penetrating injuries from needlesticks or other sharp instruments. However, data have suggested that the volume of blood transmitted via needle punctures is reduced when needles pass through gloves before contacting the skin (5). Masks and protective eyewear or face shields should reduce the incidence of contamination of mucous membranes of the mouth, nose, and eyes. It is not possible to make specific barrier precaution recommendations for every possible clinical situation and individual judgment must be used. The type of protective barrier(s) should be appropriate for the procedure being performed and the type of exposure anticipated. Universal precautions are meant to supplement, rather than replace, recommendations for routine infection control, such as handwashing and the use of gloves to prevent microbial contamination of hands (4).

SELECTION OF GLOVES (2)

Medical gloves include those marketed as sterile surgical or nonsterile examination gloves made of vinyl or latex. General purpose utility ("rubber") gloves are also used in the health care setting, but are not regulated by the FDA since they are not promoted for medical use. The type of gloves selected should be appropriate for the task being performed.

- Sterile gloves should be used for procedures involving contact with normally sterile areas of the body.

- Examination gloves should be used for procedures involving contact with mucous membranes, unless otherwise indicated, and for other patient care or diagnostic procedures that do not require the use of sterile gloves.

- Gloves should be changed between patient contacts.

- Surgical or examination gloves should not be washed or disinfected for reuse. Washing with surfactants may cause "wicking" (i.e., the enhanced penetration of liquids through undetected holes in the glove). Disinfecting agents may cause deterioration.

- General purpose utility gloves (e.g., rubber household gloves) should be used for housekeeping chores involving potential blood contact and for instrument cleaning and decontamination procedures. Utility gloves may be decontaminated and reused but should be discarded if they are peeling, cracked, or discolored, or if they have punctures, tears, or other evidence of deterioration.

Precautions for Special Situations

Precautions for HCWs who perform specialized at-risk tasks, generally include the universal precautions plus an increased emphasis on the use of surgical masks, protective eyewear, and gowns. Such special tasks may involve the splashing or aerosolizing of body fluids (4). These may include invasive procedures, dialysis, laboratory, etc. and are addressed elsewhere.

REFERENCES

1. CDC. Recommendations for prevention of HIV transmission in health care settings. MMWR 1987;36(Suppl 2):1S–18S.
2. CDC. Update: Universal precautions for prevention of transmission of human immuno-deficiency virus, hepatitis B virus, and other bloodborne pathogens in health care settings. MMWR 1988;37:377–387.
3. CDC. Guidelines for the prevention of transmission of human immunodeficiency virus, hepatitis B virus, and other bloodborne pathogens in health-care settings. MMWR 1988;37:377–82, 387–388.
4. Crutcher JM, Lamm SH, Hall TA. Procedures to protect health care workers from HIV infection: category I (health care) workers. Am Ind Hyg Assoc J 1991;52:A100–A103.
5. Mast S, Gerberding JL. Factors predicting infectivity following needlestick exposure to HIV: an in vitro model. Clin Res 1991;39:58A.

Invasive Procedures

Definition of an Invasive Procedure

An invasive procedure is defined by the CDC (1) as surgical entry into tissues, cavities, or organs or repair of major traumatic injuries a) in an operating or delivery room, emergency department, or outpatient setting, including both physician and dental offices; b) cardiac catheterization and angiographic procedures; c) a vaginal or cesarean delivery or other invasive obstetric procedure during which bleeding may occur; or

d) the manipulation, cutting, or removal of any oral or perioral tissues, including tooth structure, during which bleeding occurs or the potential for bleeding exists.

Infection Control Practices for Invasive Procedures

The application of and adherence to universal blood and body-fluid precautions (e.g., appropriate use of hand washing, protective barriers, and care in the use and disposal of needles and other sharp instruments), combined with the following precautions should be the minimum precautions taken for all invasive procedures (1,2):

- All HCWs who participate in invasive procedures must routinely use appropriate barrier precautions to prevent skin and mucous-membrane contact with blood and other body fluids of all patients. Gloves and surgical masks must be worn for all invasive procedures. Double gloving has been recommended by some to decrease the risk of blood contact in a number of surgical settings. Double gloving has been associated with decreased rates of inner glove perforations (27% to 80%) (3–7), as well as reducing blood contamination of the fingers (contamination was 7% when two gloves were worn and 51% when one glove was worn) (5). Double gloving appears to offer greater protection against damage to the inner glove as well as cutaneous exposures of the hand. Protective eyewear or face shields should be worn for procedures that commonly result in the generation of droplets, splashing of blood or other body fluids, or the generation of bone chips. Gowns or aprons made of materials that provide an effective barrier should be worn during invasive procedures that are likely to result in the splashing of blood or other body fluids. For trauma cases or procedures where a high degree of gown contamination is likely, recommendations are: wearing of a reinforced gown with a plastic urologic apron, water-resistant above-the-knee boots or shoe covers, and second sleeves that can be changed when contaminated (8). All HCWs who perform or assist in vaginal or cesarean deliveries should wear gloves and gowns when handling the placenta or the infant until blood and amniotic fluid have been removed from the infant's skin, and should wear gloves during post-delivery care of the umbilical cord (1).

- If a glove is torn or a needlestick or other injury occurs, the glove should be removed and a new glove used as promptly as patient safety permits; the needle or instrument involved in the incident should also be removed from the sterile field (1). All needlestick injuries should be reported to infection control.

- HCWs who have exudative lesions or weeping dermatitis on exposed body sites should refrain from all direct patient care and from handling patient care equipment and devices used in performing invasive procedures until the condition resolves. HCWs should also comply with current guidelines for disinfection and sterilization of reusable devices used in invasive procedures (2).

- Instruments and other reusable equipment used in performing invasive procedures should be appropriately disinfected and sterilized as part of standard infection control practices (2):
- Equipment and devices that enter the patient's vascular system or other normally sterile areas of the body should be properly sterilized before being used for each patient.
- Equipment and devices that touch intact mucous membranes but do not penetrate the patient's body surfaces should be sterilized when possible or undergo high-level disinfection if they cannot be sterilized before being used for each patient.
- Equipment and devices that do not touch the patient or that only touch the intact skin of the patient need only be cleaned with a detergent or as indicated by the manufacturer.

- Compliance with universal precautions and recommendations for disinfection and sterilization of medical devices should be closely monitored in all health care settings. Institutions are mandated to provide all HCWs with appropriate inservice education regarding infection control and safety and should establish procedures for monitoring compliance with infection-control policies. It is strongly recommended that all HCWs who might be exposed to blood in an occupational setting should receive hepatitis B vaccine, preferably during their period of professional training and before any occupational exposures could occur (2).

Considerations for Exposure-prone Invasive Procedures

Exposure-prone procedures are procedures which are likely to expose the patient to an HCW's blood. Certain invasive surgical and dental procedures which have been implicated in the transmission of HBV and HIV from infected HCWs are considered exposure prone. Examples include certain oral, cardiothoracic, colorectal, and obstetric/gynecological procedures. Based on a prospective CDC study of percutaneous injuries, a greater number of injuries occurred among surgical personnel during general surgery, gynecology, orthopedic, cardiac, and trauma operative procedures (2). Observational studies have indicated invasive procedures lasting longer than 2.5 to 3.0 hours, especially when blood loss exceeds 250 to 300 ml, and during interabdominal gynecologic procedures, vaginal hysterectomies, and major vascular procedures are associated with the highest risk of injury (9–12).

Characteristics of exposure-prone procedures include digital palpation of a needle tip in a body cavity or the simultaneous presence of the HCW's fingers and a needle or other sharp instrument or object in a poorly visualized or highly confined anatomic site (2). Injuries have occurred, particularly during manipulation of the needles and at wound closure (13). Higher rates of injury have also been reported for operations requiring manipulation of instruments deep within the wound compared to those at the surface (13). To minimize the risk of HIV or HBV transmission during exposure-prone invasive procedures, CDC has recommended the following (2):

- All HCWs should follow universal precautions, including the appropriate use of handwashing, protective barriers, and care in the use and disposal of needles and other sharp instruments. HCWs who have exudative lesions or weeping dermatitis, especially on exposed areas, should refrain from all direct patient care and from handling patient care equipment and devices used in performing invasive procedures until the condition resolves. HCWs should also comply with current guidelines for disinfection and sterilization of reusable devices used in invasive procedures.

- Exposure-prone procedures should be identified by medical/surgical/dental organizations and institutions at which the procedures are performed.

- HCWs who perform exposure-prone procedures should know their HIV antibody status. HCWs who perform exposure-prone procedures and who do not have serologic evidence of immunity to HBV from vaccination or from previous infection should know their HBsAg status and, if that is positive, should also know their HBeAg status.

REFERENCES

1. CDC. Recommendations for prevention of HIV transmission in health care settings. MMWR 1987;36(Suppl 2):1S–18S.
2. CDC. Recommendations for preventing transmission of human immunodeficiency virus and hepatitis B virus to patients during exposure-prone invasive procedures. MMWR 1991;40(RR–8).
3. Bennett B, Duff P. The effect of double gloving on frequency of glove perforations. Obstet Gynecol 1991;78:1019–1022.
4. Albin MS, Bunegin L, Duke ES, et al. Anatomy of a defective barrier: sequential glove leak detection in a surgical and dental environment. Crit Care Med 1992;20:170–184.
5. Quebbeman EJ, Telford GL, Wadsworth K, et al. Double gloving: protecting surgeons from blood contamination in the operating room. Arch Surg 1992;127:213–217.
6. Matta H, Thompson AM, Rainey JB. Does wearing two pairs of gloves protect operating theater staff from skin contamination? Br Med J 1988;297:597–598.
7. Endres D, Alun-Jones T, Morrissey MS. The effectiveness of doublegloving in otolaryngology. Clinical Otolaryngology 1990;15:535–536.
8. Schiff SJ. A surgeon's risk of AIDS. J Neurosurg 1990;73:651–660.
9. Gerberding JL, Littell C, Brown A, et al. Risk of exposure of surgical personnel to patients' blood during surgery at San Francisco General Hospital. N Engl J Med 1990; 322:1788–1793.
10. Panlilio AL, Foy DR, Edwards JR, et al. Blood contacts during surgical procedures. JAMA 1991;265:1533–1537.
11. Popejoy SL, Fry DE. Blood contact and exposure in the operating room. Surg Gynecol Obstet 1991;172:480–483.
12. Quebbeman EJ, Telford GL, Hubbard S, et al. Risk of blood contamination and injury to operating room personnel. Ann Surg 1991;213:614–620.
13. Palmer JD, Rickett JW. The mechanisms and risks of surgical glove perforation. J Hosp Infect 1992;22:279–286.

Cardiopulmonary Resuscitation (CPR) Providers

Performance of mouth-to-mouth resuscitation is most likely to result in the exchange of saliva between the rescuer and the victim. In addition, there is a possibility of blood exchange if either has had breaks in the skin on or around the lips or soft tissues of the oral cavity mucosa. Although no cases of hepatitis B (HBV) or HIV infection transmitted through CPR has been documented, there is a risk of salivary transmission of other infectious diseases (e.g., herpes simplex and Neisseria meningitis) and the theoretical risk of HIV and HBV transmission during artificial ventilation (1).

A theoretical risk of HBV/HIV transmission during the performance of CPR exists; however, the probability of a rescuer becoming HIV or HBV infected is minimal (2). Transmission of HBV or HIV is more likely if the rescuer has lesions, cuts, or sores in or around the mouth or on the hands, and has contact with the victim's blood, and/or blood-containing saliva and vomitus. Appropriate precautions should be taken to prevent exposure to blood or other body fluids (See Universal Precautions); additional guidelines to prevent transmission during CPR have been published and are summarized below (1–3).

- Mechanical ventilation or barrier devices should be accessible to those who may provide CPR in the course of employment. Masks with one-way valve devices and bag-valve devices should be available and their use instructed to those expected to provide CPR. Plastic mouth and nose covers with filtered openings may also provide some protection against transfer of oral fluids and aerosols. Handkerchiefs and masks without one-way valves should not be used.

- Disposable airway equipment or resuscitation bags should be used. Disposable resuscitation equipment and devices should be used once and disposed. If reusable, equipment and devices should be thoroughly cleaned and disinfected after each use, according to manufacturer's recommendations.

- Mechanical respiratory assist devices (e.g., bag-valve masks, oxygen demand valve resuscitators) should be available to all emergency response personnel that respond or potentially respond to medical emergencies.

- Pocket mouth-to-mouth resuscitation masks designed to isolate emergency response personnel (i.e., double lumen systems) from contact with victims' blood and blood contaminated saliva, respiratory secretions, and vomitus should be provided to all personnel who provide or potentially provide emergency treatment.

- Gloves should be worn when there is contact with blood or other body fluids.

REFERENCES

1. CDC. Guidelines for prevention of transmission of human immunodeficiency virus and hepatitis B virus to health care and public safety workers. MMWR 1989;38(S–6).
2. Standards and guidelines for cardiopulmonary resuscitation (CPR) and emergency cardiac care (ECC). JAMA 1986;255:2905–3044.
3. The Emergency Cardiac Care Committee of the American Heart Association. Risk of infection during CPR training and rescue: supplemental guidelines. JAMA 1989;262:2714–2715.

Cardiopulmonary Resuscitation (CPR) Training

Cardiopulmonary resuscitation (CPR) classes require the use of mannequins for training. During training (i.e., mouth-to-mouth ventilation), the mannequin can be contaminated with saliva. There have been no reported cases of hepatitis B (HBV) or HIV infection transmitted through CPR classes, although two cases of herpes simplex have been reported to be transmitted through the use of CPR mannequins, apparently from exposure to saliva during mannequin training (1). However, investigations have suggested that the chances of transmission under these circumstances appears to be low (2–4). HIV transmission is far less likely than hepatitis B transmission. Because tissues in and around a participant's mouth can be damaged during practice on a mannequin, CPR training does pose a theoretical risk for infection. Precautions have been recommended for the conduct of CPR classes (5–7) and are summarized as follows:

Guidelines for Class Participants and Instructors

- CPR instructors or participants with breaks in the skin on the hands or in and around the mouth (e.g., cuts; burns; cracks from eczema; chapped bleeding lips) should not use a CPR mannequin.

- Persons with dermatologic lesions (e.g., cuts, burns, eczema, or chapped and bleeding lips) on hands or the oral or circumoral areas should postpone CPR training until the skin is intact.

- Persons known to be in the active stage of an acute respiratory tract infection (e.g., a cold) or who believe they have been exposed to an infectious disease should postpone CPR training.

- Persons with chronic skin problems that are not in or around the mouth (e.g., eczema on the hands) may be able to use rubber or plastic gloves while practicing on a mannequin. If persons with chronic infections (e.g., HBV) receive or give training, precautions should be taken to protect other participants from exposure. Infected individuals should be provided with a separate mannequin for training that is not used by anyone else until it has been decontaminated according to recommended end-of-class decontamination procedures. *However, persons with an acute or chronic infection that may be transmitted by blood or saliva should first check with their physician to review the circumstances and confirm whether participation in a CPR class is appropriate, before participating in CPR training. Because course participants may not know if they have been exposed to an infection, decontamination procedures of the mannequin should be strictly followed. In addition, requests for individual mannequins should be honored, within reason.*

- CPR instructors should be thoroughly familiar with hygienic concepts and the decontamination and maintenance procedures for mannequins and accessories (e.g., face shields). Mannequins should be routinely inspected for signs of physical deterioration, such as cracks or tears in plastic surfaces, which make thorough cleaning difficult or impossible. The mannequins' clothes and hair should be washed periodically (e.g., monthly or whenever visibly soiled).

Infection Control Precautions

DURING CPR CLASSES

- Participants should wash hands thoroughly with soap and water before working with the mannequin, washing as needed during training.
- Mannequin decontamination procedures should be demonstrated before participants first use mannequins.
- Minimally, the mouths and noses of mannequins should be covered with a clean cloth or towel when not being used.
- Participants should be offered protective barriers (e.g., face shields) that avoid direct mouth-to-mouth contact.
- Students should be assigned to a specific mannequin to lessen the possible contamination of several mannequins by one student.

DURING TWO-RESCUER CPR TRAINING

During the training of two-rescuer CPR, there is no opportunity to disinfect the mannequin between students when practicing the "switching procedure." Only one student should have oral contact with the mannequin; after switching, the student taking over ventilation on the mannequin should simulate ventilation instead of blowing into the mannequin to reduce the potential for disease transmission.

DURING "OBSTRUCTED AIRWAY PROCEDURE" TRAINING

This training involves the student using his or her finger to sweep foreign matter out of the mannequin's mouth. When this procedure is practiced, the finger sweep should either be simulated or done on a mannequin whose airway was decontaminated before the procedure and will be decontaminated after the procedure.

Guidelines for Cleaning and Decontaminating CPR Mannequins

BETWEEN STUDENT USES

- Each time a different student uses the mannequin in training class, the individual protective face shield (if used) should be changed.
- Hands should be washed thoroughly before working with the mannequin.
- The mannequin's face should be dried with a clean gauze pad before the mannequin is used.

- The mannequin's face, nose, and mouth should be wiped vigorously with a clean moistened cloth or pad soaked with a solution of chlorine bleach and water, or 70% alcohol (rubbing alcohol); the pad should be placed over the mannequin's mouth and nose for at least 30 seconds.

- The mannequin should be wiped dry with a clean gauze pad.

FOLLOWING A CPR CLASS

Mannequins should be washed as soon as possible following class to keep any fluids from drying on mannequin surfaces. The following steps should be taken:

- Rubber or plastic gloves should be worn.

- The mannequin should be disassembled according to manufacturer's instructions.

- All external and internal surfaces (and any reusable face shields) should be thoroughly washed with warm soapy water and brushes.

- All surfaces should be rinsed with water.

- A fresh solution of ¼ cup chlorine bleach to one gallon of tap water (approximately 1:100 ratio) should be used to wet all surfaces for 10 minutes. Surfaces should then be immediately rinsed with fresh water and all external and internal surfaces should be dried immediately with clean towels. ¼

- After removing gloves, hands should be washed with soap and water.

REFERENCES

1. Mannis MJ, Wendel RT. Transmission of herpes simplex during CPR training. Ann Opthalmol 1984;16:64–6.
2. Glaser JB, Nadler JP. Hepatitis B virus in a cardiopulmonary resuscitation training course. Arch Intern Med 1985;145:1653–1655.
3. CDC. Lack of transmission of hepatitis B to humans after oral exposure to hepatitis B surface antigen-positive saliva. MMWR 1978; 27:247–248.
4. Osterholm MT, Bravo ER, Crosson JT, et al. Lack of transmission of viral hepatitis type B after oral exposure to HBsAg-positive saliva. Br Med J 1979;2:1263–1264.
5. American Red Cross. American Red Cross HIV/AIDS Instruction Manual. January 1990;249–260.
6. The Emergency Cardiac Care Committee of the American Heart Association. Risk of infection during CPR training and rescue: supplemental guidelines. JAMA 1989; 262:2714–2715.
7. Standards and guidelines for cardiopulmonary resuscitation and emergency cardiac care. JAMA 1986;255:2905–3044.

Clinical Laboratories

HIV has been isolated from blood, semen, saliva, tears, urine, cerebrospinal fluid, amniotic fluid, breast milk, cervical secretions, and tissue of infected persons and experimentally infected nonhuman primates. In the laboratory, the skin (especially in the presence of scratches, cuts, abrasions, dermatitis, or other lesions) and mucous membranes of the eye, nose, mouth, and possibly the respiratory tract should be considered as potential pathways for entry of virus. Guidelines have been recommended for personnel working with clinical specimens, body fluids, and human tissues in the laboratory (1–4) and are summarized below.

Universal Precautions

All blood and other body fluids from all patients should be considered infective. Universal precautions are recommended for handling all human blood specimens for hematologic, microbiologic, chemical, serologic testing. Implementation of universal blood and body-fluid precautions for all patients eliminates the need for warning labels on specimens since blood and other body fluids from all patients should be considered infective.

Collection and Transport

All blood and body fluids specimens should be placed in a well-constructed container with a secure lid to prevent leaking during transport. Care should be taken when collecting each specimen to avoid contaminating either the outside of the container or the laboratory form accompanying the specimen.

Gloves

Protective gloves should be worn by all personnel engaged in activities that may involve direct contact of skin with potentially infectious specimens, cultures, or tissues (e.g., removing tops from vacuum tubes). Gloves should be carefully removed and changed when they are visibly contaminated. Personnel who have dermatitis or other lesions on the hands and who may have indirect contact with potentially infectious specimens should also wear protective gloves.

Face Protection

Masks and protective eye wear should be worn if mucous membrane contact with blood or body fluids is anticipated.

Protective Clothing

Laboratory coats, gowns, or uniforms should be worn while working with potentially infectious materials and should be removed and placed in an appropriate designated area or container (for storage, washing, decontamination or disposal) before going to nonlaboratory areas. There is no evidence that laboratory clothing poses a risk for HIV transmission; however, clothing that becomes contaminated with HIV preparations should be decontaminated before being laundered or discarded.

Hand Washing

Hand washing with soap and water immediately after infectious materials are handled and after work is completed—*even when gloves have been worn*—should be a routine practice.

Needles

Use of needles and syringes should be avoided if possible. Extreme caution should be used when handling needles and syringes to avoid autoinoculation and the generation of aerosols during use and disposal. A needle should not be bent, sheared, replaced in the sheath or guard, or removed from the syringe following use. The needle and syringe should be promptly placed in a puncture-resistant container and decontaminated, preferably by autoclaving, before discard or reuse.

Procedures

For routine procedures, such as histologic and pathologic studies or microbiologic culturing, a biological safety cabinet is not necessary. Generation of aerosols, droplets, splashes, and spills should be avoided. A biological safety cabinet should be used for all procedures that might generate aerosols or droplets and for all infected cell culture manipulations (e.g., blending, sonicating, and vigorous mixing).

Mechanical pipetting devices should be used for manipulating all liquids in the laboratory. Mouth pipetting must not be done.

Decontamination and Environmental Considerations

Laboratory work surfaces should be decontaminated with an appropriate chemical germicide after a spill of blood or other body fluids (e.g., 1:10 dilution of 5.25% sodium hypochlorite [household bleach] with water) and when work activities are completed. Prompt decontamination of spills should be a standard practice.

- Contaminated material used in laboratory tests should be decontaminated before reprocessing or placed in bags and disposed of in accordance with institutional policies for disposal of infective waste.

- Scientific equipment that has been contaminated with blood or other body fluids should be decontaminated and cleaned before being repaired in the laboratory or transported to the manufacturer.

- All laboratory glassware, disposable material, and waste material suspected or known to contain HIV should be decontaminated, preferably in an autoclave before it is washed, discarded, etc. An alternate method of disposing of solid wastes is incineration.

- Needles, sharp instruments, broken glass, and other sharp objects must be carefully handled and properly discarded. Contaminated sharps should be discarded into sharps containers that are properly labeled, puncture resistant, leak-proof and closeable to assure containment. Care must be taken to avoid spilling and splashing infected cell culture liquid and other virus-containing materials.

- Other regulated medical waste should be placed in labeled and color-coded containers/bags which are closeable, constructed to contain all contents, and leak-proof. Prior to removal, waste bags or containers should be closed to prevent spillage or protrusion of contents during handling, storage, transport or shipping. If outside contamination occurs or is likely, the waste bags/containers must be placed in a second container that is closeable, leak-proof, labeled and color-coded.

Medical Surveillance Policies

Laboratories that test specimens, do research, or produce reagents involving HIV should have a medical surveillance program in place. Written policies should be established regarding the management of laboratory exposure to HIV; such policies should address evaluation, confidentiality, counseling, and other related issues.

REFERENCES

1. CDC. Acquired immune deficiency syndrome (AIDS): precautions for clinical and laboratory staffs. MMWR 1982 5(31): 577–80.
2. CDC. 1988 agent summary statement for human immunodeficiency virus. MMWR 1988; 37(S-4);1–22.
3. CDC. Recommendations for prevention of HIV transmission in health care settings. MMWR 1987; 36(suppl 2S):1S–18S.
4. UCLA Office of Environment, Health and Safety. Exposure control plan for compliance with Cal/OSHA Bloodborne Pathogens Standard, Section 5193 Title 8, California Code of Regulations. March 1993.

The Delivery Room and the Newborn Nursery

In the labor and operating rooms, health care workers may be exposed to infected patients' secretions and blood. Recommendations have been made to reduce the risk of HIV transmission for the health care worker, woman, and the infant during delivery and in the newborn nursery (1–9):

- Universal precautions should be observed for all patients.

- Spattering of large quantities of blood and amniotic fluid are common in deliveries. During deliveries, obstetric staff should wear fluid resistant gowns and gloves. Gloves should be worn by those who may have contact with patient secretions or blood. In all deliveries and situations where a possibility for conjunctival contact exists, goggles (eye protection) should be worn. Double gloving in the operating room has been reported to reduce the instances of skin exposure to blood after glove tears (10–13). Overshoes should be worn.

- Gloves should be used when handling the placenta or neonate until blood and secretions have been removed from the neonate's skin.

Hands should be washed immediately after gloves are removed and/or when skin surfaces are contaminated with blood. Hands should also be washed after contact with patients.

- Mechanical suction (e.g., wall or bulb suction) devices should always be used to clear the airways of newborns to lessen the risk of potential exposure to secretions of neonates; mouth suction should be avoided. Keeping pressure under 140 mm Hg will avoid damage to the neonate's oropharynx (9). If mechanical suction is not available, and mouth suction is unavoidable, double-trap isolated mouth suction is recommended.

- To limit the possibilities of intrapartum transmission, the direct contact between the vaginal secretions of an infected mother and newborn should be avoided whenever possible. Scalp blood sampling for fetal pH evaluation and scalp electrodes for monitoring the child could enhance inoculation of HIV virus into the neonate. Therefore external monitoring or auscultation should be done whenever possible. In addition, lines should not be placed into the neonate until secretions are removed.

- Most infants of known seropositive mothers may be cared for in the normal nursery and do not require isolation in a private room or cubicle, unless there are specific indications (e.g., congenital syphilis, sepsis). Gloves should be worn for contact with or potential exposure to blood or potentially infected secretions and excretions. Gloves are not required for prevention of HIV transmission while changing diapers in usual circumstances. Hand washing after changing diapers is always required to reduce the transmission of pathogens.

- Physical care of the neonates (e.g., skin, umbilical cord, eye care, administration of vitamin K) should be conducted using universal precautions. The neonate should be considered potentially uninfected, and the infant's exposure to maternal blood and body fluids on the skin as well as to other contaminating microorganisms should be minimized. Before performing a heel stick or administering a vitamin K injection, the infant's skin should first be cleaned with soap, water, and then alcohol to prevent possible contamination of the skin surface with body fluids that could be transmitted through the puncture site. Antimicrobial agents (e.g., triple dye, mupirocin) should be applied to the cord using sterile gloves. The infant should be protected from skin abrasions that can lead to infection (e.g., use mittens for infant's nails or file nails with disposable emery boards).

REFERENCES

1. Special medical reports. ACOG issues report on HIV infection in women. Am Fam Physician 1992;46:579–585.
2. Hudson CN. Nosocomial infection and infection control procedure. Bailliere's Clin Obst and Gyn 1992;6:137–148.
3. Landesman SH. Human immunodeficiency virus infection in women: an overview. Seminars in Perinatology 1989;13:2–6.

4. Minkoff HL, Feinkind L. Management of pregnancies of HIV-infected women. Clin Obstet and Gyn 1989;32:467–476.
5. Gerberding JL. University of California-San Francisco Task Force on AIDS. Recommended infection control policies for patients with human immunodeficiency virus infection: an update. N Engl J Med 1986;315:1562–1564.
6. Special Medical Reports. AAP issues statement on perinatal HIV infection. Am Fam Physician 1989;39:390–393.
7. Feinkind L, Minkoff H. HIV in pregnancy. Clin Perinatol 1988;15: 189–202.
8. Bastin N, Tamayo OW, Tinkle MB, et al. HIV disease and pregnancy part 3. Postpartum care of the HIV-positive woman and her newborn. JOGN 1992;21:105–111.
9. ACOG technical bulletin. Human immunodeficiency virus infections. Int J Gynecol Obstet 1993;41:307–319
10. Gerberding JL, Littell C, Tarkington A, et al. Risk of exposure of surgical personnel to patients' blood during surgery at San Francisco General Hospital. N Engl J Med 1990; 322:1788–1793.
11. Bennett B, Duff P. The effect of double gloving on frequency of glove perforations. Obstet Gynecol 1991;78:1019–1022.
12. Quebbeman EJ, Telford GL, Wadsworth K, et al. Double gloving: protecting surgeons from blood contamination in the operating room. Arch Surg 1992;127:213–217.
13. Endres D, Alun-Jones T, Morrissey MS. The effectiveness of double-gloving in otolaryngology. Clinical Otolaryngology 1990;15:535–536.

Dialysis Treatment

The CDC has made the following recommendations regarding precautions for dialysis treatment (1–2):

- Universal blood and body-fluid precautions should be practiced when dialyzing *all* patients

- Patients with end-stage renal disease undergoing maintenance dialysis and who are HIV infected can be dialyzed in hospital-based or free-standing dialysis units using conventional infection-control precautions.

- Strategies for disinfecting the dialysis fluid pathways of the hemodialysis machine are targeted to control bacterial contamination; this usually consists of using a solution of 500–750 parts per million (ppm) of sodium hypochlorite (household bleach) for 30–40 minutes or 1.5%–2.0% formaldehyde, overnight. There are also several commercial chemical germicides formulated to disinfect dialysis machines available. Current protocols or procedures are sufficient and do not need to be changed when dialyzing an HIV-infected patient.

- HIV-infected patients can be dialyzed by either hemodialysis or peritoneal dialysis and do not need to be isolated from other patients. The type of dialysis treatment (i.e., hemodialysis or peritoneal dialysis) should be based on the needs of the patient. The dialyzer may be discarded after each use.

- Centers that reuse dialyzers (i.e., a specific single-use dialyzer is issued to a specific patient, removed, cleaned, disinfected, and reused several times on the same patient only) may include HIV-infected patients in the dialyzer reuse program. An individual dialyzer must never be used on more than one patient.

REFERENCES

1. CDC. Recommendations for prevention of HIV transmission in health care settings. MMWR 1987;36(2S):3S–18S.
2. CDC. Recommendations for providing dialysis treatment to patients infected with human T-lymphotropic virus type III/lymphadenopathy-associated virus. MMWR 1986; 35:376–383.

Nuclear Medicine Procedures

Nuclear medicine procedures most often involve the intravenous injection or oral ingestion of radioactive materials (i.e., radiopharmaceuticals or radiotracers) for diagnostic or therapeutic purposes. HIV transmission can occur during medical procedures involving withdrawal and reinjection of blood or blood products (e.g., nuclear medicine procedures).

There have been three patients reported (two in the U.S.) who inadvertently received intravenous injections of blood or other material from patients infected with HIV undergoing nuclear medicine procedures (1–3). In two patients, the inadvertent injection of blood and blood components from an HIV-infected patient occurred (fresh whole blood in one patient (1) and white blood cells (WBCs) in a second patient [2,3]). In the first incident, a used syringe containing the blood was mistaken for another syringe containing red blood cells that had been treated (i.e., labeled) with radioactive isotope (1). In the second incident, the WBCs had been labeled with a radioactive isotope and were injected in the wrong patient when hospital personnel failed to correctly match the identification number of the recipient with that of the specimen of white blood cells. Both patients developed HIV infection despite being promptly administered zidovudine postexposure. In a third incident, a syringe that had been used during a diagnostic procedure on an HIV-infected patient was inadvertently reused; this resulted in an injection of residual material into the patient. Follow-up HIV test results were not available (3). These errors in administration of radiotracers to patients resulted from errors in the identification of the patient and/or materials to be injected. Two of the incidents also involved improper handling and disposal of used syringes.

Administration errors in nuclear medicine are relatively rare. An estimated 38 million nuclear medicine procedures were performed in 21 states in the United States, where nuclear medicine has been regulated by the U.S. Nuclear Regulatory Commission (NRC), during 1981–1990 (4). During this time, there was an overall error rate (defined by the NRC as misadministrations) of approximately 1 per 10,000 diagnostic procedures performed. Most of these reported misadministrations involved an incorrect dosage of radiopharmaceutical and/or errors in patient identification.

The CDC has developed recommendations for institutions or clinics in which nuclear medicine procedures are performed (5). Careful adherence to these procedures should minimize the risk of patient or health care worker exposure to bloodborne pathogens during nuclear medicine procedures.

- All health-care providers, including those who perform nuclear medicine procedures, should receive proper training and routine in-service education on proper infection control procedures.

- Written infection control policies and procedures specific for nuclear medicine should be promulgated, made accessible, and disseminated in departments where nuclear medicine procedures are performed. Policies should outline procedures to follow in the event of a potential emergency (e.g., administration error).

- All doses and syringes should be examined for identification and radioassayed (i.e., radiation level checked) before injection.

- All syringes should be labeled with appropriate identifying information, including the patient's name and the pharmaceutical. A unique identification number should also be used.

- Consideration should be given to implementing a system to be used when administering biologic products (e.g., labeled cells) that is similar to the system used for administering blood. Such a system requires that two persons be present to cross-check all labeling of product to be injected, the prescription, and patient identification.

- Contaminated and used syringes should be disposed of safely and appropriately. Disposal containers for syringes should be located as close as practical to the location of syringe use.

- All procedures should be documented; documentation should include at a minimum, the date, name, and amount of radiopharmaceutical, and route of administration. The name or identifying information of the person administering the dose and the exact time of administration should ideally be recorded either in the patient's or the departmental record.

- An administration error (e.g., administration involving the wrong patient or radiopharmaceutical) should be immediately reported to supervisory personnel and/or the physician in charge. Recommendations for the management of persons after a blood exposure in a health care setting should be followed. All administration errors and narrowly avoided errors in administration should be carefully evaluated to determine whether additional precautions are necessary to prevent similar potential administration errors.

- Misadministrations, as defined by the NRC or by the equivalent state agency in states that have an agreement with the NRC to carry out similar functions, should be reported to the appropriate agency as required by law. Incidents involving possible transmission of bloodborne pathogens to patients in the health care setting should also be reported through local and state health departments to CDC's HIV Infections Branch: (404) 639–1547.

REFERENCES

1. Lange JMA, Boucher CAB, Hollack CEM, et al. Failure of zidovudine prophylaxis after accidental exposure to HIV-1. N Engl J Med 1990; 19:1375–1377.
2. Davis LE, Hjelle BL, Miller VE, et al. Early viral brain invasion in iatrogenic human immunodeficiency virus infection. Neurology 1992;42:1736–1739.
3. Polder JA, Bell DM, Rutherford GW, et al. Investigation of inadvertent injection of HIV-contaminated material during nuclear medicine procedures (Abst). Vol 1. VII International Conference on AIDS. Florence, Italy, June 16–21, 1991:379.
4. United States Nuclear Regulatory Commission. Office for Analysis and Evaluation of Operational Data, 1990 annual report. Washington, DC: US Nuclear Regulatory Commission, 1991.
5. CDC. HIV exposure during nuclear medicine procedures. MMWR 1992;41:575–578.

Ophthalmology/Optometry

Although HIV has been isolated in tears, it is rare. There has been no documented cases of HIV transmission from exposure to tears, and occupational exposure to tears is unlikely to pose a risk of HIV. Adherence to universal precautions and the following precautions have been recommended to prevent HIV transmission (1):

- Professionals performing eye examinations or other procedures involving contact with tears should wash their hands immediately after a procedure and between patients. Although hand washing alone should be sufficient, disposable gloves may be worn when practical and convenient. The use of gloves is advisable when there are cuts, scratches, or dermatologic lesions on the hands. Protective measures, such as masks, goggles, or gowns are not indicated.

- Instruments that come into direct contact with external surfaces of the eye should be wiped clean and then disinfected by a 5 to 10 minute exposure to: a fresh solution of 3% hydrogen peroxide; a $\frac{1}{10}$ dilution of sodium hypochlorite (common household bleach); 70% ethanol, or 70% isopropanol. The instrument should be thoroughly rinsed in tap water and dried before being used again.

- Contact lenses used in trial fittings should be disinfected after each fitting in one of the following regimens:
  - Hard lenses can be disinfected with a commercially available hydrogen peroxide contact lens disinfecting system that is currently approved for soft contact lenses. Most trial hard lenses can also be treated with the standard heat disinfection regimen used for soft lenses, i.e., 70–80°C (172–176°F) for 10 minutes. To determine which lenses can be safely treated, suppliers of hard lenses should be consulted.
  - Rigid gas permeable (RGP) trial fitting lenses can be disinfected using the above hydrogen peroxide disinfection system. If heat-disinfected, RGP lenses may warp.
  - Soft trial fitting lenses can be disinfected using the same hydrogen peroxide system; some soft lenses have also been approved for heat disinfection.

REFERENCES

1. CDC. Recommendations for possible transmission of Human T-lymphotropic virus type III/lymphadenopathy-associated virus from tears. MMWR 1985;34(34):533–534.

Phlebotomy

The likelihood of contaminating the hands with blood containing bloodborne pathogens during phlebotomy depends on several factors:

- the skill and technique of the health care worker (HCW)

- the frequency with which the HCW performs the procedure (other factors being equal, the cumulative risk of blood exposure is higher for an HCW who performs more procedures)

- whether the procedure occurs in a routine or emergency situation (blood contact may be more likely in an emergency situation)

- the prevalence of infection with bloodborne pathogens in the patient population

Common reasons for accidental parenteral exposures include: resheathing needles and the disassembling of intravenous tubing devices, vacuum tube phlebotomy sets, and reusable cartridge injection syringes (1). The likelihood of infection after skin exposure to HIV-infected blood will depend on the virus strain and concentration, the duration of contact, and the presence of skin lesions on the hands of the HCW. Studies have shown the rate of HIV infection following accidental needlestick injuries to be about 0.4% (4 per 1000) per needlestick or other parenteral exposure (2–4), small but not insignificant. Strict adherence to universal precautions should be practiced; all blood should be considered potentially infective for bloodborne pathogens and precautions taken in handling and disposal of sharp instruments. Gloves can reduce the incidence of blood contamination of hands during phlebotomy (drawing blood samples). Although gloves cannot prevent penetrating injuries caused by needles or sharp instruments, it has been reported that when needles pass through gloves before contacting the skin, the volume of blood transmitted via needle punctures is reduced (5). Institutions that decide that routine gloving for all phlebotomies is not necessary should periodically reevaluate their policies. Gloves should always be available to health care workers who wish to use them for phlebotomy.

The CDC recommends the following guidelines concerning glove wear and phlebotomy procedures (6). Gloves should be used:

- when the HCW has cuts, scratches, or other breaks in his/her skin.

- in situations where the HCW judges that hand contamination with blood may occur (e.g., performing phlebotomy on an uncooperative patient).

- when performing finger and/or heel sticks on infants and children.

- for persons receiving training in phlebotomy.

REFERENCES

1. Jagger J, Hunt EH, Brand-Elnaggar J, Pearson RD. Rates of needlestick injury caused by various devices in a university hospital. N Engl J Med 1988;319:284–288.
2. Tokars JI, Marcus R, Culver DH, et al. Surveillance of HIV infection and zidovudine use among health care workers after occupational exposure to HIV-infected blood. Ann Intern Med 1993;188:913–919.
3. Henderson DK, Gerberding JL. Prophylactic zidovudine after occupational exposure to the human immunodeficiency virus: an interim analysis. J Infect Dis 1989;160: 321–327.
4. Becker CE, Cone JE, Gerberding J. Occupational infection with human immunodeficiency virus (HIV): risks and risk reduction. Ann Intern Med 1989;110:653–656.
5. Mast S, Gerberding JL. Factors predicting infectivity following needlestick exposure to HIV: an in vitro model. Clin Res 1991;39:58A.
6. CDC. Update: universal precautions for prevention of transmission of human immunodeficiency virus, hepatitis B virus, and other bloodborne pathogens in health care settings. MMWR 1988;37 (24)377–387.

Donor Exclusion Criteria

Blood Donors

The following donors are at risk for HIV infection and should refrain from donating blood (1–4):

- Persons with clinical or laboratory evidence of HIV infection.

- Men who have had sex with men (even once) since 1977.

- Persons with a history of injection drug use or needle sharing (past or present).

- Person with sexual contact with individuals (male or female) of countries with a high prevalence of AIDS cases.

- Persons with hemophilia or related clotting disorders who have received clotting factor concentrates.

- Men or women who have had sex in exchange for money or drugs since 1977.

- Persons who have had sexual contact in the last 12 months with any individual meeting the above description or who is at risk for HIV/AIDS.

Persons who should be deferred for 12 months include:

- Persons who have received a transfusion of whole blood, blood components, or a clotting factor concentrate in the preceding 12-month period.

- Persons who have had, or have been treated for, syphilis or gonorrhea in the preceding 12-month period, or who have had a reactive test for syphilis in the absence of a negative confirmatory test in the preceding 12-month period.

- Persons who have been raped in the preceding 12-month period.

Tissue and Organ Donation

Persons meeting any of the following exclusion criteria (5) regardless of their HIV antibody test results, should be excluded from organ or tissue donation unless the risk to the recipient of not performing the transplant is deemed to be greater than the risk of HIV transmission and disease (i.e., emergent, life-threatening illness requiring transplantation when no other organs/tissues are available and no life-saving therapies exist). In such cases, informed consent regarding the possibility of HIV transmission should be obtained from the recipient (5).

Behavior/History Exclusionary Criteria

- Men who have had sex with another man in the preceding 5 years.
- Persons who report nonmedical intravenous, intramuscular, and subcutaneous injection of drugs in the preceding 5 years.
- Persons with hemophilia or related clotting disorders who have received human-derived clotting factor concentrates.
- Men and women who have engaged in sex in exchange for money or drugs in the preceding 5 years.
- Persons who have had sex since 1977 with any person described in the four items above or with a person known or suspected to have HIV infection.
- Persons who have been exposed in the preceding 12 months to known or suspected HIV-infected blood through percutaneous inoculation or through contact with an open wound, nonintact skin, or mucous membrane.
- Inmates of correctional systems. (This exclusion is to address issues such as difficulties with informed consent and increased prevalence of HIV in this population.)

Exclusionary Criteria for Pediatric Donors

Infants and children meeting any of the exclusionary criteria listed above for adults should not be accepted as donors.

Children born to mothers with HIV infection or mothers who meet the behavioral or laboratory exclusionary criteria for adult donors (regardless of HIV status) should not be accepted as donors unless HIV infection can be definitely excluded in the child as follows:

- Children over 18 months of age who are born to mothers with or at risk for HIV infection, who have not been breast fed within the past 12 months, and whose HIV antibody tests, physical exam, and review of medical records do not indicate evidence of HIV infection can be accepted as donors.
- Infants and children under 18 months of age (born to mothers with or at risk for HIV infection) or those who have breast fed within the

past 12 months should not be accepted as donors regardless of their HIV test results.

Laboratory and Other Medical Exclusionary Criteria

Persons who cannot be tested for HIV infection because of refusal, inadequate blood samples (e.g., hemodilution that could result in false-negative tests), or any other reasons.

Persons with a repeatedly reactive screening assay for HIV-1 or HIV-2 antibody regardless of the results of the supplemental assays.

Persons whose history, medical records, autopsy reports or physical examination reveal other evidence of HIV infection or high-risk behavior such as: a diagnosis of AIDS, male-to-male sexual contact, sexually transmitted diseases, or needle tracks or other signs of drug abuse, unexplained weight loss, night sweats, blue or purple spots typical of Kaposi's sarcoma on or under the skin or mucous membranes, unexplained swollen lymph nodes (lymphadenopathy) lasting more than one month, unexplained fevers greater than 100.5°F (38.6°C) for more than 10 days, unexplained persistent cough and shortness of breath, unexplained persistent diarrhea and the presence of any opportunistic infections.

REFERENCES

1. Patijn GA, Strengers PFW, Persijn HM. Prevention of transmission of HIV by organ and tissue transplantation. Transplant International 1993;6:165–172.
2. Petersen LR, Simonds RJ, Koistinen J. HIV transmission through blood, tissues, and organs. AIDS 1993;7 (suppl 1):S99–S107.
3. Centers for Biologics and Research. Revised recommendations for prevention of human immunodeficiency virus (HIV) transmission by blood and blood products. Section I, parts A and B. Letter to registered establishments. Bethesda, MD: Food and Drug Administration, 1990.
4. WHO expert committee on biological standardization. Requirements for the collection, processing, and quality control of blood, blood components and plasma derivatives. 39th Report 1989;104–107.
5. CDC. Guidelines for prevention of transmission of HIV through transplantation of human tissue and organs. MMWR 1994;43:(RR-8).

Blood and Plasma Donors—Testing and Counseling

Blood donations in the United States have been screened for antibody to HIV type 1 (HIV-1) since March 1985 and type 2 (HIV-2) since June 1992. Only 1 in 450,000 to 1 in 660,000 donations per year are estimated to be infectious for HIV (i.e., 18–27 donations) but not detected by currently available screening tests (1). During the acute period of HIV infection, tests for p24 antigen can detect HIV infection earlier than antibody tests. p24 antigen, the core structural protein of HIV, is detectable 2–3 weeks after HIV infection during the initial burst of virus replication associated with high levels of viremia (2,3). During this time, the blood of infected persons is highly infectious and p24 antigen tests are usually positive (4–6). On average, p24 antigen is detected an estimated

6 days before antibody tests become positive (4,7). When antibodies to HIV become detectable, p24 antigen is often no longer detectable because of antigen-antibody complexing and viral clearance (4–6). As recent studies indicated that p24 screening reduced the infectious window period (7) and implementation of p24 antigen testing became logistically feasible for mass screening, the Food and Drug Administration (FDA) in August 1995 recommended that all donated blood and plasma also be screened for HIV-1 p24 antigen to further reduce the risk of HIV transmission via the receipt of donated blood and blood products (8). Donor screening for p24 antigen is expected to detect 4–6 infectious donations that would be otherwise undetected by other screening tests. Donor screening for p24 antigen is considered by the FDA as an interim measure pending the availability of technology that would further reduce the risk for HIV transmission from blood donated during the infectious window period (9).

Public Health Service (PHS) guidelines regarding interpreting p24-antigen assay results and counseling and follow-up of blood and plasma donors who have positive or indeterminate antigen-test results (9) are summarized below. These guidelines may be modified as additional information concerning antigen testing under mass screening conditions is collected and analyzed.

p24-Antigen Testing in Sites Other Than Blood Banks

Screening for the p24 antigen in settings other than blood banks (e.g., HIV counseling and testing sites, physicians' offices) is not recommended (9). Few additional infected persons would be identified by routine antigen testing in such settings because the estimated average time from detection of p24 antigen to detection of antibody is only 6 days. Moreover, recently infected persons may not have detectable levels of p24 antigen. Circumstances where antigen testing may be appropriate may be in the diagnosis of perinatally exposed children (10,11). Diagnostic testing for HIV infection in children 18 months and older and adults should routinely consist of an HIV-1 antibody screening test and Western blot or immunofluorescent assay to confirm antibodies to HIV-1.

p24-Antigen Testing and Interpretation of Test Results

The p24-antigen screening assay is an enzyme immunosorbent assay (EIA) performed on serum or plasma. If the first screening test is nonreactive, the test result is reported as negative. If the first screening test is reactive, the p24 EIA is repeated in duplicate. If both duplicate tests are nonreactive, the test result is reported as negative. If at least one of the repeated p24 EIA tests is reactive, the test is considered repeatedly reactive; the donation is then discarded, the donor is deferred from donating blood, and a more specific assay (the neutralization assay) is performed to verify the presence of p24 antigen. The neutralization-assay should be performed before informing donors of test results. Donations collected within 3 months of a repeatedly reactive p24-antigen test (re-

Table 8.1.
Definitions Used in Interpreting HIV-1 p24 Antigen Tests*

p24-Antigen Test Result	Definition
Initially reactive	Initial p24 EIA test is reactive
Repeatedly reactive	One or both duplicate p24 EIA retests is (are) reactive
Negative	Initial p24 EIA test is not reactive or initial p24 EIA test is reactive and both duplicate p24 EIA retests are not reactive
Positive	p24 EIA test is repeatedly reactive and the neutralization test is positive (i.e., neutralizing).
Indeterminate	p24 EIA test is repeatedly reactive and the neutralization test is either negative (i.e., non-neutralizing) or invalid.

*According to FDA recommendations
From CDC. US Public Health Service Guidelines for testing and counseling blood and plasma donors for human immunodeficiency virus type 1 antigen. MMWR 1996;45:RR-2.

gardless of neutralization-assay results) should be quarantined pending results of repeat donor testing for antigen and antibody to HIV (8). Definitions used in interpreting HIV-1 p24-antigen tests according to FDA recommendations are shown in Table 8.1.

Donor Counseling, Follow-up, and Deferral

Blood and plasma donors in the blood-bank setting who have positive or indeterminate HIV-test results should be counseled regarding information for follow-up diagnostic evaluation and available services (e.g., medical, preventive, and psychosocial). Infected persons should also be counseled in preventing transmission to others. Counseling should be done in accordance with PHS standards and guidelines (12,13). The PHS guidelines for notification and counseling of donors who have repeatedly reactive antigen-test results are based on available data. As additional information concerning antigen testing under mass screening conditions are collected and analyzed, these guidelines may be modified.

POSITIVE p24-ANTIGEN-TEST RESULTS

Donors who have negative HIV-antibody test results but whose screening-test results for HIV antigen are repeatedly reactive and neutralization-assay results are positive, should be counseled that they are probably infected with HIV (Figure 8.1). Donors who have such test results should be notified promptly after a positive neutralization test. Prompt notification is important because persons who are newly infected with HIV and do not have antibodies often have high viral titers and may be at high risk for transmitting HIV infection (2). According to FDA recommendations, donors who repeatedly have reactive and neutralizing p24-antigen tests should be advised that they are permanently deferred from future blood and plasma donation.

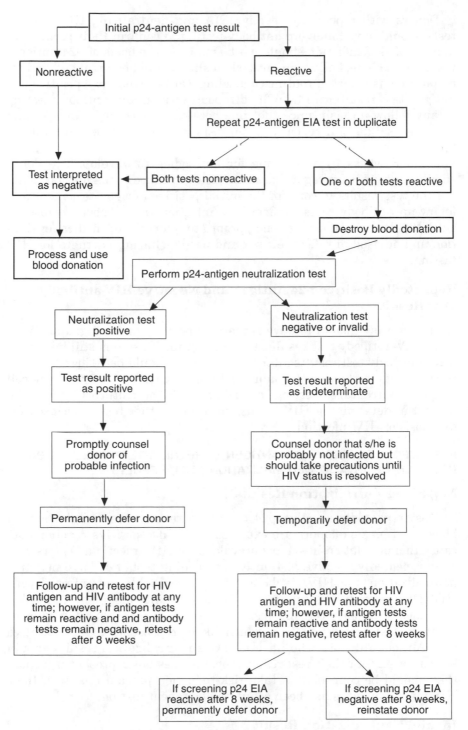

Figure 8.1.   Algorithm for p24-antigen testing, donor notification and counseling, unit disposition, follow-up evaluation, and deferral of blood and plasma donors who have negative HIV-antibody-test results. Source: CDC. US Public Health Service Guidelines for testing and counseling blood and plasma donors for human immunodeficiency virus type 1 antigen. MMWR 1996;45(RR-2).

Donors with repeatedly reactive EIA and neutralizing HIV antigen tests should have follow-up antibody testing to confirm their results; diagnosis of HIV infection should not be made on the basis of p24 antigen-test results alone. Follow-up antibody testing should be arranged and incorporated as a part of routine counseling. Donors who have positive p24 antigen test results can be offered repeat antigen and antibody testing at any follow-up visit since the time between detection of antigen and antibody is 6 days. If repeat antigen tests remain reactive and antibody tests remain negative, antibody testing should be repeated after a minimum of 8 weeks to allow time for antibodies to develop. The donor should be counseled regarding strategies to reduce transmission pending the test results to confirm the initial positive antigen-test results. If follow-up antibody tests confirm HIV infection (i.e., a positive test result), the donor should be given appropriate referrals for medical evaluation and advised to refer their sex and needle-sharing partners for HIV testing.

Repeatedly Positive p24 Antigen and Negative HIV-antibody Test Results

Although it is unusual to have repeatedly positive p24 antigen and negative HIV-antibody test results, this may occur. If persons still have negative antibody test results after 8 weeks, they should be referred for further medical evaluation, including determining CD4+ T-lymphocyte cell count or percentage. Testing for HIV by PCR or culture also may be helpful in determining HIV status; however, neither test is licensed for diagnosis of HIV infection.

REPEATEDLY REACTIVE p24 ANTIGEN SCREENING-TEST RESULTS BUT NEGATIVE OR INVALID NEUTRALIZATION TEST RESULTS

Negative Neutralization Results

Most repeatedly reactive p24 antigen screening test results among blood- and plasma-donors are expected to be false-positive reactions because this population has a low prevalence of HIV infection. Donors who have repeatedly reactive p24 antigen screening tests but have negative neutralization and HIV antibody tests are probably not infected with HIV. Donors with negative neutralization results should be counseled that their antigen screening tests were reactive but that their supplementary tests were negative, which likely represents a false-positive test. Although donors who have negative neutralization results should be reassured that their test result probably does not represent infection, they should be counseled to take risk-reduction precautions until their HIV-infection status has been confirmed by repeat testing.

Invalid Neutralization Result

An invalid neutralization result occurs when a sample is repeatedly reactive in the initial screening test, but in the neutralized assay, the neutralized sample and unneutralized control both fall below the cutoff level. Invalid results most frequently occur when a screening test value is low or borderline reactive in an uninfected person; however, invalid results can also occur when a screening test value is low or borderline reactive in an infected person (14). Sample deterioration or antigen-antibody complex formation during storage may also result in an invalid result. Donors with invalid neutralization results should be counseled that their antigen screening tests were reactive but their supplementary tests were inconclusive due to the invalid neutralization-test results. Although these donors are probably not infected with HIV, infection cannot be excluded. These donors should be counseled to take HIV risk-reduction precautions until their HIV-infection status is confirmed. Retesting a fresh sample may clarify the result.

Excluding HIV Infection

Donors with repeatedly reactive p24 antigen screening test results, invalid or negative neutralization test results, and negative HIV-antibody test results can be offered repeat antigen and antibody test at any follow-up visit to exclude HIV infection. A negative antigen and antibody test result at the time of follow-up indicates that the donor was not infected with HIV at the time of the initial test.

For donor reentry purposes, or for diagnostic purposes among donors with continued reactive antigen screening-test results and negative antibody test results, repeat antigen and antibody testing should be performed a minimum of 8 weeks after the initial repeatedly reactive antigen screening test. Antigen and antibody tests that are negative and are performed 8 weeks or longer after the initial repeatedly reactive antigen screening tests indicate the donor was uninfected at the time of the initial test. If the donor's screening antigen test remains repeatedly reactive, neutralization tests remains negative, and HIV-antibody tests are negative or indeterminate, the donor is probably uninfected with HIV. Further follow-up and additional testing (i.e., CD4+ T-lymphocyte cell count or percentage, HIV PCR, and culture) may clarify the infection status, although these tests are not licensed for diagnosis of HIV infection.

Donors whose blood samples are repeatedly reactive by the p24 screening test and negative or invalid on the neutralization test should be temporarily deferred from donating blood or plasma for a minimum of 8 weeks according to FDA recommendations. These donors should be counseled that donor deferral does not indicate infection, because the screening test on which the deferral was based was most likely a false-positive result. Such donors are not infected and can be reinstated as blood or plasma donors if their samples test negative by screening tests for p24 antigen and HIV antibodies after 8 weeks. However, if, after 8 weeks, their samples test repeatedly reactive on the screening test for HIV antigen or are positive for antibody, the donors should be permanently deferred from donating blood or plasma—regardless of HIV-antigen neutralization-test results.

REFERENCES

1. Lackritz EM, Satten GA, Aberle-Grasse J, et al. Estimated risk of transmission of the human immunodeficiency virus by screened blood in the United States. N Engl J Med 1995;333:1721–1725.
2. Daar ES, Moudgil T, Meyer RD, Hoo DD. Transient high levels of viremia in patients with primary human immunodeficiency virus type 1 infection. N Engl J Med 1991; 324:961–964.
3. Clark SJ, Saag MS, Decker WE, et al. High titers of cytopathic virus in plasma of patient with symptomatic primary HIV-1 infection. N Engl J Med 1991;324:954–960.
4. Gallarda JL, Henard DR, Liu D, et al. Early detection of antibody to human immunodeficiency virus type 1 by using an antigen conjugate immunoassay correlates with the presence of immunoglobulin M antibody. J Clin Microbiol 1992;30:2379–2384.
5. Zaaijer HL, v Exel-Oehlers P, Kraaijeveld T, Altena E, Lelie PN. Early detection of antibodies to HIV-1 by third generation assays. Lancet 1992;340:770–772.
6. Henrard DR, Phillips J, Windsor I, et al. Detect of human immunodeficiency virus type 1 p24 antigen and plasma RNA: relevance to indeterminate serologic tests. Transfusion 1994;34:376–380.
7. Busch MP, Lee LLJ, Satten GA, et al. Time course of detection of viral and serologic markers preceding human immunodeficiency virus type 1 seroconversion: implications for screening of blood and tissue donors. Transfusion 1995;35:91–97.
8. Food and Drug Administration, Center for Biologics Evaluation and Research. Recommendations for donor screening with a licensed test for HIV-1 antigen [memorandum]. August 8, 1995.
9. CDC. US Public Health Service Guidelines for testing and counseling blood and plasma donors for human immunodeficiency virus type 1 antigen. MMWR 1996; 45:RR-2.
10. Early HIV Infection Guideline Panel. Clinical Practice Guideline Number 7: evaluation and management of early HIV infection. Washington DC: US Department of Health and Human Services, Public Health Service, Agency for Health Care Policy and Research, 1994; DHHS publication no. (AHCPR)94-0572.
11. CDC. 1994 Revised classification system for human immunodeficiency virus infection in children less than 13 years of age. MMWR 1994;43(RR-12).
12. CDC. HIV counseling, testing, and referral standards and guidelines. Atlanta, GA: US Department of Health and Human Services, Public Health Service, CDC, 1994.
13. CDC. Recommendations for HIV testing services for inpatients and outpatients in acute-care hospital settings; and technical guidance on HIV counseling. MMWR 1993;42(RR-2).
14. Alter HJ, Epstein JS, Swenson SG, et al. Prevalence of human immunodeficiency virus type 1 p24 antigen in US blood donors—an assessment of the efficacy of testing in donor screening. N Engl J Med 1990;323:1312–1317.

Artificial Insemination and Semen Banking

Most transmission of HIV by artificial insemination occurred before 1985, prior to the implementation of donor screening recommendations. HIV has been transmitted through unprocessed infected semen during artificial insemination (1,2). There are procedures to process semen which attempt to eliminate HIV from semen, however there is a lack of evidence that any procedure can completely eliminate HIV from semen (3). A possible case of HIV transmission to a woman was reported following artificial insemination with processed semen from her HIV-infected husband (3). For the insemination, fresh ejaculate was processed in an attempt to remove virus from spermatozoa to avoid HIV transmission. Although sexual transmission from the woman's husband cannot be excluded, it is also possible that the insemination procedures may have resulted in transmission; infected leukocytes of free virus may not have been removed from the husband's semen with the procedures used (3). However, there have also been recent reports of conception without HIV transmission following insemination with processed semen from HIV-infected males (4). One investigation of 29 discordant couples (HIV-negative female, HIV-positive male) undergoing intrauterine insemination with processed semen from the husband, reported none of the 29 women seroconverted after 6 months. Processed semen was used, with the absence of HIV antibodies confirmed before each insemination. None of the 10 babies to date was seropositive, the oldest child being 3 years old (4). Further evidence of the safety of this approach is needed. Currently, the Centers for Disease Control (CDC) recommends against insemination with semen from HIV-infected men (3,5). The following compiles the recommendations regarding artificial insemination, donor screening, and semen banking (5–8).

Recipients

- All couples initiating an infertility workup should be offered HIV testing. HIV testing should be encouraged for all recipients of donated eggs, sperm, and/or embryos.

Donors

- All prospective donors should be screened for behavioral risk factors for HIV infection; donors who present with behavioral risk factors for HIV infection should be excluded. The donor should also have a physical examination as close as possible prior to donation; special attention should be given to physical signs of HIV disease and injecting drug use. The exam should be properly documented by a licensed physician at the time of donation, showing no obvious evidence of HIV infection. Prospective donors should be tested for antibody to HIV-1 and HIV-2 at the time the semen is collected. The American Fertility Society also encourages donors and their partners to be required to undergo HIV testing (7).

- Prospective donors should be provided information about HIV transmission modes and risks for HIV infection, emphasizing that HIV can be transmitted via semen. They should be told a negative HIV antibody test does not guarantee that the donor is free of HIV infection because of the "window period" (i.e., donation prior to seroconversion). A donor having behavioral risk factors which place him at risk for HIV infection will be excluded. Direct questions regarding high-risk behavior should be asked.

- Semen donors found to be acceptable after careful screening should sign a consent statement indicating that they have reviewed and understand the provided information regarding the spread of HIV and have agreed not to donate should they be at potential risk for spreading HIV. The statement should also indicate that the prospective donor understands that HIV testing will be performed as part of the donor screening process, and if found to be HIV-positive, the donor will be notified.

- The donor should be tested for HIV-1 and HIV-2 at the time the semen is collected. The semen collection from donors should be placed in frozen quarantine for a minimum of six months. Before frozen semen is used for artificial insemination, the donor should be retested for HIV-1 and HIV-2 antibodies six months after the donation. Responsible medical personnel must be certain that the blood samples are from the same donor, and the donor's identity must be assured. Frozen semen should be used only if both tests are negative for HIV antibody (3,6).

- The use of fresh semen for artificial insemination is not recommended. Because HIV can be transmitted before the donor has become seropositive (during the "window" period), the potential for HIV transmission by fresh semen cannot be entirely eliminated. The use of fresh semen for donor insemination may be appropriate when the semen is from a donor in a mutually monogamous marriage/relationship with the recipient (3). Otherwise, semen from all other donors should be frozen and quarantined for a minimum of 6 months, and the semen used only if both HIV tests are negative (i.e., at the time of collection, and 6 months later).

- Because there is no evidence that any procedure can reliably eliminate HIV from semen, the CDC currently recommends against insemination with semen from HIV-infected men.

Additional Guidelines for Oocyte Donation

Additional guidelines for oocyte donation have also been made by the American Fertility Society (7):

The screening of oocyte donors are similar to the procedure for sperm donors (e.g., medical history and serological testing for HIV 1 and 2). Donors presenting with risk factors for HIV infection should be disqualified. All donors (of eggs and/or embryo) and their partners should be required to undergo HIV testing. All recipients are also encouraged to be tested for HIV.

Currently there is no practical procedure to freeze and quarantine oocytes prior to use. Embryo freezing is practical, but embryo cryopreservation and quarantining is not currently required. Couples entering an oocyte donor program should be given the following choices:

- Whether they wish to assume the low risk of acquiring HIV by using fresh embryos.

- Whether they wish to have the donated oocytes fertilized, the embryos frozen and quarantined, the donor recalled and retested for HIV six months later, and only if negative to then undergo embryo transfer.

REFERENCES

1. Stewart GJ, Tyler JPP, Cunningham AL, et al. Transmission of human T-cell lymphotropic virus type III (HTLV-III) by artificial insemination by donor. Lancet 1985;2:581–584.
2. Chaisson MA, Stoneburner RL, Joseph SC. Human immunodeficiency virus transmission through artificial insemination. J AIDS 1990;3:69–72.

3. CDC. HIV infection and artificial insemination with processed semen. MMWR 1990;39:249,255.
4. Semprini AE, et al. Insemination of HIV-negative women with processed semen of HIV-positive partners. Lancet 1992;340:1317–1319.
5. CDC. Semen banking, organ and tissue transplantation and HIV antibody testing. MMWR 1988;37:57–63.
6. CDC. Guidelines for prevention of transmission of HIV through transplantation of human tissue and organs. MMWR 1994;43(RR-8).
7. American Fertility Society. Guidelines for gamete donation:1993. Fertility & Sterility 1993;59 (Suppl 1):1S–9S.
8. American Medical Association. Prevention and control of acquired immunodeficiency syndrome: an interim report (board of trustees report). JAMA 1987;258:2097–2103.

Organ and Tissue Transplantation

Routine HIV antibody screening for all potential blood, organ, and tissue donors in the United States was implemented in 1985 (1). Since then, several cases have been reported via transplanted organ and tissue allografts. In these cases, a false negative screening test result was caused either by multiple blood transfusions during the donor procedure resulting in the dilution of the anti-HIV antibody titer below a detectable level, or HIV infection during the time period between infection and antibody seroconversion (window period) (2–4), a period ranging from four to 26 weeks from the primary infection to seroconversion (5). In another case, an organ from an HIV-infected donor was transplanted under emergency conditions before HIV/antibody test results were known (6).

Transmission of HIV has been reported through transplantation of kidney, liver, heart, pancreas, bone, and possibly skin (2–4,7). Viable HIV has been recovered from bone, marrow, and tendons of patients with AIDS suggesting HIV transmission via grafting of these tissues could take place (2). Although the exact risk of HIV transmission from various tissues is not known, some organs and tissues present higher risk of HIV transmission than others (3). The risk of transmission from an HIV-infected donor appears to be almost 100% (8). Fresh-frozen, unprocessed bone appears to carry a high risk of transmission, particularly if marrow elements and adherent tissue are not removed (8). Relatively avascular solid tissue, some of which is also processed using techniques that might inactivate HIV appears to be of lower risk for HIV transmission. Although HIV has been isolated from tears, corneal tissue, aqueous humor, and conjunctival epithelium, there have been no reported cases of HIV transmission from corneal transplants from HIV-infected donors (9,10). HIV transmission via corneal graft transplantation is currently considered unlikely (2).

The use of routine HIV screening cannot rule out HIV with a false-negative test result during the window period or by the dilution of anti-HIV antibody titer caused by a massive transfusion. Preventing HIV transmission from organ/tissue donors must consider several factors: differences between living, brain-dead, and cadaveric donors with respect to donor screening; time constraints due to tissue/organ viability that may preclude performing certain screening procedures; differences in the risk of transmission of HIV from various organs and tissues; differences in systems for procuring and distributing organs and tissues; how screening practices may affect the limited availability of organs and tissues; and the benefit of the transplant to the recipient (8). Published CDC recommendations for the prevention of HIV transmission through transplantation of human tissue and organs with respect to donor screening and testing, and quarantine of tissue from living donors are summarized below (8):

Recommendations for Organ and Tissue Transplantation (8)

DONOR SCREENING

- All prospective donors, or next-of-kin or significant life partners accompanying brain-dead or cadaveric donors, and parents of potential pediatric donors should be informed of the general nature of the donor evaluation process, including a review of medical and behavioral history, physical examination, and blood tests to exclude infectious agents that might be transmitted by organ or tissue transplant.

- Prospective living donors or next of kin or significant life partners accompanying brain-dead or cadaveric donors should be informed about modes of transmission and risk factors for HIV infection, emphasizing that HIV can be transmitted via transplanted organs and tissues. They should be told that a negative test for HIV antibody does not guarantee that the donor is free of HIV infection because of the rare situation of donation after infection but before seroconversion. Therefore, organs and tissue must not be transplanted from persons who may have engaged in activities that placed them at increased risk for HIV infection. This information should be presented in simple language to ensure that the donor, next of kin, or significant life partner understands what is considered high-risk behavior and the importance of excluding persons who have engaged in this behavior. Persons soliciting the donation should not place undue pressure to donate on potential living donors and those persons providing permission for potential brain-dead or cadaveric donors who might otherwise decline to donate or give permission because of high-risk behavior.

- To ascertain risk factors, all prospective living donors should be interviewed in a confidential and sensitive manner by a health care professional competent to elicit information about behaviors that place persons at risk for HIV infection.

- For potential pediatric donors for whom maternal transmission of HIV is a consideration, the mother and, if possible, the father should be interviewed about behaviors that may have placed the parents at risk of acquiring HIV infection that could have been transmitted to their child.

- For brain-dead or cadaveric donors, except where retrieval occurs by legal authorization, the next of kin or significant life partner should be interviewed in a confidential and sensitive manner by a health care professional regarding potential HIV risk factors in the donor. If available, other family members, friends, and sex partners may also need to be interviewed. When consent for removal of organs/tissue is required, at minimum, the person signing the consent should be interviewed. Other possible sources of information about behavioral risk factors may include the hospital, police, and coroner's records, if available. When an interview is not performed, as allowed by legal authorization, the transplant surgeon should be fully informed that the donation was accepted, even though a direct interview with the next of kin or significant life partner was not performed.

- If available, the medical records, including autopsy reports of all donors, should be reviewed for signs and symptoms associated with HIV infection and for evidence of high-risk behavior (e.g., male-to-male sexual contact, acquisition of sexually transmitted diseases, exchange of sex for money or drugs, injecting-drug use, or birth to a mother either at risk or infected with HIV.)

- All prospective donors of organs and solid tissue should undergo a thorough physical examination as close as possible prior to donation, with special attention to physical signs of HIV disease and injecting drug use. The extent of the physical exam should be determined by the responsible medical officers according to the context of organ/tissue donation. Human milk banks should obtain a release from the primary health care provider certifying that the prospective donor is in good health and does not constitute a risk to potential recipients.

- Prospective living organ, tissue and milk donors found to be acceptable for donation after careful screening should sign a consent statement indicating that they have reviewed and understand the information provided regarding the spread of HIV and have agreed not to donate should they be a potential risk for transmitting HIV. The consent should also indicate that the prospective donor understands that he/she will be tested for HIV as part of the donor screening process and will be notified of positive results as specified by any existing state statutes, regulations, or guidelines.

- For acceptable brain-dead or cadaveric donors, it should be documented that a careful attempt has been made to eliminate high risk individuals through available information (e.g., interview of family members or significant life partners, physical examination, review of medical records, autopsy findings, and any other records that might provide information about high-risk behavior or possible HIV infection). For either donor type, this statement should be included in the transplant records or record of the procuring agency (e.g., as part of a general checklist or donor evaluation form covering all important aspects of the donor evaluation). All records generated by the interview should be kept confidential.

DONOR TESTING (8)

- For all prospective donors, a blood sample should be obtained before any transfusions were administered (during the current hospitalization) and as close to the time of retrieval of tissue as possible. Bone marrow donors must provide blood samples far enough in advance of marrow harvest to permit the tests to be performed and the results reported before the recipient's preparative regimen (marrow ablatement) is begun. Samples should be tested for antibodies to both HIV-1 and HIV-2 using FDA-licensed tests (separate or a combination test). All antibody screening tests should be performed by enzyme immunoassay (EIA) unless the recipient's or donor's condition dictates a more rapid donor evaluation.

- Transfusions and infusion of other fluids to the prospective donor might produce false-negative results because of hemodilution. Efforts should be made to perform HIV antibody testing on the most recent pretransfusion specimen for which the identity and quality can be assured. Specimens should not be drawn immediately downstream from an intravenous site to prevent significant dilution with intravenous fluids.

- Posttransfusion specimens may be considered for testing after all efforts to obtain a pretransfusion/infusion sample have been exhausted and posttransfusion samples have been assessed for evidence of significant dilution. The suitability of posttransfusion/infusion samples must consider: a) the volume of the material transfused as a percentage of the patient's total blood volume, and b) the amount of time between the last transfusion/infusion and the collection of the sample to be tested. An exchange of one total blood volume will reduce the concentration of an intravascular substance such as IgG to 35% of initial levels if there is no replacement from the extravascular space. More than 50% of total body IgG is extravascular, and reequilibration to normal levels of IgG should be nearly complete within 24 hours of a total blood volume exchange of albumin (11).

- The HIV p24-antigen assay may identify the rare HIV-infected, but antibody-negative donor. However, because of the limited number of studies examining the utility of this assay for screening organ/tissue donors, there is currently no definitive recommendation on the use of this test by the U.S. Public Health Service. Institutions choosing to use the HIV-1 p24-antigen assay should be aware that in populations with low prevalence (e.g., organ/tissue donors), a large percentage of persons who test repeatedly positive (without confirmation with the neutralization assay) will be false positives. Potential problems concerning decreased specificity when using the assay to test postmortem samples should also be considered.

- The testing algorithm for HIV antibody assays should be performed as described in the package insert with an initial test and if reactive, a retest on the same specimen. In extreme cases when time constraints of some situations do not allow the delay caused by repeat testing by EIA as described in the package insert, the sample should be set up in triplicate in the initial EIA. A repeatedly reactive result (positive screening test) is defined as reactivity above the test cutoff in two or more of the three assays. When testing by EIA is impractical, a more rapid licensed test should be performed in triplicate. Testing by the conventional algorithm should be performed as early as possible, even if it follows the procurement and/or transplant of the organs or tissues.

- A repeatedly reactive screening assay should be confirmed with more specific supplemental tests. An aliquot of the original sample should be analyzed using the following more specific tests. For repeatedly reactive HIV-1 antibody EIAs, an HIV-1 Western blot or immunofluorescence assay should be performed. For repeatedly reactive HIV-1 antigen assays (if performed), a neutralization procedure must be performed. For HIV-2, no licensed supplemental test is available; however, consideration may be given to the use of research assays such as Western blot, immunofluorescence, radioimmune precipitation, and synthetic peptide made with the state or local health department. For repeatedly positive combination HIV-1 and -2 assays, the published testing algorithm should be followed. When the results of any of these supplemental tests are unclear, use of research assays should be considered.

- HIV test results for organ and tissue donors should be handled in a confidential manner, consistent with general medical practices and applicable federal and state statutes, regulations, and guidelines.

- A prospective donor found to be HIV positive during the screening process should be notified, but not before the repeatedly reactive screening assay has been confirmed by using the following, more specific supplemental tests. An aliquot of the original sample should be analyzed by using more specific and appropriate tests (e.g., Western blot, immunofluorescence assay, neutralization procedure, radioimmune precipitation). For repeatedly reactive HIV-1 antibody EIAs, an HIV-1 Western blot or immunofluorescence assay should be performed. For repeatedly reactive HIV-1 antigen assays (if performed), a neutralization procedure must be performed. For HIV-2 antigen assays (if performed), a neutralization procedure must be performed. For HIV-2, no licensed supplemental test is available; however, consideration may be given to the use of research assays such as Western blot, immunofluorescence, radioimmune precipitation, and synthetic peptide-based EIA. Arrangements for HIV-2 supplemental testing may need to be made with either the state or local health department. For repeatedly reactive combination HIV-1 and HIV-2 assays, the CDC testing algorithm should be followed (8). When the results of any supplemental tests are unclear, the use of research assays should be considered.

- Notification of prospective living donors who are found to be HIV-infected through the screening process and the spouse or known sex partners of cadaveric or brain-dead donors should be done in accordance with state law. All notifications should be handled in a manner congruent with current recommendations regarding counseling, testing, and partner notification. Before notification of these persons, transplant and procurement organizations should consult with their state health department concerning local notification policies. Notification should be done in a confidential and sensitive manner by staff competent in counseling and discussing positive HIV results and their implications. If such staff is unavailable in the organ/tissue procurement organization, arrangements should be made with other organizations (e.g., health departments, clinics) to provide appropriate notification.

- When possible, one or more of the following samples from the donor should be saved for at least 5 years after the expiration date of the tissue: dried-blood spots, a frozen buffy coat, spleen cells, lymph node cells, bone marrow, and an aliquot of serum. These samples can be examined in the event that subsequent information indicates that the donor may have donated during the period after infection and prior to antigen/antibody seroconversion.

- Confirmed positive HIV test results in a prospective organ/tissue donor should be reported to state health agencies if required by state law or regulation.

DONOR EXCLUSION CRITERIA

The exclusion criteria for donors of organ and tissue are similar to those used in the blood bank setting. Criteria include behavioral risks, laboratory, and medical indications of being at risk to HIV (See Donor Exclusion Criteria). Persons meeting any of the criteria should be excluded from organ or tissue donation unless the risk to the recipient from not performing the transplant is judged to be greater than the risk of HIV transmission. In such a case, informed consent regarding the possibility of HIV transmission should be obtained from the recipient.

INACTIVATION OF HIV IN ORGANS/TISSUES

Currently there are no definitive recommendations regarding inactivation of HIV in organs and tissues (8). Until more is known, it is prudent to process bone and bone fragments and carefully evacuate all marrow components from whole bone whenever feasible.

QUARANTINE

When possible, tissue donations from living donors should be placed in frozen quarantine and the donor retested for HIV-1 and HIV-2 antibodies after six months. The quarantined material should be released only if the follow-up test results are obtained and are negative.

TESTING AND REPORTING OF RECIPIENTS

Transplant recipients and their health providers should be aware of the small but potential risk of infections, including HIV, from transplanted organs and tissues. The recipient's informed consent to the transplant should include acknowledgment of the risks, including HIV transmission.

Until the risk for IIIV transmission from screened donors has been clarified, recipients of solid organs should be advised routinely to be tested for HIV immediately prior to and at three months following the transplantation. Testing of recipients should be voluntary and done with the consent of the recipient. Recipients of tissues other than solid organs do not require routine testing for HIV following receipt of the tissue from appropriately screened donors. Results of HIV testing of organ recipients should be collected and analyzed by the Scientific Registry for Transplant Recipients. This recommendatioin for recipient testing may be omitted in a revision of these guidelines should data show no benefit for recipient testing.

If a transplant recipient is determined to have HIV infection, consistent with state law, the transplant center or healthcare provider should immediately notify the state health department and the organization from which the tissue was obtained. HIV infection in a recipient of a solid organ should also be reported to the Scientific Registry for Transplant Recipients.

TRACKING OF RECIPIENTS AND TISSUES AND RECALL OF STORED TISSUES

Also important is the timely detection, reporting, and tracking of potentially infected organs, tissues and recipents, and recall of stored tissues from donors found to be infected after donation. This involves having a graft identification system and accurate record keeping that allows the tracking of organs and tissues from the donor source to the recipient institution and vice versa. Once an organ/recipient is found to be infected with HIV, the organ/tissue collection center should be notified and, in collaboration with the state and local health department and with assistance from the CDC, they should determine whether the donor was HIV infected. This is done by determining the HIV-infection status of other recipients of organs/tissues and by laboratory testing of stored donor material. If evidence suggests HIV infection, all other recipients of that donor's tissue and organs should be notified through their transplanting physician and informed of the liklihood of HIV exposure and the recipients should be advised to undergo HIV testing. All stored organ/tissues from a donor found to be HIV-infected should be retrieved and quarantined immediately and either used only for research purposes or destroyed, except when the transplantation of an indispensable organ/tissue is necessary to save the patient's life

A summary of strategies to prevent HIV transmission through organ and tissue transplantation (8,12) is shown in Table 8.2.

Table 8.2.

Strategies to Prevent HIV Transmission from Organ and Tissue Transplantation

Donor screening for HIV-associated risk behaviors
Physical examination of donor for signs of HIV disease and injecting drug use
Laboratory testing of donors for antibody to HIV-1 and HIV-2
Quarantine of tissues from living donors and repeat donor testing after 6 months
Inactivation or removal of HIV in allograft processing
Timely detection, reporting, and tracking of potentially infected organs, tissues, and recipients
Recall of stored tissue from donors found to be infected after organ and tissue donation

REFERENCES

1. CDC. Testing donors of organs, tissues, and semen for antibody to human T-lymphotropic virus type III/lymphadenopathy-associated virus. MMWR 1985;34:294.
2. Patijn GA, Strengers PFW, Persijn HM. Prevention of transmission of HIV by organ and tissue transplantation. Transplant International 1993;6:165–172.
3. Simonds RJ, Holmberg SD, Hurwitz RL, et al. Transmission of human immunodeficiency virus type 1 from a seronegative organ and tissue donor. N Engl J Med 1992; 326(11):726–732.
4. CDC. Human immunodeficiency virus infection transmitted from an organ donor screened for HIV antibody—North Carolina. MMWR 1987;36:306–308.
5. Horsburgh CR Jr, Ou CY, Jason J, et al. Duration of human immunodeficiency virus infection before detection of antibody. Lancet 1989;2:637–640.
6. Samuel D, Castaing D, Adam R, et al. Fatal acute HIV infection with aplastic anaemia, transmitted by liver graft. Lancet 1988;1:1221–1222.
7. CDC. Transmission of HIV through bone transplantation: case report and public health recommendations. MMWR 1988;37(39):597–599.
8. CDC. Guidelines for prevention of transmission of HIV through transplantation of human tissue and organs. MMWR 1994;43:(RR-8).
9. Prepose JS, MacRae S. Quinn TC, Ward JW. Serologic markers after transplantation of corneas from donors infected with human immunodeficiency virus. Am J Opthalmol 1987; 103:798–801.
10. Schwarz A, Hoffman F. L'age-Stehr J, et al. Human immunodeficiency virus transmission by organ donation: outcome in cornea and kidney recipients. Transplantation 1987;44:21–24.
11. Chopek M, McCullough J. Protein and biochemical changes during plasma exchange. In Berkman EM, Umlas J, eds. Therapeutic hemapheresis. Washington DC: American Association of Blood Banks, 1980:13–52.
12. Petersen LR, Simonds RJ, Koistinen J. HIV transmission through blood, tissues, and organs. AIDS 1993;7(Suppl 1):S99–S107.

The Dental Setting

Dental patients and dental health care workers (DHCWs) may be exposed to a variety of microorganisms via blood or oral or respiratory secretions. These microorganisms may include cytomegalovirus, hepatitis B virus (HBV), hepatitis C virus (HCV), herpes simplex virus types 1 and 2, HIV, *Mycobacterium tuberculosis,* staphylococci, streptococci, and other viruses and bacteria, specifically those that infect the upper respiratory tract. Infections may be transmitted in the dental operatory through several routes, including direct contact with blood, oral fluids, or other secretions; indirect contact with contaminated instruments, operatory equipment, or environmental surfaces; or contact with airborne contaminants present in either droplet spatter or aerosols of oral and respiratory fluids. Universal precautions must be observed routinely in the care of all dental patients (1). To reduce the risk of disease transmission among DHCWs and their patients, the Centers for Disease Control (CDC) has recommended infection control practices (2) applicable to all settings where dental treatment is provided. These recommended practices are summarized below and should be observed in addition to the practices and procedures for worker protection required by the Occupational Safety and Health Administration (OSHA) final rule on Occupational Exposure to Bloodborne Pathogens (29 CFR 1910.1030) (3) published in the Federal Register, Dec 6, 1991.

Vaccines for Dental Health Care Workers

Although HBV infection is uncommon among adults in the U.S. (1%–2%), serologic surveys have indicated that 10%–30% of health care workers or DHCWs show evidence of past or present HBV infection (4,5). The OSHA bloodborne pathogens final rule requires that employers make hepatitis B vaccinations available without cost to their employees who may be exposed blood or other infectious materials. The CDC also recommends that all workers, including DHCWs, who might be exposed to blood or blood-contaminated substances in an occupational setting be vaccinated for HBV. DHCWs also are at risk for exposure to and possible transmission of other vaccine-preventable diseases; therefore, vaccination against influenza, measles, mumps, rubella, and tetanus may be appropriate for DHCWs.

Protective Attire and Barrier Techniques

GLOVES

To protect personnel and patients in dental care settings, medical gloves (latex or vinyl) must always be worn by DHCWs when there is a potential for contacting blood, blood-contaminated saliva, or mucous membranes. Nonsterile gloves are appropriate for examinations and other nonsurgical procedures; sterile gloves should be used for surgical procedures. Before the treatment of each patient, DHCWs should wash their hands and put on new gloves. Following the treatment of each patient or before leaving the dental operatory, DHCWs should remove and discard gloves, then wash their hands. DHCWs always should wash their hands and reglove between patients. Surgical or examination gloves should not be washed before use; nor should they be washed, disinfected, or sterilized for reuse. Washing of gloves may cause "wicking" (penetration of liquids through undetected holes in the gloves) and is not recommended. Deterioration of gloves may be caused by disinfecting agents, oils, certain oil-based lotions, and heat treatments, such as autoclaving.

FACE PROTECTION

When splashing or spattering of blood or other body fluids is likely (which is common in dentistry), chin length plastic face shields or surgical masks and protective eyewear should be worn. When using a mask, it should be changed between patients or during patient treatment if it becomes wet or moist. Face shields or protective eyewear should be washed with an appropriate cleaning agent and, when visibly soiled, disinfected between patients.

PROTECTIVE CLOTHING

Protective clothing (e.g., reusable or disposable gowns, laboratory coats, or uniforms) should be worn when clothing is likely to be soiled with blood or other body fluids. Reusable protective clothing should be washed, using a normal laundry cycle, according to the instructions of detergent and machine manufacturers. Protective clothing should be changed at least daily or as soon as it becomes visibly soiled. Protective garments and devices (including gloves, masks, and eye and face protection) should be removed before personnel leave the areas of the dental office used for laboratory or patient care activities.

SURFACE COVERS

Impervious, backed paper, aluminum foil, or plastic covers should be used to protect items and surfaces (e.g., light handles, x-ray unit heads) that may become contaminated by blood saliva during use and that are difficult or impossible to clean and disinfect. Between patients, the coverings should be removed (while DHCWs are gloved), discarded, and replaced (after ungloving and washing of hands) with clean material.

OTHER

Appropriate use of rubber dams, high-velocity air evacuation, and proper patient positioning should minimize the formation of droplets, spatter, and aerosols during patient treatment. In addition, splash shields should be used in the dental laboratory.

Handwashing and Hand Care

DHCWs should wash their hands before and after treating each patient (i.e., before glove placement and after glove removal) and after barehanded touching of inanimate objects likely to be contaminated by blood, saliva, or respiratory secretions. Hands should be washed after removal of gloves because gloves may become perforated during use, and DHCWs hands may become contaminated through contact with patient material. Soap and water will remove transient microorganisms acquired directly or indirectly from patient contact; for many routine dental procedures (e.g., examinations and nonsurgical techniques), handwashing with plain soap is adequate. For surgical procedures, an antimicrobial surgical handscrub should be used.

When gloves are torn, cut, or punctured, they should be removed as soon as patient safety permits. DHCWs then should wash their hands thoroughly and reglove to complete the dental procedure. DHCWs who have exudative lesions or weeping dermatitis, particularly on the hands, should refrain from all direct patient care and from handling dental patient care equipment until the condition resolves.

Sharp Instruments and Needles

Sharp items (e.g., needles, scalpel blades, wires) contaminated with patient blood and saliva should be considered as potentially infective and handled with care to prevent injuries. Used needles should never be recapped or otherwise manipulated utilizing both hands or any other technique that involves directing the point of a needle toward any part of the body. Either a one-handed "scoop" technique or a mechanical device designed for holding the needle sheath should be employed. Used disposable syringes and needles, scalpel blades, and other sharp items should be placed in appropriate puncture-resistant containers located as close as is practical to the area in which the items were used. Bending or breaking of needles before disposal requires unnecessary manipulation and is therefore not recommended.

Before attempting to remove needles from nondisposable aspirating syringes, DHCWs should recap them to prevent injuries. Either of the two acceptable techniques may be used. For procedures involving multiple injections with a single needle, the unsheathed needle should be placed in a location where it will not become contaminated or contribute to unintentional needlesticks between injections. If the decision is made to recap a needle between injections, a one-handed "scoop" technique or a mechanical device designed to hold the needle sheath is recommended.

Sterilization or Disinfection of Dental Instruments

Dental instruments are classified into three categories: critical, semicritical or noncritical, depending on their risk of transmitting infection and the need to sterilize them between uses. Every dental practice should classify instruments as follows:

CRITICAL

Surgical and other instruments used to penetrate soft tissue or bone are classified as critical and should be sterilized after each use. These devices include forceps, scalpels, bone chisels, scalers, and burs.

SEMICRITICAL

Semicritical instruments do not penetrate soft tissues or bone but contact oral tissues (e.g., mirrors and amalgam condensers). These devices should be sterilized after each use. If sterilization is not feasible because the instrument will be damaged by heat, the instrument should receive, at the minimum, high-level disinfection.

NONCRITICAL

Instruments or medical devices such as external components of x-ray heads that come into contact only with intact skin are classified as noncritical. Because these noncritical surfaces have a relatively low risk of transmitting infection, they may be reprocessed between patients with intermediate-level or low-level disinfection (See Cleaning and Disinfection of Dental Unit) or detergent and water washing, depending on the nature of the surface and the degree and nature of the contamination.

Sterilization or Disinfection Methods of Dental Instruments

Before sterilization or high-level disinfection, instruments should be cleaned thoroughly to remove debris. Persons involved in cleaning and reprocessing instruments should wear heavy-duty (reusable utility) gloves to lessen the risk of hand injuries. After using instruments, they should be placed into a container of water or disinfectant/detergent as soon as possible to prevent drying of patient material and make cleaning easier and more efficient. Cleaning may be accomplished by thorough scrubbing with soap and water or a detergent solution, or with a mechanical device (e.g., ultrasonic cleaner). The use of covered ultrasonic cleaners, when possible, is recommended to increase efficiency of cleaning and to reduce handling of sharp instruments.

All critical and semicritical dental instruments that are heat stable should be sterilized routinely between uses by steam under pressure (autoclaving), dry heat, or chemical vapor, following sterilizer and instrument manufacturers' instructions. Critical and semicritical instruments that will not be immediately used should be packaged before sterilization.

Proper functioning of sterilization cycles should be verified by the periodic use (at least weekly) of biologic indicators (i.e., spore tests). Heat-sensitive chemical indicators (e.g., those that change color after exposure to heat) alone do not ensure adequacy of a sterilization cycle but may be used on the outside of each pack to identify packs that have been processed through the heating cycle. A simple and inexpensive method to confirm heat penetration to all instruments during each cycle is using a chemical indicator inside and in the center of either a load of unwrapped instruments or in each multiple instrument pack; this procedure is recommended for use in all dental practices. Instructions provided by the manufacturers of medical/dental instruments and sterilization devices should be followed closely.

In all dental and other health care settings, indications for the use of liquid chemical germicides to sterilize instruments (i.e., cold sterilization) are limited. For heat-sensitive instruments, this procedure may require up to 10 hours of exposure to a liquid chemical agent registered with the U.S. Environmental Protection Agency (EPA) as a "sterilant/disinfectant." This sterilization process should be followed by aseptic rinsing with sterile water and drying. If the instrument is not used immediately, it should be placed in a sterile container.

EPA-registered "sterilant/disinfectant" chemicals are used to attain high-level disinfection of heat-sensitive semicritical medical and dental instruments. The product manufacturers' directions regarding appropriate concentration and exposure time should be closely followed. The EPA classification of the liquid chemical agent (i.e., "sterilant/disinfectant") will be shown on the chemical label. Liquid chemical agents that are less potent than the "sterilant/disinfectant" category are not appropriate for reprocessing critical or semicritical dental instruments.

Cleaning and Disinfection of Dental Unit and Environmental Surfaces

After treatment of each patient and at the completion of daily work activities, countertops and dental unit surfaces that may have become contaminated with patient material should be cleaned with a disposable towel, using an appropriate cleaning agent and water as necessary. Surfaces then should be disinfected with a suitable chemical germicide.

A chemical germicide registered with the EPA as a "hospital disinfectant" and labeled for "tuberculocidal" (i.e., mycobactericidal) activity is recommended for disinfecting surfaces that have been soiled with patient material. These intermediate level disinfectants include phenolics, iodophors, and chlorine-containing compounds. Because mycobacteria are among the most resistant groups of microorganisms, germicides effective against mycobacteria should be effective against many other bacterial and viral pathogens. A fresh solution of sodium hypochlorite (household bleach) prepared daily is an inexpensive and effective intermediate-level germicide. A solution concentration ranging from 500 to 800 ppm of chlorine (a 1:100 dilution of bleach and tap water, or $\frac{1}{4}$ cup of bleach to 1 gallon of water) is effective on environmental surfaces that have been cleaned of visible contamination. Caution should be exercised, since chlorine solutions are corrosive to metals, especially aluminum.

Low level disinfectants—EPA-registered "hospital disinfectants" that are not labeled for "tuberculocidal" activity (e.g., quaternary ammonium compounds) are appropriate for general housekeeping purposes such as cleaning floors, walls, and other housekeeping surfaces. Intermediate and low-level disinfectants are not recommended for reprocessing critical or semicritical dental instruments.

Disinfection and the Dental Laboratory

Lab materials and other items that have been used in the mouth (e.g., impressions, bite registrations, fixed and removable prostheses, orthodontic appliances) should be cleaned and disinfected before being manipulated in the laboratory, whether an onsite or remote location. These items also should be cleaned and disinfected after being manipulated in the dental laboratory and before placement in the patient's mouth. Because of the increasing variety of dental materials used intraorally, DHCWs are advised to consult with manufacturers regarding the stability of specific materials relative to disinfection procedures. A chemical germicide having at least an intermediate level of activity (i.e., "tuberculocidal hospital disinfectant") is appropriate for such disinfection. Communication between dental office and dental laboratory personnel regarding the handling and decontamination of supplies and materials is important.

Handpieces and Antiretraction Valves

Routine between-patient use of a heating process capable of sterilization (i.e., autoclaving, dry heat, or heat/chemical vapor) is recommended for all high-speed dental handpieces, low-speed handpiece components used intraorally, and reusable prophylaxis angles. Manufacturers' instructions for cleaning, lubrication, and sterilization procedures should be followed closely to ensure both the effectiveness of the sterilization process and the longevity of these instruments. According to manufacturers, virtually all high-speed and low-speed handpieces in production today are heat tolerant, and most heat-sensitive models manufactured earlier can be retrofitted with heat-stable components.

Internal surfaces of high-speed handpieces, low-speed handpiece components, and prophylaxis angles may become contaminated with patient material during use. This retained patient material then may be expelled intraorally during subsequent uses. Restricted physical access—particularly to internal surfaces of these instruments—limits cleaning and disinfection or sterilization with liquid chemical germicides. Surface disinfection by wiping or soaking in liquid chemical germicides is not an acceptable method for reprocessing high-speed handpieces, low-speed handpiece components used intraorally, or reusable prophylaxis angles.

Because retraction valves in dental unit water lines may cause aspiration of patient material back into the handpiece and water lines, antiretraction valves (one-way flow check valves) should be installed to prevent fluid aspiration and to reduce the risk of transfer of potentially infective material. Routine maintenance of antiretraction valves is necessary to ensure effectiveness; the dental unit manufacturer should be consulted to establish and appropriate maintenance routine.

High-speed handpieces should be run to discharge water and air for a minimum of 20–30 seconds after use on each patient. This procedure is intended to aid in physically flushing out patient material that may have entered the turbine and air or water lines. Use of an enclosed container or high-velocity evacuation should be considered to minimize the spread of spay, spatter, and aerosols generated during discharge procedures. Additionally, there is evidence that overnight or weekend microbial accumulation in water lines can be reduced substantially by removing the handpiece and allowing water lines to run and to discharge water for several minutes at the beginning of each clinic day. Sterile saline or sterile water should be used as a coolant/irrigator when surgical procedures involving the cutting of bone are performed.

Intraoral Devices Attached to Air and Water Lines of Dental Units

Other reusable intraoral instruments attached to, but removable from, the dental unit air or water lines—such as ultrasonic scaler tips and component parts and air/water syringe tips—should be cleaned and sterilized after treatment of each patient in the same manner as handpieces (as described above). Manufacturers' directions for reprocessing should be followed to ensure effectiveness of the process as well as longevity of the instruments.

Some dental instruments have components that are heat sensitive or are permanently attached to dental unit water lines. Some items may not enter the patient's oral cavity, but are likely to become contaminated with oral fluids during treatment procedures (e.g., handles or dental unit attachments of saliva ejectors, high-speed air evacuators, and air/water syringes). These components should be covered with impervious barriers that are changed after each use or, if the surface permits, carefully cleaned and then treated with a chemical germicide having at least an intermediate level of activity. As with high-speed dental handpieces, water lines to all instruments should be flushed thoroughly after the treatment of each patient; flushing at the beginning of each clinic day also is recommended.

Single-Use Disposable Instruments

Single-use disposable instruments (e.g., prophylaxis angles; prophylaxis cups and brushes; tips for high-speed air evacuators, saliva ejectors, and air/water syringes should be used for one patient only and discarded appropriately. These items are neither designed nor intended to be cleaned, disinfected, or sterilized for reuse.

Handling of Biopsy Specimens

In general, each biopsy specimen should be put in a sturdy container with a secure lid to prevent leaking during transport. Care should be taken when collecting specimens to avoid contamination of the outside of the container. If the outside of the container is visibly contaminated, it should be cleaned and disinfected or placed in an impervious bag.

Extracted Teeth

Persons handling extracted teeth should wear gloves. Gloves should be disposed and hands washed after completion of work activities. Extracted teeth used for the education of DHCWs should be considered infective and classified as clinical specimens because they contain blood. The collection, transport or manipulation of extracted teeth should be handled with the same precautions as a specimen for biopsy. Universal precautions should be adhered to whenever extracted teeth are handled. All persons handling extracted teeth in dental educational settings should receive hepatitis B vaccine.

Disposal of Waste Materials

Blood, suctioned fluids, or other liquid waste may be poured carefully into a drain connected to a sanitary sewer system. Disposable needles, scalpels, or other sharp items should be placed intact into puncture-resistant containers before disposal. Solid waste contaminated with blood or other body fluids should be placed in sealed, sturdy impervious bags to prevent leakage of the contained items. All contained solid waste should then be disposed of according to requirements established by local, state or federal environmental regulatory agencies and published recommendations.

Implementing Recommended Infection Control Practices

Emphasis should be focused on the consistent adherence to recommended infection control strategies, including use of protective barriers and appropriate sterilization, disinfection of instruments and environmental surfaces. Each dental facility should develop a written protocol for instrument reprocessing, operatory cleanup and management of injuries.

REFERENCES

1. CDC. Recommendations for prevention of HIV in health care settings. MMWR 1987;36:(2S)
2. CDC. Recommended infection-control practices for dentistry. MMWR 1993;42(RR-8):1–12.
3. Department of Labor, Occupational Safety and Health Administration. 29 CFR Part 1910.1030, Occupational exposure to bloodborne pathogens; final rule. Federal Register 1991;56(235):64004–64182.
4. CDC. Guidelines for prevention of transmission of human iimmunodeficiency virus and hepatitis B virus to health-care and public-safety workers. MMWR 1989;28 (suppl No. S-6):1–37.
5. Siew C, Gruninger SE, Mitchell EW, Burrell KH. Survey of hepatitis B exposure and vaccination in volunteer dentists. J Am Dent Assoc 1987;114:457–459.

Environmental Precautions: Sterilization, Disinfection and Housekeeping

No environmentally mediated mode of HIV transmission has been documented. An extensive study performed on HIV survival in the environment found HIV to be detectable by tissue-culture techniques one to three days after drying (1). However, the study used HIV samples which were much more concentrated than those normally found in the blood of HIV-infected persons (i.e., 100,000 times greater). Even though HIV could be detected for up to three days, the rate of inactivation was very rapid. CDC studies have shown that drying causes a 90 to 99% reduction in HIV concentration within several hours (2). In tissue-culture fluid, cell-free HIV could be detected up to 15 days at room temperature, up to 11 days at 37°C (98.6°F) and up to one day if the HIV was cell-associated (2).

Inactivation of HIV and Germicides

HIV has been demonstrated to be rapidly inactivated after being exposed to commonly used chemical germicides at concentrations much lower than used in practice (2). Embalming fluids are similar to the types of chemical germicides that have been tested and found to completely inactivate HIV. A solution of sodium hypochlorite (household bleach) prepared daily is an inexpensive and effective germicide. Concentrations ranging from approximately 500 ppm (1:100 dilution of household bleach) sodium hypochlorite to 5000 ppm (1:10 dilution of household bleach) are effective, depending on the amount of organic material (e.g., blood, mucus) present on the surface to be cleaned and disinfected. Commercially available chemical germicides may be more compatible with certain medical devices that might be corroded by repeated exposure to sodium hypochlorite, especially at the 1:10 dilution (2). Recommendations regarding the use of bleach to disinfect drug injection equipment have been updated (3). However, CDC recommendations for disinfecting environmental surfaces contaminated with blood are unchanged (3). The CDC recommendations for disinfecting environmental surfaces continues to include use of a 1:100 dilution of household bleach (or ¼ cup bleach to one gallon tap water) and other appropriate disinfectants (3). For decontaminating objects soiled with blood or body fluids, contact times of 20 to 30 minutes with the appropriate disinfectant have been recommended (4).

Although the likelihood of environmentally mediated HIV transmission is probably very small, there is a theoretical possibility that exposure to HIV in the environment could result in infection. Consequently, the precautions have been designed to prevent such transmission from occurring. Standard sterilization and disinfection procedures for patient care equipment recommended for use in a variety of health care settings (e.g., hospitals, medical clinics and offices, hemodialysis centers, emergency care facilities, long-term nursing care facilities) are adequate to sterilize or disinfect instruments, devices, or other items contaminated with blood or other body fluids from persons infected with blood borne pathogens, including HIV (2). The following precautions have been recommended for sterilization, disinfection, and housekeeping techniques and should be followed routinely for the care of all patients (2–5). Sterilization and disinfection techniques for the dental setting are described separately.

Sterilization and Disinfection Techniques

Instruments or devices that enter sterile tissue or the vascular system of any patient or through which blood flows should be sterilized before reuse. Devices or items that contact intact mucous membranes should be sterilized or receive high-level disinfection, a procedure that kills vegetative organisms and viruses but not necessarily large numbers of bacterial spores. Chemical germicides that are registered with the EPA as "sterilants" may be used either for sterilization or for high-level disinfection, depending on contact time (5). Table 8.3 describes the methods and applications for cleaning, disinfecting, and sterilizing equipment in the prehospital setting and also apply to surfaces for housekeeping and other cleaning tasks (5). In general, large amounts of blood or fluids should be removed before the object is sterilized. The ef-

Table 8.3.

Reprocessing Methods for Equipment Used in Prehospital Health Care Settings

	Effective Against	Methods	Use
Sterilization	Destroys all forms of microbial life including high numbers of bacterial spores	Steam under pressure (autoclave), gas (ethylene oxide), dry heat, or immersion in EPA-approved chemical "sterilant" for prolonged periods of time, e.g., 6–10 hours or according to manufacturers' instructions. Note: liquid chemical "sterilants" should be used only on those instruments that are impossible to sterilize or disinfect with heat	For those instruments or devices that penetrate skin or contact normally sterile areas of the body, e.g., scalpels, needles, etc. Disposable invasive equipment eliminates the need to reprocess these types of items. When indicated, arrangements should be made with a health care facility for reprocessing of reusable invasive instruments
High-level disinfection	All forms of microbial life except high numbers of bacterial spores	Hot water pasteurization (80–100°C, 30 minutes) or exposure to an EPA-registered "sterilant" chemical, except for short exposure time (10–45 minutes or as directed by the manufacturer)	For reusable instruments or devices that come into contact with mucous membranes (e.g., laryngoscope blades, endotracheal tubes, etc.)
Intermediate-level disinfection	Mycobacterium tuberculosis, vegetative bacteria, most viruses, and most fungi, but does not kill bacterial spores	EPA-registered "hospital disinfectant" chemical germicides that have a label claim for tuberculocidal activity; commercially available hard-surface germicides or solutions containing at least 500 ppm free available chlorine (a 1:100 dilution of common household bleach approximately ¼ cup bleach per gallon of tap water)	For those surfaces that come into contact only with intact skin, e.g., stethoscopes, blood pressure cuffs, splints, etc., and have been visibly contaminated with blood or bloody body fluids. Surfaces must be precleaned of visible material before the germicidal chemical is applied for disinfection
Low-level disinfection	Most bacteria, some viruses, some fungi, but not Mycobacterium tuberculosis or bacterial spores	EPA-registered ("hospital disinfectants" (no label claim for tuberculocidal activity)	These agents are excellent cleaners and can be used for routine housekeeping or removal of soiling in the absence of visible contamination
Environmental disinfection	Environmental surfaces which have become soiled should be cleaned and disinfected using any cleaner or disinfectant agent which is intended for environmental use. Such surfaces include floors, woodwork, ambulance seats, countertops, etc.		

Adapted from CDC. MMWR 1989;38 (No S-6)
NOTE: To assure effectiveness of any sterilization or disinfection process, equipment and instruments must first be thoroughly cleaned of all visible soil.

fectiveness of chemical germicides may be markedly decreased if objects are not first cleaned of large amounts of body fluids.

Medical devices or instruments that require sterilization or disinfection should be thoroughly cleaned before being exposed to the germicide, according to manufacturer's instructions for germicide use. It is important to closely follow the manufacturer's specifications for compatibility of the medical device with chemical germicides. Information on specific label claims of commercial germicides can be obtained by writing to: Disinfectants Branch, Office of Pesticides, EPA, 401 M Street, SW, Washington, DC 20460.

Housekeeping Strategies

In the context of environmental condition, health care facilities currently recommended cleaning, disinfection, or housekeeping strategies are as follows (2):

Environmental surfaces such as walls, floors, and other surfaces are not associated with transmission of infections to patients or HCW. Routine cleaning and removal of soil should be done, although extraordinary efforts to disinfect or sterilize these environmental surfaces are not necessary. Cleaning schedules and methods vary according to the area of the hospital or institution, the type of surface to be cleaned, and the amount and type of soil present. Horizontal surfaces (e.g., bedside tables and hard-surfaced flooring) in patient care areas are usually cleaned on a regular basis, when soiling or spills occur, and when a patient is discharged. Cleaning of walls, blinds, and curtains is recommended only if they are visibly soiled. Disinfectant fogging is an unsatisfactory method of decontaminating air and surfaces and is not recommended. Disinfectant-detergent formulations registered by EPA can be used for cleaning environmental surfaces, in accordance with manufacturer's instructions. The actual physical removal of microorganisms by scrubbing is probably as important as any antimicrobial effect of the cleaning agent used.

Cleaning and Decontaminating Spills of Blood and Other Body Fluids (2–5)

All spills of blood and blood-contaminated fluids should be promptly cleaned up while wearing gloves, and using an EPA-approved germicide (i.e., "hospital disinfectants" and ones that are tuberculocidal when used at recommended dilution) or a 1:100 solution of household bleach (2,3). The procedure for cleaning spills or objects contaminated with blood or body fluids varies with different situations. In patient care areas, visible material should first be removed and then the area should be decontaminated. Disposable towels or other appropriate means should be used to avoid direct contact. The effectiveness of chemical germicides may be markedly decreased if objects or surfaces are not first cleaned of gross amounts of body fluids. If splashing is anticipated, protective eyewear and an impervious gown should be also worn. With large spills of cultured or concentrated infectious agents in the laboratory, the contaminated area should be flooded with a liquid germicide before cleaning, then decontaminated with a fresh germicidal chemical. Gloves should be worn during the cleaning and decontaminating procedures and hands washed following removal of gloves. Soiled cleaning equipment should be cleaned and decontaminated or disposed of appropriately. Plastic bags should be available for removal of contaminated items from the spill site.

Laundry (2,5)

The risk of actual disease transmission through soiled linen is negligible. Hygienic and common sense storage and processing of clean and soiled linen are recommended. Soiled linen should be handled as little as possible and with minimum agitation to prevent gross microbial contamination of the air of persons handling the linen. All soiled linen should be bagged at the location where it is used, it should not be sorted or rinsed in patient care areas.

Linen soiled with blood or body fluids should be placed and transported in bags that prevent leakage. Personnel involved in the bagging, transport, and laundering of contaminated clothing should wear gloves. In hot water laundry cycles, linens should be laundered with detergent at a minimum of 71°C (160°F) for 25 minutes. If low-temperature ($\leq 70°$C [158°F]) laundry cycles are used, chemicals suitable for low-temperature washing at the proper concentration should be added.

Infective Waste (2,5)

Those wastes with the potential for causing infection during handling and disposal, and for which some special precautions appear prudent, should be identified. Wastes for which special precautions appear prudent include microbiology laboratory waste, pathology waste, and blood specimens or blood products. Although any item that has had contact with blood, exudates, or secretions may be potentially infective, it is not usually considered practical or necessary to treat all such waste as infective. Infective waste, in general, should either be incinerated or should be autoclaved before disposal in a sanitary landfill. Bulk blood, suctioned fluids, excretions, and secretions may be carefully poured down a drain connected to a sanitary sewer. Sanitary sewers may also be used to dispose of other infectious wastes capable of being ground and flushed into the sewer.

REFERENCES

1. Resnik L, Veren K, Salahuddin SZ, Tondreau S, Markham PD. Stability and inactivation of HTLV-III/LAV under clinical and laboratory environments. JAMA 1986; 255:1887–1891.
2. CDC. Recommendations for prevention of HIV transmission in health-care settings. MMWR 1987;36:(No.2S).
3. CDC. Use of bleach for disinfection of drug injection equipment. MMWR 1993; 42:418–419.
4. Crutcher JM, Lamm SH, and Hall TA. Procedures to protect health care workers from HIV infection: category I (health-care) workers. Am Ind Hyg Assoc J 1991;52: A100–A103

5. CDC. Guidelines for prevention of transmission of human immunodeficiency virus and hepatitis B virus to health-care and public safety workers. MMWR 1989;38(No S–6).

Infection Control in the Era of Tuberculosis

Recent hospital outbreaks of multidrug-resistant tuberculosis (MDR-TB) have refocused attention on the transmission of tuberculosis in hospitals and other health care settings. Transmission has occurred in such institutions as jails, hospitals, homeless shelters, AIDS hospices long-term residential facilities and drug treatment facilities (1–5). Institutional spread of tuberculosis (TB) may occur from unsuspected cases of TB within a facility, infectious cases recently initiated on antituberculous treatment, and patients treated with inadequate or ineffective therapy. Clearly, the lack of adherence to infection control guidelines to prevent institutional spread of tuberculosis has also played a role in recent outbreaks (4). Multiple outbreaks of tuberculosis occurring in health care settings, including outbreaks of MDR-TB, have been associated with high rates of mortality in HIV-infected individuals and pose additional risks to health care workers (1,5).

The etiologic agent of tuberculosis, *Mycobacterium tuberculosis,* may be spread by small airborne droplets produced by patients with pulmonary or laryngeal TB. Infectious TB patients produce large respiratory droplets (5 microns) and smaller droplet nuclei (1–5 microns). The larger respiratory droplets are less infectious since they do not remain suspended in the air, and when inhaled tend to settle in the upper airways where they do not produce infection. Droplet nuclei remain suspended in the air and may be carried long distances by air currents throughout rooms and within a building. These smaller droplet nuclei are carried past the mucociliary blanket of the upper respiratory tract into the lower respiratory tract where they reach alveoli and can establish infection (6–8). Respiratory droplets containing *M. tuberculosis* are produced primarily by coughing, although sneezing, singing, laughing and speaking may also produce infectious droplets (9). Patients with extrapulmonary tuberculosis (e.g., meningitis, lymphadenitis) are not infectious and generally do not need to be isolated once pulmonary disease has been excluded. Patients with abscesses or fistulas should have routine bodily fluid precautions. Additionally, patients with open wounds draining material with high concentrations of acid-fast bacilli or wounds subjected to procedures resulting in aerosolization should be placed on respiratory isolation (6).

Table 8.4 lists risk factors associated with transmission of tuberculosis. Contacts of infectious TB cases are at increased risk of tuberculous infection if they have had prolonged exposure (e.g., household members or coworkers). The environmental factors associated with transmission in an exposure setting include the volume of air (e.g., size of the room), the presence of ultraviolet (UV) light and the frequency of air exchanges (i.e., dilution of infectious particles) that occur through natural or artificial means (8). Consequently, household contacts of an infectious family

Table 8.4.

Risk Factors Associated with Transmission of Tuberculosis

Positive AFB sputum smears[a]
Cavitary disease
Presence of cough
Laryngeal disease

[a]acid-fast bacilli

member are more likely to be infected if crowding and poor ventilation exist in the home. Institutional outbreaks of TB have been associated with the lack of isolation of infectious patients, delays in initiating therapy, inadequate treatment and the placement of TB patients in rooms with ventilation that directed airflow carrying infectious droplets into other rooms or hallways. HIV coinfection has not been shown to increase the infectivity of TB patients (10).

The risk of infection with TB is proportional to the duration of exposure to an infectious case and the concentration of airborne infectious droplets (6). TB is less contagious than other airborne infections such as measles or varicella; about 30% of close contacts of newly diagnosed cases of pulmonary TB will be infected with *M. tuberculosis* (11). Individuals with latent infection may be identified by tuberculin skin testing. Immunocompetent tuberculin reactors have about a 10% risk of developing active tuberculosis over their lifetime if no preventive therapy is given, the risk being greatest in the first one to two years after initial infection. In contrast, HIV-infected individuals with tuberculous infection have an 8–10% risk per year of developing active TB (12,13). Much of the heightened concern regarding TB transmission is directed towards HIV-infected individuals, because of their increased risk of developing active tuberculosis either from reactivation of a previous infection or newly acquired infection (primary TB).

The resurgence of tuberculosis in the past decade, along with the development of MDR-TB, has led to the review of TB policies in health care settings and the recommendation at local, state and federal levels of specific actions to reduce the risk of TB transmission in these settings (6,14). Transmission of TB can be reduced by: a) methods that reduce the infectivity of the source case, b) environmental modifications that reduce the concentration of infectious droplet nuclei in the exposure setting; and c) active surveillance of personnel for tuberculous infection.

Decreasing the Infectiousness of TB Patients

The most effective intervention to halt the transmission of TB is the early identification of infectious cases and initiation of anti-tuberculous therapy. Transmission of TB in institutional settings has frequently been associated with unrecognized cases of pulmonary tuberculosis. Therefore, a high index of suspicion for TB needs to be maintained in

Table 8.5.
Groups at Increased Risk for Tuberculosis

Close contacts of tuberculosis cases
Persons born in high prevalence countries[a]
Persons with HIV infection
Low-income, high-risk minority populations[b]
Intravenous drug users and alcoholics
Homeless persons
Persons with certain medical conditions[c]
Residents of long-term facilities (e.g., prisons, nursing homes)

[a]Asia, Africa and Latin America
[b]African-Americans, Hispanics, Native Americans
[c]Diabetes, silicosis, certain malignancies, renal failure, immunosuppressive therapy, postgastrectomy, malnutrition

Table 8.6.
Environmental Approaches to Control Spread of TB

Patient isolation
Ventilation
Negative-pressure isolation
Air filtration (HEPA)[a]
Ultraviolet air disinfection
Particulate respirators

[a]High efficiency particle air filters

health care settings and other institutions caring for populations at increased risk for tuberculosis (Table 8.5).

The current recommendations for the *initial* treatment of pulmonary tuberculosis is a 6-month regimen consisting of isoniazid (INH), rifampin (RIF), pyrazinamide (PZA) and ethambutol (EMB) given for 2 months followed by INH and RIF for 4 months. Although adequate treatment of drug-sensitive TB normally requires six months of therapy, longer regimens are necessary in individuals with multiple drug resistance (15). Details about antituberculous treatment are discussed in the section, Tuberculosis and HIV infection. Effective antituberculous therapy rapidly decreases infectiousness of TB cases by reducing concentrations of acid-fast bacilli (AFB) in sputum, the amount of sputum and cough frequency (16). Although patients with multidrug-resistant TB are not more infectious than other TB patients, they will remain infectious for longer periods of time.

Environmental Control

Environmental approaches to control of TB include patient isolation, ventilation, directional airflow, air filtration, ultraviolet air disinfection and particulate respirators (Table 8.6).

PATIENT ISOLATION

Respiratory isolation of suspected TB cases in appropriately venti-lated rooms is necessary for inpatient facilities. Suspected or known TB cases should be instructed to cover their mouth and nose when coughing or sneezing, which will reduce respiratory droplet generation. Although masks are recommended when patients are outside of their room, surgi-cal masks do not filter out droplet nuclei, therefore all but essential studies should be discouraged until the patient has been on antitubercu-lous therapy for 2 to 3 weeks (14). Infectivity decreases with time on ef-fective therapy, although the length of time until a person is no longer infectious varies. Although many authors have quoted two weeks of anti-tuberculous therapy as being the time period when cases with pul-monary TB are no longer infectious, over 50% of patients may have posi-tive sputum cultures at the end of four weeks of therapy with isoniazid and rifampin (16). Decisions regarding the infectiousness of a given pa-tient should be individualized considering the type of disease (e.g., ad-vanced cavitary, drug-resistant), the clinical and microbiologic (AFB smears) response to therapy, the environmental setting and the relative susceptibility of those who may be potentially exposed to the patient. In general, patients who have received effective therapy and have three consecutive morning sputum specimens negative for AFB, and have demonstrated clinical improvement are unlikely to be infectious (14). While two or three weeks of therapy may be adequate to decrease the in-fectiousness of a TB case, decisions regarding the discontinuation of res-piratory isolation should be made with caution.

VENTILATION AND DIRECTIONAL AIR FLOW

Droplet nuclei generated by the cough of a patient with pulmonary TB may remain suspended in room air for long periods of time (7,8). The concentration of infectious droplet nuclei may be reduced or eliminated by appropriate ventilation. Ventilation serves to reduce TB transmission by decreasing the concentration of droplet nuclei using the introduction of outside or recirculated air and by removal of infectious particles (8,14). Air is removed from the room by one of two methods: direct ex-haust to the outside or by recirculation through the general ventilation system. If air containing droplet nuclei is recirculated into other rooms, individuals may become infected with tubercle bacilli without being di-rectly exposed to TB cases. Vents that exhaust air to the outside should be located away from intake vents and pedestrian traffic. Adequate air mixing within a room is important for ventilation efficiency and is de-pendent on the location of the air-supply and exhaust vents. Ventilation rate standards for air changes per hour (ACH), the replacement of the quantity of air contained by a room are set by the American Society of Heating, Refrigerating and Air Conditioning Engineers (ASHRAE) and the federal Health Resources and Services Administration (HRSA) (17,18). Currently, ventilation rates of six air changes or greater are rec-ommended in TB isolation rooms in existing facilities and ≥ 12 ACH are recommended in new or renovated facilities (14).

The direction of air flow in a room relative to surrounding areas is also an important factor in preventing TB transmission. Recent hospital outbreaks of MDR-TB have been associated with high transmission rates in HIV-infected patients and skin test conversions among health care workers. Investigation of these outbreaks found incomplete adherence to isolation procedures and TB infection control guidelines, including the placement of patients into hospital rooms with positive air-pressure differential, so that air flow was directed from the hospital rooms into adjacent corridors (4). Isolation rooms need to be maintained under negative air pressure, which requires the rate of air exhaust to exceed the rate of air intake, to prevent airborne spread of infectious particles into adjacent areas. Doors to isolation rooms should remain closed and isolation rooms need to be inspected on a regular basis by trained staff. The use of flutter strips or smoke-tube testing are simple and rapid methods to assess direction of air flow. Additional measures, including air filtration and germicidal ultraviolet irradiation, may be used to supplement ventilation as a means of reducing TB transmission (8,14).

AIR FILTRATION

Air filtration in ventilation systems via high-efficiency particle air (HEPA) filters that effectively removes particles ≥ 0.3 microns in diameter with 99.7% efficiency has been used to prevent nosocomial spread of *Aspergillus* infection and may prove useful in an adjunctive role for TB infection control (8). For many health facilities, HEPA filtration and recirculation of air may be more economical than direct exhaust to the outside, although HEPA filtration systems are not currently recommended for filtration of air from TB isolation rooms back into the general air circulation (14). Portable HEPA filter units are now available, and may play a supplementary role to standard environmental controls for local air disinfection, although their effectiveness has not been adequately tested. Portable units are relatively inexpensive and easy to use. The difficulty of moving enough room air through HEPA filtration systems to conduct effective air changes is one major limitation. The use of HEPA filtration may be most useful in the recirculation of air in waiting rooms or emergency rooms where an increased risk of TB exposure exists (8,14).

ULTRAVIOLET AIR DISINFECTION (UVGI)

Ultraviolet germicidal irradiation is an effective means of air disinfection for airborne infections, such as tuberculosis, that are spread via respiratory droplets (14,19). Ultraviolet (UV) lamps have been recommended as a supplement to ventilation systems in high-risk settings (14). UV lamps are usually installed on ceilings within a room or corridor; however, adequate air mixing is important for their effectiveness since they provide local disinfection for upper room air. Ultraviolet lamps may also be installed in ventilation ducts, but UV treatment alone is currently not recommended to recirculate air from TB isolation rooms back into the general ventilation system (14). The use of UV lamps has been controversial because of concerns for safety. Overexposure has been associated with keratoconjunctivitis, redness of the skin and may be associated with skin cancers (6). The risks of UVGI are low when properly used and maintained; and the potential benefits in preventing TB transmission probably outweigh these risks.

PARTICULATE RESPIRATORS

Standard surgical masks do not provide adequate protection against infectious droplet nuclei produced by persons with pulmonary TB. The use of respiratory protective devices (particulate respirators), which filter particles 1 μm in size (≥95% efficiency), has been recommended for individuals in the following settings: 1) rooms in which patients with known or suspected TB are isolated; 2) during cough-inducing procedures; and 3) other settings with increased risk for TB exposure (14). Despite published CDC and OSHA guidelines regarding the use of respiratory protective devices in health care facilities, then use has been limited because of high costs and inconvenience (20). Particulate respirators (PRs) appear to play an important role in certain settings with a high risk of TB transmission, such as medical procedures (e.g., bronchoscopy) that produce large amounts of infectious droplets and in settings where appropriate ventilation is unavailable. Respirators with HEPA filters are the only PRs currently certified for use. Valveless PRs or surgical masks should be used by TB patients when being transported outside of their isolation room (8,14). Respiratory protector devices used in health care settings must be certified by the National Institute for Occupational Safety (NIOSH). Additional information on PRs may be obtained in the NIOSH Guide to Industrial Respiratory Protection (21).

PROCEDURES

Medical procedures which carry additional risk of TB transmission due to generation of large amounts of infectious respiratory droplets are listed in Table 8.7. Procedures, such as sputum induction and aerosolized pentamidine (AP) treatments, which induce coughing in patients who may have TB should be conducted in a separate room or booth with local exhaust ventilation. Negative air pressure in these booths or rooms should be maintained respective to surrounding areas. UVGI and HEPA filters are possible adjunctive measures for these areas. Ideally, patients should be screened for active tuberculosis before initiating AP therapy. Bronchoscopy should be performed in well-ventilated, negative-

---

Table 8.7.

High Risk Procedures for Transmission of Tuberculosis

Sputum induction
Aerosolized pentamidine treatment
Bronchoscopy
Endotracheal intubation and suctioning

pressure rooms with air exhausted to the outside or recirculated through HEPA filters in accordance with state and federal regulations. Health care workers should wear PRs when present in areas where these procedures are performed on patients at increased risk for tuberculosis (8,14).

Surveillance for Tuberculous Infection

The most important means of reducing the transmission of TB is early identification of persons with tuberculous infection or active tuberculosis, and the initiation of an appropriate treatment regimen. Screening for tuberculous infection using Mantoux skin testing and current guidelines for interpretation (Table 8.8) is necessary for any health care facility providing services for high risk populations (Table 8.5) (11,12,14). Chest radiographs should be obtained in high-risk individu-

---

Table 8.8.
Interpretation of Tuberculin Skin Tests

1. An induration of ≥ 5 mm is classified as positive in:
   Persons with HIV infection or risk factors for HIV infection with unknown HIV status;
   Persons who have had recent close contact[a] with persons with active TB;
   Persons who have abnormal chest radiographs consistent with old, healed TB.
2. An induration of ≥ 10 mm is classified as positive in all persons who do not meet any of the criteria above but who have other risk factors for TB including:
   High-risk groups
      Intravenous drug users known to be HIV seronegative;
      Persons with other medical conditions associated with an increased risk of progressing from latent TB infection to active TB (e.g., silicosis; gastrectomy, jejuno-ileal bypass surgery; being 10% or more below ideal body weight; chronic renal failure; diabetes mellitus; high dose corticosteroid and other immunosuppressive therapy; some hematologic disorders, e.g., leukemias and lymphomas; and other malignancies)
      Children < 4 years of age
   High-prevalence groups
      Foreign-born persons from high-prevalence countries in Asia, Africa, and Latin America;
      Persons from medically underserved low income populations;
      Residents from long-term care facilities (e.g., correctional institutions, nursing homes);
      Persons from high-risk populations in their communities, as determined by local public health authorities.
3. An induration of ≥ 15 mm is classified as positive for persons who do not meet any of the above criteria.
4. Recent converters are defined on the basis of both induration and age:
   ≥ 10 mm increase within a 2-year period is classified as a recent conversion for persons < 35 years of age;
   ≥ 15 mm increase within a 2-year period is classified as positive for persons ≥ 35 years of age
   ≥ 5 mm increases under certain circumstances (#1, above)
5. PPD skin-test results in health-care workers (HCWS)
   In general, the recommendations in Sections 1, 2, and 3 should be followed. In facilities where TB patients receive care, an induration of ≥ 10 mm in HCWs who have no other risk factors is a suitable cut-off point.
   ≥ 10 mm increase in induration within a 2-year period is classified as a recent conversion for HCWs.

Adapted from MMWR 1994; 43 (No RR-13)
[a]Recent close contact implies household contact or unprotected occupational exposure similar in intensity and duration to household contact.

als presenting in acute care settings, and in populations where tuber-culin testing may not be feasible (e.g., correctional facilities). The recent outbreaks of tuberculosis in hospitals and residential facilities have demonstrated rapid progression of tuberculous infection to disease in HIV-infected persons and the health care risks posed to employees (1–4). Health care facilities need to provide active surveillance pro-grams to screen for TB among personnel. The frequency of tuberculin screening should be dictated by the exposure risk to infectious TB pa-tients in an area or occupational group within a facility. The assessment of risk in a faculty is based on the prevalence of TB in the community, the number of TB patients seen in the facility, and the frequency of health care worker PPD test conversions. Employees who perform cough-inducing procedures (Table 8.7) or who work in settings (e.g., emergency room that place them at increased risk of exposure to infec-tious TB patients need to be screened most frequently every 3–6 months) (14). Health care workers with positive skin tests or skin test conversions should be evaluated for active tuberculosis by clinical and radiographic examinations. In the absence of clinical and radiologic evi-dence of TB, persons with positive skin tests should be offered preven-tive therapy according to current guidelines recommended by the Cen-ters for Disease Control (11,14). All persons with a positive skin test should be evaluated for risk factors for HIV infection and offered HIV testing if necessary. HIV testing, along with pre- and posttest counsel-ing, should be performed on any person diagnosed with tuberculosis.

Health care workers and patients will need to be evaluated following a documented exposure to an infectious TB patient. Persons with initial negative Mantoux skin tests after exposure should receive follow-up tu-berculin testing in twelve weeks. Contacts with a previous positive Man-toux test do not need repeat skin testing and a chest radiograph is rec-ommended only for those who are clinically symptomatic (14).

Health care workers with medical conditions causing immune suppres-sion, including HIV infection, should be counseled regarding their risks for TB infection. Ideally, these individuals should work in areas at the lowest risk for occupational TB exposure and screened every 6 months (14).

The transmission of tuberculosis in health care facilities poses new chal-lenges to medical and engineering staff in implementing existing guide-lines and in the development of better methods for preventing airborne in-fections. In health care facilities where nosocomial outbreaks of TB have occurred, institution of existing infection control measures was associated with decreases in TB transmission (14,22). The development and imple-mentation of an active, integrated TB infection control plan in any facility caring for TB patients is fundamental in the prevention of tuberculosis.

REFERENCES

1. CDC. Nosocomial transmission of multidrug-resistant TB to healthcare workers and HIV-infected patients in an urban hospital—Florida. MMWR 1990;39:718–722.
2. CDC. Nosocomial transmission of multidrug-resistant tuberculosis among HIV-infected persons—Florida and New York, 1988–1991. MMWR 1991;40:585–591.

3. CDC. Transmission of multidrug-resistant tuberculosis from an HIV-positive client in a residential substance-abuse treatment facility—Michigan. MMWR 1991; 40:129–131.
4. Pearson ML, Jereb JA, Frieden TR, et al. Nosocomial transmission of multidrug-resistant Mycobacterium tuberculosis: a risk to patients and health care workers. Ann Intern Med 1992;117:191–196.
5. McGowan JE. Nosocomial tuberculosis: New progress in control and precaution. Clin Infect Dis 1995;21(3):489–505.
6. CDC. Guidelines for preventing transmission of tuberculosis in health care settings, with special focus on HIV-related issues. MMWR 1990;39(RR-17).
7. Riley RL. Airborne infection. Am J Med 1974;57:466–475.
8. Nardell EA. Environmental control of tuberculosis. Med Clin North Am 1993;77: 1315–1325.
9. American Thoracic Society, CDC. Diagnostic standards and classification of tuberculosis. Am Rev Respir Dis 1990;142:725–735.
10. Klausner JD, Ryder RW, Baende E, et al. Mycobacterium tuberculosis in household contacts of human immunodeficiency type 1-seropositive patients with active pulmonary tuberculosis in Kinshasa, Zaire. J Infect Dis 1993;168:106–111.
11. CDC. Screening for tuberculosis and tuberculosis infection in high risk populations, and the use of preventive therapy for tuberculosis infection in the United States: recommendations of the Advisory Committee for Elimination of Tuberculosis. MMWR 1990;39(RR-8).
12. CDC. Purified protein derivative (PPD)-tuberculin anergy and HIV infection: guidelines for anergy testing and management of anergic persons at risk of tuberculosis. MMWR 1991;40(RR-5).
13. Selwyn PA, Hartel D, Lewis VA, et al. A prospective study of the risk of tuberculosis among intravenous drug users with human immunodeficiency virus infection. N Engl J Med 1989;320:546–550.
14. CDC. Guidelines for preventing the transmission of Mycobacterium tuberculosis in health-care facilities, 1994. MMWR 1994;43 (no RR-13).
15. American Thoracic Society. Treatment of tuberculosis and tuberculosis infection in adults and children. Am J Respr Crit Care Med 1994;149:1359–1374.
16. Noble RC. Infectiousness of pulmonary tuberculosis after starting chemotherapy: Review of the available data on an unresolved question. Assoc Pract Infect Control 1981;9:6–10.
17. American Society of Heating, Refrigerating and Air Conditioning Engineers. Ventilation for acceptable indoor air quality. Standard 62–1989. Atlanta, Georgia: ASHRAE, Inc., 1989.
18. Health Resource and Services Administration. Guidelines for construction and equipment of hospital and medical facilities. Rockville, Maryland: US Department of Health and Human Services, Public Health Service, 1984; PHS publication (HRSA)84–145.
19. Riley RL, Nardell EA. Clearing the air: the theory and application of ultraviolet air disinfection. Am Rev Respir Dis 1989;139:1286–1294.
20. Adal KA, Anglim AM, Palumbo CL, et al. The use of high-efficiency particulate air-filter respirators to protect hospital workers from tuberculosis, a cost-effectiveness analysis. N Engl J Med 1994;331:169–173.
21. NIOSH. Guide to industrial respiratory protection. Morgantown, WV. U.S. Department of Health and Human Services, Public Health Service, CDC, 1987, DHS Publication no. (NIOSH) 87–116.
22. Blumberg HM, Watkins DL, Berschling JD, et al. Preventing nosocomial transmission of tuberculosis. Am Int Med 1995;122:658–663.

Post-HIV Exposure Management

Although universal infection control precautions, safer use of needles, and other innovations may substantially reduce the incidence of occupational exposure, the risk is not completely eliminated and accidental exposures through needlestick injuries and other contact with bodily fluids do occur. Guidelines have been developed to address occupational exposures to possible HIV-infected bodily fluids.

Risk Factors in Health Care Settings

The risk of HIV from discrete exposures is lower than that associated with HBV exposure. In one surveillance project of occupationally exposed healthcare workers (HCWs), percutaneous injury accounted for the largest amount (89%) of occupational exposures, predominantly caused by needles (i.e., syringe, intravenous, suture and other needles) and other sharp instruments (e.g., scalpels, lancets) (1). Common reasons reported for accidental parenteral exposures are: resheathing needles and the disassembling of intravenous tubing devices, vacuum tube phlebotomy sets, and reusable cartridge injection syringes (2). HIV is transmitted to about 0.3%–0.4% (1,3) of HCWs who sustain percutaneous injuries with HIV-infected blood. Large amounts of injected blood, hollow-bore needlesticks, and deep needlesticks are also associated with infection. A recent retrospective case-control study of HCWs who had a documented occupational percutaneous exposure to HIV revealed an increased risk of HIV infection following percutaneous exposures to HIV-infected blood with certain characteristic of the exposure and source patient (4). If the exposure involved a larger quantity of blood, there was an increased risk for HIV transmission; this was indicated by a deep injury to the HCW, visible contamination with the source patient's blood on the device causing the injury, or a procedure involving a needle placed directly in a vein or artery. Exposure to blood from source patients who died within 60 days as a result of AIDS also increased the risk of transmission; this most likely reflects the higher titer of HIV in blood late in the course of AIDS or other factors (e.g., presence of syncytia-inducing strains of HIV) (5,6). Identification of these risk factors in the case-control study suggests that risk for HIV infection exceeds 0.3% for percutaneous exposures involving a larger blood volume and/or higher titer in blood (7). The risk from mucosal and nonintact cutaneous exposure is not zero (on average, approximately 0.1% and >0.1%, respectively [8]), but too low to be reliably estimated in studies performed to date (1,8). A large prospective study evaluating cutaneous exposures detected no infections after 2712 instances of HIV exposure to intact skin (9). Anecdotal case reports have suggested that mucous membrane exposure or splashes might result in infection, especially when the duration of exposure or quantity of blood involved is large (10). The risks following mucous membrane and skin exposures to HIV-infected blood probably also depend on the blood volume and titer of HIV; a higher risk is likely for prolonged skin contact, the involvement of an extensive area or where skin integrity is visibly compromised, and/or involves a higher HIV titer (7).

Definition of an Occupational Exposure

As defined by the Centers for Disease Control (3), an occupational exposure that may place a worker at risk for HIV infection is a percutaneous injury, contact of mucous membranes, or contact of skin (especially when the exposed skin is chapped, abraded, or afflicted with dermatitis, or the contact is prolonged or involving an extensive area) with blood, tissues, or other body fluids to which universal precautions apply. These include: semen, vaginal secretions, or other body fluids contaminated with visible blood, because these substances have been implicated in the transmission of HIV infection; cerebrospinal fluid, synovial fluid, pleural fluid, peritoneal fluid, pericardial fluid, and amniotic fluid, because the risk of transmission of HIV from these fluids has not yet been determined; and laboratory specimens that contain HIV (e.g., suspensions of concentrated virus).

Post-exposure Management

Guidelines regarding the post-exposure management of workers who have occupational exposures that place them at risk for HIV infection have been published and can provide a framework regarding initial action (3,7,8–14). A system for prompt evaluation, counseling, and follow-up after a reported occupational exposure should be initiated immediately after an occupational exposure occurs. A program should also test protocols and mechanisms to assure the availability of confidential and free administration of initial doses of post-exposure prophylaxis (PEP); in some situations a plan for 24-hour, 7-day-a-week access to a program might be appropriate (3,10,11,13). Although the effectiveness is uncertain, if PEP is used; it should be started as quickly as possible. As part of job orientation and ongoing job training, workers who might be reasonably considered at risk for occupational exposure to HIV should be familiarized with the principles of post-exposure management; ongoing educational programs, posters, wallet-sized cards or file cards containing information and instructions for accessing post-exposure services are other ways to inform HCWs (3,10,12). HCWs should be educated to know what to do immediately if they have an accidental exposure (i.e., perform initial decontamination by washing the wound or rinsing the exposed mucous membrane) and to report exposures immediately after they occur for a risk assessment (4,11). Immediate reporting of exposures is important because certain interventions that are appropriate (e.g., zidovudine or hepatitis B prophylaxis) must be initiated promptly to be effective (3). The following compiles post-exposure management guidelines recommended by the Public Health Service (PHS), National Institutes of Health (NIH), and UC San Francisco/San Francisco General Hospital (UCSF/SFGH) (3,7,10–13).

Following an Occupational Exposure

WOUND DECONTAMINATION

Following an exposure, the wound should be cleansed as soon as patient safety permits. Puncture wounds and other cutaneous injuries should be washed with soap and water, and wounds with visible defects should be irrigated with sterile saline, a disinfectant, or other suitable solution (8). Exposed oral and nasal mucosa should be flushed vigorously with water, and eyes irrigated with clean water, normal saline, or sterile irrigants designed for this purpose. If the wound requires suturing, emergency care should be provided by personnel who are expert at wound decontamination and repair. Human bite wounds may necessitate antibiotic prophylaxis, depending on the site or exposure and the severity of the wound. Existing guidelines for wound management should, if appropriate, be followed by tetanus prophylaxis (8).

REPORTING EXPOSURES

A mechanism to facilitate the reporting of exposures and provision of follow-up care should be available and communicated to all employees at risk. Reporting systems should ideally allow prompt access to expert consultants as well as anonymity of the exposed worker. San Francisco General Hospital has established a 24 hours-a-day hotline for confidential reporting, with expert clinicians coordinating reporting and initial management of exposed persons (11).

HEPATITIS PROPHYLAXIS

After an occupational exposure, both the exposed worker and the source individual should be evaluated to determine the possible need for the exposed worker to receive prophylaxis against hepatitis B. Hepatitis B vaccine should be offered to any susceptible health care worker who has an occupational exposure and has not previously been vaccinated with hepatitis B vaccine. Hepatitis B immune globulin (HBIG) may also be indicated, particularly if the source patient or material is found to be positive for hepatitis B surface antigen (HBsAg). Hepatitis B prophylaxis with HBIG must be given as soon as possible and definitely within 48 hours of exposure. It has also been suggested that the source patient also be evaluated for evidence of HCV infection (8,11). Workers who sustain parenteral injuries and are exposed to HCV are recommended to have liver function tests and baseline testing for HCV antibody; retesting should be performed at 3 and 6 months after the injury (8,11).

EXPOSURE HISTORY

An accurate history is necessary to document an occupational exposure to blood or body fluids and to identify the severity of accident. This information may be useful in evaluating the transmission risk and determining the appropriate management protocol. Descriptive data can also be used for surveillance purposes and assist in identifying high-risk activities and targets for intervention (e.g., noncompliance with institutional policies, defective infection control procedures, deficiencies in the availability of materials). Elements of an exposure history (3,8) are summarized in Table 8.9.

Table 8.9.
Occupational HIV Exposure History

Date and time of exposure
Job duty or activity being performed by worker at time of exposure
Description of accident and exposure
Location and type of exposure -needle stick, puncture, laceration, abrasion, mucosal
    inoculation, contamination of nonintact skin, bite
Description of source fluid/material involved (e.g., blood, blood products, bloody body fluids,
    and tissues, inflammatory exudates, amniotic fluids, semen, etc.) Fluids not associated with
    risk of HIV transmission (as regarded by CDC) should also be reported and evaluated to
    determine the need of post-exposure care (e.g., saliva, stool, urine).
Whether the source material contained HIV or HBV, (if known)
Severity of exposure
    Percutaneous exposure: the depth of penetration, and volume of fluid injected (if any); type
        of needle (hollow-bore, surgical, or other), gauge of needle, if gloves used, whether
        needle passed through gloves en route to skin
    Skin or mucous-membrane exposure: the extent and duration of contact, the condition of
        the skin (e.g., existing dermatitis; chapped, abraded, or intact skin), volume of body
        fluid involved, mechanism used for decontamination
Identification of device/instrument responsible for exposure (if any)
Use of protective equipment used (e.g., gloves, eye protection, masks)
Demographic information about the exposed worker
Information about source patient
    Is HIV status known?
    If HIV positive, clinical stage of illness and CD4 count (if possible)
    HIV risk factors present/not present
    HBV risk assessment
Characteristics of work environment (e.g., level of staffing at that time, number of hours and
    consecutive shifts worked, impact of patient cooperation as a factor contributing to the
    exposure, whether the procedure was an emergency)

EVALUATION OF SOURCE PATIENT

Efforts should be made to identify the source patient of the substance involved in the exposure. The source patient should be informed of the incident and tested for HIV antibody with consent, along with HBsAg. When the patient is unable to participate in the decision process, where permitted, consent may be obtained by the next of kin, the individual assigned power of attorney by the patient, or other party legally allowed to make medical decisions. When consent cannot be obtained, policies should be developed for testing source individuals that are in compliance with applicable state and local laws. In some states (e.g., California), a person cannot be tested for HIV without that person's informed consent, although some states do allow testing of source patients without consent (11). Confidentiality of the source patient should be maintained at all times. Rapid turnaround time for source-patient testing is important since the decision to initiate prophylaxis may depend on the test result.

BASELINE HIV TESTING

The HCW should receive baseline HIV testing as soon as possible following potential exposure to HIV. HIV testing at the time of occupational exposure is a way of documenting baseline HIV status and, should transmission occur, is important in establishing that seroconversion occurred as an outcome of an exposure incident. A positive baseline HIV test result defines an earlier infection with HIV. The HCW may wish to have anonymous HIV testing, because of concern that an HIV antibody test result would be included in their record and result in negative consequences. However, anonymous testing provides no documentation and is not helpful if the HCW wants to document HIV status at the time of exposure. HCWs with occupational exposures should receive counseling and be tested for HIV antibody as soon as possible, with baseline testing done within the first 2 weeks of exposure. If the HCW chooses to defer baseline testing, a serum sample should be submitted to the blood bank so that testing can be performed at a later date for medical, legal, or other purposes.

FOLLOW-UP

If the source patient is HIV infected or refuses testing, the PHS recommends a clinical and serological evaluation of the HCW for evidence of HIV infection as soon as possible after exposure (baseline) and if negative, follow-up HIV testing at 6 weeks, 3 months, and 6 months after exposure to document the presence or absence of infection. Delayed seroconversion (i.e., when the HIV antibody first appears later than 6 months after exposure) is rare among HCWs, and continued testing beyond 6 months is not recommended, unless symptoms of HIV infection appear or the HCW is involved in experimental treatment protocols. Persons with occupational exposures should be advised to return for medical evaluation if symptoms or signs compatible with acute retroviral infection develop within the follow-up period. Illness, particularly if characterized by fever, rash, myalgia, fatigue, malaise, or lymphadenopathy, may be indicative of acute HIV infection, drug reaction, or another medical condition and should prompt a thorough clinical and laboratory evaluation. As ELISA results may be negative at the onset of acute illness, Western Blot (14), p24 (14), or PCR testing could be performed if HIV infection is suspected.

If the source individual is seronegative and has no clinical manifestations of AIDS or HIV infection, no further HIV follow-up of the exposed worker is necessary unless epidemiologic evidence suggests that the source individual may have been recently exposed to HIV or if testing is desired by the HCW or recommended by the health care provider. In these instances, the guidelines may be followed as described for those of the HIV-positive source. If the source individual cannot be identified, decisions regarding PEP should be individualized, based on factors such as exposure risk and whether potential sources are likely to include a person at increased risk of HIV infection (3,7,10). Those who receive PEP should be closely monitored for signs of drug-induced toxic effects.

COUNSELING

An occupational exposure will result in stress and should be recognized as part of the spectrum of morbidity in the HCW. Psychological reactions such as anger, denial, anxiety, depression, fear, sexual dysfunction, sleep disturbances, and psychosis have been reported as a result of occupational exposure (8,11). Initial counseling should focus on issues related to HIV testing as a routine component of post-exposure care. This may help diminish any negative reactions precipitated by the suggestion that the HCW seek counseling. The first counseling task should help workers cope with their reactions to the exposure by encouraging them to talk about the accident and express their feelings (15). Counseling should provide information available regarding PEP (7) and also assist in developing plans for coping with the possibility that the worker has been infected (15). During the follow-up period, especially for the first 6 to 12 weeks after the exposure when most infected persons are expected to seroconvert, exposed workers should be counseled regarding the importance of adhering to recommendations for preventing the HIV transmission. Recommendations include avoiding blood, semen, or organ donation, and abstaining or using measures to prevent HIV transmission during sexual intercourse (e.g., condom use, avoid exchange of body fluids, defer pregnancy). In addition, exposed women should not breastfeed infants during the follow-up period in order to prevent the infant's possible exposure to HIV in breast milk. Risk reduction counseling regarding preventing future occupational exposures should also be given. During all phases of follow-up, confidentiality of the worker's identification should be protected. The needs of third parties (e.g., sexual partners, family, friends, household contacts) affected by the exposure should also be addressed (8). Provision of supportive counseling by trained clinicians and access to consult experts skilled in crisis intervention and stress management are essential to a post-exposure program; these should be available when baseline results are given and on follow-up visits (8).

Documentation and Confidentiality

If an occupational exposure occurs, circumstances surrounding the exposure should be recorded in the worker's confidential medical record and the hospital epidemiologist should be notified. Relevant information includes: exposure history, details about counseling, post-exposure management, and follow-up. Maintaining confidentiality of the exposed worker is extremely important. Records of occupationally-exposed employees should be filed separately from patient records and routine employee health records and access to these records should be strictly controlled. The employee's name or other associated identifiers should not be sent with lab samples for HIV, HBV, and HCV tests; documentation by a number system rather than personal identifiers may be used (8,11). An anonymous system can also be used with pharmacy services, e.g., pharmacy personnel are only aware that an HCW is coming in for zidovudine and do not know the individual's name or any other information (11). The employee should be informed of the procedures used to ensure confidentiality and reassured that records will not be released without his/her consent.

Use of Antiretroviral Drugs

Although studies of HIV-infected patients have provided information regarding the potency and toxicity of antiretroviral drugs, it is uncertain to what extent these can be applied to uninfected persons receiving PEP (7). Combination therapy with the nucleosides ZDV and lamivudine (3TC) has greater antiretroviral activity than ZDV alone in HIV-infected patients, and is active against many ZDV-resistant HIV strains without significantly increased toxicity (16). There are greater increases in antiretroviral activity with the addition of a protease inhibitor; indinavir (IDV) is more potent than saquinavir at currently recommended doses among protease inhibitors, and appears to have fewer drug interactions and short-term adverse effects than ritonavir (16). There are little data that assess the possible long-term (i.e., delayed) toxicity resulting from the use of these drugs in persons uninfected with HIV (7).

ZDV PEP is usually tolerated well by HCW in currently recommended doses; short-term toxicity primarily includes gastrointestinal symptoms, fatigue, and headache, and is associated with higher doses (1,14). The toxicity of other antiretroviral drugs in persons uninfected with HIV has not been well characterized. The use of 3TC in HIV-infected persons can cause gastrointestinal symptoms and, rarely, pancreatitis. IDV toxicity includes gastrointestinal symptoms and, usually, after prolonged use, mild hyperbilirubinemia and kidney stones (16). The concurrent use of IDV and certain other drugs, including some nonsedating antihistamines, is contraindicated (7). Limited data have shown that the use of ZDV in the second and third trimesters of pregnancy and early infancy was not associated with serious adverse effects in mothers or infants; data are limited regarding the safety of ZDV during the first trimester of pregnancy or of other antiretroviral agents during pregnancy (7). The use of 3TC has been associated with pancreatitis in HIV-infected children (17,18), although it is not known whether 3TC causes fetal toxicity (16).

Although failures of ZDV PEP have occurred (1), a CDC retrospective case-control study of HCWs with a documented occupational percutaneous exposure to HIV-infected blood suggested that postexposure use of ZDV may be protective (4). After controlling for other factors associated with HIV transmission risk, the HIV risk among HCWs who used ZDV was reduced approximately 79% (4). This recent CDC study suggested that postexposure use of ZDV may be protective for HCWs prompted a PHS interagency working group with expert consultation to update its recommendations regarding the use of post-exposure antiretroviral therapy (4,7).

The PHS has made provisional recommendations regarding the use of PEP based on limited data regarding efficacy and toxicity of PEP and risk for HIV infection after different types of exposure; these are summarized below (7). At present, ZDV should be considered for all PEP regiments because ZDV is the only agent which data support the efficacy of PEP in the clinical setting since most occupational exposures to HIV do not result in transmission of the infection. Changes in drug regimens may be appropriate, based on factors such as probable antiretroviral drug resistance profile of HIV from the source patient; local availability of drugs; and medical conditions, concurrent drug therapy, and drug toxicity in the exposed worker (7). These recommendations were not developed to address nonoccupational (e.g. sexual) exposures.

PHS Recommendations Regarding Post-exposure Prophylaxis (PEP) for Occupational Exposures to HIV (7)

RISK OF HIV INFECTION FOLLOWING EXPOSURE

Factors that may increase or decrease the probability of HIV transmission after an occupational exposure should be assessed. Chemoprophylaxis should be recommended to exposed workers after occupational exposures are associated with the highest risk for HIV transmission. For exposures with a lower, but nonnegligible risk, PEP should be offered, balancing the lower risk against the use of drugs having uncertain efficacy and toxicity. For exposures with negligible risk, PEP is not justified (Table 8.10).

INTERVAL BETWEEN EXPOSURE AND INITIATION OF PROPHYLAXIS (IF GIVEN)

PEP should be initiated promptly, preferably within 1–2 hours postexposure (7). Although animal studies suggest that PEP probably is not effective when started later than 24–36 hours post-exposure (14,19) the interval after which there is no benefit from PEP for humans is undefined. Initiating therapy after a longer interval (e.g., 1–2 weeks) may be considered for the highest risk exposures; even if infection is not prevented, early treatment of acute HIV infection may be beneficial (20). The optimal duration of PEP is unknown; because 4 weeks of ZDV appeared protective (4), PEP should be administered for 4 weeks if tolerated. Since it is important to start administering PEP as soon as possible, the source patient status is not always known before initiation of prophylaxis (11). If the source patient or the patient's HIV status is unknown, initiating PEP should be decided on a case-by-case basis, based on the exposure risk and likelihood of HIV infection in known or possible source patients. If additional information becomes available, decisions can be modified regarding PEP (7).

COUNSELING AND FOLLOW-UP

Workers with occupational exposures to HIV should be informed that (a) the knowledge regarding the efficacy and toxicity of PEP is limited; (b) for agents other than ZDV, limited data exist concerning toxicity in persons without HIV infection or who are pregnant; and (c) any or all drugs for PEP may be declined by the exposed worker. Exposed workers should receive follow-up counseling and medical evaluation, including

Table 8.10.

Provisional PHS Recommendations for Chemoprophylaxis After Occupational Exposure to HIV, by Type of Exposure and Source Material—1996

Type of Exposure	Source Material[a]	Antiretroviral Prophylaxis[b]	Antiretroviral Regimen[c]
Percutaneous	Blood[d]		
	Highest risk	Recommend	ZDV plus 3TC plus IDV
	Increased risk	Recommend	ZDV plus 3TC, ± IDV[e]
	No increased risk	Offer	ZDV plus 3TC
	Fluid containing visible blood, other potentially infectious fluid,[f] or tissue	Offer	ZDV plus 3TC
	Other body fluid (e.g., urine)	Not offer	
Mucous membrane	Blood	Offer	ZDV plus 3TC, ± IDV[e]
	Fluid containing visible blood, other potentially infectious fluid,[f] or tissue	Offer	ZDV, ± 3TC
	Other body fluid (e.g., urine)	Not offer	
Skin, Increased risk[g]	Blood	Offer	ZDV plus 3TC, ± IDV[e]
	Fluid containing visible blood, other potentially infectious fluid,[f] or tissue	Offer	ZDV, ± 3TC
	Other body fluid (e.g., urine)	Not offer	

[a]Any exposure to concentrated HIV (e.g., in a research laboratory or production facility) is treated as percutaneous exposure to blood with highest risk.

[b]Recommend—Postexposure prophylaxis (PEP) should be recommended to the exposed worker with counseling. Offer—PEP should be offered to the exposed worker with counseling. Not offer—PEP should not be offered because these are not occupational exposures to HIV.

[c]See text for antiretroviral regimens.

[d]Highest risk—exposure to both larger volume of blood (e.g., deep injury with large diameter hollow needle previously in source patient's vein or artery, especially involving an injection of source-patient's blood) AND blood containing a high titer of HIV (e.g., source with acute retroviral illness or end-stage AIDS; viral load measurement may be considered, but its use in relation to PEP has not been evaluated). Increased risk—EITHER exposure to larger volume of blood OR to blood with a high titer of HIV. No increased risk—NEITHER exposure to larger volume of blood NOR blood with a high titer of HIV (e.g., solid suture needle injury from source patient with asymptomatic HIV infection).

[e]Possible toxicity of additional drug may not be warranted (see text).

[f]Potentially infectious fluids include semen; vaginal secretions; cerebrospinal, synovial, pleural, peritoneal, pericardial, and amniotic fluids.

[g]For skin, risk is increased for exposures involving a high titer of HIV, prolonged contact, an extensive area, or an area in which skin integrity is visibly compromised. For skin exposures without increased risk, the risk for drug toxicity outweighs the benefit of PEP.

Adapted from CDC Update: Provisional Public Health Service Recommendations for chemoprophylaxis after occupational exposure to HIV. MMWR 1996;45:22:468–472.

HIV-antibody tests at baseline and periodically for at least 6 months post-exposure (e.g., 6 weeks, 12 weeks, and 6 months), and should observe precautions to prevent possible secondary transmission (7). For HCWs who decide to initiate PEP, a written consent should be obtained (3). The consent document should reflect information presented in the counseling session, emphasizing the need for follow-up medical evaluations and taking precautions to prevent the transmission of HIV infection during the follow-up period. Those HCWs who decide to take PEP should be closely monitored for drug-toxicity. HCWs who become infected with HIV should receive appropriate medical care.

POST-EXPOSURE PROPHYLAXIS (PEP) REGIMENS AND FOLLOW-UP

ZDV should be considered for all PEP regimens because ZDV is the only agent for which data support the efficacy of PEP in the clinical setting. 3TC should usually be added to ZDV for increased antiretroviral activity and activity against many ZDV-resistant strains. A protease inhibitor (preferably IDV) should be added for exposures with the highest risk for HIV transmission (see Table 8.10). Adding a protease inhibitor may also be considered for lower risk exposures if ZDV-resistant strains are likely, although it is uncertain whether the potential additional toxicity of a third drug is justified for lower risk exposures. An HIV strain is more likely to be resistant to a specific antiretroviral agent if this is derived from a patient who has been exposed to the agent for a prolonged period of time (e.g., 6–12 months or longer). In general, resistance develops more readily in persons with more advanced HIV infection (e.g., CD4+ T-lymphocyte count of <200 cells/mm^3), reflecting the increasing rate of viral replication during later stages of the illness. For HIV strains resistant to both ZDV and 3TC or resistant to a protease inhibitor, or if these drugs are contraindicated or poorly tolerated, the optimal PEP regimen is uncertain; expert consultation is advised.

Antiretroviral regimens provisionally recommended by the PHS are shown in Table 8.10; regimen dosages are as follows:

- zidovudine (ZDV): 200 mg three times a day.
- lamivudine (3TC): 150 mg two times a day.
- indinavir (IDV): 800 mg three times a day (if IDV is unavailable, saquinavir may be used, 600 mg three times a day).

Prophylaxis should be given for 4 weeks. Refer to package inserts for full prescribing information.

If PEP is used, drug-toxicity monitoring should include a complete blood count and renal and hepatic chemical function tests at baseline and 2 weeks after starting PEP. If subjective or objective toxicity is noted, dose reduction or drug substitution should be considered with expert consultation, and further diagnostic studies may be indicated.

Information for Exposed Health Care Workers

- Concerning questions or information regarding occupational exposure, the State Occupational Safety and Health Administration (OSHA) Office or the CDC should be contacted. Telephone (404) 639-1547.

- Health care providers in the United States are encouraged to enroll all workers who receive PEP in an anonymous registry being developed by CDC, Glaxo Wellcome Inc., and Merck & Co., to assess toxicity. Telephone (888) 737-4448, (888) PEP-4HIV.

- Updated information about HIV PEP will be available beginning in early 1997 from the following sources:
  - Internet at CDC's home page: http://www.cdc.gov
  - CDC's FAX information service: telephone (404) 332-4565; Hospital Infections Program Directory: telephone (800) 458-5231.
  - National AIDS Clearinghouse: telephone (800) 458-5231.
  - HIV/AIDS Treatment Information service: telephone (800) 448-0440.

REFERENCES

1. Tokars JI, Marcus R, Culver DH, Schable CA, et al. Surveillance of HIV infection and zidovudine use among health care workers after occupational exposure to HIV-infected blood. Ann Intern Med 1993;118:913–919.
2. Jagger J, Hunt EH, Brand-Elnaggar J, Pearson RD. Rates of needlestick injury caused by various devices in a university. N Engl J Med 1988;319:284–288.
3. CDC. Public health service statement on management of occupational exposure to human immunodeficiency virus, including considerations regarding zidovudine postexposure use. MMWR 1990;39:(RR-1).
4. CDC. Case-control study of HIV seroconversion in health-care workers after percutaneous exposure to HIV-infected blood—France, United Kingdom, and United States, January 1988–August 1994. MMWR 1995;44:929–933.
5. Ho DD, Mougil T, Alam M. Quantification of HIV type in the blood of infected persons. N Engl J Med 1989;321:1621–1625.
6. Richman DD, Bozzette S. The impact of syncytium-inducing phenotype of human immunodeficiency virus on disease progression. J Infect Dis 1994;169:968–974.
7. CDC. Update: Provisional Public Health Service recommendations for chemoprophylaxis after occupational exposure to HIV. MMWR 1996;45:468-472.
8. Geberding JL, Henderson DK. Management of occupational exposures to bloodborne pathogens: hepatitis B virus, hepatitis C virus, and human immunodeficiency virus. Clin Infect Dis 1992;14:1179–1185.
9. Henderson DK, Fahey BJ, Willy M, et al. Risk for occupational transmission of human immunodeficiency virus type 1 (HIV-1) associated with clinical exposures. A prospective evaluation. Ann Intern Med 1990;113:740–746.
10. Goldschmidt RH. Current Report—HIV accidental exposure to HIV infection by health care workers. J Am Board Fam Pract 1990;3:129–131.
11. Fahrner R. Implementation of a hospital policy for health care workers exposed to hepatitis or the human immunodeficiency virus. Am J Hosp Pharm 1993;50:269–275.
12. Gerberding JL. Managing HIV exposure in health care settings. Focus 1990;5:1–2.
13. Henderson DK, Beekmann SE, Gerberding J. Post-exposure antiviral chemoprophylaxis following occupational exposure to the human immunodeficiency virus. AIDS Updates 1990;3:1–7.
14. Gerberding JL. Management of occupational exposures to blood-borne viruses. N Engl J Med 1995;332:444–451.
15. Dilley JW. Counseling health workers after accidental exposure. Focus 1990;5:3.
16. Marcus R, CDC Cooperative Needlestick Surveillance Group. Surveillance of health care workers exposed to blood from patients infected with the human immunodeficiency virus. N Engl J Med 1988;319:1118–1123.
17. Connor EM, Sperling RS, Gelber R, et al. Reduction of maternal-infant transmission of human immunodeficiency virus type 1 with zidovudine treatment. N Engl J Med 1994;331:1173–1180.
18. Connor EM, Sperling R, Shapiro D, et al. Long-term effect of zidovudine exposure among uninfected infants born to HIV-infected mothers in pediatric AIDS Clinical Trials Group protocol 076. In: Abstracts of the 35th interscience conference on antimicrobial agents and chemotherapy. Washington, DC: American Society for Microbiology, 1995;205.
19. Niu MT, Stein DS, Schnittman SM. Primary human immunodeficiency virus type 1 infection: review of pathogenesis and early treatment interventions in humans and animal retrovirus infections. J Infect Dis 1993;168:1490–1501.

20. Kinloch-de Loës S, Hirschel BJ, Hoen B, et al. A controlled trial of zidovudine in primary human immunodeficiency virus infection. N Engl J Med 1995;333:408–413.

Management of HIV-infected Health Care Workers

Health care workers (HCWs) with HIV infection are at increased risk of acquiring or having serious complications of infectious disease. There is the risk of severe infection following exposure to patients with infectious diseases that are easily transmitted if appropriate precautions are not taken (e.g., measles, varicella). Health care workers with impaired immune system should be counseled regarding the potential risk associated with caring of patients with any transmissible infection and should follow existing infection control recommendations to minimize risk of exposure to other infectious agents. Recommendations for vaccination requirements should be considered.

The risk of HIV transmission from an infected health care provider to a patient is extremely low. The risk of dying from HIV or HBV infection acquired during an invasive procedure performed by an infected surgeon has been estimated to be 2.4 to 24 deaths per million, similar to the risk of becoming HIV-infected from a transfused unit of screened blood (1). The Centers for Disease Control (CDC) have made the following recommendations regarding HIV-infected workers (2,3). Currently, available data provide no basis for recommendations to restrict the practice of HCWs infected with HIV or HBV who perform invasive procedures not identified as exposure-prone, provided the infected HCWs practice recommended surgical or dental technique and comply with universal precautions and current recommendations for sterilization/disinfection. The CDC recommends that HCWs who are infected with HIV or HBV (and are HBeAg positive) should not perform exposure-prone procedures unless they have sought counsel from an expert review panel and been advised under what circumstances, if any, they may continue to perform these procedures. Such circumstances would include notifying prospective patients of the HCW's seropositivity before they undergo exposure-prone invasive procedures. In practice, this negates their ability to do any exposure-prone procedure.

The review panel should include experts who represent a balanced perspective and might include all of the following: the HCW's personal physician(s); an infectious disease specialist with expertise in the epidemiology of HIV and HBV transmission; a health professional with expertise in the procedures performed by the HCW; and state or local public health official(s). If the HCW's practice is institutionally based, the expert review panel might also include a member of the infection-control committee, preferably the hospital epidemiologist. HCWs who perform exposure-prone procedures outside the hospital/institutional setting should seek advice from appropriate state and local public health officials regarding the review process. This panel of experts must recognize the importance of confidentiality and the privacy rights of infected HCWs.

Mandatory testing of HCWs for HIV antibody, HBsAg, or HBeAg is not recommended. The current assessment of the risk that infected HCWs will transmit HIV or HBV to patients during exposure-prone procedures does not support the resources required to implement mandatory testing programs. Compliance by HCWs with recommendations can be increased through education, training, and appropriate confidentiality safeguards.

HCW with HIV/HBV and whose practices are modified, should be provided opportunities to continue appropriate patient care activities whenever possible. Career counseling and job retraining should be encouraged to promote the continued use of the HCW's talents, knowledge, and skills. HCWs whose practices are modified because of HBV infection and are HBeAg-positive should be reevaluated periodically to determine whether their HBeAg status changes due to resolution of infection or as a result of treatment.

REFERENCES

1. Bell DM, Shapiro CN, Culver DH, Martone WJ, Curran JW, Hughes JM. Risk of hepatitis B and human immunodeficiency virus transmission to a patient from an infected surgeon due to percutaneous injury during an invasive procedure: estimates based on a model. Infect Agents Dis 1992;1:263–269.
2. CDC. Recommendations for preventing transmission of human immunodeficiency virus and hepatitis B virus to patients during exposure-prone invasive procedures. MMWR 1991;40:(RR-8).
3. CDC. Recommendations for prevention of HIV transmission in health care settings. MMWR 1987;36:2S.

CHAPTER 9

Risk Reduction and Prevention

Risk Reduction

Risk reduction strategies focus on initiating and sustaining behavior change that reduce a person's chance of acquiring or transmitting HIV. To provide focused risk reduction strategies, an individual's risk behaviors and the consistent practice of risk reduction behavior should first be assessed (see *Risk Assessment*). Guidelines regarding risk reduction approaches have been published (1–7).

Risk reduction strategies will be more relevant if they are tailored to each individual's behaviors, educational level, culture, race/ethnicity, age, social and economic background, personal circumstances, knowledge, skills, and desires. Information should be understandable, appropriate for each individual's educational level, age and culture; this requires the use of appropriate vocabulary, using slang, street or descriptive terms when necessary. Written materials should be given to reinforce all information. Counseling and discussion should be interactive, open, non-judgmental, and responsive to the individual's concerns and needs. Individuals should be encouraged to freely express their feeling as this is important in developing appropriate and personalized risk reduction goals and strategies.

Risk reduction should assist persons in making the most appropriate choices to reduce risk. This includes helping the individual accurately perceive his or her risk of acquiring or transmitting HIV, providing training in specific skills (e.g., negotiation, assertiveness) necessary to implement risk reduction behaviors, and help motivating individuals to use those skills (8). Assisting an individual in building and practicing learned skills (e.g., role playing) may help the individual develop solutions for specific or anticipated situations. Interventions directed at specific behaviors (e.g., always using a condom for vaginal sex with my primary partner, telling my partner to use a condom) may be more effective than those directed at broader behavioral categories (e.g., practicing safe sex, negotiating condom use) or at outcomes or goals (e.g., avoiding AIDS) (9).

Prevention goals and risk reduction strategies should be developed together with the individual to achieve behavior change. A realistic and incremental plan with specific steps or actions to reduce the individual's risk should be negotiated. Identify one or two behavior changes that the individual would be willing to make to reduce his/her risk and discuss how these changes could be implemented. There should be a focus on the barriers, difficulties, or circumstances which interfere with risk reduction efforts (past and present), as well as how these circumstances might be resolved or avoided (e.g., "What would make it easier for you to use a condom every time you have sex?") (6).

Because changing behavior is difficult and takes time, any positive actions taken should be recognized, praised, reinforced, and supported. Any previous actions taken to reduce risk (e.g., successful condom negotiation with a new sex partner) provides an opportunity for reinforcement and support of safe behavior choices.

It is important that the risk reduction plan be consistent with the individual's expressed or implied intentions to change behaviors, and the specific options available to the individual for reducing his/her risks outlined and discussed. The plan must be realistic and feasible, otherwise it will fail. Counseling should actively help the individual plan how risk reduction behaviors will be integrated into the context of his/her life.

Once the individual establishes safer behaviors, counseling should focus on maintaining safer behaviors to prevent relapse into unsafe practices.

REFERENCES

1. Breuer NL. A guide to self care for HIV infection, 2nd ed. Los Angeles: Los Angeles AIDS Project, 1993.
2. CDC. 1993 sexually transmitted diseases treatment guidelines. MMWR 1993;42(RR-1).
3. CDC. Technical guidance on HIV counseling. MMWR 1993;42(RR-2):11–17.
4. CDC. Recommendations for assisting in the prevention of perinatal transmission of human t-lymphotropic virus type III/lymphadenopathy-associated virus and acquired immunodeficiency syndrome. MMWR 1985;34:721–726,731–732.
5. Holman S, Sunderland A, Berthaud M, et al. Prenatal HIV counseling and testing. Clin OB & GYN 1989;32:334–455.
6. Kassler WJ, Wu AW. Addressing HIV infection in office practice. Primary Care 1992:19:19–33.
7. CDC. HIV counseling, testing and referral standards and guidelines. May 1994. US Dept of Health and Human Services.
8. Nolte S, Sohn MA, Koons B. Prevention of HIV infection in women. JOGNN 1993; 2:128–134.
9. Fishbein M. Developing effective interventions to reduce HIV transmission: lessons learned from behavioral research (abstr). Presented at IXth International Conference on AIDS. Berlin, June 1993:842.

Safer Sex

Reducing the risk of sexual transmission focuses on promoting safer sex behaviors. Safer sex is a term used to define those sexual practices which have a lower probability of HIV transmission from one sexual partner to another. HIV is found in semen, blood, and vaginal/cervical secretions. Although HIV has been documented in tears, saliva, and urine, the risk of HIV transmission appears to be lower with these body fluids. Safer sexual practices avoid the exchange of genital secretions and blood from one sexual partner to another. However, it is important to realize that although safer sex practices reduce the risk of HIV transmission, they do not eliminate the risk of transmission from one sex partner to another. Practices that are completely "safe" from HIV transmission are abstinence, and sexual intercourse between two mutually monogamous and uninfected partners. As long as the relationship is mutually monogamous, both partners are uninfected, and no other risk behaviors exist, there is no risk for HIV transmission. Lower risk activities are less clear, because they involve some risk of contact between mucous membranes and bodily fluids other than blood and semen. Safer sex guidelines have been published (1–7) and vary somewhat in the degree of risk attributed to certain behaviors; these are summarized below and in Table 9.1. *It is important to remember that sexual activities cannot be strictly categorized, but fall into a continuum of risk and depend on a number of factors:* presence of blood; whether a partner's semen or vaginal fluids enter the other partner's body; exposure of mucous membrane to potentially infectious blood, semen, vaginal fluids; and the presence of broken/torn skin or tissue. Because intimate behaviors are varied and

Table 9.1.
Safer Sex Guidelines

No risk
   Abstinence from sexual contact
   Monogamous relationship, both partners uninfected
   Voyeurism/sharing fantasies/phone sex
   Self-masturbation
   Masturbation with partner (intact skin, no cuts, lesions)
   Touching, massaging, hugging, stroking
   Dry kissing
   Use of own unshared sexual toys
Lower risk
   Deep (French) kissing
   Oral-genital contact with a condom or oral dam[a]
   Vaginal intercourse with condom (and water lubricant)[a]
   Anal intercourse with condom (and water lubricant)[a]
   Oral-anal contact ("rimming") with an oral dam[a]
   Water sports (urination on partner's intact skin)
Higher risk
   Vaginal/anal intercourse without a condom
   Oral-anal contact ("rimming") without an oral dam
   Oral-genital contact without a condom or oral dam
   Rectal douching in combination with anal sex
   Rectal fisting/rectal trauma followed by anal sex
   Urination on broken skin or inside body
   Sharing sex devices

[a]Condom/oral dam breakage or leakage would make this a higher risk activity.

unique to each relationship, the individual must decide where behaviors fall along the continuum of risk.

No Risk Activities

Activities which involve no contact between bodily fluids and mucous membranes or skin have no risk for HIV infection. Abstinence, hugging, social kissing, self-masturbation, massage, body rubbing, shared fantasies, and erotic talking are examples of behaviors that are considered to be "no risk" activities.

Contact between body fluids and intact skin is unlikely to cause infection. However, there is a theoretical risk of transmission in the presence of open lesions, or cuts in the mouth or skin. Case reports of HIV transmission via mucocutaneous contact with body fluids of HIV-infected persons indicate that infection is possible when there are breaks in the mucous membranes or skin. In this respect, mutual masturbation could pose a risk for HIV infection in the presence of cuts or open lesions unless condoms or gloves are worn.

Lower Risk Activities

Lower risk activities usually involve a barrier (e.g., condom, dental dam) between potentially infective blood or body fluids and mucous membranes. The degree of risk for many behaviors is uncertain since they have not been studied independently. However, these behaviors present a *theoretical* risk of transmission by mucous membrane contact with bodily fluids, particularly in the presence of broken skin, tears, or lesions. Some fluids (e.g., saliva, urine) may contain a low concentration of HIV and, although it is *possible* that these fluids may transmit the virus, that is much less likely (1,5,6,8). Options under lower risk activities include vaginal and anal (anal-genital) sex with condoms, oral-anal contact (rimming) with a dental dam, oral sex (fellatio and cunnilingus) with a condom or a dental dam, and French kissing (1,4–6,8).

ANAL/VAGINAL INTERCOURSE WITH A CONDOM

The use of latex condoms during anal or vaginal intercourse reduces the risk of HIV transmission (9). Latex condoms are an effective mechanical barrier to HIV, herpes simplex virus, hepatitis B virus, Chlamydia trachomatis, and Neisseria gonorrhea (9). Studies of couples discordant for HIV infection demonstrated that the consistent and correct use of condoms are highly effective in preventing HIV transmission (10,11). However, sex with a condom is not risk free. It is important that condoms are used correctly and consistently. If the condom breaks or leaks during sex, there is a risk of infection.

ORAL-GENITAL AND ORAL-ANAL SEX WITH A LATEX BARRIER

A latex barrier (i.e., condom, dental dam) is recommended for oral-genital (fellatio, cunnilingus) and oral-anal (rimming) contact. Unprotected oral sex on an infected male without ejaculation is not safe because seminal fluid (pre-ejaculatory fluid, "pre-cum") may contain virus (1,5). It is important that the latex barrier (condom, dam) is placed on the partner's penis, anus, or over the partner's vaginal area before there is any oral contact.

OTHER SEXUAL PRACTICES

If sexual practices involve urine (i.e., urination on or in the partner's body, "water sports"), it should not be allowed to enter the mouth, rectum, eyes, or contact any open cuts on the skin (5).

The role of deep or French kissing in HIV transmission has not been clarified. However, HIV has been isolated in low amounts from saliva, and transmission via microlesions in the oral mucosa from deep kissing is theoretically possible (3). Therefore, deep or French kissing is not considered risk free for HIV-discordant couples (12,13).

Higher Risk Activities

Sexual behaviors generally involve contact between blood, semen, vaginal secretions, or urine with a mucous membrane (e.g., linings of the rectum, vagina, mouth, urethra) have a higher risk of transmitting HIV. In addition, sexual practices causing tissue trauma, lacerations, or small fissures involving the rectum appear to facilitate HIV transmission (e.g., "fisting," anal sex) (4,6,14). There has been some evidence suggesting transmission can occur during oral contact with the genital or anal area (i.e., fellatio, cunnilingus, or anilingus without a latex barrier) (15–19). Limited information is available on sexual practices causing vaginal trauma and HIV transmission.

VAGINAL/ANAL SEX WITHOUT A CONDOM

Sexual intercourse with ejaculation and without a condom exposes the mucous lining of the vagina or rectum to potentially infected semen. During receptive anal intercourse, the rectal mucosa is particularly vulnerable to tearing and may facilitate entry of HIV into the blood stream. Although the receptive partner has the highest risk of HIV infection during unprotected rectal or vaginal intercourse, the insertive partner is also at risk. Unprotected anal or vaginal intercourse can expose the penis (urethra) of the insertive partner to potentially infected vaginal fluids or blood. Repeated unprotected intercourse, even between infected partners, is also considered unsafe as the repeated exposures possibly increases the viral load, and potentially introduces coinfection with other STDs (e.g., hepatitis) or more virulent strains of HIV. Unprotected intercourse should be considered only after both partners agree to be monogamous and do not have any other risk for HIV exposure (e.g., injection drug use). Both partners should undergo HIV testing and, if both are negative, they can consider having unprotected intercourse. However, in the event that either partner had behaviors or partners "at risk", HIV testing should be repeated 6 months after the last "at risk" behavior to insure that seroconversion does not occur (20). Until the results of the repeat test are known, only safer sex behaviors should be practiced during this interim.

ORAL-GENITAL CONTACT WITHOUT A CONDOM/ORAL DAM (FELLATIO, CUNNILINGUS)

HIV infection following oral-genital sex has been reported (15, 21–22). Although initially, little or no risk was associated with oral (orogenital) sex (23), it does appear to have a small risk, particularly for the receptive partner (14). A small risk has been associated with orogenital sex, with case reports implicating oral-genital contact as the source of HIV infection (14–19). Fellatio (oral contact with the penis and swallowing the semen) is a higher risk activity if the lining of the partner's mouth is exposed to semen (including pre-cum) (6,14). Since there is a possibility that virus is present in the semen and could enter the bloodstream via small tears in the lining of the mouth, stomach, or gastrointestinal tract, swallowing semen is considered unsafe. Cunnilingus (oral contact with a woman's genital areas) is also considered risky because vaginal and cervical secretions may contain virus.

ORAL-ANAL CONTACT WITHOUT AN ORAL DAM (RIMMING)

Rimming is considered to be a higher risk activity because blood may be present in the rectum or feces and may come in contact with the lining of the mouth. This poses a potential risk of infection, particularly to the receptive partner (5,6,24–26). As HIV-1 has been shown to be present in pre-ejaculatory fluid (27,28), oral-genital sex without intraoral ejaculation is probably not risk free. Although oral-anal activity has not been identified as an independent risk factor for HIV in studies concerning male-to-male transmission (29–31), oral-anal contact may be a marker for other high-risk behaviors (30).

RECTAL DOUCHING/RECTAL TRAUMA

Rectal douching (31–33) and fisting (penetration of the anus with the hand) (29,33) have been shown to increase the risk of HIV transmission during male-to-male sex. These types of practices may disrupt the mucosal barrier of the rectum, facilitating HIV entry into the bloodstream during subsequent exposure to infectious fluids. In one study, a greater degree of rectal trauma (i.e. use of enema; receptive fisting; evidence of scarring, fissure, or fistula during examination, and reported presence of blood in the rectum area) was associated with a higher risk for HIV infection (34).

Use of Barrier Protection

MALE CONDOMS

The U.S. Public Health Services currently recommends the use of latex condoms with or without spermicides (35). The consistent and proper use of latex condoms significantly reduces the risk of HIV transmission during sexual intercourse, although it does not provide 100% protection against HIV. Condom failure can occur (e.g., tearing, slipping off, leakage, improper usage), causing a risk of infection. Condom breakage usually occurs with inexperience and can be reduced with practice and after recognizing the likely causes for breakage. Since condom breakage is more common when the vagina is not well lubricated, the use of water-based lubricants and longer foreplay may be helpful. Condom efficacy may be influenced by type of intercourse; condom breakage has been shown to occur more frequently during anal rather than vaginal intercourse (8). Newer condoms have been designed for anal sex and are less likely to break than condoms designed for contraception (36).

Using two condoms with enough lubrication has also been suggested to decrease the risk of HIV transmission during anal sex (1). Since condoms are often used incorrectly, descriptive handouts might be helpful.

Most condom failures are due to inconsistent use, often from not having one when needed; therefore individuals should have condoms readily accessible (e.g., next to the bed). Recommendations regarding condom use have been published and are summarized in Table 9.2 (5,37,38). Because condom self-efficacy and attitudes towards condom use are important predictors of condom use, it is important not only to know how to use a condom correctly but to associate condoms with pleasure. Assisting individuals in developing skills which enhance the enjoyment of condoms may facilitate condom use (39).

Table 9.2.

Effective and Proper Condom Use

- Latex condoms should be used since natural skin (e.g., sheep skin) condoms may allow the passage of HIV.
- Condoms should not be used beyond their expiration date. Condoms in damaged packages or those that appear old (e.g., brittle, sticky, discolored) should not be used.
- Condoms should be stored in a cool, dry place out of direct sunlight. Condoms should not be stored in a hot glove compartment or carried in hip wallets for long periods of time since heat can damage the condom.
- A new condom should be used with each act of sexual intercourse.
- Condoms should be handled carefully to avoid damaging it with fingernails, teeth, or other sharp objects.
- The condom should be unrolled directly on the penis as soon as it is erect ("hard"), before the penis comes in contact with the vagina or the anus. Roll the condom all the way down to the base of the penis.
- When putting on a condom, pinch about one-half inch of the condom's tip to leave a small air-free space—this will collect the semen and prevent the condom from bursting upon ejaculation.
- The condom should fit snugly so that it does not slip off during intercourse. If needed, water-based lubricants should be used. Oil-based lubricants should not be used, since they weaken latex.
- After ejaculation, the penis should be withdrawn promptly from the vagina or rectum before the penis becomes soft. The rim of the condom should be held firmly against the base of the penis during withdrawal so that the condom cannot slip off and no semen escapes.
- If a condom breaks, it should be replaced immediately. If ejaculation occurs after the condom breaks, the immediate use of spermicide has been suggested, although its protective value post-ejaculatively is unknown.
- Condoms should be used only once; they should not be reused.

FEMALE CONDOMS

The female condom (marketed in the United States as the Reality™ condom) consists of a lubricated polyurethane pouch with a ring on each end. One ring (at the closed end of the pouch) is used to anchor the device internally; the other ring forms the external opening of the pouch and remains outside the vagina after insertion. During sex, the condom covers the labia and the base of the penis (40). The female condom has been shown to be an effective mechanical barrier against sexually transmitted diseases (STDs), including HIV, hepatitis B, and cytomegalovirus (36,40,41). The availability of female or vaginal condoms allow women more control in their own protection. Currently, the female condom is costly and may be prohibitive for most women. Female condoms are available in one size and intended for one-time use. It is not necessary to have it fitted by a health professional, and it does not need to be placed precisely over the cervix. Instructions regarding the correct usage of the female condom (40) are found in Table 9.3.

ORAL/DENTAL DAMS

The use of oral dams during oral-genital contact and oral-anal contact lowers the risk of HIV transmission by creating a barrier between bodily secretions and the partner's lips, tongue, and mouth lining. Oral dams

---

Table 9.3.
Using the Female (Reality™) Condom

- Insert the condom up to eight hours before intercourse (although in clinical trials, most people inserted it two to 20 minutes prior to intercourse)
- Although the condom is prelubricated, extra lubricant can be applied inside or outside the sheath.
- Squeeze the inner ring of the female condom and push it upward in the vagina as far as it can go (similar to a diaphragm).
- Using the index finger, check that the inner ring has been placed just past the pubic bone.
- The outer ring and approximately one inch of the sheath should remain outside the body, lying against the labia.
- Although the outer ring may move from side to side or the sheath may slip up and down inside the vagina during intercourse, this does not reduce protection.
- If the outer ring is pushed inside the vagina or if the penis can be felt underneath or beside the sheath, intercourse should be stopped, the device removed and relubricated, and then reinserted.
- Following intercourse, squeeze and twist the outer ring to keep the sperm inside the sheath. It should then be pulled out and discarded.

(a.k.a. dental dams from use in dental surgery) are sold in dental supply stores but may be expensive. Plastic wrap or a condom can be used as alternatives. The tip of an unlubricated condom can be cut off and then the condom cut lengthwise; it will unroll into a square of latex. Oral dams should be used only once.

Nonoxynol-9

Nonoxynol-9 is a spermicide which inactivates HIV and other sexually transmitted diseases (23,35). Although condoms are also recommended to be used in combination with spermicides (35), this is based on hypothetical considerations. The effectiveness of spermicides in the prevention of HIV transmission is unknown (35). Spermicides may reduce the risk of gonorrhea and chlamydia (42). However, there have been no reports which indicate that nonoxynol-9 used alone without condoms is effective in preventing HIV transmission during sexual intercourse nor that the use of nonoxynol-9 with a condom increases the protection against HIV infection provided by condom use alone (35). No data exist to substantiate the potential benefits of spermicides in preventing HIV transmission. It has been suggested that spermicides may potentially increase the risk of HIV transmission through irritation of the genital epithelium or rectal mucosa (43,44). The use of spermicides alone is inadequate to protect against HIV, and if used, should be used in combination with a condom.

Lubricants

Using lubricants with condoms may help avoid breakage of the condom or abrading body tissue. A water-based lubricant (e.g., surgical lubricants, K-Y Jelly, or diaphragm jelly) should be used. Oil-based lubricants (e.g., hand and body lotion, Vaseline, Crisco, butter, baby oil, vegetable oil, mineral oil, suntan lotion, petroleum jelly, massage oils) should never be used because they weaken the latex. A drop of lubricant should be placed inside the tip of the condom before it is put on the penis; too much lubricant inside the condom may result in condom slippage during intercourse. A generous amount of lubricant can be used on the outside of the condom.

Contraceptive Methods

It is important to discuss contraceptive methods in relation to HIV-risk reduction, because preventing pregnancy does not necessarily prevent HIV transmission. The use of oral contraceptives, and other non-barrier techniques (e.g., IUD) without barrier protection may result in the transmission of HIV. Sterilization does not provide any protection against HIV transmission. The use of a latex condom with or without spermicides provides the best protection against HIV transmission during sexual intercourse, however, pregnancies can occur if this is the sole birth control method. (See also *Contraceptive Methods and Effectiveness against HIV Infection.*)

Strategies for Sexually Active Persons

For sexually active individuals, it is essential to minimize the risk of HIV transmission to oneself as well as to others. Individuals should be assisted to identify their risks and to make appropriate choices for risk reduction. Realistic strategies should be developed together with the individual, discussing obstacles to risk reduction and feasible solutions which are consistent to the individual's intentions. Individuals should be supported in their commitment to practice and maintain safer behaviors. Aside from the provision of knowledge and skills, an individual's behavior choices and risk reduction steps should be reinforced. Specific risk reduction strategies for the sexually active person include decreasing the number of sexual partners, avoiding infected partners, practicing safer sex behaviors, using barrier methods correctly and consistently during sex, and avoiding alcohol and other substances that may impair judgment.

AVOID MULTIPLE AND INFECTED PARTNERS

Having multiple sexual partners has been associated with increased rates of HIV infection, particularly in areas with a high prevalence of HIV (4,20,30–32). The more sexual partners an individual has, the greater the probability of having contact with an HIV-infected person. Anonymous or casual sex should be eliminated or limited. Limiting sexual contact to one partner offers no protection if the partner is already HIV infected or has multiple partners. Individuals should be encouraged to choose their sexual partners carefully. Since many HIV-infected persons are asymptomatic and look healthy, partners should know about each other (i.e., sexual and drug history) before initiating sex. A partner who has had previous STDs, multiple sexual partners, used crack cocaine or injection drugs, or has lived or is living in geographic areas with high HIV prevalence may be at risk for HIV infection (20).

COMMIT TO SAFER SEX BEHAVIORS

Risk reduction should assist the individual in making informed decisions regarding sexual practices, particularly those that will minimize the risk for HIV infection. Individuals should be given information regarding: potentially risky sexual practices, factors associated with increased rates of HIV infection during sexual intercourse (e.g. receptive anal intercourse, having sex when either partner has genital ulcer disease, nonulcerative STDs, ulcerations, sores, or abrasions on the genitals, anus or mouth) (23,45); and the protection condoms provide against HIV infection and other STDs. Sex toys (dildos, vibrators, etc.) should not be shared and should be cleaned thoroughly with soap and water (5). Healthy behaviors should also be discussed: avoiding/limiting the use of alcohol and recreational drugs (particularly cocaine) since their use can lead to impaired judgment and unsafe behaviors; and when appropriate, obtaining family-planning assistance and early diagnosis and treatment of STDs (46). Strong predictors of condom use include prior successful attempts to use condoms, commitment to using condoms, verbal communication skills, and perceived sexual enjoyment (39,47–51). Therefore, risk reduction should also promote greater commitment to safer sex practices—discussing barriers to condom use and strategies to increase condom use, building sexual communication skills, and teaching how condoms can be a pleasurable part of sex. Condoms must be used correctly and consistently to be effective in preventing HIV infection. The importance of consistent condom use and maintaining this behavior should emphasized and reinforced.

PLAN FOR RISK REDUCTION (1,4,5,20)

Planning ahead for risk reduction may increase the commitment to use condoms, since an individual may be more emotionally prepared, carry condoms, and assert his or her intentions of having safer sex to a partner before any sexual involvement occurs. It might be necessary to teach persons new sexual scripts that include (52): (a) acknowledging that a new relationship may include sex or that sex may occur in unexpected circumstances, (b) preparing for sex even if the probability for occurrence is perceived to be low (e.g., always carrying a condom, defining self-limits), and (c) discussing safe sex and sexual limits with potential sex partners.

Before deciding to have sex, an individual should know his/her partner well and discuss risk reduction, preferably before sexual excitement interferes. Issues concerning sexual activity should be thought through well in advance to avoid impulsive decisions and to send clear and consistent messages to the partner. Risk reduction decisions should be made with partners; there should be agreement on practicing safe sex and on which types of sexual activities are acceptable to both partners. Social and negotiation skills training as well as role playing may be helpful.

For condoms to be effective, they must be used correctly and consistently. Condoms should be readily accessible if an individual is planning to have sex. When possible, situations which place an individual at risk (e.g., drinking alcohol) should be avoided and no decisions about sexual activity should be made while under the influence of alcohol and drugs.

REFERENCES

1. Breuer NL. A guide to self care for HIV Infection. 2nd ed. Los Angeles: Los Angeles AIDS Project, 1993
2. Holman S, Sunderland A, Berthaud M, et al. Prenatal HIV counseling and testing. Clin OB & GYN 1989;32:334–455.
3. Kassler WJ, Wu AW. Addressing HIV infection in office practice. Primary Care 1992; 19:19–33.
4. Raisler J. Safer sex for women. NAACOG's Clinical Issues in Perinatal and Woman's Health Nursing 1990;1:28–32.
5. Pinsky L, Douglas PH, Metroka C. The HIV treatment fact book. New York: Pocket Books, 1992:89–118.
6. Owen WF Jr. The clinical approach to the male homosexual patient. Med Clinics North America 1986;70:499–535.
7. Glasel M. High-risk sexual practices in the transmission of AIDS. In DeVita VT Jr, Hellman S, Rosenberg SA, eds. AIDS: Etiology, diagnosis, treatment, and prevention. Second edition. Philadelphia: JB Lippincott Co, 1988:355-367.
8. Nolte S, Sohn MA, Koons B. Prevention of HIV infection in women. J of Obstet Gynecol Neonatal Nursing 1993;2:128–134.
9. CDC. Update Barrier Protection Against HIV Infection and other Sexually Transmitted Diseases. 1993;42:589–591, 597.
10. Saracco A, Musicco M, Nicolosi A, Angarano G, Arici C, Gavazzeni G, et al. Man-to-woman sexual transmission of HIV: Longitudinal study of 343 steady partners of infected men. J Acquired Immune Deficiency Syndromes 1993;6:407–502
11. DeVincenzi I and the European Study Group on Heterosexual Transmission of HIV. Heterosexual Transmission of HIV in a European Cohort of Couples. IXth International conference on AIDS. Berlin, June 1993. (abs WSC02-1).
12. Wofsy C. Prevention of HIV transmission. In: Sande MA, Volberding PA, eds. The Medical Management of AIDS. Philadelphia: WB Saunders,1990:29–53.
13. Piazza M, Chirianni A, Picciotto L, et al. Passionate kissing and microlesions of the oral mucosa: possible role in AIDS transmission. JAMA. 1989;261:244–245.
14. Caceres CF, van Griensven GJP. Male homosexual transmission of HIV-1. AIDS 1994;8:1051–1061.
15. Lifson AR, O'Malley PM, Hessol NA, Buchbinder SP, Cannon L, Rutherford GW. HIV seroconversion in two homosexual men after receptive oral intercourse with ejaculation: implications for counseling concerning safe sexual practices. Am J Public Health 1990, 80:1509–1511.
16. Murray AB, Greenhouse PR, Nelson WL, Norman JE, Jeffries DJ, Anderson J. Coincident acquisition of *Neisseria gonorrhoeae* and HIV from fellatio [letter]. Lancet 1991;2:830
17. Lane HC, Holmberg SC, Jaffe HW. HIV seroconversion and oral intercourse [letter]. Am J Public Health 1991;81:658.
18. Goldberg DJ, Green ST, Kennedy DH, Emslie JAN, Black JD. HIV and orogenital transmission. Lancet 1988;2:1363.
19. Spitzer PG, Weiner NJ. Transmission of HIV infection from a woman to a man by oral sex. N Engl J Med 1989;320:251.
20. Peterman TA, Cates W, Wasserheit JN. Prevention of the sexual transmission of HIV. In: Devita VT, Hellman S, Rosenberg SA, eds. AIDS: etiology, diagnosis, treatment and prevention, 3rd ed. Philadelphia: JB Lippincott Co, 1992:443–451.
21. Marmor M, Ewiss LR, Lyden M, et al: Possible female-to-female transmission of human immunodeficiency virus. Ann Intern Med 1986;105:969.
22. Mayer KH, DeGruttola V: Human immunodeficiency virus and oral intercourse. Ann Intern Med 1987;107:428–429.

23. Kingsley LA, Detels R, Kaslow R, et al. Risk factors for seroconversion to human immunodeficiency virus among male homosexuals. Results from the Multicenter AIDS Cohort Study. Lancet 1987;1:345–349

24. Samuel M, Hesso N, Shiboski S, Engel R, Speed T, Winkelstein W. Factors associated with human immunodeficiency virus seroconversion in homosexual men in three San Francisco cohort studies, 1984–1989. J Acquir Immune Defic Syndr 1993;6:303–312

25. Keet IPM, Albrecht van Lent N, Sandfort TGM, Coutinho RA, van Griensven GJP. Orogenital sex and the transmission of HIV among homosexual men. AIDS 1992;6:223–226.

26. Keppman JS, Longini IM, Jacquez JA, et al. Assessing risk factors for transmission of infection. Am J Epidemiol 1991;133:1199–1209.

27. Ilaria G, Jacobs JL, Polsky B, et al. Detection of HIV-1 DNA sequences in pre-ejaculatory fluid. Lancet 1992;340:1469.

28. Pudney J, Oneta M, Mayer, Seaage G, Anderson D. Pre-ejaculatory fluid as a potential vector for sexual transmission of HIV-1. Lancet 1992;340:1470.

29. Jeffries E, Willoughby B, Boyko WJ, et al. The Vancouver Lymphadenopathy-AIDS Study: 2. Seroepidemiology of HTLV-III antibody. Can Med Assoc J 1985;132:1373–1377.

30. Darrow WW, Echenberg DF, Jaffe HW, et al. Risk factors for human immunodeficiency virus (HIV) infections in homosexual men. Am J Public Health 1987;77:479–483.

31. Moss AR, Osmond D, Bacchetti P, et al. Risk factors for AIDS and HIV seropositivity in homosexual men. Am J Epidmiol 1987;125:1035–1047.

32. Winkelstein W Jr, Lyman DM, Padian N, et al. Sexual practices and risk of infection by the human immunodeficiency virus. JAMA 1987;257:321–325.

33. Coates RA, Calzavar LM, Read SE, et al. Risk factors for HIV infection in male sexual contacts of men with AIDS or an AIDS-related condition. Am J Epidemiol 1988;128:729–739.

34. Chmiel JS, Detels R, Kaslow RA, et al. Factors associated with prevalent human immunodeficiency virus (HIV) infection in the Multicenter AIDS Cohort Study. Am J Epidemiol 1987;126:568–577.

35. CDC. Update: Barrier protection against HIV infection and other sexually transmitted diseases. MMWR 1993;42:589–591, 597.

36. Wigersma I, Oud R. Safety and acceptability of condoms for use by homosexual men as a prophylactic against transmission of HIV during anogenital sexual intercourse. Br Med J. 1987;295:94.

37. CDC. Condoms for prevention of sexually transmitted diseases. MMWR 1988;37:133–137.

38. CDC. 1993 sexually transmitted diseases treatment guidelines. MMWR 1993;42 (RR-1).

39. Malow RM, Corrigan SA, Cunningham SC, et al. Psychosocial factors associated with condom use among African-American drug abusers in treatment. AIDS Education and Prevention 1993;5:244–253.

40. Anastasi JK. What to tell patients about the female condom. Nursing 1993;23:71–73.

41. Drew WL, Blair M, Miner RC, Conant M. Evaluation of the virus permeability of a new condom for women. Sexually Transmitted Diseases 1990;17:110–112.

42. Cates W, Stone KM. Family planning, sexually transmitted diseases, and contraceptive choice: a literature update. Fam Plann Perspect 1992;24:75–84.

43. Jeffries DJ. Nonoxynol 9 and HIV infection. British Medical Journal 1988;296:1798.

44. Gollub EL, Stein Z. Nonoxynol-9 and the reduction of HIV transmission in women. AIDS 1992;6:559–601.

45. Cameron DW, Padian NS. Sexual transmission of HIV and the epidemiology of other sexually transmitted diseases. AIDS 1990;4(Suppl 1):S99–S103.

46. CDC. HIV Counseling, Testing and Referral Standards and Guidelines. May 1994. US Dept of Health and Human Services. Atlanta, Georgia

47. Catania JA, Coates TJ, Golden E, et al. Correlates of condom use among black, Hispanic, and white heterosexuals in San Francisco: The AMEN Longitudinal Survey. AIDS Educ Prev 1994;6:12–26.

48. Catania J, Coates TA, Kegeles S. et al. Condom use in multi-ethnic neighborhoods of San Francisco: The population-based AMEN (AIDS in Multi-Ethnic Neighborhoods) study. Am J Public Health 1992;82:284–287.

49. Catania J, Kegeles S, Coates T. Towards an understanding of risk behavior: an AIDS risk reduction model (ARRM). Health Education Quarterly 1990;17:381–399.

50. MacDonald N, Wells G, Fisher W, et al. High-risk STD/HIV behavior among college students. JAMA 1990;263:3155–3159.

51. Valdiserri R, Lyter D, Leviton L, Callahan C, Kingsley L, Rinaldo C. AIDS prevention in homosexual and bisexual men: results of a randomized trial evaluating two risk reduction interventions. AIDS 1989;3:21–26.
52. Fischer W. Understanding and preventing adolescent pregnancy and sexually transmissible disease/AIDS. In: Edwards J, ed. Applying social influence processes in preventing social problems. Beverly Hills: Plenum Press, 1989.

Contraceptive Methods and Effectiveness Against HIV

Discussing contraceptive methods in relation to HIV-risk reduction is important, because preventing pregnancy does not necessarily prevent HIV transmission. Contraceptive methods and their effectiveness in protecting against HIV are summarized below.

Male Condom

The use of latex condoms has been shown to substantially reduce the risk for HIV transmission among sero-discordant heterosexual couples (i.e., one partner is HIV positive, and the other is HIV negative) in several studies (1–5). The importance of consistent (i.e., using a condom with each act of intercourse) and correct condom use was emphasized in two studies of sero-discordant couples (3,4). In one study of sero-discordant couples, none of the 123 partners using condoms consistently seroconverted, while 12 (10%) of 122 seronegative partners who used condoms inconsistently became infected (3). Another study of sero-discordant couples, in which the male partners were HIV infected, three (2%) of 171 consistent condom users seroconverted, compared to eight (15%) of 55 inconsistent condom users (4). Considering person-years at risk, this correlated to a rate of HIV transmission among couples reporting consistent condom use at 1.1 per 100 person-years of observation, compared to 9.7 among inconsistent users (4). A study of discordant couples in which the female partner was seropositive, no seroconversions occurred in men using condoms during most or all intercourse (5).

An intact latex condom provides a mechanical barrier to HIV, HSV, hepatitis B virus, *Chlamydia trachomatis,* and *Neisseria gonorrhoea.* In addition, using latex condoms reduces the risk for sexual transmitted diseases (e.g., gonorrhea, herpes simplex virus infection, genital ulcers, and pelvic inflammatory disease) (1).

Natural-membrane condoms do not offer the same level of protection against sexually transmitted diseases (STDs) as latex condoms. Natural-membrane condoms have naturally occurring pores that are small enough to prevent passage of sperm but large enough to allow passage of viruses in laboratory studies (1).

Condoms are regulated as medical devices and subject to random sampling and testing by the Food and Drug Administration (FDA). Each latex condom manufactured in the United States is tested electronically for holes before packaging. Condom breakage rates during use are low in the United States (two or fewer per 100 condoms tested) (6). Studies have shown that with proper use, condoms are unlikely to break or slip (7). Reported breakage rates were reported to be 2% or less for vaginal or anal intercourse (1). Slippage of the condom during intercourse and during withdrawal was reported for 1 (0.4%) of 237 condoms in each instance (8). Condom failure usually results from inconsistent or incorrect use rather than condom breakage.

Data from the 1988 National Survey of Family Growth point out the importance of consistent and correct use of contraceptive methods in pregnancy prevention (9). The typical failure rate during the first year of male condom use was 15%, compared to 8% for oral contraceptives, and 26% for periodic abstinence. This compares to a 15% failure rate for people who consistently use male condoms, a 2% failure rate for women who always use oral contraceptives (0.1%), and a zero failure rate for those who always abstain (10).

Female Condom

A condom has been developed for use by women. The female condom is a lubricated polyurethane sheath with a ring on each end that is inserted in the vagina. Laboratory studies indicate that the female condom (Reality™) is an effective mechanical barrier to viruses, including HIV or other STDs (7). An evaluation of its effectiveness in preventing pregnancy was conducted during a six-month period for 147 women in the United States; the estimated 12-month failure rate for preventing pregnancies was 26%; for the 86 women who used this condom consistently and correctly, the estimated 12-month failure rate was 11%.

Vaginal Spermicides (Nonoxynol-9)

Nonoxynol-9 is a spermicide and has been shown to inactivate HIV and other sexually transmitted pathogens (7). Studies have demonstrated that among women, vaginal use of nonoxynol-9 without condoms reduced risk for gonorrhea; by 89% in one study, and 24% in another; it also reduced the risk of chlamydial infection by 22% in one study (1). However, spermicides have also been reported to cause vaginal irritation (11), and may facilitate HIV transmission by disrupting the vaginal mucosa. Whether the use of vaginal spermicides (i.e., film, gel suppositories; contraceptive foam has not been studied) alone without condoms is effective in preventing sexual transmission of HIV has not been established in human studies (6). No data exist which indicate that condoms lubricated with nonoxynol-9 are more effective against HIV infection and other STDs than by condom use alone (7). Therefore, use of latex condoms with or without spermicides are recommended (7).

Diaphragm

Women using the diaphragm alone as a contraceptive should not assume protection against HIV infection. Although diaphragm use has been shown to protect against cervical gonorrhea, chlamydia, and trichomoniasis in cross sectional and case-control studies, no cohort studies have been done. In addition, the portal of entry among women with gonorrhea and chlamydia usually involves the cervix, whereas HIV may infect women through the vagina or vulva, as well as the cervix (6).

Nonbarrier Methods of Contraception

Nonbarrier methods for contraception include hormonal contraception (oral contraceptives, Norplant™, Depo-Provera™), surgical sterilization, or hysterectomy. Nonbarrier contraceptive methods offer no protection against HIV or other STDs. Women who are using nonbarrier contraceptive methods may wrongly perceive themselves to be at no risk for HIV infection; they should be counseled regarding the use of condoms, safer sexual practices, and the risk for HIV (6).

There have been data which suggest the possible interaction of HIV disease and oral contraception, however current information appears to be insufficient to contraindicate oral contraceptives for HIV-seropositive women (12). Similarly, available information on longer-acting hormonal contraceptives (e.g., Norplant™, Depo-Provera™) has not suggested any risk in their use in women with HIV infection, although more data are needed. Oral contraceptives (OCs) have been shown to influence the pharmacokinetics of other drugs through their effect on protein-binding patterns and metabolism. There have also been reports of reduced efficacy of OCs in patients receiving antibiotic therapy. However, there are no interactions yet identified between zidovudine and OCs; only rifampin has been reported to interact with OCs (12).

The intrauterine device (IUD) is not recommended for HIV-infected women because it poses a potential risk of causing abrasions and may provide a port of entry for HIV. The woman may be more susceptible to ascending infections and pelvic inflammatory disease (PID) (13). The tail of the IUD may cause microabrasions on the head of the penis during intercourse, facilitating blood-to-blood contact. The IUD could also theoretically modify the course of other sexually transmitted infections (14).

Surgical sterilization is the most common contraceptive method for women over 30 years old in the U.S. and is used by 28% of women age 15 to 44 years old (15). It is also more common among women of color, and women who reside in low socioeconomic, inner city communities (15). In one study, more women who had been surgically sterilized reported never using condoms (78%) compared to nonsterilized women (46%) (16). Similar findings have been reported among sterilized women in drug treatment programs. This points to the importance of educational efforts regarding the importance of condom use in preventing STDs. Women planning surgical sterilization should be counseled before and after sterilization regarding the need for continued barrier protection.

REFERENCES

1. Cates W, Stone KM. Family planning, sexually transmitted diseases, and contraceptive choice: a literature update. Fam Plann Perspect 1992;24:75–84.

2. Weller SC. A meta-analysis of condom effectiveness in reducing sexually transmitted HIV. Soc Sci Med 1993;1635–1644.
3. DeVincenzi I. European Study Group on Heterosexual Transmission of HIV. Heterosexual transmission of HIV in a European cohort of couples. IXth International Conference on AIDS. 1993. (abstr. WE-CO2-1:83).
4. Saracco A, Musicco M, Nicolosi A, et al. Man-to-woman sexual transmission of HIV: longitudinal study of 343 steady partners of infected men. J Acquir Immune Defic Syndr 1993;6:497–502.
5. Nicolosi A, Musicco M, Saracco A, Lazzarin A. Insertive peno-anal intercourse is a risk factor in HIV female-to-male sexual transmission. IXth International Conference on AIDS. Berlin, June 1993. abstract PO-C11-2854:p693
6. CDC. 1993 Sexually Transmitted Diseases Treatment Guidelines. MMWR 1993;42(RR-1)
7. CDC. Update: Barrier Protection against HIV infection and other sexually transmitted diseases. MMWR 1993:42:589–591, 597.
8. Trussell JE, Warner DL, Hatcher R. Condom performance during vaginal intercourse: comparison of Trojan-Enz™ and Tactylon™ condoms. Contraception 1992;45:11–19.
9. Jones EF, Forrest JD. Contraceptive failure rates based on the 1988 NSFG. Fam Plann Perspect 1992;24:12–19.
10. Trussell J, Hatcher RA, Cates W, Stewart FH, Kost K. Contraceptive failure in the United States: an update. Stud Fam Plann 1990;21:51–54.
11. Peterman TA, Cates W, Wasserheit JN. Prevention of the Sexual Transmission of HIV. In Devita VT, Hellman S, Rosenberg SA(eds) AIDS: Etiology, Diagnosis, Treatment and Prevention, Third Edition. JB Lippincott Co; Philadelphia. 1992. 443–451.
12. Minkoff HL, DeHovitz JA. Care of women infected with the human immunodeficiency virus. JAMA 1991;266:2253–2258.
13. Senanayake P, Kramer DG. Contraception and the etiology of pelvic inflammatory disease: new perspectives. Am J Obstet Gyneol. 1980;138:852–860.
14. Nanda D, Minkoff HL. Pregnancy and women at risk for HIV infection. Primary Care 1992;19:157–169.
15. Mosher WD. Contraceptive practice in the United States, 1982–1988. Fam Plann Perspect 1990;22:198–205.
16. CDC. Surgical sterilization among women and use of condoms—Baltimore, 1989–1990. MMWR 1992;41:568–569,575.

Risk Reduction—Injecting Drug and Substance Use

All persons using drugs should be encouraged to restrict if not terminate their drug use. This may require enrollment in a drug treatment program. Unfortunately, there are not enough treatment programs to accommodate the majority of injection drug users (IDUs). In the interim, HIV risk reduction involves avoiding exposure to contaminated needles; avoiding shooting galleries; cleaning the skin; and consistently and thoroughly cleaning drug injection equipment ("works," "gimmicks," "sets," "rigs") if one re-uses injection equipment (1–6). Drug injection equipment includes needles and syringes, cookers, cotton, and the water used to mix drugs and rinse out syringes (6). Sterile needles and syringes are safer than bleach-disinfected, previously used needle and syringes. Needle and syringe exchange programs are a means of providing sterile equipment to IDUs and decreasing multiple persons using the same injection equipment. Bleach disinfection is to be used when never-used, sterile injection equipment is unavailable. However, due to the limitations in the availability of sterile needles and syringes, and of drug abuse treatment, adequate disinfection of equipment will likely continue to be important in HIV prevention efforts (7).

The client should be informed of the available drug treatment programs in the area, support groups, etc., and encouraged to enroll. For IDUs who are waiting to enter treatment programs or unable to stop using drugs, risk reduction should emphasize the following (5,6,8):

- Substance use by injection should be discouraged.

- Those who cannot stop injecting drugs should use sterile needles and syringes, ideally only once and then safely disposing of them. Avoid re-using equipment that has been previously used by someone else. Drug equipment including syringes, rubber bulbs, needles, cookers, and cotton should never be shared, passed along, or left behind.

- Injection equipment should not be bought or rented since it may have been used by someone else. If works are bought, they should be thoroughly disinfected before they are used.

- If works must be shared or re-used they should be thoroughly disinfected before and after each person uses them.

Disinfection of Needles and Syringe

Recent studies have cast doubt on the efficacy of bleach cleaning of needles and syringes under the method recommended since 1986. In this method, the needle and syringe are filled with full-strength bleach for a few seconds and flushed with water, and then the procedure is repeated (9). One study reported a 10% bleach solution was ineffective in removing blood from syringes when the solution was used in a six-second rinse followed by two six-second rinses with water; clotted blood was more difficult to remove than fresh blood (10). Full-strength household bleach has been shown to inactivate pelleted HIV after 30 seconds, but a 10% bleach solution only after 2 hours (11). Further studies which evaluated the efficacy of bleach to inactivate HIV-infected blood in needles and syringes also demonstrated that bleach concentration and exposure time were critical to HIV disinfection (12). Consistent with earlier findings, HIV was inactivated within 30 seconds of exposure to undiluted household bleach. To optimize the effects of disinfectants, it is important to flush out the blood and other debris in the syringe through mechanical cleaning (e.g., flushing with water) prior to disinfecting with bleach (13).

NEW RECOMMENDATIONS FOR EQUIPMENT STERILIZATION

New recommendations have been made to enhance the effectiveness of bleach disinfection when cleaning injection equipment were issued jointly by Centers for Disease Control (CDC), the Center for Substance Abuse Treatment (CSAT), and the National Institute on Drug Abuse (NIDA) in 1993 (14–16). The guidelines advocate extended bleach contact times. Inactivation of virus occurs when it is exposed to full-strength bleach for at least 30 seconds (11,12). To increase the exposure time, AIDS education programs now recommend (a) completing the old

Table 9.4.

Disinfecting Drug Injection Equipment

- Disinfect the equipment twice—once immediately after using it and again just before re-use.
- Before using bleach, wash out the needle and syringe by filling them three times with clean water (to reduce the amount of blood and other debris in the syringe). Presence of blood reduces the effectiveness of bleach.
- Use full-strength liquid household bleach (NOT diluted).
- Completely fill the needle and syringe with bleach at least three times. DO NOT RE-USE THE BLEACH. The syringe should be full with bleach for at least 30 seconds each time. The longer the syringe is full of bleach, the more likely HIV will be inactivated.
- After using bleach, rinse the syringe and needle at least three times with clean water. Do not re-use water used in the pre-bleach washing; it may be contaminated.
- Each time the needle and syringe are filled (with pre-wash water, bleach, and rinse water), fill the syringe completely to the top.
- Shaking and tapping the syringe are recommended when the syringe is filled with pre-bleach wash water, bleach, and rinse water. Shaking the syringe should improve the effectiveness of all steps.
- Taking the syringe apart (removing the plunger) may improve the cleaning/disinfection of parts (e.g., behind the plunger) that might not be reached by solution in the syringe.
- Never share rinse water or bleach.

Adapted from California Department of Health Services Office of AIDS. New guidelines on bleach disinfectant of needles and syringes. California HIV/AIDS update 1993;6(3):37–38.

bleach/water cycle five times instead of twice, or (b) filling the needle and syringe with full-strength bleach and then shaking or tapping the barrel of the syringe for 30 seconds (14,16,17). These recommendations with clarifications made by the California Health Department of Health Services Office on AIDS (14,16) are shown in Table 9.4.

The individual should be assisted to develop adequate techniques that enable thorough disinfection of the drug equipment. Compliance with the recommended procedure is necessary if it is to be effective in reducing HIV transmission among IDUs (12) and should be a focus for risk reduction efforts. Despite IDUs' being knowledgeable about basic element of bleach cleansing procedures in one study, compliance was demonstrated to be limited (18). More than 80% of IDUs who use bleach for disinfection have been reported to use it for less than 30 seconds (19). Individuals may need assistance in accurately "judging" the contact time (duration that bleach is inside the syringe). IDUs should be aware that the re-use or sharing of equipment carries a risk for transmitting HIV; consistent and thorough cleaning with disinfectants should reduce but may not eliminate the risk of HIV transmission (1,16,18–20).

Drugs, Alcohol, and Increased Risk Behaviors

Because of the occurrence of sexual and perinatal HIV transmission among IDUs and the association of unsafe sexual activity with crack use, risk reduction efforts for IDUs should also emphasize safer sex guidelines (e.g., condom use, reduction in number of sex partners) (21–24). The use of drugs or alcohol can impair judgment, leading to unprotected sex or sharing dirty needles. It should be explained that all drugs (e.g., heroin, crack, cocaine, alcohol, marijuana, "uppers," "downers") can place a person at risk for HIV. Suggestions which might help the individual include (25,26): deciding in advance the number of drinks he or she will have; switching to sparkling water, juices, or soft drinks after one alcoholic drink; and avoiding situations where drugs or alcohol might be a temptation. In addition, referral to self-help programs (Narcotics Anonymous, Alcoholics Anonymous) might be helpful.

REFERENCES

1. Marmor M, DesJarlais DC, Friedman et al. The epidemic of acquired immunodeficiency syndrome (AIDS) and suggestions for its control in drug abusers. J Subs Abuse Treat 1984;1:237–247.
2. Chaisson RE, Moss A, Onishi R, et al. Human immunodeficiency virus infection in heterosexual intravenous drug users in San Francisco. Am J Public Health 1987;77:169–171.
3. Sorensen JL, Wermuth LA, Gibson DR, Choi KH, Guydish JR, Batki SL. Preventing AIDS in Drug Users and their Sexual Partners. 1991. Guilford Press, New York.
4. Miller HG, Turner CF, Moses LE. AIDS: The Second Decade. 1990. National Academy Press, Washington, DC.
5. Brown BS, Beschner GM. Handbook on Risk of AIDS: Injection Drug Users and Sexual Partners. 1993. Greenwood Press, Westport, CT.
6. Haverkos HW, Jones TS. HIV, Drug-use paraphernalia, and bleach. J Acquir Immun Defic Synd 1994;7:741–742.
7. Watters, JK. Historical perspective on the use of bleach in HIV/AIDS prevention. J Acquir Immun Defic Synd 1994;7:743–746.
8. American Medical Association, Council on Scientific Affairs. Reducing transmission of human immunodeficiency virus (HIV) among and through intravenous drug abusers (Resolution 164, A-87). Chicago:AMA 1988.
9. Newmeyer J. Why bleach? Development of a strategy to combat HIV contagion among San Francisco intravenous drug users. In Battjes R, and Pickens RW, eds. Needle Sharing among Intravenous Drug Users: National and International Perspectives. Rockville, MD: National Institute on Drug Abuse, 1988;151–159.
10. Contoreggi C, Jones SW, Simpson PM, Lange WR, Meyer WA. A model of syringe disinfection as measured by polymerase chain reaction for human leukocyte antigena and HIV genome. Presented at the Eighth International Conference on AIDS 1992 (abstr PC-4280) Amsterdam.
11. Shapshak P, McCoy CB, Rivers JE, et al. Inactivation of human immunodeficiency virus-1 at short time intervals using undiluted bleach. J Aquir Immune Defic Syndr 1993;6:218–219.
12. Shapshak P, McCoy CB, Shah SM, et al. Preliminary laboratory studies of inactivation of HIV-1 in needles and syringes containing infected blood using undiluted household bleach. J Acquir Immun Defic Syndr 1994;7:754–759.
13. Vlahov D, Astemborski J, Solomon L, Nelson KE. Field effectiveness of needle disinfection among injecting drug users. J Aquir Immune Defic Syndr 1994;7:7660–7666.
14. California Department of Health Services Office of AIDS. New guidelines on bleach disinfection of needles and syringes. California HIV/AIDS Update. 1993;6(3):37–38.
15. CDC. Use of bleach for disinfection of drug injection equipment. MMWR 1993;42:418–419.
16. Curran JW, Scheckel LW, Milstein RA. HIV/AIDS prevention bulletin. Rockville, MD: Centers for Disease Control, Center for Substance Abuse Treatment, and National Institute on Drug Abuse, April 19, 1993.
17. Watters J, Jones TS, Shapshak P, et al. Household bleach as disinfectant for use by injecting drug users. Lancet 1993;342:742–743.
18. McCoy CB, Rivers JE, McCoy HV, Shapshak P, Weatherby NL, Chitwood DD, Page JB, Inciardi JA, McBride DC. Compliance to bleach disinfection protocols among injecting drug users in Miami. J Aquir Immune Defic Syndr 1994;7:773–776.
19. Gleghorn AA, Doherty MC, Vlahov D, Celentano DD, Jones TS. Inadequate bleach contact times during syringe cleaning among injection drug users. J Aquir Immune Defic Syndr 1994;7:767–772.
20. Millstein RA. NIDA community alert bulletin. Rockville, MD: National Institute on Drug Abuse, March 25, 1993.

21. CDC. Update: Reducing HIV transmission in intravenous-drug users not in drug treatment—United States. MMWR 1990;39:529,535–538.
22. CDC. Update: Acquired immunodeficiency syndrome associated with intravenous drug use—United States, 1988. MMWR 1989;38:165–170.
23. Schoenfisch S, Ellerbrock T, Harrington P et al. Risk of HIV infection and behavioral changes associated with crack cocaine use in prenatal patients. (abstr) Presented at the Ninth International Conference on AIDS. Berlin June 1993. (PO-C15-2920).
24. Longshore D, Anglin MD. Number of sex partners and crack cocaine use. Is crack an independent marker for HIV risk? Journal of Drug Issues 1995;25:1–15.
25. Breuer NL. A Guide to Self Care for HIV Infection, Second Edition. 1993. AIDS Project Los Angeles; Los Angeles.
26. Leigh BC, Stall R. Substance use and risky sexual behavior for exposure to HIV. Am Psychologist 1993;48:1035–1045.

Prevention Considerations and Approaches

In the absence of a cure or vaccine for HIV infection, the prevention and education remain the primary strategies against HIV transmission. However, it has been shown that knowledge alone does not determine behavioral change. To develop successful AIDS prevention programs, a greater understanding of factors which determine risk-taking as well as preventive behaviors is needed. Interventions should also address the socio-environmental influences on preventive behaviors and the beliefs of individuals (i.e., beliefs about norms, values, and self-efficacy). Cultural attitudes may influence sexual behaviors, injecting practices, and gender roles, affecting the effectiveness of an intervention. Educational materials cannot always be simply translated for different populations; the content may not be appropriate for populations where education, terminology, and cultural attitudes differ. Different population segments have different educational needs, requiring input from members of targeted population to develop sensitive, relevant, language appropriate, and effective programs and materials (1).

In addition, once behavioral change has been adopted, there may be difficulty in maintaining these changes, resulting in the relapse into unsafe sexual or drug injecting practices. It has been suggested that the kind of motivation necessary to initiate behavior change differs from that to maintain behavioral change (2). A mix of techniques may be needed to encourage both the adoption of and long-term adherence to risk reduction behaviors (2). Prevention efforts, therefore, must consider not only communicating knowledge effectively and understandably, but consider the factors which motivate and maintain behavioral change, and assist in developing skills necessary to carry out such changes. Methods for prevention can be varied and innovative to best suit the targeted audience; role playing, skill-provision training, individual and group approaches, peer outreach and counseling, social activities, novellas, video, and plays are examples of intervention methods utilized.

Several theoretical models have been used to help understand behavioral risk reduction and to serve as an approach for prevention programs. These include the health belief model (3) which proposes that an individual is more likely to adopt actions to avoid a disease if s/he believes that they are personally susceptible to it; that the consequences of having the disease would be severe; and that taking preventive actions would be beneficial and outweigh the barriers. According to social cognitive theory (4), the appraisal of one's self-competence (i.e., self-efficacy) relative to preventive behaviors creates the self-confidence necessary to carry out these behaviors. A model of social influence based on the reference group hypothesizes that there is an interaction between behavioral norms (beliefs how people typically act) and values (beliefs about how people should act), generating a normative standard to which persons aspire to conform (5). This normative standard influences the adoption and maintenance of preventive behaviors.

The Ajzen-Fishbein model (AFM) addresses the relationship of attitudes and behaviors, proposing that the intention to perform a specific act is a function of the attitude toward the act (e.g., condom use provides less satisfying sex), the "subjective (perceived) norm" of that act, and the motivation to comply (6).

Behavioral research findings have suggested that intention, ability, and the presence or absence of environmental constraints are necessary and sufficient to predict a given behavior (7). Additional variables which may also explain variation in a given intention include attitudes, norms, self-standards, emotional reactions, and self-efficacy (7). The relative importance of these variables in determining behavior will vary from behavior to behavior and between populations. It is therefore important that interventions are behavioral and population specific, culturally relevant, and focus on variables that serve as the primary determinants in a given population (7).

Until a vaccine or cure is developed for HIV infection, prevention and education are the most promising strategies to prevent HIV transmission. Developing effective educational and prevention programs requires an understanding of the diversity of populations, and the factors which may motivate and facilitate behavioral change.

REFERENCES

1. Report of the Presidential Commission on the Human Immunodeficiency Virus Epidemic. Washington D.C.: 1988 (June 24)
2. Stall R, Ekstrand M. Implications of relapse from safe sex. Focus 1989;4:3.
3. Becker M. The health belief model and personal health behavior. Health Educ Monogr. 1974;2(special issue).
4. Bandura A. Social Foundations of Thought and Action: A Social Cognitive Theory. Englewood cliffs, NJ: Prentice-Hall; 1986.
5. Fisher JD. Possible effects of reference group-based social influence on AIDS—risk behavior and AIDS prevention. Am Psychol 1988;43:914–920.
6. Zimmerman RS, Olson K. AIDS-related risk behavior and behavior change in a sexually active, heterosexual sample: a test of three models of prevention. AIDS Educ and Prev 1995;6:189–205.
7. Fishbein M. Developing effective interventions to reduce HIV transmission: lessons learned from behavioral research. (abstr) Presented at IXth International Conference on AIDS. Berlin June 1993. PO-D13-3748.

Men Who Have Sex with Men

Homosexual and bisexual men may live in a variety of social structures; they may be celibate, married to or have a relationship with a woman, be involved in a monogamous relationship with one man, involved in sexually open relationships with another man, or have a series of encounters without a primary relationship (1,2). Men who have sex with men (MSM) consist of many subcultures and sexual identities: a) men who identify themselves as homosexual/bisexual; b) men who identify as heterosexuals but who have sex with men and women; and c) gay/bisexual males who are closeted. Gay and bisexual men may be geographically isolated with little access to gay-sensitive AIDS prevention services or peer support, or have other risk factors for AIDS (e.g., drug use, heterosexual contact with an injecting drug user). Moreover, there is also a diversity of culture, social norms, and support networks among gay and bisexual men. To be effective, prevention programs for men engaging in same-sex activities must consider the age, social, behavioral and cultural characteristics of each population and their impact on behavior.

Epidemiological Trends

Although the majority of cumulative AIDS cases are attributed to male-male sexual contact, the proportion of reported AIDS cases in homosexual and bisexual men has been declining. During 1981–1987, male-male sexual contact accounted for 64% of AIDS cases in the United States, decreasing 45% during 1994 to October 1995 (3). AIDS cases attributed to male-male contact have been relatively stable in the Northeastern United States for several years but increasing in other regions, particularly in the South (4). A steady decline in the seroconversion rate among homosexual and bisexual men has also been observed (5–9) and has corresponded with a decline in risky sexual behaviors (7,9,10).

Although preventive sexual behaviors have been adopted among homosexual and bisexual men, risk behaviors continue to be practiced. Homosexual men in small cities outside the epicenters, as well as young gay and bisexual men have reported high rates of at-risk behaviors (11–14). Recent surveys of homosexual and bisexual men in the United States have also shown a relapse from safer sex to riskier practices, i.e., those who stopped anal sex and started again (12,15–19). There has also been a trend in the type of HIV risk from a large number of partners to that with steady sexual partners (10); homosexual men have reported lower rates of condom use with steady partners than with casual partners (20,21). Using the estimated incidence of AIDS-defining opportunistic illnesses (AIDS-OIs), the CDC evaluated trends in AIDS incidence in the U.S. from 1989 to June 1994 (22). Although the level of increase in AIDS cases among MSM is smaller than earlier in the epidemic, rates of AIDS-OIs continue to increase among MSM (22). From 1989 to mid-1994, AIDS-OIs rates increased 31%, from 12.1 to 15.9 cases per 100,000 males 13 years of age and older (22). Rates of increase varied by geographic region with the greatest increase found in the Midwest (49%) and the South (51%), and smaller increases in the West (21%) and Northeast (13%) (22). In addition, rural areas (i.e., population less than 50,000) and areas with populations of 50,000 to 1 million demonstrated the highest percentage increase. Rates of increase also varied by race and ethnicity, with highest increases reported among African-American (79%) and Latin-American (61%) men (22).

Risk Profile

Sexual risk factors for HIV transmission among men who have sex with men include unprotected anal sex and multiple sex partners, particularly anonymous ones (22,23). Unprotected anal intercourse presents a greater risk of HIV transmission to the receptive partner than to the insertive partner (23–26). Other factors associated with HIV infection among homosexual men have been rectal trauma, history of sexually transmitted disease (STD) and gonorrhea, use of nitrates ("poppers"), history of hepatitis B, heavy drinking, use of cocaine, and younger age (25,27–29). Recent evidence has also suggested a small risk of HIV transmission associated with receptive oral sex (28,30,31).

Although gay men who continue to practice high-risk behaviors (i.e., unprotected anal intercourse with multiple partners or partners of unknown serostatus) generally have high factual knowledge of risk behaviors, many have been unknowledgeable about the appropriate types of condoms and lubricants (32). Unprotected anal intercourse has been associated with low self-efficacy, low sexual impulse control, low condom commitment, riskier perceived norms, and poor communication skills (33). Inconsistent or noncondom use has also been associated with greater pleasure of sexual activity (12,34). Although knowledge of HIV status has been associated with reducing risk behaviors, it has also been associated with reduced condom use among partners with identical serostatus (21,35). AIDS incidence has been also correlated with socioeconomic status, including level of education, employment status, and income (36).

Once adopting safer health behaviors, individuals may lapse to unsafe sexual behaviors (12,15,17–19,37). Among homosexual and bisexual men, predictors of relapse to unprotected anal intercourse have been associated with younger age (18,37,38); history of high-risk sexual behaviors (18); having a primary sex partner (38); being bisexual (38); and having sex under the influence of alcohol or drugs (18,38,39). In one study among homosexual men, safer sex behaviors were maintained for a median of 30 months before relapse to unsafe behaviors (i.e., unprotected insertive or receptive anal intercourse) (40). Homosexual men who were younger, HIV infected, and used poppers were more likely to lapse from safer behaviors sooner (40).

ALCOHOL AND DRUG USE

Men who have sex with men and inject drugs (MSM IDUs) constitute 25% of cumulative AIDS cases through mid-1995 in the United States (41). HIV infection rates of 54% and 24% have been reported for behaviorally homosexual and bisexual male injection drug users, respectively (42).

The use of alcohol and drug has been associated with unsafe behaviors (29,33,39,43,44). Substance use can indirectly result in unsafe sex by disinhibiting sexual restraints, affecting risk perception and impairing the social skills necessary to negotiate safer sex (40,44). It may also lead to the exchange of sex to finance drug use (45). A high prevalence of risky drug injection and sexual practices was reported among MSM IDUs in one study including recent sharing of injection equipment, trading sex for money or drugs, engaging in anal sex, and having multiple sex partners (46). Eighty-six percent of MSM IDUs reported sharing drug equipment when preparing or injecting drugs, with less than one-third using bleach to clean their needle or syringe the last time they shared injection equipment (46). Frequency of alcohol and drug use among gay and bisexual youth has been related to a greater number of male sexual partners and engaging in oral or anal sex (29). Combining alcohol or drug use with sex is more likely to result in high-risk sexual behaviors (43,47,48). Gay men engaging in unprotected anal sex were more likely to drink heavily before sex and perceive sex as better after drinking (43). Rates of unprotected anal intercourse among gay and bisexual men in substance-abuse treatment are higher compared to a community-based cohort of gay and bisexual males (49). Substance abusing gay men who have a pattern of alcohol and drug use in conjunction with sex may find the idea of "sober sex" to be discomforting (49).

AGE

Young MSM continue to be at risk for HIV infection. HIV seroprevalence among MSM aged 18–23 years in San Francisco was 4.8% during 1992–1993 (50) and, 9% among MSM aged 18–24 years in New York City (51). The overall rates of new HIV infections among MSM in San Francisco and New York City during the same time period were 1.2% and 2%, respectively (50,51). Geographic patterns of AIDS trends also indicate that a greater proportion of cases among adolescent and young adult (aged 13–29 years) MSM are occurring in small (50,000–499,999 population) metropolitan statistical areas (MSAs) and rural areas in the South (25%) and the Midwest (21%) (3). Recent surveys have reported HIV seroprevalence among young homosexual and bisexual men in the San Francisco areas to be 9.4% to 11% (52,53). Young gay men, even those who are HIV seropositive for (54) report levels of emotional distress and self-esteem similar to the norms for their heterosexual peers. Youths exhibit many positive coping styles, and continue to have romantic relationships. However, young gay HIV-positive youths report frequent stressful life events, primarily the death/illness of friends and violent crimes, and their social support networks often include people who engage in sexual- and substance abuse-acts.

In one survey, 70% of young HIV-infected homosexual/bisexual men (17 to 22 years old) did not know they were HIV seropositive and only 23% were receiving medical care (53). Adolescent gay and bisexual youths are at risk for HIV for several reasons. Sexual partners of adolescent gay/bisexual youth may include gay adult males (55), a group with a high prevalence of AIDS. In addition, younger gay males engage in more sexual risk behaviors than older gay men (12,29). Among gay and bisexual male youth in one study, condom use was inconsistent, typically initiated one year after sexual activity began (with both male and female partners), more common with male than female partners, and used more often during anal sex than oral sex (29). Over half of adolescent gay and bisexual male adolescents in one survey reported a history of unprotected anal intercourse and/or injection drug use, despite demonstrating accurate knowledge and beliefs about HIV (56). Unprotected sex among these youths was associated with substance abuse, having a steady partner, noncommunication with partners about risk reduction, frequent intercourse and perceiving they were likely to acquire HIV (56).

Compared to heterosexual male youths, substance use is higher among homosexual/bisexual male youths (29). Homeless and runaway adolescents may be especially at risk. One study reported 90% of homeless runaway youth were sexually active, 82% used alcohol or other drugs, and 25% exchanged sex for money, food, clothes or a place to stay (57). Moreover, because gay adolescent males may not identify with the gay community, they may not be exposed to HIV prevention (58).

Unlike their heterosexual peers, many young men who are attracted to other men face extreme social pressures to deny or reject that attraction. Not only do they face the possibility of verbal abuse and discrimination, but also the chance of rejection by friends and family, or being violently attacked (gay-bashed) (59–61). For adolescents, the stress related to the process of "coming out," or acknowledging and accepting homosexual feelings in oneself and then disclosing it to others, has been positively correlated to unprotected oral and anal sex, suicide attempts, and alcohol and drug use (62). Unlike many adults, young people generally lack personal resources (e.g., financial independence), have few or no positive role models, and have less developed coping abilities, therefore making the coming-out process more stressful, which possibly leads to these problem behaviors.

BISEXUAL MALES

It has been estimated that 14% of all men with AIDS in the United States are bisexual (63). Although homosexual and bisexual men are often grouped together, HIV risk behaviors have been reported to differ between men reporting exclusively homosexual activity and those reporting bisexual activity (63–65). Among men with AIDS, bisexual men were more likely than homosexual men to report injection drug use (63,65,66) and to have received money for sex (65). In one study, bisexuals who inject drugs report higher rates of prostitution, and half the bi-sexual men engaging in prostitution report noncondom use with their clients (65).

Sexual identity does not necessarily predict sexual behavior. Men who have sex with men or both men and women may conceal their sexual orientation or may not self-identify as bisexual or homosexual (66). In a survey of injection drug users in San Francisco, almost half of the behaviorally bisexual males identified themselves as heterosexual (42). In a survey of MSM IDUs from three U.S. cities, nearly two-thirds self-identified as bisexual, 33% as heterosexual, and 5% as homosexual (46). Risk behaviors may also vary by self-identification. Men who are behaviorally sexual or homosexual but do not self-identify as such report higher risk behaviors than self-identified homosexual and bisexual men (67,68). In another study, MSM but self-identified as being bisexual or heterosexual were more likely to use injection drugs, have a substantial HIV seroprevalence and to report more female partners than men who self-identified as being homosexual (68). Another survey demonstrated that among men who had anal sex with men, lower rates of condom use were reported for men who self-identified as being heterosexual compared to self-identified homosexual or bisexual men (67). Prevention efforts which focus on perceived sexual identity may miss men who are married or who are not connected to the homosexual/bisexual culture.

Men who are behaviorally bisexual may not disclose this behavior to their female partners, placing them also at risk. Married men who had sex with men were less likely than unmarried men to inform their partner of their behavior (69). Preliminary data linking AIDS surveillance and death certificate information revealed that 3% of homosexual men and 24% of bisexual men with AIDS were currently married (63). Consequently, many women may be unaware of their partner's bisexual behavior (63,70).

AFRICAN-AMERICAN AND LATIN-AMERICAN MEN

Male-male sexual contact is the most frequently reported mode of HIV exposure among African-American and Latin-American men with AIDS, accounting for 40% and 45% of cases through mid-1995, respectively (41). 1989–1994 trends in AIDS among MSM reveal rates of AIDS-OIs increased disproportionately among African- and Latin-Americans compared to Whites (22). Higher HIV seroprevalence rates also reflect the racial and ethnic disparities among gay and bisexual men. Among homosexual/bisexual men in a cohort study, HIV-seroprevalence was significantly higher among African-American (47%) and Latin-American (50%) than White (35%) men (71). Similarly, among men visiting STD clinics who reported male-male sex, HIV seroprevalence was higher for African-Americans (median 43.6%) than for white men (median 23.2%) (72). Higher HIV seroprevalence rates have also been reported among minority youths compared to their White counterparts (53,73). AIDS and HIV seroprevalence rates among Latin-Americans in the U.S. vary by geographical region and place of birth (74–76). Among

1994 AIDS cases reported among Latin-Americans in the United States, male-to-male sexual contact accounted for 36% of those born in the United States; 53% of those born in Central/South America; 60% of those born in Mexico; and 17% of those born in Puerto Rico (77).

African-American and Latin-American homosexual/bisexual men are also more likely to report other risk behaviors (e.g., injection drug use [IDU], heterosexual contact with an IDU) compared to white homosexual/bisexual males (78). A greater proportion of homosexual/bisexual African and Latin Americans also report unsafe anal sex practices (13,71,79,80) as well as a history of STD (71). Among men with AIDS who report male-male sex, ethnic minority males are significantly younger and more likely to also report sex with a female and injection drug use than whites (81). Among gay and bisexual youth, African-Americans initiate intercourse at an earlier age (29) and have a higher prevalence of unprotected anal intercourse (79) than other ethnic/racial groups. Furthermore, among men with AIDS who report male-male sex, African- and Latin-Americans report higher rates of bisexual activity (63,66,82). In one study, 22% of bisexual Latin American men with AIDS in one study were married (65). Higher rates of bisexuality reported among African-American men have also been reported by others (66,82). This higher rate of bisexual activity also places ethnic/racial women at risk. Among women with AIDS in 1989, the rate of AIDS due to sexual contact with a bisexual man was three and five times higher for Latin-American and African-American women, respectively, than for white women (63).

Cultural aspects, country of origin, as well as the degree of acculturation may also play a role in sexual behavior for persons born outside the United States. Cultural differences exist in the definition of "homosexuality" and gay identity (83,84). For example, many Mexican men who practice the insertive role in male-to-male sex and who also have sex with women, view themselves as heterosexuals (85). Studies in Mexico have reported up to 30% of men age 15–25 years old engage in bisexual activity (85). Increased acculturation is associated with increased flexibility about sexual roles and adoption of Anglo cultural patterns (85). Latin Americans who have not lived long in the U.S. are less likely to be acculturated and may demonstrate behavior patterns similar to their country of origin (65). Among men with AIDS in one study, the highest proportion of bisexual activity was reported by Latin Americans, especially those born outside the U.S. (primarily Mexico) and living in the U.S. less than 10 years (65). Of men with AIDS born in the U.S., African-Americans reported a higher rate of bisexual behavior compared to whites and Latin-Americans (65). It has been suggested that African-American men may adopt a bisexual lifestyle because of the negative attitudes toward homosexuality in the African-American community (86).

SOCIAL CONTENT

Lifestyle and social influences may also play a role in behaviors. Gay males frequenting bars may have a higher lifestyle risk, as higher rates of unprotected anal sex with nonmonogamous partners are reported, compared to community samples of gay men (33). Men in steady relationships may also be at increased risk. Lower rates of consistent condom use among homosexual men have been reported with primary partners rather than with one-time/occasional partners (20–21). Having sex in a steady relationship has been found to be a consistent predictor of unprotected oral and anal sex among homosexual men (80). Behaviors within primary partnerships may be based on knowledge of HIV serostatus (87,88). It has been found that 74% of HIV-positive youths disclose their serostatus to their sexual partners (89). Persons in steady relationships may believe that their sexual activities are safe, even though the relationships are often not mutually monogamous and the partners may not have similar HIV infection status (80). Also influential on behavior is peer support; there are strong associations between risk behavior levels and perception of peer acceptability of condom use (14,90). High risk behaviors have been associated with the perception that among friends, safer sex was unacceptable and condoms were not always used (32). Conversely, gay male substance abusers who had only protected anal intercourse were more likely to perceive safe sex as the community norm, and receive encouragement from friends to practice safe sex (91).

Prevention Strategies

Health care providers and public health practitioners are increasingly endorsing routine counseling and antibody testing for HIV (92), particularly for those who engage in high-risk acts (93). However, it is unclear at this time how effective HIV testing is as a prevention strategy (94, 95). Nationally, testing is not occurring at a high rate, even though it is believed that early detection of HIV is beneficial to the individual and society (96,97). Knowing that one is HIV-positive may permit better medical management of HIV disease (e.g., prophylactic treatment for opportunistic infections, monitoring health status), provide an opportunity for reducing perinatal transmission, and promote adoption of safer sexual and drug-use practices in order to reduce the risk of future HIV transmission (98,99). While HIV testing hypothetically provides these benefits, is is unclear whether individuals change their behaviors in response to the testing (35,100).

In a study of 272 adolescents recruited from community-based agencies that serve high-risk youths in AIDS epicenters, almost two-thirds had been tested for HIV (97). Unfortunately, most also apeared to be continuing to engage in sexual and substance abuse acts that place them at risk for HIV. Youths who engaged in HIV-related risk acts, both sexual and injecting drug use, were those most likely to be tested and retested for HIV. Those who perceived themselves at risk and, in fact, were at risk, continued to be tested for HIV over time. It appears that when youths engage in multiple high-risk acts and test negative for HIV multiple times, they may be reinforced for unrealistic and misinformed attributions for their negative test. The test result may serve to reinforce risky behavior patterns rather than serve as a motivator for changing risk acts. It is critical that future strategies for HIV testing examine strategies for focusing testing on person at risk.

Behavioral change and the decline in the incidence of HIV have been well documented among the homosexual community. Among homosexual and bisexual men, prevention efforts have been associated with a reported decrease in the number of sex partners and unprotected anal sex (101–103), increased condom use for insertive anal sex (103,104), increased overall condom use (33,103), and a steady decline in the seroconversion rate among homosexual and bisexual men (6,9). Prevention efforts have been directed towards lifestyle risk characterized by unprotected sex and multiple partners, especially anonymous ones. There has been an emphasis in personal responsibility and protection of partners, discouraging at-risk behaviors and encouraging the adoption of preventive measures. Sexual behavior change has been correlated with education and knowledge about AIDS, adequacy of social support, peer norms regarding AIDS and sexual behavior, affective states, alcohol and drug use, perceived risk of AIDS, and expectations concerning the difficulty and effectiveness of efforts to avoid HIV infection (105–107). Demographic, socioeconomic variables and past sexual behavior patterns have also been reported to be strong predictors of observed behavior change (108). Bartering sex is a key factor in maintaining high-risk behavior among young MSM (29).

Emphasizing the high risks associated with unprotected anal intercourse in HIV transmission (26) as well as believing that safer sex reduces risk is considered an important element of motivating risk reduction behavior (109). However, education should also include provision of safer sex skills, enhancing confidence in practicing those skills (i.e., perceived self-efficacy), and promoting and developing peer and social support which encourages HIV risk reduction (91,104,109–114).

This involves not only providing basic skills for condom use and proper choice of lubricants but the ability to discuss sex and condom use with sex partners. Condom use among male homosexuals has been associated with greater assertiveness in negotiating condom use (112, 115,116). Negotiating safer sex skills is especially important for men who have sex with occasional and one-time partners. Skill provision should also be directed towards men who engage in receptive anal intercourse (21). Men should have the perceived self-efficacy to practice safer sex behaviors in difficult situations (e.g., under the influence of drugs, alcohol) (109–111). As greater pleasure of unprotected sexual activity is associated with inconsistent or noncondom use (12,34), it is important to assist men in developing sexual communication skills and teaching how condoms can be a pleasurable part of sex. Risk reduction should also assist individuals to control impulses. Interventions should consider the personality types of men; men with assertive communication styles may have more success in changing condom-use behavior with partners than men with unassertive personalities (21). Among those populations where perceived risk is not associated with adoption of safer behaviors, skills should be directed to eroticize condoms to enhance their use, increase the perception that condoms can prevent disease, and modify norms about condom use (79). Because men may have multiple risks for HIV infection (e.g., injection drug use, bisexual activity, commercial sex), each risk behavior should be addressed. Prevention efforts should address both drug-related and sexual risk factors particularly for MSM IDUs. It is important that HIV-prevention activities are culturally appropriate when addressing ethnic/racial populations.

The differences between sexual identity and sexual behavior should be considered in prevention and counseling. Because some MSM will not self-identify as homosexual or bisexual, risk assessment for HIV infection and prevention efforts should focus on behaviors (having sex with a man) regardless of self-identification. For men who do not self-identify as homosexual, a variety of settings may be necessary to implement interventions as messages that appear to be directed towards homosexual men may be ignored or resisted. Interventions for bisexual men may require different strategies than those involved in exclusive homosexual behavior and should consider the female partner (sexual roles, venues for coed socializing) in prevention strategies (79).

HIV prevention may be enhanced by strategies or programs which introduce new behavioral standards and social norms that encourage the avoidance of high-risk activities and the adoption of risk reduction practices (117). The use of structural interventions are generally effective, e.g., only safe sex clubs. Using peer outreach and group methods may maximize the social influence, facilitating the redefinition of social norms that support safer behaviors. The expectation and acceptance of safer sexual behaviors as social norm may encourage their adoption in practice (117).

Special Considerations for Prevention

SUBSTANCE ABUSE

Among substance-abusing gay and bisexual men, abstinence from alcohol and drugs appears to be important in reducing sexual-risk behaviors (49). Decreasing drug use has been paralleled with a decline in unprotected anal intercourse (118). Gay and bisexual men recovering from alcohol or drug abuse may be vulnerable to drug relapse, especially if there is an association between substance use and sex (49). Interventions will need to address not only preventing drug usage but breaking the pattern of sex and drugs among this population (49). Gay and bisexual men who use alcohol or drugs in sexual situations must learn how to have "sober sex" (49). Gay and bisexual males with substance abuse histories will need follow-up support and skill reinforcement. Assistance in developing skills such as personal efficacy (i.e., raising self-esteem, ability to cope with a given situation or problem), social skills (e.g., assertiveness skills, stress and anger management), and social support is especially important (119–121).

MEN WITH PRIMARY PARTNERS

Although condom use among male homosexuals has been associated with having more than one sexual partner (12,115), condom use is more often practiced outside the primary relationship (20,21). Interventions should therefore focus on preventing transmission between steady partners, promoting safer sexual behavior within the primary relationship. Condom use messages should target sexual behavior within primary relationships where partners do not know their HIV status, partners are discordant for HIV infection, or one or more partners engage in other at-risk activities (e.g., needle sharing, multiple sex partners).

YOUTH

For gay and bisexual youth, early interventions appear to be critical (before the age of 12) (29). A youth's history of sexual behaviors and abstinence appears to be a strong predictor of current HIV risk acts and number of sexual partners (101). Prevention programs should not only focus on preventing unprotected anal intercourse, but also address heterosexual behaviors and the consistent use of condoms during oral and vaginal intercourse. The adolescent should be assisted to cope in stressful situations, to identify personal cues and triggers which place him at risk, and to practice behavior-coping responses to such situations (101). Strategies might include decision-making exercises, communication and negotiation skills, peer counseling and discussions, and promoting "norms" supportive of condom use.

MAINTENANCE OF SAFE BEHAVIORS

Prevention programs must also address the maintenance of safer behaviors. Motivating behavior change may be different than those to maintain changes, and interventions should differentiate between adoption of and long-term adherence of safer-sex practices. Relapse from safe to unsafer sex behaviors (e.g., unprotected anal sex) has been associated with individual motivation, attitudes and normative beliefs (122), younger age (18,38), use of poppers (amyl nitrates) (40,118), use of cocaine (29) and history of high-risk behaviors and intoxication preceding sex (18). Individuals should also be assisted to control their impulses and develop social support which encourages a safer sex lifestyle (91). Supporting the individual's personal decision-making process and having outcomes which agree with the individual's preference may improve motivation in maintaining safe behaviors (122). Follow-up interventions should reinforce prevention messages, skill provision training, and the self-confidence of men who have made positive behavior changes. Relapse prevention efforts should be focused on younger men (38,40), men with primary partners (38), bisexuals (38), HIV-infected homosexual men (40), men who use poppers (40), and persons who have sex under the influence of drugs and alcohol (38).

INTERVENTION DESIGN

The diversity of populations, lifestyle and associated risk behaviors should be considered when designing interventions. For example, as higher risk-taking behaviors among gay male bar patrons have been reported (32), programs for men who frequent bars should focus on communication skills, safer sex commitment, and high risk situations (33). For hard-to-reach populations, interventions should be innovative. The use of a risk-reduction counseling group via telephone (toll free) has been used for closeted and/or geographically isolated gay and bisexual males (123). Peer-run community mobilization prevention programs have been shown to decrease rates of unsafe sex (i.e., unprotected anal intercourse) among young gay and bisexual men (96,102,124). Social and outreach events (project center drop-in, dance parties, bar outreach) have been effective in reaching the young (124), and safe-sex workshops have increased encouragement of safe sex among participants with their friends (124). To be effective, prevention programs must consider the full range of behaviors that place individuals at risk, but also consider the cultural differences, community norms, and the social network among men involved in same-sex activity.

REFERENCES

1. Owen, WF. The clinical approach the male homosexual patient. Medical Clinics of North America. 1986;70:499–535.
2. Roffman R, Ryan R, Downey L, Beadnell B. A telephone group intervention can overcome barriers to enrolling isolated gay and bisexual males in AIDS risk-reduction counseling. Presented at the IXth International Conference on AIDS. Berlin, June 1993 (abstr PO-C23-3166).
3. CDC. First 500,00 AIDS Cases—United States. MMWR 1995:44:849–853.
4. Centers for Disease Control. Update: Acquired immunodeficiency syndrome—United States, 1991. MMWR;1992;41:463–468.
5. Weinstock HS, Sidhu J, Gwinn M, Karon J, Petersen LR. Trends in HIV seroprevalence among persons attending sexually transmitted disease clinics in the United States, 1988–1992. J Acquir Immune Defic Syndr Hum Retrovirol 1995;9:514–522.
6. Kellogg TA, Reardon J, Ruiz J, et al. Trends in HIV-1 seroprevalence among gay and bisexual men in the San Francisco Bay area. Presented at IXth International Conference of AIDS. Berlin, June 1993 (abstr PO-C12-2882).
7. Winkelstein W, Wiley JA, Padian NS, et al. The San Francisco Men's Health Study: Continued decline in HIV seroconversion rates among homosexual/bisexual men. Am J Public Health 1988;78:1472–1474.
8. Hoover DR, Munoz A, Carey V, Chmiel JS, Taylor JMG, Margolick JB, et al. Estimating the 1978–1990 and future spread of human immunodeficiency virus type 1 in subgroups of homosexual men. Am J Epidemiol 1991;134:1190–1205.
9. Winkelstein W Jr., Wiley JA, Padian NS, et al. The San Francisco Men's Health Study: III. Reduction in human immunodeficiency virus transmission among homosexual/bisexual men, 1982–1986. Am J Public Health 1987;77:685–689.
10. Coutinho RA, van Griensven GJP, Moss A. Effects of preventive efforts among homosexual men. AIDS 1989;3:S53–S56.
11. Dean L, Meyer I. Rates of unprotected anal and oral sex in a cohort of young gay men in New York City, 1990–1991. Presented at the IXth International Conference of AIDS. Berlin, June 1993 (abstr PO-C12-2884).
12. Hays RB, Kegeles SM, Coates TJ. High HIV risk taking among young gay men. AIDS 1990; 4:901–907.
13. Hirozawa AM, Givertz D, Lemp G, et al. Prevalence of HIV-1 among young gay and bisexual men in San Francisco and Berkeley, CA: The second young men's survey.

Presented at the IX International Conference of AIDS. Berlin, June 1993 (abstr PO-C12-2875).

14. Kelly JA, Lawrence JS, Brasfield TL, Stevenson LY, Diaz Y, Hauth AC. AIDS risk behavior patterns among gay men in small southern cities. Am J Public Health 1990; 80:416–418.

15. Stall R, Ekstrand M, Pollack L, McKusick L, Coates TJ. Relapse from safer sex: the next challenge for AIDS prevention efforts. J Acquir Immune Defic Syndr 1990;3: 1181–1187.

16. Dean L, Gallaher P. Trends in sexual behavior practices of a panel of New York City Gay Men:1981–1991. Presented at the IXth International Conference of AIDS. Berlin, June 1993 (abstract PO-D06-3603)

17. Adib SM, Joseph HG, Ostrow DG, Tal M, Schwartz SA. Relapse in sexual behavior among homosexual men: a 2 year follow-up from the Chicago MACS/CCS. AIDS 1991;5:757–760.

18. Kelly KA., Lawrence JS, Brasfield TL. Predictors of vulnerability to AIDS risk behavior relapse. J Consult Clinic Psychol 1991;59:163–166.

19. McCusker J, Stoddard AM, McDonald M, Zapka JG, Mayer KH. Maintenance of behavioral change in a cohort of homosexually active men. AIDS 1992;6:861–868.

20. Stall RD, Coates TJ, Hoff C. Behavioral risk reduction for HIV infection among gay and bisexual men: a review of results from the United States. Am Psychol 1988; 43:878–885.

21. CDC. Changes in sexual behavior and condom use associated with a risk-reduction program—Denver, 1988–1991. MMWR 1992;41:412–415.

22. CDC. Update: Trends in AIDS among men who have sex with men—United States, 1989–1994. 1995;44:401–404

23. Moss AR, Osmond DH, Bacchetti PB, et al. Risk factors for AIDS and HIV seropositivity in homosexual men. Am J Epidmiol 1987;125:1035–1047

24. Winkelstein W Jr, Lyman DM, Padian N, et al. Sexual practices and risk of infection by the AIDS-associated retrovirus. The San Francisco Men's Health Study. JAMA 1987;257:321–325.

25. Darrow WW, Echenberg DF, Jaffe HW, et al. Risk factors for human immunodeficiency virus infections in homosexual men. Am J Public Health 1987;77:479–483.

26. Detels R, English P, Visscher BR, et al. Seroconversion, sexual activity and condom use among 2915 seronegative men followed for up to 2 years. J Acquir Immune Defic Syndr , 1989:2:77–83.

27. Chmiel JS, Detels R, Kaslow RA, Van Raden M, Kingsley LA, Brookmeyer R. Factors associated with prevalent human immunodeficiency virus (HIV) infection in the Multicenter AIDS Cohort Study. Am J Epidemiol 1987;126:2167–2172.

28. Cecares CF, van Griensven GJP. Male homosexual transmission of HIV-1. AIDS 1994; 8:1051–1061.

29. Rotheram-Borus MJ, Rosario M, Heino FL, Meyer-Bahlburg, Koopman C, Dopkins SC, Davies M. Sexual and substance use acts of gay and bisexual male adolescents in New York City. J Sex Research 1994;31:47–57.

30. Samuel M, Hessol N, Shiboski S et al. Factors associated with human immunodeficiency virus seroconversion in homosexual men in three San Francisco cohort studies, 1984–1989. J Acquir Immune Defic Syndr 1993;6:303–312.

31. Keet IPM, Albrecht van Lent N, Sanfort TEM, et al. Orogenital sex and the transmission of HIV among homosexual men. AIDS 1992;6:223–226.

32. Bahr GR, Sikkema KJ, Kelly JA, et al. Attitudes and characteristics of gay men who remain at continued risk for contracting HIV infection. Presented at the IXth International Conference on AIDS. Berlin, June 1993 (abstr PO-C12-2880).

33. Ekstrand ML, Stall R, McKusick L, et al. Two worlds of risk-gay male bar patrons need special AIDS prevention interventions. Presented at the IXth International Conference on AIDS. Berlin, June 1993 (abstr WS-D07-3).

34. McKusick L, Coates TJ, Morin SF et al. Longitudinal predictors of reductions in unprotected anal intercourse among gay men in San Francisco: The AIDS behavioral research project. Am J Public Health 1990;80:978–983.

35. Higgins DL, Galavotti C, O'Reilly KR, et al. Evidence for the effects of HIV antibody counseling and testing on risk behaviors. JAMA 1991;266:2419–2429.

36. Hu DJ, Frey R, Costa S, et al. AIDS rates and sociodemographic variables in the Newark, New Jersey, metropolitan area. Presented at the IXth International Conference on AIDS. Berlin, 1993 (abstr WS-C04-2).

37. Ekstrand ML, Coates TJ. Maintenance of safer sexual behaviors and predictors of

risky sex. The San Francisco Men's Health Study. Am J Public Health 1990; 180: 973–977.

38. Valleroy L, O'Reilly K, Rolfs R. Predictors of lapse to unprotected anal intercourse in a cohort of homosexual and bisexual men in the USA. Presented at the IXth International Conference on AIDS. Berlin, June 1993 (abstr POC23-3170).

39. Stall R, McKusick L, Wiley J, et al. Alcohol and drug use during sexual acitivity and compliance with safe sex guidelines for AIDS: The AIDS behavioral research project. Health Education Quarterly 1986;13:359–371.

40. de Witt JBF, van Griensven GJP. Time from safer to unsafe sexual behavior among homosexual men. AIDS 1994;8:123–126.

41. Centers for Disease Control. HIV/AIDS Surveillance Report. 1995 Mid-year edition; 1995;7 (1). CDC:Atlanta, GA

42. Lewis DK, Watters JK. Sexual behavior and sexual identity in male injection drug users. J Acquir Immune Defic Syndr 1994;7:190–198.

43. Hauth AC, Perry MJ, Solomon LJ, et al. Alcohol use is strongly associated with continued risky sex among gay men: risk behavior patterns and alcohol-sex attributions. Presented at the IXth International Conference on AIDS. Berlin, June 1993 (abstr PO C23).

44. Siegel K, Mesagno FP, Chen J, Christ G. Factors distinguishing homosexual males practicing risky and safer sex. Social Science in Medicine 1989;6:561–569.

45. Fullilove R, Fullilove M, Bowser B, Gross S. Risk of sexually transmitted disease among Black adolescent crack users in Oakland and San Francisco, Calif. JAMA 1990;263:851–855.

46. CDC. HIV Risk Practices of Male Injecting-Drug Users who have sex with men. MMWR 1995;44:767–769.

47. Robertson J, Plant M. Alcohol, sex and risk of HIV infection. Drug and Alcohol Dependence 1988; 22:75–78.

48. Stall R, Ostrow D. Intravenous drug use, the combination of drugs and sexual activity and HIV infection among gay and bisexual men: The San Francisco Men's Health Study. Journal of Drug Issues 1989;19:57–73.

49. Paul JP, Stall R, Davis F. Sexual Risk for HIV Transmission among gay/bisexual men in substance-abuse treatment. AIDS Education and Prevention 1993;5:11–24.

50. Osmond DH, Page K, Wiley J, et al. HIV infection in homosexual and bisexual men 18 to 29 years of age: the San Francisco young men's health study. Am J Public Health 1994;84:1993–1997.

51. Dean L, Meyer I. HIV prevalence and sexual behavior in a cohort of New York City gay men (aged 18–24). J Acquir Immune Defic Syndr 1995;8:208–211.

52. Winkelstein JR, Wiley JA, Osmond D, Coates T, Sheppard HW, Page K, et al. The San Francisco Young Men's Health Study. Presented at the IX International Conference on AIDS, Berlin, June 1993. (abs WS-CO-73).

53. Lemp GF, Hirozawa AM, Givertz D, Nieri GN, Anderson L, Lindegren ML, et al. Seroprevalence of HIV and risk behaviors among young homosexual and bisexual men. The San Francisco/Berkeley Young Men's Survey. JAMA 1994;272:449–454.

54. Rotheram-Borus MJ, Murphy DA, Reid HM, Coleman C. Correlates of emotional distress among HIV+ youths: health status, stress, and personal resources. Annals of Behavioral Medicine In press.

55. Remafedi G. Adolescent homosexuality: Psychosocial and medical implications. Pediatrics 1987;79:331–337.

56. Remafedi G. Predictors of unprotected intercourse among gay and bisexual youth: knowledge, beliefs, and behavior. Pediatrics 1994; 94:163–168.

57. Cohen E, Mackenzie RG, Yates GL. HEADSS, a pschosocial risk assessment instrument: implications for designing effective intervention programs for runaway youth. J Adolesc Health 1991;12:539–544.

58. Remafedi G. Fundamental issues in the care of the homosexual youth. Med Clin North Am 1990;71:1169–1179.

59. Rotheram-Borus MJ, Fernandez MI. Sexual orientation and developmental challenges experienced by gay and lesbian youths. Journal of Suicide and Life Threatening Behavior 1995;25:1–10.

60. Rotheram-Borus MJ, Hunter J, Rosario M. Coming-out as lesbian or gay in the era of AIDS. In: Herek G & Greene B, eds. AIDS, identity, and community: The HIV epidemic and lesbians and gay men. Contemporary perspectives on lesbian and gay psychology. Washington DC: American Psychological Association Press, 1995; Vol 2: 150–168.

61. Hunter J. Violence against lesbian and gay male youths. Journal of Interpersonal Violence 1990;5:295–300.

62. Rosario M, Rotheram-Borus MJ, Reid HM. Gay-related stress and its correlates among gay and bisexual male adolescents of predominantly Black and Hispanic background. Journal of Community Psychology, in press
63. Chu SY, Peterman TA, Doll LS, et al. AIDS in bisexual men in the United States: epidemiology and transmission to women. Am J Public Health 1992;82:220–224.
64. Doll LS, Peterson LR, White C, et al. Homosexually and non-homosexually identified men who have sex with men: a behavioral comparison. J Sex Res 1992;29:1–14.
65. Diaz T, Chu SY, Frederick M, et al. Sociodemographics and HIV risk behaviors of bisexual men with AIDS: results from a multistate interview project. AIDS 1993; 7:1227–1232.
66. Lever J, Kanouse DE, Rogers WH et al. Behavior patterns and sexual identity of bisexual men. J Sex Res 1992;29:141–167.
67. CDC. Condom use and sexual identity among men who have sex with men—Dallas, 1991. MMWR 1993;42:7,13–14.
68. Wood RW, Kreueger LE, Pearlman TC, Goldbaum G. HIV transmission: Women's risk from bisexual men. Am J Public Health 1993;83:1757–1759.
69. Earl WL. Married men and same sex activity: a field study of HIV risk among men who do not identify as gay or bisexual. J Sex Marital Ther 1990;16:251–257.
70. Hays D, Samuels A. Heterosexual women's perceptions of their marriages to bisexual or homosexual men. J Homosex 1989;18:81–100.
71. Easterbrook PJ, Chmiel JS, Hoover DR, Saah AZ, Kaslow RA, Kingsley LA, Detels R. Racial and ethnic differences in human immunodeficiency virus type 1 (HIV-1) seroprevalence among homosexual and bisexual men. The Multicenter AIDS Cohort Study. Am J Epidemiol 1993;138:415–429.
72. Centers for Disease Control. National HIV serosurveillance summary-results through 1992. Publication No. HIV/NCID/11–93/036. Atlanta, GA: U.S. Department of Health and Human Services, Public Health Service, 1992.
73. Burke D, Brundage J, Goldenbaum M, Gardner L, Peterson M, Visintine R et al. Human immunodeficiency virus infections in teenagers. Seroprevalence among applicants for U.S. military service. JAMA 1990;263:1074–1077.
74. Diaz T, Buehler JW, Castro KG, Ward JW. AIDS trends among Hispanics in the United States. Am J Public Health 1993;83:504–509.
75. Centers for Disease Control. AIDS among racial/ethnic minorities—United States, 1993. MMWR 1994;43:644–647, 653–655.
76. Selik RM, Castro KG, Pappaioanou M, Buehler JW. Birthplace and the risk of AIDS among Hispanics in the United States. Am J Public Health 1989;79:836–839.
77. Centers for Disease Control. HIV/AIDS 1994 Surveillance Report Year-end Edition, 1994:6 (2).
78. MacQueen KM, Ciesielski C. Race/ethnicity differences among homosexual/bisexual men with AIDS who have multiple modes for HIV transmission. IXth International Conference on AIDS. Berlin, June 1993. (abstr PO-D06-3591).
79. Peterson JL, Coates TH, Catania JA, Middleton L, Hilliard B, Hearst N. High-risk sexual behavior among gay and bisexual African-American men. Am J Public Health 1992;82:1490–1494.
80. Doll LS, Byers RH, Bolan G, Douglas JM, Moss PM, Weller PD, et al. Homosexual men who engage in high-risk sexual behavior. A multicenter comparison. Sex Transmitted Disease 1991;18:170–175.
81. Fleming PL, Ward JW, Dean HD, et al. AIDS in minority men who report male-to-male sex, United States. Presented at the IXth International Conference on AIDS. Berlin, June 1993 (abstr PO-C12-2879).
82. Kramer MA, Aral SO, Curran JW. Self-reported behavior patterns of patients attending a sexually transmitted disease clinic. Am J Public Health 1980;70:997–1000.
83. Tan ML. Recent HIV/AIDS Trends among men who have sex with men. Presented at the Xth International Conference on AIDS. Yokohama 1994. (PL-13).
84. Wellings K. et al. Sexual Diversity and Homosexual Behaviour. In Anne M. Johnson et al. (eds) Sexual Attitudes and Lifestyles. 1994: Oxford: Blackwell Scientific Publications.
85. Carrier JM. Mexican male bisexuality. In Klein F, Wolff TJ, eds. Bisexualities: Theory and Research New York, Haworth Press; 1985.
86. Doll LS, Peterson J, Magan JR, Carrier JM. Male bisexuality and AIDS in the United States. In R. Tielman, M. Carballo, A. Hendriks, eds. Bisexuality and HIV/AIDS. 1991 Buffalo, NY: Prometheus Books; 1991.
87. Valdiserri RO, Lyter DW, Leviton LC, Callahan CM, Kingsley LA, Rinaldo CR. Variables influencing condom use in a cohort of gay and bisexual men. Am J Public Health 1988;78:801–805.

88. Van Griensven GJ, de Vroome EM, Tielman, et al. Effect of human immunodeficiency virus (HIV) antibody knowledge on high-risk sexual behavior with steady and non-steady sexual partners among homosexual men. Am J Epidemiol 1989;129:596–603.
89. Rotheram-Borus MJ. HIV+ youths. Presentation at the American Psychological Association Office on AIDS Conference, Behavioral and Social Science Consultation with Three HIV Prevention Community Planning Groups, Washington DC, May 1996.
90. Kelly JA, St Lawrence JS, Brasfield TL et al. Psychological factors which predict AIDS high-risk and AIDS precautionary behavior. J Consult Clin Psychol. 1990; 58:117–120.
91. Crosby GM, Paul J, Barrett D, et al. Gay male substance abusers who only have safer sex. Presented at the IX International Conference of AIDS. Berlin, June 1993 (abstr PO-C12-2873).
92. Anonymous. Publicly funded HIV counseling and testing: United States, 1990. Patient Education & Counseling 1990;19:219–222.
93. Hein K. Evolution or revolution: reforming health care for adolescents in America. J Adolesc Health 1993;14:533–539.
94. Rotheram-Borus MJ, Gillis R, Reid, Fernandez I, Gwadz M. HIV testing, behaviors, and knowledge among adolescents at high risk. Submitted for publication.
95. Beardsell S. Should wider HIV testing be encouraged on the grounds of HIV prevention? AIDS Care 1994;6:5–19.
96. Bayer R, Levine C, Wolf SM. HIV antibody screening: an ethical framework for evaluating proposed programs. JAMA. 1986;256:1768–1774.
97. Levine C, Bayer R. The ethics of screening for early intervention in HIV disease. Am J Public Health 1989;79:1661–1667.
98. Rotheram-Borus MJ, Murphy D, Coleman C. Interventions for adolescents living with HIV: routines, relationships, roles, and stages of adaptation. In: Chesney MA, Antoni MH, eds. Health psychology and HIV disease: from transmission to treatment. Washington DC: The American Psychological Association Division of Health Psychology, In press.
99. Rotheram-Borus MJ, Murphy DA, Reid H, Coleman C. Correlates of emotional distress among HIV+ youths: health status, stress, and personal resources. Ann Behav Med. In press.
100. Friedman LS, Strunin L, Hingson R. A survey of attitudes, knowledge, and behavior related to HIV testing of adolescents and young adults enrolled in alcohol and drug treatment. International Association for Adolescents Health, Fifth Congress. J Adolesc Health 1993;14:442–445.
101. Rotheram-Borus JH, Reid H, Rosario M. Factors mediating changes in sexual HIV risk behaviors among gay and bisexual male adolescents. Am J Public Health 1994;84:1938–1946.
102. Becker MH, Joseph JG. AIDS and behavioural change to reduce risk. Am J Public Health 1988;78:394–410.
103. Rotheram-Borus MJ, Reid HM, Rosario M. Factors mediating changes in sexual HIV risk behaviors among gay and bisexual adolescents. Am J Public Health 1994;84: 1938–1946.
104. Valdiserri RO, Lyter DW, Leviton LC, et al. AIDS prevention in homosexual and bisexual men: results of a randomized trial evaluating two risk reduction interventions. AIDS 1989;3:21–26.
105. Beltran ED, Ostrow DG, Joseph JG. Predictors of sexual behavior change among men requesting their HIV-1 antibody status: The Chicago MACS/CCS cohort of homosexual/bisexual men, 1985–1986. AIDS Educ and Prev 1993;5:185–195.
106. Rotheram-Borus MJ, Rosario M, Reid HM, Koopman C. Predicting patterns of sexual acts among homosexual and bisexual youths. The American Journal of Psychiatry 1995;152:588-595.
107. Rosario M, Rotherum-Borus MJ, Reid HM. Gay-related stress and its correlates among gay and bisexual male adolescents of predominantly Black and Hispanic backgrounds. Journal of Community Psychology. In press.
108. Montgomery SB, Joseph JG, Becker MH, Ostrow DG, Kessler RC, Kirscht JP. The Health Belief Model in understanding compliance with preventive recommendations for AIDS: How useful? AIDS Education and Prevention 1989;1:303–323.
109. CDC. Patterns of Sexual behavior change among homosexual/bisexual men—selected U.S. Sites, 1987–1990. 1991;40:792–794.
110. Darrow WW, Echenberg DF, Jaffe HW, et al. Risk factors for human immunodeficiency virus infections in homosexual men. Am J Public Health 1987;1:345–349.
111. Kingsley LA, Kaslow R, Rinaldo CR Jr, et al. Risk factors for seroconversion to human immunodeficiency virus among male homosexuals. Lancet 1987;1:345–349.

112. Miller S, Hunter J, Rotherum-Borus MJ. Adolescents living safely: AIDS awareness, attitudes, and actions for gay, lesbian and bisexual youths. New York: HIV Center for Clinical and Behavioral Studies, New York State Psychiatric Institute, 1991.
113. Rotheram-Borus MJ, Rosario M, Koopman C. Minority youths at high risk: Gay males and runaways. In: Gore S, Colten ME, eds. Adolescent stress: causes and consequences. New York: Aldine de Gruyter. 1991:181–200.
114. Rotheram-Borus MJ, Reid HM, Gwadz M. Risk for HIV among homosexual, bisexual, and heterosexual male and female adolescents. Submitted for publication.
115. Adib SM, Joseph JG, Ostrow, DG, James SA. Predictors of relapse in sexual practices among homosexual men. AIDS Ed and Prev 1991;3:293–304.
116. Rotheram-Borus MJ, Murphy DA, Srinivasan S, Reid HM. Changing sexual risk acts among adolescents. AIDS Education and Prevention, in press.
117. Kelly JA, St. Lawrence JS, Stevenson Y, Hauth AC, Kalichman SC, Diaz YE, et al. Community AIDS/HIV risk reduction: the effects of endorsements by popular people in three cities. Am J Public Health; 1992:82:1483–1489.
118. Ostrow DG, Beltran ED, Joseph JG, et al. Recreational drugs and sexual behavior in the Chicago MACS/CCS cohort of homosexually active men. Chicago Multicenter AIDS Cohort Study (MACS)/Coping and Change Study. J Subst Abuse 1993;5: 311–325.
119. Bandura A. Perceived self-efficacy in the exercise of control over AIDS infection. In V. Mays, G. Albee, J. Jones, J. Schneider (eds), Psychological Approaches to the Prevention of AIDS. 1989; Beverly Hills, CA: Sage Publications.
120. Catania J, Gibson D, Chitwood D, Coates T. Implications of the AIDS risk reduction model for the gay community: The importance of perceived sexual enjoyment and help seeking behaviors. In V Mays, G. Albee, J. Jones, J. Schneider (eds), Psychological Approaches to the Prevention of AIDS. 1989 Beverly Hills, CA: Sage Publications.
121. Catania J, Kegeles S, Coates T. Towards an understanding of risk behavior: An AIDS risk reduction model (ARRM). Health Education Quarterly 1990;17:53–72.
122. de Wit JBF, van Griensven GJP, Kok G, Sandfort TGM. Why do homosexual men relapse into unsafe sex? Predictors of resumption of unprotected anogenital intercourse with casual partners. AIDS 1993;1113–1118.
123. Roffman R, Ryan R, Downey L, Beadnell B. A telephone group intervention can overcome barriers to enrolling isolated gay and bisexual males in AIDS risk-reduction counseling. Presented at the IXth International Conference on AIDS. Berlin, June 1993 (abstr PO-C23-3166).
124. Hays RB, Kegeles S, Coates T. Community mobilization promotes safer sex among young gay and bisexual men. Presented at the IXth International Conference on AIDS-Berlin, June 1993 (abstr WS-C07-1).

Prevention Considerations for Injection Drug Users

Injection drug use is an important factor in HIV transmission, accounting for 25% of AIDS cases in the United States (1). Injection drug use also contributes indirectly to HIV transmission via sex with an injection drug user (IDU) and perinatal transmission from an infected mother to her child. Because injection drug use has been associated with explosive growth in HIV in the several East coast cities, prevention efforts directed towards IDUs play an important role in areas of relatively low seroprevalence. Drug abuse treatment has been shown to be effective in reducing drug use and behaviors that risk HIV transmission among IDUs (2–5). IDUs not in treatment have been shown to have a higher incidence of HIV infection than those who remain in treatment (2). However, approximately 85% of injection drug users (IDUs) are not in drug treatment programs (6). There is a need to expand the capacity of drug treatment programs and improve the quality of treatment, design better approaches to recruit and retain IDUs in treatment programs, and develop and promote alternative prevention strategies for those IDUs not in treatment (2,7,8).

Prevention efforts directed towards IDUs are challenging for a number of reasons. IDUs are difficult to reach and influence with traditional modes of health service delivery or public health education and interventions. Governmental approaches towards drug dependency tend to further isolate and alienate this population (9). Persons dependent on drugs are unorganized and leaderless, often having poor self-image and a low sense of self worth. IDUs not in drug treatment are at high risk for HIV, as the sharing of drug injection equipment with another IDU, condom non-use during sexual activity, and multiple sexual partners are common (10). Drug use patterns may vary, ranging from occasional users who function well in society to those who must support their habit through crime or through the exchange of sex for money and drugs. Prevention strategies should consider this continuum of drug use patterns, as well as have an understanding of social and ritual aspects of drug use (11). In addition, the high frequency of unsafe sexual practices among injection drug users requires an emphasis on safer sex among IDUs and their partners.

Dynamics of Injection Drug Use

The injection drug of choice for IDUs was previously heroin; today a variety of drugs are injected (e.g., cocaine, amphetamines). Injecting drugs, which can also be snorted or smoked, may be a preferred route of administration for a number of reasons (12). Injection is more economical, requiring less to achieve the same "high"; there is a quicker release from withdrawal; and the initiation into injection practices is usually through a social contact (12). Almost all IDUs are introduced into the practice by friends, lovers, or dealers, who may supply them with the drug and the injection equipment (13). IDUs may work together in pairs or "friendship groups" to obtain money and drugs, and sharing resources (e.g., drugs, equipment) among friends supports the ethic of cooperation within friendship groups (14). These social dynamics may hinder preventive efforts. As needle sharing may occur in friendship groups, refusing to share drug injection equipment with another IDU may signal mistrust or suspicion (15). The subject of bleach use to prevent virus transmission is difficult to raise, having been reported to be socially disruptive and interfering with the pleasures of getting high (16). A person who brings bleach into a circle of users may be suspected of having AIDS (16).

Risk Activities

UNSAFE INJECTION PRACTICES

Risk factors associated with exposure to HIV infection among IDUs include frequency of drug injection, sharing injection equipment, backloading, and injecting in shooting galleries (14,15). Of approximately

17,000 IDUs not in drug treatment in the U.S. and Puerto Rico, 78% reported sharing drug injection equipment with another IDU and 20% sharing with strangers (10). Of those IDUs who reported sharing drug injection equipment, only 14% always cleaned the equipment with bleach before injecting, and 60% cleaned with bleach some of the time (10). Backloading, a form of drug sharing which is syringe-mediated, has also been associated with seropositivity (17). The IDU uses the syringe to mix drugs and then gives measured shares to other IDUs by squirting the drug solution into the syringes of other IDUs (17). Shooting galleries, places to shoot drugs with injection equipment that is borrowed or rented, are believed to facilitate the transmission of HIV. Even among low prevalence cities, IDUs who use shooting galleries demonstrate higher rates of HIV infection than those who do not (18,19). IDUs may prefer to rent rather than carry their own injection equipment because of the likelihood of getting arrested when on their way to purchase drugs or in the neighborhood of shooting galleries. Other reasons cited for using shooting galleries include access (e.g., the shooting gallery is close to the user's home, drugs are available at the shooting gallery or nearby, or injection equipment is available) and IDUs' desire to conceal drug use from the people with whom they live (20,21). However, injection equipment may be contaminated and successively used by a large number of drug injectors frequenting the same gallery, thus facilitating HIV transmission. In addition, certain behaviors associated with shooting galleries may also increase the risk of transmission. IDUs who attended shooting galleries have reported disinfecting needles inconsistently or not at all (16,20). Some studies (20,22,23), but not others (24,25), have found that cocaine injectors engage in more needle sharing than other IDUs. Although there is methadone treatment for heroin dependence, no specific therapy exists for treating cocaine dependence (22).

Preventive behaviors have been reported to be increasing among IDUs. Needle sharing, use of shooting galleries, and use of potentially contaminated syringes have reportedly decreased, and needle cleaning with bleach/alcohol has increased (14,20,26–28). However, although a large proportion of IDUs have reported modifying their needle use behaviors to reduce risk of HIV infection, many continue to report high-risk needle practices (e.g., needle sharing and use of shooting galleries) (28,29).

SEXUAL ACTIVITY

Unsafe sexual activity is prevalent among IDUs. Many have multiple sex partners and use condoms inconsistently if at all (10). In a survey of IDUs not in drug treatment in the United States, the majority reported never using a condom during sexual activity (10). Condom use varied with the type of activity; a majority of male IDUs reported never using condoms during vaginal insertive intercourse (70%), heterosexual anal insertive sex (78%), and homosexual/bisexual anal insertive sex (53%). Fifty-seven percent of female IDUs reported never using condoms during vaginal receptive intercourse; 68% reported never using condoms during anal receptive sex (10). In another survey of IDUs in New York City, 43% reported never using condoms, 31% always using condoms, and 26% using condoms some of the time (30). Although nonmonogamous sex has not decreased among IDUs, reported condom use has increased among IDUs in recent years (28). However, among IDUs who have both steady and casual sex partners, condoms are more often used with casual rather than with steady partners (30,31).

Risk behavior may also be affected by the type of drug used. High-risk sexual behavior has been reported to be higher among those injecting cocaine compared to those injecting heroin (32). Increased sexual activity is also linked to the noninjection use of cocaine (e.g., crack) (22). The potential for sexually transmitted diseases and HIV is increased as crack use is associated with the exchange of sex and money for drugs and an increase in unprotected sexual contact (22,33,34). Among persons with AIDS, the highest rates of prostitution and other risky sexual behaviors have been reported for men who injected drugs and used crack and for women who used crack (35). Among male IDUs with AIDS, trading sex for money was more likely to be reported among bisexuals compared to homosexuals; heterosexual male IDUs were the least likely to report this behavior (36).

Considerations for Prevention Strategies

SAFER SEXUAL PRACTICES

Risk reduction (e.g., using condoms) rather than risk elimination (e.g., mutual monogamy) appears to be a more feasible strategy for IDUs, particularly because nonmonogamous relationships and multiple sex partners appear to be common. Barriers to condom use include reduced penile sensitivity and sexual enjoyment (37,38). Condoms are also associated with the perception of partner unfaithfulness, particularly among crack users (39). Associated with condom use among African-American IDUs were: higher levels of self-efficacy, sexual communication skills, condom-use skills and the belief that condoms do not decrease pleasure (32). Nonusers of condoms were more likely to state that condoms decrease pleasure. HIV-risk reduction information and skills training (e.g., communication skills in negotiating safer sex behavior and condom use) should develop the cognition and skills which will enhance the enjoyment of condoms (32). Higher rates of consistent condom use have been correlated with practicing safe injecting behaviors; therefore, messages should link prevention for both injection drug use- and sex-related transmission (30). Larger risk reductions have been observed in drug use behaviors than in sexual risk behaviors among IDUs (40). Studies have shown that IDUs appear to have modified their drug-using behavior more than their sexual practices (20,41). Although safer sex behaviors should be a priority, it may be easier to focus on altering injection practices.

SOCIAL SUPPORT AND NETWORK

The social support and network appear to be important for the IDU. Risk reduction has been reported to be the greatest when peer group norms support risk reduction, and when one has close social ties to non-injectors (31,42–45). Improved drug use behavior among IDUs in short-term treatment programs was associated with decreased number of friends who inject drugs (social network), increased number of persons to talk with when upset (social support), and increased argumentative skills concerning safe drug use (46). Individual condom use has been associated with peers practicing safer sex (i.e., condom use, restriction to safer sex activities) as well as drug injection HIV-risk reduction (i.e., cleaning needles, or using only new needles) (30). Risk behaviors of IDUs are also related to their peers' efforts to avoid needle sharing and to perceptions that peers would be offended by the refusal to share needles (11). Talking about AIDS with drug-using friends and sexual partners has also been reported as a predictor of risk reduction (47). The use of peer outreach and group methods may help to maximize the impact of social influence (30). Enhancing specific family protective variables may also result in less needle sharing. In a survey of male IDUs, sibling support, child support and significant other support was associated with less frequent drug use or multiple drug use (48).

For recovering drug users, long term maintenance of behavior changes may be difficult because of the IDU's social environment; relapse is more likely to occur when persons influence them to use drugs (11,46). Long term monitoring, follow-up, and repeated contact with IDUs who have returned to the community after drug treatment are necessary, since peers may influence former drug users to use drugs. It has also been suggested that recovering drug users replace network members with peers who do not support drug use. Reinforcement of risk reduction behaviors and ongoing support for changes are integral to relapse prevention.

PARTNERS OF IDUs

Although most sex partners of women IDUs also use drugs, most partners of chemically dependent men do not inject drugs and may be unaware of the partner's drug use (49–51). Some women may be unaware of a partner's drug use if she, herself, does not use drugs, or if the partner's drug use is concealed (52). Among female partners, there is often a sense of powerlessness, low self-esteem, and social isolation. In addition, they may be economically and emotionally dependent, as well as subjected to physical abuse (52). There may be an imbalance of power within the relationship and women may be afraid to confront their partner regarding risk behaviors and/or initiate discussions regarding risk assessment and safer sex. Requesting the use of condoms might also imply a lack of trust between partners. Although some women may avoid sex as a strategy to reduce risk (53), this may threaten the relationship.

The seroprevalence among non-IDUs who are sex partners of IDUs can be as high as 14% (10). Therefore, education efforts should also be focused on this population. Partners of IDUs must be aware of the risk posed by a partner who injects drugs and the need to protect themselves. Given the lower rates of consistent condom use reported by IDUs with their steady partners (i.e., primary relationships) than with casual partners (30,31), interventions should particularly focus on the primary relationship. Condom use messages should target sex behaviors within primary relationships where partners do not know their HIV status, are discordant for HIV infection, or one or more partners are continuing at-risk activities (30). Women partners should be assisted not only in reducing risk of sexual transmission, but perhaps also in reducing her partner's risk of transmission by injection drug use. Spouses and partners may be able to persuade IDUs to become involved in prevention programs and seek drug treatment, try to change their partners' drug use patterns, encourage their partners to stop sharing needles, or clean their partners' needles (11,52). "Domesticating" the drug habit has also been reported, i.e., negotiating changes that allow better control and scrutiny of drug using behaviors (e.g., male partners may inject drugs only at home) (52). Domestication may be less threatening to both members of the relationship because it supports the traditional role of women as care giver and is less conflictive than negotiating safer sex. Although domestication seems to reinforce stereotypical roles of women, it may be a reasonable adaptation for women in these situations (52).

NEW GUIDELINES FOR DISINFECTION OF DRUG EQUIPMENT

The recommended protocol of using bleach to clean needles and syringes in 1986 was to fill needles and syringes twice with bleach followed with two water rinses (54–56). Since then, the use of bleach to disinfect shared and used drug equipment has been a fundamental component of many HIV prevention programs (40,57) and is the principal AIDS prevention objective (by the US Public Health Service) for IDUs not enrolled in drug abuse treatment (58,59).

Recently, the effectiveness of bleach in activating HIV as well as the recommended bleach disinfecting procedure has been investigated. Laboratory studies concluded that HIV in blood within the needles and syringes shared by IDUs is more difficult to disinfect that previously believed (60), and may not be as effective when applied under "street" conditions (61–63). Studies suggest that bleach-cleansed equipment should not be relied upon to prevent new HIV incidence among IDUs (61,64). Disinfecting drug equipment, as practiced in 1991, did not eliminate HIV risk among drug users who reported using it all the time (64). 1993 guidelines regarding disinfection of drug equipment (59,65,66) recommended that full strength liquid bleach be used to disinfect equipment (60) and that the contact time between the bleach and all contaminated parts of the syringe be at least 30 seconds (62,63) Furthermore, among IDUs, there is a lack of compliance to syringe cleaning strategies (67) and insufficient bleach contact times (<30 secs) during syringe cleaning (68). Therefore, if these protocols are to significantly affect HIV transmission risk, increased compliance and sufficient exposure times of infected needles and syringes to bleach solutions will be required. The revised 1993 bleach disinfection protocol has also raised a new dilemma (60). Syringes have been shown to become damaged after a relatively few rinses with undiluted bleach (60). Cleaning the syringe as recommended may make the syringe inoperable more quickly than if it is rinsed only with water, and would require that the IDU purchase a new syringe, a potential disincentive to disinfect with bleach. Although equipment disinfection is an adjunctive method to reduce risk (53), it is not a substitute for drug cessation or use of sterile equipment (2,60,64).

Intervention Programs for IDUs

Street outreach programs have been the major nontreatment approach for IDUs in the United States. Most programs in the U.S. involve distribution of bleach and condoms, and sometimes include syringe and/or needle exchange and distribution. For IDUs unable or unwilling to enter drug treatment programs, access to sterile needles (e.g., needle exchange or needle distribution programs) is one way to reduce risk among IDUs, and are a safer alternative than previously used bleach-disinfected equipment. However, this has been met with social, legal and political resistance. Although the National Commission on AIDS recommended the removal of legal barriers to purchasing and possessing needles and syringes (69), it is illegal in most states to possess and distribute needles and syringes, and prohibited in several states to sell needles and syringes (70). Syringe exchange programs (SEPs) in some U.S. cities may function semi-legally, illegally but are tolerated, or illegal/underground. Syringe exchange programs may also offers services such as provision of latex condoms, HIV counseling and testing, tuberculin skin testing, primary health care, and directly observed tuberculosis therapy (71). Most give counseling regarding medical hygiene standards when injecting illegal drugs (i.e., prepare the injection site with an alcohol swab; use a new sterile needle and syringe for each injection; avoid reuse of syringes, even by the same person; use clean, ideally sterile water to prepare drugs for injection; and return used syringes to the SEP for safe disposal) (71). The number of SEPs operating in the U.S. increased 82% from that in 1993 (71), with the number of syringes exchanged by SEPs increasing threefold from 2.4 million in 1992 (72) to 8 million in 1994 (71).

Opposition to programs which promote safer injection behaviors primarily centers on whether such practices promote or condone injection drug use. However, studies demonstrate the effectiveness of SEPs and other interventions that increase access to sterile in preventing HIV infection. Participation of IDUs in SEPS was associated with substantial lower risk for hepatitis B and hepatitis C among IDUs (sixfold and sevenfold lower, respectively) (73). Evaluation of syringe exchange programs have demonstrated that reduced needle risk behaviors are associated with IDUs who participate (i.e., exchangers) compared to nonexchangers (23,72,74,75). In many but not all studies, exchangers have reported lower rates of sharing contaminated equipment; a decrease in sharing equipment, borrowing used needles, renting or buying used needles; a decrease in frequency of injection; and a higher likelihood to clean equipment and use alcohol pads (23,72,74,75). Exchangers were also more likely to report condom use, although they were also more likely to have multiple sexual partners (76). Undesirable side effects (e.g., new persons initiating injection drug use, higher frequency of injection) have not been reported (23,77–79). Research suggests that in addition to reducing risk behaviors, syringe exchange programs may broaden the reach of intervention. Such programs may facilitate the entry of IDUs into drug treatment by attracting IDUs who otherwise would not seek drug treatment (20). The National Academy of Sciences recently reviewed research on SEPs and in 1995 concluded that SEPs should be regarded as an effective component of a comprehensive strategy to prevent infectious disease (80). Following a partial repeal of a Connecticut law that required a prescription to purchase syringes and a law the regarded possession of syringes as illegal, purchasing of syringes from pharmacies by IDUs increased and sharing of injection equipment decreased (73,81).

Interventions directed towards IDUs and their sex partners have demonstrated an overall reduction in high-risk behaviors and facilitated entry into drug treatment programs (40). IDUs reported a decrease in borrowing and sharing of drug injection equipment, an increased use of bleach for disinfection of drug equipment, and increased condom use with steady partners as well as multiple partners (40). In addition, 14% to 35% of IDUs had entered a drug treatment program in five U.S. cities (40). Social networks of IDUs have been targeted to maximize reinforcement of individual's behaviors, using ex-addicts in a street-based program; this has been shown to reduce unsafe injecting behaviors dramatically (82). Programs have also tried to influence the IDU subculture to incorporate bleach use as a normative standard. Thus, outreach programs may also affect the behaviors of IDUs who do not participate directly in the interventions (83). Cross sectional samples of IDUs recruited during 1986 and 1989 revealed that the introduction of outreach programs to IDUs in 1986 corresponded with the start of community-wide increases in bleach use (3% in 1986 to 86% in 1989) (83). Linking drug treatment, HIV, STD and other infectious disease prevention with primary care has also helped substance abusers to access primary care services, substance abuse treatment, and related disease care (84). Through the linkage of services, 41% consented to HIV testing and 14% received early intervention for HIV infection. Of the populations reached through linking services, 60% were persons of color, 40% women, and 14% adolescents (84).

Prevention programs can be effective if behavioral interventions are combined with the use of nontraditional outreach workers. Street-based outreach models are effective models for promoting behavior change in IDUs (60); as evidenced by significant changes in high-risk behavior reported among IDUs participating in such programs (85–87). Programs should be multifaceted, involve the use of peers, and provide skill training and social support resources. The availability of counseling and support services is especially important for people who experience denial in reaction to a positive result and for those who need to notify their drug and sexual partners (88,89). Reported predictors of risk reduction among IDUs include educational levels, knowing a person can be HIV-infected and still look healthy, and previously being tested for HIV (47). Strategies should help the IDU personalize his or her risk for HIV infection but also avoid raising perceived risk to such a high level that it results in fatalism, which could undermine risk reduction. Strategies should also motivate and assist IDUs to enroll into treatment settings and emphasize the importance of terminating drug use. For those unable or unwilling to stop injecting drugs, risk reduction strategies (i.e., safer injection behaviors, bleach cleansing technique, safer sex), skills, and training should be given and reinforced. Distributing supplies (e.g., bleach, condoms, syringe exchanges) and providing follow-up to reinforce and support behavioral change might facilitate risk reduction.

Because individuals who use crack are more likely to engage in atrisk sexual behaviors, preventing sexual transmission of HIV should be emphasized. Basing risk assessment and prevention efforts on behaviors is particularly important for IDUs who have sex with men (MSM), many of whom may not self-identify as homosexual or bisexual. Training should not only enhance communication skills in negotiating safer sex behavior and condom use but should enhance the enjoyment of condoms (32). Building peer support for behavioral change, monitoring and providing ongoing support, as well as addressing the cultural norms of the drug user subculture are also important components of prevention. Referrals to abstinence-oriented peer support groups (e.g., Narcotics Anonymous) may be helpful to prevent relapse (90).

REFERENCES

1. CDC. HIV/AIDS Surveillance Mid-End Edition 1995;Vol 7:No 1.
2. Haverkos HW, Jones TS. HIV, drug-use paraphernalia, and bleach. J Acquir Immune Defic Syn 1994;7:741–742.
3. Yancovitz SR, Des Jarlais DC, Peyser NP, et al. A randomized trial of an interim methadone maintenance clinic. Am J Public Health 1991;81:1185–1191.
4. Batki S, Sorensen J, Coates C, et al. Methadone maintenance for AIDS-affected IV drug users: treatment outcome and psychiatric factors after three months. In: Harris LS, ed. Problems of drug dependence 1988. NIDA Res Mongr 1989;90:343.
5. Ball JC, Lange WR, Myers CP, et al. Reducing risk of AIDS through methadone maintenance treatment. J Health Soc Behav 1998;29:214–216.
6. Hahn RA, Onorato I, Jones TS, Dougherty J. Prevalence of HIV infection among intravenous drug users in the United States. JAMA 1989;18:2677–2684.
7. Report of the Second Public Health Service AIDS Prevention and Control Conference. Workgroup report: Intravenous drug abuse. Public Health Reports; 1988: 103 (suppl 1 revised):66–71.
8. Martinez B. Needle exchange programs: are they effective? Washington, DC: Office of National Drug Control Policy Bulletin No. 7. 1992.
9. Karan LD. Primary Care for AIDS and Chemical Dependence. In Addiction Medicine [Special Issue]. West J Med 1990;152:538–542.
10. CDC. Risk Behaviors for HIV Transmission among IVDUs not in drug treatment—U.S., 1987–1989. MMWR 1990;39:273–276.
11. Schilling RF, Schinke SP, Nichols SE, et al. Developing strategies for AIDS prevention research with black and Hispanic drug users. Public Health Reports 1989;104:2–11.

12. Stryker J. IV Drug Use and AIDS: Public policy and dirty needles. J Health Politics, Policy and Law 1989;14:719–740.
13. Des Jarlais DC, Friedman SR, Strug D. AIDS and needle sharing within the IV drug use subculture. In Feldman DA and Johhnson TM (eds) The Social Dimensions of AIDS: Methods and Theory. Praeger: NY,1986:11–125.
14. Friedman SR, DesJarlais DC, Neaigus A. AIDS among drug injectors: the first decade. In DeVita VT, Hellman S, Rosenberg SA (eds) AIDS: Etiology, Diagnosis, Treatment, and Prevention JB Lippincott C: Philadelphia, 1992:453–461.
15. Conviser R, Rutledge J. The need for innovation to halt AIDS among intravenous drug users and their sexual partners. AIDS and Public Policy Journal 1988;3:43–50.
16. Connors MM. Risk perception, risk taking and risk management among intravenous drug users: Implications for AIDs prevention. Social Science and Medicine 1992;34: 591–601.
17. Jose B, Friedman SR, Neaigus A, et al. Syringe-mediated drug-sharing (backloading): a new risk factor for HIV among injecting drug users. AIDS 1993;7:1653–1660.
18. Chaisson RE, Bacchetti P, Osmond D, et al. Cocaine use and HIV infection in intravenous drug users in San Francisco. JAMA 1989;261;561–565.
19. Des Jarlais DC. The first and second decades of AIDS among injecting drug users. British J of Addiction 1992;87:347–353.
20. Longshore D, Anglin D, Henson KD, Annon K. HIV Transmission and Risk Behavior among drug users in Los Angeles County: 1993 Update. Los Angeles: UCLA Drug Abuse Research Center, 1993.
21. Waldorf D, Reinarman C, and Murphy S. Needle sharing, shooting galleries, and AIDS risk among intravenous drug users in San Francisco: Criminal justice and public health policy. Criminal Justice Policy Review 1989;3:391–406.
22. CDC. Update: Acquired Immunodeficiency Syndrome associated with intravenous drug use—United States, 1988. MMWR 1989;38:165–170.
23. Watters JK, Estilo MJ, Clark GL, Lorvick J. Syringe and needle exchange as HIV/AIDS prevention for injection drug users. JAMA 1994;271:115–120.
24. Booth RE. Predictors of unsafe needle practices: Injection drug users in Denver. Journal of Acquired Immune Deficiency Syndromes 1994;7:504–508.
25. Longshore D, Anglin MD, Hsieh SC, Annon K. Drug-related HIV risk behaviors and cocaine preference among injection drug users in Los Angeles. Journal of Drug Education 1993;23:259–272.
26. DesJarlais DC, Friedman SR, Sotheran JL, et al. Continuity and change within an HIV epidemic. Injecting drug users in New York City, 1984 through 1992. JAMA 1994;271:121–127.
27. Battjes R, Pickens R. Trends in HIV infection and AIDS Risk Behaviors among injecting drug users in selected US Cities. (abstr) Presented at IXth International Conference on AIDS. Berlin, June 1993. PO-C15-2950.
28. Longshore D, Anglin MD, Annon K, Hsieh SC. Trends in self-reported HIV risk behavior: Injection drug users in Los Angeles. Journal of Acquired Immune Deficiency Syndromes 1993; 6:82–90.
29. Lehman JS, Nahlen B, Green TA, et al. Needle-use behaviors in injection drug users (IDUs) entering drug treatment in the United States (USA). (abstr) Presented at IXth International Conference on AIDS. Berlin, June 1993. PO-C15-2951.
30. CDC. Condom use among male injecting-drug users—New York City, 1987–1990. MMWR 1992;41:617–620.
31. Abdul-Quadar AS, Tross S, Friedman SR, et al. Street-recruited intravenous drug users and sexual risk reduction in New York City. AIDS 1990;4:1075–1079.
32. Malow RM, Corrigan SA, Cunningham SC, et al. Psychosocial factors associated with condom use among African-American drug abusers in treatment. AIDS Education and Prevention. 1993; 5:244–253.
33. Schoenfisch S, Ellerbrock T, Harrington P, et al. Risk of HIV infection and behavioral changes associated with crack cocaine use in prenatal patients. (abstr) Presented at IXth International Conference on AIDS. Berlin, June 1993. PO-C15-2920.
34. Longshore D, Anglin MD. Number of sex partners and crack cocaine use: Is crack an independent marker for HIV risk? Journal of Drug Issues 1995;25:1–15.
35. Diaz T, Chus S, Sanchez C, et al. Sexual practices among crack/cocaine users with AIDS: Supplement to HIV/AIDS Surveillance. (abstr) Presented at IXth International Conference on AIDS. Berlin, June 1993. PO-C15-2953.
36. Diaz T, Chu SY, Frederick M, et al. Sociodemographics and HIV risk behaviors of bisexual men with AIDS: results from a multistate interview project. AIDS 1993;7: 1227–1232.
37. Valdisseri R, Arena V, Proctor D, Bonati F. The relationship between women's attitudes

about condoms and their use: Implications for condom promotion programs. Am J Public Health 1989;79:499–501.

38. Magura S, Shapiro JL, Siddiqi Q, Lipton DS. Variables influencing condom use among intravenous drug users. American J Public Health 1990;80:82.
39. Gunter D, Wettrich M. Client-reported condom attitudes and perceptions among crack-using clients in sexually transmitted disease clinics U.S. 1991. (abstr) Presented at IXth International Conference on AIDS. Berlin, June 1993. PO-C24-3192.
40. CDC. Update: Reducing HIV transmission in treatment—United States. MMWR 1990;39:31:529,535–538.
41. Curtis JL, Crummey FC, Baker SN, et al. 1989. HIV screening and counseling for intravenous drug abuse patients: Staff and patient attitudes. Journal of the American Medical Association 1989; 261:258–262.
42. Friedman SR, Des Jarlais DC, Sotheran JL, et al: AIDS and self-organization among intravenous drug users. Int J Addict 1987;22:201–219.
43. Magura S, Grossman JI, Lipton DS, et al. Determinants of needle sharing among intravenous drug users. Am J Public Health, 1989;79:459.
44. Neaigus A, Sufian M, Friedman SR, et al. Effects of outreach intervention risk reduction among intravenous drug users. AIDS Educ Prevent, 1990; 2:253–280.
45. Klee H. Faugier J, Hayes C, et al. Factors associated with risk behavior among injecting drug users. AIDS Care 1990;2:133.
46. Zapka JG, Stoddard AM, McCusker J. Social network, support and influence: relationships with drug use and protective AIDS behavior. AIDS Educ Prev 1993; 5:352–366.
47. Des Jarlais DC. Cross cultural similarities in AIDS risk reduction among injecting drug users. (abstr) Presented at IXth International Conference on AIDS. Berlin, June 1993. WS-D09-3.
48. Masci JR, Brook DW, Roberto J, et al. Interactive effects of family protective factors on needle-sharing behavior. (abstr) Presented at IXth International Conference on AIDS. Berlin, June 1993. PO-D22-4069.
49. Mondanaro J. Chemically Dependent Women: Assessment and Treatment. Lexington, Massachusetts: Lexington Books. 1989.
50. Turner C, Miller H, Moses L. eds. AIDS: Sexual Behavior and Intravenous Drug Use. Washington, DC: National Academy Press.
51. Cohen JB, Hauer LB, Wofsy CB. Women and IV drugs: Parental and heterosexual transmission of human immunodeficiency virus. J Drug Issues 1989;19(10):39–56.
52. Miller C. Reducing risk among female partners of injection drug users. Focus 1991; 7(1):1–8.
53. Sibthorpe B. The social construction of sexual relationships as a determinant of HIV risk perception and condom use among injection drug users. Medical Anthropology Quarterly 1992; 6:255–270.
54. Watters JK, Newmeyer JA, Feldman HW, Biernacki P. Street-based AIDS prevention for intravenous drug users in San Francisco: prospects, options, and obstacles. In: Community Epidemiology Work Group proceedings, June 1986. Vol II. Selected issues: acquired immunodeficiency syndrome (AIDS), drug abuse and crime, ethnographic research, international research. Rockville, MD: National Institute on Drug Abuse, 1986:I:37–43.
55. Newmeyer JA, Feldman HW, Biernacki P, Watters JK. Preventing AIDS contagion among intravenous drug users. Med Anthropol 1989;10:167.
56. Newmeyer J. Why bleach? Development of a strategy to combat HIV contagion among San Francisco intravenous drug users. In Battjes R, and Pickens RW, eds. Needle sharing among intravenous drug users: national and international perspectives. Rockville, MD: National Institutes on Drug Abuse, 1988;151–159.
57. Watters JK, Jones TS, Shapshak P, et al. Household bleach as disinfectant for use by injecting drug users. Lancet 1993;342:742–743.
58. United States Public Health Service. Healthy people 2000. U.S. Department of Health and Human Services Publication PHS 91-50212. Washington, DC: U.S. Government Printing Office, 1991.
59. CDC. Use of bleach for disinfection of drug injection equipment. MMWR 1993;42: 418–419.
60. Flynn N, Jain S, Keddie EM, et al. In vitro activity or readily available household materials against HIV-1: is bleach enough? J Acquir Immune Defic Syndr 1994;7:747–753.
61. Vlahov D, Munoz A, Celentano DD, et al. HIV seroconversion and disinfection of injection equipment among intravenous drug users, Baltimore, Maryland. Epidemiology 1991;2:442–444.
62. Shapshak P, McCoy CB, Rivers JE, et al. Inactivation of human immunodeficiency virus-1 at short time intervals using undiluted bleach. J Acquir Immune Defic Syndr 1993;6:218–219.

63. Shapshak P, McCoy CB, Shah SM, et al. Preliminary laboratory studies of inactivation of HIV-1 in needles and syringes containing infected blood using undiluted household bleach. J Acquir Immun Defic Syndr 1994;7:754–759.

64. Vlahov D, Astemborski J, Solomon L, Nelson KE. Field effectiveness of needle disinfection among injecting drug users. J Acquir Immun Defic Syndr 1994;7:7660–7666.

65. California Department of Health Services Office of AIDS. New guidelines on bleach disinfection of needles and syringes. California HIV/AIDS Update. 1993;6(3):37–38.

66. Curran JW, Scheckel LW, Milstein RA. HIV/AIDS prevention bulletin. Rockville, MD: Centers for Disease Control, Center for Substance Abuse Treatment, and National Insitute on Drug Abuse. April 19, 1993.

67. McCoy CB, Rivers JE, McCoy HV, Shapshak P, Weatherby NL, Chitwood DD, Page JB, Inciardi JA, McBride DC. Compliance to bleach disinfection protocols among injecting drug users in Miami. J Acquir Immun Defic Syndr 1994;7:773–776.

68. Gleghorn AA, Doherty MC, Vlahov D, Celentano DD, Jones TS. Inadequate bleach contact times during syringe cleaning among injection drug users. J Acquir Immun Defic Syndr 1994;7:767–772.

69. AIDS National Commission on Acquired Immune Deficiency Syndrome. The twin epidemics of substance use and HIV. Washington, DC: National Commission on Acquired Immune Deficiency Syndrome, July 1991:10–11.

70. Gostin L. The needle-borne epidemic: causes and public health responses. Behavioral Sciences and the Law 1991;9:287–304.

71. CDC. Syringe Exchange Programs—United States, 1994–1995. MMWR 1995;44:684–685, 691.

72. Lurie P, Reingold AL. The public health impact of needle exchange programs in the United States and abroad. Berkeley: Institute for Health Policy Studies, University of California, San Francisco. 1993.

73. Valleroy LA, Weinstein B, Jones TS, et al. Impact of increased legal access to needles and syringes on community pharmacies' needle and syringe sales—Connecticut, 1992–1993. J Acquir Immun Defic Syndr 1995;10:73–81.

74. Harris N, McGought J, Shapiro E, et al. The impact of a syringe exchange program on drug injection behavior associated with HIV in Seattle, Washington, USA. (abstr) Presented at IXth International Conference on AIDS. Berlin, June 1993. PO-C24-3179.

75. Paone D, Des Jarlais DC, Caloir S, et al. AIDS risk reduction behaviors among participants of syringe exchange programs in New York City, USA. (abstr) Presented at IXth International Conference on AIDS. Berlin, June 1993. PO-C24-3188.

76. Harris N, McGough J, Shapiro E, Fields J, Weiss N. The impact of a syringe exchange program on HIV-associated sexual behavior among drug injectors in Seattle, Washington, USA. (abstr) Presented at IXth International Conference on AIDS. Berlin, June 1993. PO-C24-3179.

77. Buning EC. Effects of Amsterdam needle and syringe exchange. The International J Addictions 1991;26:1303:1311.

78. Grund JC, Blanken P, Adriaans NF, et al. Reaching the unreached: targeting hidden IDU populations with clean needles via known user groups. J Psychoactive Drugs 1992;24:41–47.

79. Kaplan EH, O'Keefe E. Let the needles do the talking! Evaluating the New Haven needle exchange. Interfaces 1993;23:7–28.

80. Normand J, Vlahov D, Moses LE, eds. Preventing HIV transmission: the role of sterile needles and bleach. Washington, DC: National Academy Press, 1995.

81. Groseclose SL, Weinstein B, Jones TS, et al. Impact of increased legal access to needles and syringes on practices of injecting-drug users and police officers—Connecticut, 1992-1993. J Acquir Immun Defic Syndr 1995;10:82–89.

82. Wiebel W, Jiminez A, Johnson W, et al. Positive effect on HIV seroconversion of street outreach intervention with IDU in Chicago, 1988–1992. (abstr) Presented at IXth International Conference on AIDS. Berlin, June 1993. WS-C15-2.

83. Watters J. Observations on the importance of social context in HIV transmission among intravenous drug users. J Drug Issues 1989;19:9–26.

84. Holloway J, Trent S. Lerner H, et al. Integrating primary health care and substance abuse treatment. (abstr) Presented at IXth International Conference on AIDS. Berlin, June 1993. PO-D18-3936.

85. van den Hoek JAR, van Haastrecht HJA, Coutinho RA. Risk reduction among intravenous drug users in Amsterdam under the influence of AIDS. Am J Public Health 1989;79:1355–1357.

86. Watters JK, Downing M, Case P, Lorvick, Cheng Y-T, Fergusson B. AIDS Prevention for intravenous drug users in the community: street-based education and risk behaviors. Am J Commun Psychol 1990;18:587–596.

87. McCoy CB, Chitwood DD, Khoury EL, Miles CE. The implementation of an experimen-

tal design in the evaluation of an intervention to prevent AIDS among IV drug users. J Drug Issues 1990;20:215–222.

88. Magura S, Siddiqi Q, Shaprio J et al. Outcomes of an AIDS prevention program for methadone patients. The International J Addictions 1991;26:629–655.

89. Rhodes F, Corby NH, Wolitski RJ et al. Risk behaviors and perceptions of AIDS among street injection drug users. J Drug Education 1990;20:271–288.

90. Selwyn PA. Issues in the clinical management of intravenous drug users with HIV infection. AIDS 1989;3(suppl 1): S201–S208.

Prevention Considerations for African-Americans and Latin Americans

HIV infection disproportionately affects ethnic minority communities, particularly African-Americans and Latin Americans. Although African-Americans and Latin Americans constitute only 12% and 6% of the U.S. populations, respectively, they collectively represent approximately 51% of the AIDS cases in the United States (1). Injecting drug use, either by direct use of drugs or through heterosexual contact with an injecting drug user (IDU), plays a major role in HIV transmission, accounting for 39% of male and 68% of female AIDS cases among African-Americans and Latin Americans (1). Heterosexual contact with a person at-risk or with HIV infection plays a significant role in HIV transmission among racial/ethnic women and accounts for 33% and 44% of cumulative AIDS cases among African-American and Latin American women (1). Among the 94% of African American and Latin American children who are perinatally infected, 60% had mothers with a risk linked to injecting drug use (1). African-American and Latin American IDUs have higher rates of AIDS, frequenting "shooting galleries," and sharing drug injection equipment, compared to white IDUs (2–7). Condom use among African-American and Latin American women has been reported to be lower than whites (8–10) and unsafe sex practices are prevalent among homosexual/bisexual men (11–13). Male-male sexual contact also plays a major role in HIV transmission among racial/ethnic males, accounting for 40% and 45% of AIDS cases among African-American and Latin American men, respectively (1). In racial/ethnic communities, lack of knowledge about HIV prevention has been reported to be more common (14–16) and misconceptions regarding HIV transmission are prevalent (14). Knowledge levels may be influenced by the degree of acculturation, with more recent immigrants being less informed regarding HIV transmission (17–18). In addition, many African-Americans and Latin Americans may not perceive themselves at risk for AIDS, viewing AIDS as a problem primarily of the white gay community (16,18–19). A lack of perceived risk may result in practicing risky behaviors. AIDS prevention for ethnic populations require targeted strategies as socioeconomic factors, lack of access to health care, cultural diversity, and language and cultural differences present special challenges for these populations.

Economic, Social, and Cultural Factors

Economic, social, and cultural factors can play an important role in educational efforts and should be integrated into prevention programs for African-Americans and Latin Americans. Many African-Americans and Latin Americans have low incomes, which may prevent them from seeking care (e.g., lack of access, transportation, or child care) (20). Lower income levels are also associated with greater misinformation on AIDS and a greater tendency to underestimate personal risk (21). Immediate concerns, such as employment or daily survival, may also have greater priority than AIDS prevention. Poverty may lead to drug use (as an escape from the problems of poverty), drug dealing (as a source of income), and survival sex (sex exchanged for money, drugs, or shelter). Persons of color may underuse the health care system because of lack of access, fears of inadequate treatment, and cultural insensitivity within the health care system (17,22,23). Poor education and language difficulties, as well as a reluctance to go beyond the family unit or ethnic community, may also be barriers in seeking health care (23). There may be a distrust of government and public agencies, given the experiences of discrimination and economic disadvantages by racial/ethnic minorities (22). Less likely than whites to seek assistance from formal organizations, African-Americans and Latin Americans may feel that white-, gay-, or lesbian-oriented agencies cannot meet their needs or understand their ethnic beliefs (22–24). In addition, medical practices from cultural traditions may be used in combination with contemporary biomedicine (17). Because prescription medicines (including injectables) are available over the counter in many Latin American countries, Latin Americans may use needles and syringes for activities other than drug use (25). Other barriers which make prevention efforts difficult in African-American and Latin American communities include the imbalance of power between genders and the strong stigma associated with AIDS and the behaviors associated with HIV transmission. Being HIV infected may mean loss of family support, rejection, and isolation (26).

It is important to remember that within African-American and Latin American communities, there is heterogeneity and diversity relative to culture, values, language, national origins, health practices, and community setting (e.g., rural versus urban versus border community). Individuals may originate from varying countries (e.g., Haiti, Africa, Mexico, United States) and a common language will not always equate to homogeneity—dialects and cultural values may be dependent on the country of origin (e.g., Puerto Rico versus Mexico versus Cuba). Cultural values, health practices, attitudes, and ideas may also change with degree of acculturation, depending on the length of time a family lives in the United States (i.e., number of generations), age, sex, education, and economic status (17). For example, high-acculturated Latin American women are more likely to be at risk for HIV infection via sex with multiple partners, and both injection and noninjection drug use compared to low-acculturated Latin American women, who are more likely to become HIV infected through their husbands or partners (27).

Cultural Aspects of Sex

In many Latin American communities, sexuality appears to be very private and personal. Sex is generally a taboo subject and sex education may be lacking. Because discussing sex may not be appropriate, especially for women (15,25–26,28–31), sexual partners and practices (e.g., condom use and birth control) may not be discussed, even between sexual partners. Latin Amerian women are often unaware of a partner's bisexuality and/or drug use behavior. In addition, machismo (values relating to virility) and marianismo (values relating to virginity) are prevalent beliefs in Spanish-speaking cultures and influences how men and women view and interact with each other (18,26). Latin American men are considered superior to women, and expected to be highly sexual, with sex outside the marriage allowed (18,28). In the traditional Latin American culture, a "good" woman should not know about sex, be sexually inexperienced and naive, having sex only within the context of marriage (26,29). Consequently, it is inappropriate for a woman to bring up subjects like AIDS and condoms. Latin American women carrying or requesting the condom use may be stigmatized as experienced, loose, and, therefore, less desirable (26).

Although the public dialogue about sex may be open among African-Americans, effective communication about sexual practices between a man and woman may be lacking (31). Sexual behaviors also differ by gender. A male's nonmonogomous sexual behavior may be acceptable within the cultural norms (24). African-American men are more likely to have more sexual partners and sex outside the marriage compared to women (31). A "bad" woman might be characterized in the African-American community as someone having simultaneous multiple sexual relationships, being sexually aggressive, or having a disregard for her partner or relationship (31).

HOMOSEXUALITY/BISEXUALITY

Because of the strong attitudes against bisexuality and homosexuality which exist in racial/ethnic communities, many African-American and Latin American men who have sex with women but also engage in same sex activities may not self-identify as being homosexual or bisexual; these include men who have sex in prison or who have the insertor (and perceived masculine) role in oral and anal sex (29,32–34). Men who do not self-identify as being homosexual or bisexual have reported high risk activities (35), placing themselves at greater risk for HIV infection. The strong value of the family in the Latin American culture may make choosing a homosexual lifestyle inconceivable because of the potential alienation from the family; this may force some homosexuals to lead bisexual lives (29). Of men with AIDS who were born in the U.S, African-American men had higher rates of bisexual behavior than white and Latin American men (33,36–37). Reasons hypothesized for African-American men adopting bisexual behavior includes the unacceptability of homosexuality in the African-American community and the perception of betraying the African-American community by being involved with the gay white community (38).

Higher proportions of bisexuality activity among racial/ethnic men also have implications for racial/ethnic women. Rates of AIDS due to sexual contact with bisexual men are highest among African-American and Latin American women (39). Many African-American and Latin American women may be unaware of their partner's bisexual behavior. It has also been demonstrated that married men who have sex with men are less likely than unmarried men to inform their regular partner of their behavior (40). In one study, 22% of Latin Americans with AIDS who reported bisexual activity were married (33).

IMBALANCE OF POWER BETWEEN GENDERS

Most African-American and Latin American women will be in unequal relationships and unable to make decisions and changes regarding safer sexual behaviors. The male is usually dominant in the areas of sexual behavior and contraceptive practices (41). Poor women, in particular, may be economically dependent on men and may not be in the position to insist on condom use. Lower income African-American and Latin American women have reported a perceived sense of powerlessness, characterized by intense concerns, low self-esteem, and a loss of control (27). Among Latin American couples, cultural values may influence gender roles, playing a major role in the imbalance of power. Although Latin American women may be responsible for birth control, contraceptive use may need to be authorized by the man. Among African-Americans, economic factors also play a role. The ratio of single men to single women is lower in the African-American community compared to the white community (30). The instability in adult sexual relationships as suggested by the decline in stable adult relationships (measured by out-of-wedlock births, divorces, single parent families) facilitates the imbalance of power toward men (31). The imbalance between the number of marriageable men (heterosexual, employed, and not incarcerated) to women is further exacerbated by the increasing unemployment among African-Americans (31). For African-American men, attitudes related to sexuality and gender roles may be tied to their relative lack of power in controlling events in other domains (22).

CHILDBEARING AND CONTRACEPTION

Childbearing is highly valued for both African-American and Latin American women and the suggestion of delaying or terminating a pregnancy may be completely unacceptable to them or their partner (42–43). Children may be considered an important contribution to the community and may be the only means to achieve a sense of identity and status, particularly for women whose opportunities have been limited by poverty and racism (28). Pregnancy is related to elevated self-esteem and children to heightened status among family members and within the community (41). The ability to reproduce is seen in the African-American community as a powerful tool for liberation and against racism (16); contraception and family planning may be seen as an attempt to eliminate African-Americans (44,45). Religion may also play a role in contraception; Catholicism, a dominant religion in the Latin American culture opposes contraception methods and abortion. Ethnic/

racial women are less likely to report the use of barrier contraceptives (8–10,46). African-American women are more likely to favor contraceptive methods that do not depend on the partner's behavior (e.g., condom use, withdrawal of penis) (16). In addition, heterosexual anal intercourse may be used by both African-American and Latin American women as an alternative method for birth control or to maintain vaginal virginity (47).

Safer Sex

Adopting safer sex practices can be complicated by childbearing issues, gender roles, and the imbalance of power present in the relationship among racial/ethnic women. The cultural association of condoms with prostitution and uncleanliness, perceived diminished sensation, discomfort, inconvenience, as well as the lack of information concerning the protection condoms provide, may also attribute to the low condom use among African-American and Latin American women (15). Condom use is also more likely to be associated with distrust (48). Because many Latin American men believe that condoms should not be used with "good women" such as their wives or steady partners, a Latin American woman who requests condom use by her partner or husband may be implying a message of distrust (30). In a culture which places high value on marriage and family, a Latin American who suggests using condoms may be perceived as desiring sex only for pleasure without any intention for marriage and a family (26). Among Haitians, a condom is perceived as a foreign object which devalues a woman (23). A woman who raises the issue of condom may be suspected of adultery (24). Physical abuse or abandonment may result from African-American and Latin American women requesting condom use by their partner (16,24). African-American women are also not likely to advocate safer sex practices regardless of their partners' sexual practices or drug habits (49–50).

Family and Social Support

Among racial/ethnic communities of color, the care giving provider is often the family unit, and the kinship network (e.g., parents, siblings, friends) may be a dominant influence on health behavior, support, and information (16–17). Social support may also help reinforce a person's own coping skills (17,22). Familismo, an important cultural characteristic among Latin Americans, emphasizes the family as the primary social unit and source of support. The strong familial orientation of the Latin American culture also creates a number of obligations. Other family members may be consulted before a decision is made, and family members may provide economic and emotional assistance. However, familismo may also mean Latin Americans avoid sharing their problems outside the family circle. Drug programs, for example, are generally designed to substitute for the absent family. Because Latin American drug users are more likely to access their own families for support and less likely to seek solutions to their problems in group settings, most drug treatment programs may be inappropriate (25).

Medical and Alternative Health Practices

Alternative healing practices may be common among Latin Americans. Using spiritual practices (espiritismo/santeria) and alternative healers (e.g. santeros, cuanderos) may be preferred to health institutions. Providers should be aware of the prevalence of folk beliefs and healing practices in Latin American population and assess any incompatibilities between folk and biomedical treatment practices (51). In one survey of Latin Americans, 57% were involved in spiritual practices, 40% in conventional religion, and/or 41% new age practices to manage and treat their HIV infection along with medical care (51). Needles and syringes used by Latin Americans for ear piercing and vitamin and medication injections may not be perceived as a mode of HIV transmission (25).

Other Aspects That May Affect Prevention Efforts (18,25)

Other aspects in the Latin American culture which should be considered in prevention efforts are as follows:

Simpatia is the importance of smooth social relations, mandating politeness and respect, and avoiding assertiveness, direct negative responses and criticism. Simpatia avoids confrontation, so any AIDS prevention activities that involve confrontation, e.g., insisting on condom use with a sexual partner, will seem inappropriate. In addition, Latin American listeners may appear to agree with a message, even though they do not understand it or have no intention of following the advice.

Respeto refers to the importance of maintaining personal integrity in interactions with others. Patients receiving drug treatment, for example, must feel they are being treated with respect and value, otherwise the treatment will be rejected. Another dimension of respeto is not questioning an authority figure, even if something is not understood. Questions should be asked to assure that AIDS information and behavior change messages have been correctly understood.

Implications for Prevention Programs

For interventions to be effective, they must be culturally sensitive, anticipating and responding to specific needs and concerns. Experienced and skilled members of the targeted community should be included as partners in planning, educators, and peer leaders of prevention programs. Interventions delivered by community members and peers may influence social norms as well as provide an effective means to educate difficult-to-reach groups of the community (19). Because language skills, beliefs, knowledge, and behavior may vary, interventions should consider the degree of the client's educational level and degree of acculturation. Culturally relevant materials and content should be used, and interventions should be personalized and integrated into the individual's lifestyle. The intervention medium (e.g., theater skits, rap) and site (e.g., church, bars, clubs, student organizations, private homes) should be culturally appropriate and comfortable to convey messages effectively. Because of the lack of perceived risk which may exist among persons of color, education should also help the individual assess his or her risk. Programs should anticipate and respond to concerns, such as genocide theories, ideally through skilled members of the community (22). Any given behavior should neither be accepted nor rejected without understanding its cultural significance (22).

The importance of social support and the family among African-Americans and Latin Americans can have a positive impact on AIDS prevention efforts. Messages that emphasize the man's responsibility of protecting the family from AIDS or social responsibility to the community may be more effective (16,22). The negative impact of AIDS on the family and especially on children may be used in motivating behavior change (e.g., condom use) or initiating drug treatment. Interventions might involve the spouses and the extended kinship network to reinforce efforts to adopt safer sex practices, and assist against drug use relapse pressures (22). AIDS prevention activities that involve confrontation for women, such as insisting on condom use with a sexual partner, assertiveness skills, or negotiating new sexual behaviors, may be inappropriate for women in unequal relationships (e.g., low-acculturated Latin American women). A more appropriate approach might be to aim messages about condom use to the male partner, or include both partners in the intervention (28–29). Focusing on the protection of the family may make it more acceptable that both partners be included in discussion (16). Ideally both partners should be fully educated at the same time; first separately with same-gender counselors, and then together to establish dialogue between them (28). When possible, risk reduction should also assist in providing skills which enhance sexual communication, commitment to condom use, and the enjoyment of condoms (52–53). The use of the female condom may provide an alternative for women, allowing control over safe sex practices without challenging the power of the male partner (54). Couple-focused intervention may also promote longer lasting behavior change with respect to safer drug use behaviors. Fostering group pride may serve not only to empower people to respond constructively but also to develop pride within the individual; this may be done by including culturally relevant content, setting and media (19). Women should be assisted to "empower" themselves as much as possible, setting personal goals and discussing what actions may achieve them. Techniques for enhancing self-esteem and feelings of control should be taught. African-American and Latin American women with high self-esteem and a stronger sense of coherence report less emotional distress and fewer high-risk behaviors (27). Problem-focused forms of coping are associated with lower emotional distress and better health behaviors (55–57). Problem-focused coping responses, such as ways to seek information or support, steps in decision making, and reducing stress should be discussed (55–57). Focusing on issues such as self help, economic hardship, and exercising control on the environment have also been reported to be helpful (22).

Reaching racial/ethnic bisexual/homosexual men may be difficult. Prevention messages directed specifically at homosexual/bisexuals may be ignored by a large proportion who do not self-identify as being homosexual or bisexual. It is important that prevention efforts focus on risk behaviors versus groups.

For racial/ethnic communities access to information, services, and AIDS education may be difficult due to cultural and language differences, and economic, educational and social factors. Prevention efforts should consider that risk behaviors for HIV may be only one part of a constellation of behaviors that define an individual's lifestyle. Priorities such as unemployment and poverty that influence an individual's lifestyle also may need to be addressed and accommodated. Providing assistance in job skills, housing, and food may be just as important as culturally sensitive and appropriate education and skill training. Understanding the various cultural, social, and economic factors that impact African-American and Latin American communities can lead to more effective prevention efforts for this population.

REFERENCES

1. CDC. HIV/AIDS Surveillance Report. 1995 Mid-year Edition 1995:7(No. 1).
2. CDC. Human immunodeficiency virus infection in the United States: a review of current knowledge. MMWR 1987;36(Supp No.S-6).
3. Chaisson RE, Moss AR, Onishi R, et al. Human immunodeficiency virus infection in heterosexual intravenous drug users in San Francisco. Am J Pub Health 1987;77:169–172.
4. Friedman S, Des Jarlais D, Sotheran J. AIDS education for intravenous drug users. Health Education Quarterly 1986;13:383–393.
5. Friedman SR, Des Jarlais SR, Novice DM, et al. HIV-1 infection among intravenous drug users in Manhattan, New York City, from 1977–1987. JAMA 1989;261:1008–1012.
6. Lange WR, et al. The geographic distribution of human immunodeficiency virus markers in parental drug abusers. Am J Public Health 1988;78:443–446.
7. Sufian M, Friedman S, Neaigus A, et al. Impact of AIDS on Puerto Rico intravenous drug users. His J Behav Sci 1990;12:122–134.
8. Fordyce EJ, Balanon A, Stoneburner R, Rautenberg E. Women and AIDS: a survey of knowledge, attitudes and behaviors. New York: New York City Dept of Health, Division of AIDS Program Services, 1989.
9. CDC. Heterosexual behaviors and factors that influence condom use among patients attending a sexually transmitted clinic—San Francisco. MMWR 1990;39:685–688.
10. Mosher WE, Bachrach CA. Contraceptive use in the United States, 1982. Vital Health Statistics, 1986; 23 (12), Department of Health and Human Services Publication No. 86-1988, National Center for Health statistics. Washington, DC: Goverment Printing Office.
11. Carballo-Diequez A, Dolezal C. Barriers to condom use among Puerto Rican men who have sex with men. (abstr) IXth International Conference on AIDS. Berlin, June 1993 (PO-D23-4113).
12. Hays RB, Kegeles SM, Coates TJ. High HIV risk taking among young gay men. AIDS 1990;4:901–907.
13. Mays VM, Cochra SD. High risk HIV-related sexual behaviors in a national sample of US black gay and bisexual men. IXth International Conference on AIDS. Berlin, June 1993 (WS-C07-2).
14. DiClemente RJ, Boyer CB, Morales ES. Minorities and AIDS: knowledge, attitudes and

misconceptions among Black and Latin American adolescents. Am J Public Health 1988;78:55–57.

15. Marin G. AIDS prevention among Hispanics: Needs, risk behaviors and cultural values. Public Health Reports 1989;104(5):411–415.

16. Mays VM, Cochran SD. Issues in the perception of AIDS risk and risk reduction activities by black and Hispanic/Latin American women. Am J Psychol 1988;43:949–957.

17. Hahn RE, Castro KG. The health and health care status of Latino populations in the U.S.; a brief review. In: Marinez-Maza O, Shin DM, Banks HE, eds. Latin Americans and AIDS: A National Strategy Symposium. 1989. CIRID at UCLA; Los Angeles.

18. Marin B. Hispanic Culture. Hispanic culture: effects on prevention and care. Focus 1991;6:1–2.

19. Croteau JM, Nero CI, Prosser DJ. Social and cultural sensitivity in group-specific HIV and AIDS programming. J Counseling & Develop 1993;7:290–295.

20. CDC. AIDS among racial/ethnic minorities—United States, 1993. MMWR 1994;43: 644–647,653–655.

21. Kalichman SC, Hunter TL, Kelly JA. Perceptions of AIDs susceptibility among minority and nonminority women at risk for HIV infection. J Consult Clin Psych 1992; 60:725–732.

22. Schilling RF, Schinke SP, Nichols SE, et al. Developing strategies for AIDS prevention research with black and Hispanic drug users. Public Health Reports 1989;104;2–11.

23. Stuntzner-Gibson D. Women and HIV disease: an emerging social crisis. Social Work 1991;36(1):22–28.

24. Andriote J. For women at risk prevention begins with self-esteem. The NAN Monitor 1988;3:12–14.

25. Marin B, Hispanic Culture: Implications for AIDS prevention (handout). Presented at HIV/AIDS: Advanced Nursing Management Conference. Los Angeles. 1993.

26. Worth D, Rodriguez R. Latin American women and AIDS. Siecus Rep 1987; Jan–Feb: 5–7.

27. Nyamathi AM. A research trajectory on health promotion among impoverished women of color. University of California/Health Net Wellness Lecture Series. October 17, 1994; 1–18.

28. Nyamathi A, Shin D. Designing a culturally sensitive AIDS educational program for black and Hispanic women of childbearing age. NACOOG's Clinical Issues in Perinatal and Woman's Health Nursing 1990;1:86–98.

29. de la Vega E. Considerations for reaching the Latino population with sexuality and HIV/AIDS information and education. Siecus Report 1990;18:1–8.

30. Anastos K, Palleja SM. Caring for women at risk of HIV infection. J Gen Int Med 1991;6:S40–S46.

31. Fullilove MT, Fullilove RE, Haynes K, Gross S. Black women and AIDS prevention: A view towards understanding the gender rules. J Sex Res 1990;27:47–64.

32. Peterson JL, Gerado M. Issues in the prevention of AIDS among black and Hispanic men. Am Psychol 1988;43:871–877.

33. Diaz T, Chu SY, Frederick M, et al. Sociodemographics and HIV risk behaviors of bisexual men with AIDS: results from a multistate interview project. AIDS 1993; 7:1227–1232.

34. Carrier J. Mexican male bisexuality. In: Klein F, Wolf T, eds. Bisexualities: Theory and Research. New York: Haworth Press; pp. 75–85.

35. CDC. Condom use and sexual identity among men who have sex with men—Dallas, 1991. MMWR 1993;42:7,13–14.

36. Lever J, Kanouse DE, Rogers WH, et al. Behavior patterns and sexual identity of bisexual men. J Sex Res 1992;29:141–167.

37. Kramer MA, Aral SO, Curran JW. Self-reported behavior patterns of patients attending a sexually transmitted disease clinic. Am J Public Health 1980;70:997–1000.

38. Doll LS, Peterson LR, White C, et al. Homosexually and non-homosexually identified men who have sex with men: a behavioral comparison. J Sex Res 1992;29:1–14.

39. Chu SY, Peterman TA, Doll LS, et al. AIDS in bisexual men in the United States: epidemiology and transmission to women. Am J Public Health 1992;82:220–224.

40. Earl WL. Married men and same sex activity: a field study of HIV risk among men who do not identify as gay or bisexual. J Sex Marital Ther 1990;16:251–257.

41. Mitchell JL, Heagarty M. Special considerations for minorities. In: Pizzo PA, Wilfert CM, eds. Pediatric AIDS. Williams and Wilkins; Baltimore; 1991:704–713.

42. Bouknight RR, Bouknight LG. Acquired immunodeficiency syndrome in the black community: focusing on education and the black male. NY State J Med 1988;88:232–235.

43. Holman S. Berthaud M, Sunderland A, Moroso, et al. Woman infected with human im-

munodeficiency virus: Counselng and testing during pregnancy. Semin Perinatol 1989;13:7–15

44. Population Reference Bureau Selection No. 37. Race consciousness and fears of black genocide as barriers to family planning. 1971:6.
45. Turner CB, Darity WA. Fears of genocide among Black Americans as related to age, sex, and region. Am J Public Health 1973;63:1029–1034.
46. Kapila R, Koser P. Women and AIDS: an overview. Med Aspects Hum Sex 1988;22: 92–103.
47. Thomas SB, Gilliam AG, Iwrey CG. Knowledge about AIDS and reported risk behaviors among black college students. J Amer Coll Health 1989;38:61–66.
48. Choi KH, Rickman R, Catania J. What do U.S. heterosexual adults believe about condoms. IXth International Conference on AIDS. Berlin June 1993 (PO-C22-3146).
49. Flaskerud JH, Rush CE. AIDS and traditional health beliefs and practices of black women. Nursing Research 1989;38:210–215.
50. Njeri N. A new sexuality? Essence 1989;January:114–118.
51. Suarez M, Raffaelli M, O'Leary A, LoConte J. Use of alternative healing practices among HIV-infected Hispanics. IXth International Conference on AIDS. Berlin, June 1993 (PO-D22-4089).
52. Malow RM, Corrigan SA, Cunningham SC, et al. Psychosocial factors associated with condom use among African-American drug abusers in treatment. AIDS Education and Prevention 1993;5:244–253.
53. Catania JA, Coates TJ, Golden E. et al. Correlates of condom use among black, hispanic, and white heterosexuals in San Francisco: The AMEN Longitudinal Survey. AIDS Education and Prevention 1994;6:12–26.
54. Shervington DO. The acceptability of the female condom among low-income African-American women. J Natl Med Assoc 1993;85:341–7 (published erratum appears in J Natl Med Assoc 1993;85:497,564).
55. Fawzy FI, Cousins N, Fawzy NW, Kemeny ME, Elashoff R, Morton D. A structured psychiatric intervention for cancer patients: Changes over time in methods of coping and effective disturbance. Arch Gen Psych 1990;47:720–725.
56. Gass K, Chang A. Appraisals of bereavement, coping, resources, and psychosocial health dysfunction in widows and widowers. Nursing Research 1989;38:31–36.
57. Namir S, Wolcott D, Fawzy F, Alumbaugh M. Coping with AIDS: psychological and health implications. J App Soc Psych 1987;17:309–328.

CHAPTER 10

Self-Care for Persons with HIV

Precautions for Persons Living with HIV

For the person living with HIV, it is important to take care of one's health. This section contains recommendations to decrease the risk of infections and promote health (e.g., adhering to treatment and visiting the physician regularly). The following measures provide guidelines to reduce the risk of opportunistic infection in the immunosuppressed individual and decrease the risk of HIV transmission through blood or other bodily fluids.

Daily Hygiene (1–3)

GENERAL HYGIENE

- Bathe regularly, using a mild soap and rinse well.
- Use body lotions or creams to restore moisture to dry skin.
- Do not share razors.
- Keep fingernails and toenails clean. Keep nails short.
- Avoid excessive hair washing, using only gentle shampoos (e.g. baby shampoo).
- Wash hands before and after contact with contaminated materials, contact with own body fluids (e.g. semen, mucus, blood), after using the bathroom, before eating, and before cooking.
- Unwashed hands should be kept away from eyes, nose and mouth.

DENTAL HYGIENE (1–4)

- Maintain good dental hygiene.
- Brush with a soft toothbrush after meals; do not share toothbrushes, toothpicks, dental floss or water picks. Wash glasses used for rinsing the mouth in hot, soapy water, or use paper cups.
- Schedule regular dental checkups every 3 to 6 months.
- Use rinses of diluted hydrogen peroxide to kill bacterial infection and promote healing (1 part peroxide to 10 parts water).

Housekeeping (1–3)

- Wash dishes and silverware in dishwasher or hot soapy water.
- Do not use dirty sponges to wash dishes or clean food preparation areas.
- Clean bathroom and kitchen floors at least weekly. For disinfection of floors, sink, bathtubs, showers, and toilet bowl, clean the surface of debris and disinfect with bleach solution (1 part bleach, 9 parts water).
- Clean mops and sponges by soaking them in a bleach solution (1 part bleach, 9 parts water) for 5 minutes.
- Wash clothes and bed linens as usual unless soiled with body fluids (e.g., urine, feces, semen); they should then be washed separately.
- Spills of body fluids or waste (blood, urine, stool, vomitus, etc.) should be cleaned with paper towel and disposed of properly. Disinfect the surface with bleach solution (1 part bleach, 9 parts water).
- Trash can be handled normally. Tampons, sanitary napkins, and trash containing tissue or bandages with large amount of sputum, wound drainage, blood, etc., should be disposed of in a lined container with a disposable plastic bag.

Food Safety

Persons with HIV are vulnerable to pathogens caused by eating contaminated foods. Infectious organisms include salmonella, campylobacteria, shigella, *Clostridium perfringens, Staphylococcus aureus,* and *Clostridium botulinum.* These infections occur more frequently, are more severe, and last longer in people who are HIV infected (4). Food safety is an important issue for persons with HIV infection. Guidelines concerning the purchase and safe preparation of food have been developed (4–6) and are compiled in Table 10.1.

Travel

Travelers are often exposed to pathogens uncommon or absent in the resident country. When traveling to some countries, risks for certain infectious diseases may be higher due to tropical climate or inadequate hygiene and sanitation (4,7). A CDC International Traveler's Hotline, (404) 332-4555, is available for up-to-date health information for travelers, including current areas of infectious disease and vaccination requirements. In addition, some countries may impose travel restrictions to HIV-infected persons; they may not be allowed to travel in some countries. Call the local consulate office for further information.

Enteric infections (related to the gastrointestinal tract) appear to pose the greatest risk to HIV-infected travelers (7). The presence of microorganisms in food and water may be prevalent, increasing risk to enteric infections. Enteric infections include *E. coli* diarrhea, hepatitis A,

Table 10.1.

Food Precautions for Persons Living with HIV

Grocery Shopping
- Shop for non-perishable before perishable items.
- Check the expiration date (e.g., "sell by") of items.
- Buy only items with intact safety seals and canned items that are not dented.
- Buy fruits and veggies with unbroken skins

Storage & Refrigeration
- Freeze perishables promptly when returning home from the market. Cold foods should be kept below 40°F and hot foods above 140°F.
- Double-bag raw meats, poultry, and seafood in plastic and keep in lower compartments of the freezer and refrigerator to prevent contamination of other foods by drippings.
- Refrigerate or freeze, label and date cooked foods in small sealed containers while they are still hot.
- Keep cooked foods for a maximum of 3 days in the refrigerator and 30 days in the freezer (if the freezer is separate), otherwise for a maximum of 2 weeks.
- Foods containing protein, like fish, poultry, lean meat, cheese, eggs, and ready made salads or sandwich fillings should be refrigerated immediately. Keep all foods covered.
- Do not refreeze food that has been defrosted or partially thawed.
- Used packaged luncheon meats within 2–5 days after opening.

Cooking
- Meats, poultry, fish, and eggs should be cooked thoroughly. Pre-cook all meats before grilling. Use a meat thermometer, the temperature of meat, poultry, fish should reach 165° to 212°F.
- Leftovers should be heated thoroughly to an internal temperature of 165°F (use a meat thermometer).

Eating Precautions
- Don't eat raw meat, chicken, shell fish, or eggs. (e.g., steak tartar, uncooked oysters or clams, homemade mayonaise or other dishes made with uncooked eggs). Avoid raw eggs, unless commercially pasteurized (e.g., Egg Beaters® or Scramblers®)
- Avoid undercooked meat, chicken, poultry, fish and shellfish, and eggs. Avoid raw (unpasteurized) milk.
- Avoid salads and raw vegetables at restaurants, particularly when the T-cell count is low. Choose hot soups instead.
- Take caution with food that may have been outside for a long time or carelessly prepared (e.g., picnic foods or food purchased from street vendors).

Food Preparation
- Do not thaw food at room temperature; thaw frozen foods in the refrigerator or microwave oven (on the defrost/low setting). Cook foods as soon as possible after thawing.
- Use paper or cloth towel once daily.
- Throw away any food that is or suspected to be spoiled.
- Use only pasteurized milk, cheese, and other dairy products.
- Keep all utensils in contact with food clean.
- During preparation of food, care should be taken not to contaminate cooked foods with raw meat, fish, or poultry. Examples: Do not cut cooked meat on a cutting board that has just been used for raw meat.
- Do not stuff meats or poultry in advance.
- Use a cutting board made of hard plastic or marble (easier to clean) and not wood.
- Frequently wash hands when cooking and always after handling raw meat, chicken, or fish.
- Fresh fruits and vegetables should be washed thoroughly with cold water before and after peeling
- If T-cell count is low, the following solution has been suggested to wash fruits and vegetables:
Mix a solution of water (one gallon) and 2% iodine tincture (20 drops) and let stand for 10 or more minutes before washing fruits or vegetables. The reaction between the carbohydrates and iodine may turn the water blue, but the fruits and vegetables are safe to eat. The used water should be discarded. *Note:* Iodine tincture can be found in most drug stores, bleach (2 tbsp/gallon water) or iodine tablets (found in outdoor sporting goods stores) can also be used as an alternative. Consult the physician or dietician regarding the correct product to use before starting.

Washing, Cleaning, & Hygiene
- Hygiene should be emphasized. Hands should be thoroughly washed in hot, soapy water and rinsed before and after handling food, before eating food, and after using the toilet.
- Cover hand cuts with bandaids.
- All utensils, cutting boards, and appliances should be thoroughly washed with soap and hot water (or diluted bleach solution). Any utensil or equipment in contact with raw meat, fish, eggs or poultry should be washed after use and before being exposed to cooked products or other foods.
- Wash dishes in hot, soapy water with clean cloth or sponge. It is suggested to soak the cleaning cloth or sponge in a mixture of household bleach and water (1 to 9 parts) for 5 min. This solution can also be used to clean counters, floors, and appliances.

salmonella, and shigella. Respiratory tract infections are also common (e.g. influenza, measles, histoplasmosis, and coccidioidomycosis) among travelers. Vectorborne infections include malaria, yellow fever, and babesiosis. Other routes of possible infections include percutaneous penetration (i.e., through the skin) by certain parasites (e.g., rabies, schistosomiasis, and hookworm) (7).

Preventive strategies include utilizing hygiene measures to avoid exposure (e.g. do not eat raw vegetables and fruits, drink bottled water), immunization, and prevention of illness through the use of antibiotics, prophylactic antimicrobial therapy, immunizations, or immune globulins (4,7). If possible, travel to areas where coccidioidomycosis and histoplasmosis are endemic should be avoided. Travel plans and available preventive medications should be discussed with the physician. An adequate supply of condoms and lubricant should be packed, as condoms in some countries may be in short supply or of inferior quality (4). Plans for emergency and routine health care should be made prior to travel. This may include additional insurance for a return flight home in the event any major medical care is needed and the preference to be treated in the home city (4).

Recommended immunizations for HIV-infected adult travelers (7) are summarized in Table 10.2; the information given assumes a history of routine childhood immunization with vaccine against diphtheria-tetanus, measles-mumps-rubella, and polio. Contraindicated vaccines contain live organisms. Immune globulin should be given to all travelers to developing countries to protect against hepatitis A infection, unless the individual is already known to be immune (8). Immune globulin should be given either 2 weeks after or 3 months before live vaccines, such as measles (7,8), since immune globulins can interfere with the response to live vaccines. Additional required immunizations and prophylaxis will largely depend upon the destination of travel (e.g., areas endemic for malaria) and should be discussed with the health provider.

Table 10.2.
Immunizations for Adult Travelers Infected with HIV to Developing Countries

	Indicated Immunizations	Contraindication
Standard immunizations	• Inactivated parenteral polio vaccine (single booster dose for adults) • Inactivated parenteral typhoid vaccine (booster interval, 3 years) • Immune globulin (effective duration, 3 to 5 months, depending on dose) • Measles-mumps-rubella (single dose for adults)*	Live oral polio vaccine Live oral typhoid vaccine

*May be omitted if patient has physician-diagnosed measles or serologic evidence of measles immunity.
MODIFIED from Wilson ME, von Reyn FC, and Fineberg HV. Infections in HIV-infected travelers: Risks and Prevention. Ann Int Med 1991;144:588.

Vaccines and Immunizations

Routine immunizations for adults with HIV-infection having normal childhood immunization series include the following (7,9–14):

Diphtheria, tetanus (booster interval, 10 years)
Mumps, measles, and rubella (MMR)
Influenza (repeat annually)
Pneumococcus (single dose)
Hepatitis B series (unless patient is already immune as indicated by presence of hepatitis B antibody)
Haemophilus influenza type B (Hib) (single dose for adults)

Routine immunizations of individuals infected with HIV have been the standard of care. Live vaccines (except MMR) are contraindicated, but other immunizations have been generally recommended, regardless of HIV status. However, recent evidence suggests that vaccination may stimulate HIV replication, at least temporarily, theoretically accelerating HIV disease progression (15). This has led to a reevaluation of routine immunizations of HIV-infected individuals. The clinical efficacy of immunizations on HIV-infected adults is uncertain due to the limited data available. Routine immunization against pneumococcus for all HIV-infected patients, and hepatitis B immunization for susceptible HIV-infected individuals who engage in high-risk behaviors have been recommended (15). The benefits of influenza and *H. influenza* vaccines should be discussed with your physician before a decision is reached, especially when an individual's CD4 cell counts are lower than 100. Some physicians do not recommend influenza or *H. influenza* vaccine with low CD4 cells (15).

Pets (1,4,16)

Animals may harbor organisms that are transmissible, including cats (*Toxoplasma gondii*), birds (e.g. *Chlamydia psittaci, Histoplasma capsulatum*), turtles (*salmonella*), and tropical fish (*mycobacterium*). Pet birds and cats should be checked by a veterinarian. Wash hands with soap and water after handling pets, especially after cleaning their litter or living areas; wear gloves and a mask when cleaning. Litter boxes should be emptied (not sifted) daily. Gloves should be worn when cleaning aquariums and handling fish. Sick pets should be seen promptly by a veterinarian; neither sick pets nor their litter should be handled by the person with HIV infection.

Other (16)

- Avoid persons with chickenpox or shingles until the chicken pox/shingles have completely crusted over. Also avoid persons who have been recently exposed to chickenpox (particularly from the 10th to 21st day after exposure).

- If exposed to measles, chicken pox or shingles, contact your physician within 24 hours.

REFERENCES

1. Shin DM, Avers JA, eds. AIDS/HIV Reference Guide for Medical Professionals, Third Edition. Los Angeles: CIRID at UCLA. 1988
2. Breuer NL. A Guide to Self Care for HIV Infection, Second Edition. 1993. AIDS Project Los Angeles; Los Angeles.
3. Moffatt B, Spiegel J, Parrish S, Helquist M. AIDS: A Self-Care Manual. 1987. AIDS Project Los Angeles; Los Angeles.
4. Pinsky L, Douglas PH, Metroka C. The Essential HIV Treatment Fact Book. New York: Pocket Books; 1992; 89–118.
5. Cowell C, Rubin KW. Children with AIDS living at home: A Challenge for a Community Support Team. 1080 Nutrition Focus 4(5);1–5
6. Wong G. HIV Disease Nutrition Guidelines 1993. Chicago: Physicians Association for AIDS Care
7. Wilson ME, Fordham von Reyn F, Fineberg HV. Infections in HIV-infected travelers: risks and prevention. Ann Intern Med 1991; 114:582–592.
8. CDC. Health information for international Travel, 1990. Atlanta, Georgia: Centers for Disease Control; 1990. HHS Publication No. (CDC)90-8290.
9. Jewett JF and Hecht FM, Preventive health care for Adults with HIV. JAMA 1993; 269:1144–1153.
10. CDC. Protection against viral hepatitis: recommendations for the Immunization Practices Advisory Committee (ACIP). MMWR 1990;39(RR-5):5–22.
11. CDC. Recommendations of the Immunization Practices Advisory Committee: pneumococcal polysaccharide vaccine. MMWR 1989;38:64–76.
12. CDC. Prevention and control of influenza recommendations of the immunization practices advisory committee (ACIP). MMWR 1992;41(RR-9):1–17.
13. USPHS/ISDA. Guidelines for prevention of opportunistic infections in persons infected with human immunodeficiency virus: an overview. Clin Infect Dis 1995;21(Suppl 1):S12-S31.
14. Recommendations of the advisory committee on immunization practices (ACIP): use of vaccines and immune globulins in persons with altered immunocompetence. MMWR 1993;42 (RR-4).
15. Singer M, Sax P. Routine Immunization in HIV: Helpful or harmful. AIDS Clinical Care. 1996;8:1,12,13,15.
16. U.S. Dept Health and Human Services. Caring for someone with AIDS. May 1994 Inv. #498.

Nutritional Management of Symptoms

People living with HIV may eat less because of side effects from medication, the effects of other diseases, and a lack of appetite. Anorexia, nausea, and vomiting may also lead to lowered intake, and symptoms such as mouth sores, swallowing problems and taste alterations can make eating difficult. Suggested interventions (1–5) that may assist in these complications are outlined below.

Lack of Appetite

- Eat small, frequent meals of favorite foods.
- Maximize calorie intake by eating foods high in protein and calories, nutrient-dense snacks and drinking shakes or high-calorie nutritional supplements (e.g., dried fruit, cheese and crackers, peanut butter and jelly sandwich, fruit nectar).
- Try eating in a pleasant environment and with friends or family.
- Get together with other people for social activities that may spark an interest in eating.

- Take a short walk before eating to boost appetite.
- Ask someone to prepare food for you. Buy convenience foods low in fat: low-fat entrees and ready-to-eat snacks. Prepare a large amount of food when feeling well and freeze in individual packages.
- Avoid food odors when not eating. Minimize food odor by ventilating the home well, particularly the kitchen.

Diarrhea

- Eat small, frequent meals.
- Drink large amounts of liquid. Have drinks and foods with sodium and potassium (e.g., bouillon, fruit juices, commercial or home-prepared salt-sugar solutions). Potassium is found in meat, dairy products, and most fruits and vegetables (bananas, tomatoes, potatoes, apricots and peaches).
- Continue eating and drinking plenty of fluids (approximately eight glasses each day) to prevent dehydration and weakness. If increasing calorie intake, have drinks with calories throughout the day instead of plain water (e.g., diluted pectin-containing juices [apple, pear, peach, nectarine, grape], or electrolyte solutions, like Pedialyte®, Gatorade®, Exceed®).
- Increase intake of soluble fiber (e.g., white rice, oatmeal, mashed potatoes, cooked fruits and vegetables without the skin).
- Have a low-lactose diet. Some high-lactose foods are milk, milk powder, ice cream, and milk-containing desserts, soups, and baked goods. Low-lactose dairy products include yogurt, aged cheeses, and specially-treated lactose-free or low-lactose milk. Non-dairy calcium rich foods include: canned sardines or salmon with bones, corn tortillas, tofu, calcium-fortified soy milk, cooked collard greens, turnip or beet leaves, 100% Natural® or Total® cereal, calcium-fortified. An alternative to a low-lactose diet is to take lactase (Lact-Aid™), the enzyme that allows digestion of lactose.

Avoid the following foods and drinks:

- Citrus fruits and juices (orange, tangerine, grapefruit, lemon, lime)
- Caffeine (e.g., coffee, tea, some carbonated beverages, and chocolate)
- Alcohol and gas-forming foods (kidney beans, lentils, broccoli, corn, onion, garlic)
- Fatty and greasy foods (e.g., cream, creamy sauce, luncheon meats, bacon, sausage, regular cheeses, oil, nuts, avocados, olives, salad dressings, butter, and margarine)
- Insoluble fiber grains (e.g., wheat bran, brown rice, popcorn, cornmeal, bran-type cold cereal, granola, wheat germ, nuts and seeds, vegetables and fruits with the skin)
- Sorbitol (a sweetener) and too many sweets

Nausea

- Use trial and error to establish which foods are tolerable.
- Eat easily digested, soft (e.g., rice, pureed foods, eggs) and salty (saltine crackers, pretzels) foods. Eat crackers, dry cereal, or toast in the morning.
- Drink clear liquids or carbonated beverages between meals, avoiding fluids (including soup) during meals. Drink cold or icy beverages: lemon, lime or ginger ale.
- Eat small frequent meals to avoid an empty stomach. Eat foods that are cold or at room temperature.
- Eat slowly and chew thoroughly.
- Avoid greasy, fatty, sweet, and spicy foods.
- Avoid foods with strong aromas. Try to avoid food odors when not eating. To disperse cooking odors, allow plenty of fresh air in home.
- If taking medication, discuss with the physician the possible altering of the timing of medication doses to after meals. If being treated with radiation or chemotherapy, eat a small meal at least two hours before treatment; favorite foods should be saved for later in the day (to minimize aversion to those foods). Request antiemetic medication.
- Avoid reclining immediately after a meal. Allow an hour or two after a meal before going to bed (elevating head, and supporting back with a flat pillow).

Mouth Sores and Problems Swallowing

- Have frequent small meals. Have snacks such as high-calorie and protein milk shakes, ice cream, or commercial dietary supplements.
- Drink large amount of fluids; use a straw for drinking.
- Eat soft and moist foods (e.g., mashed potatoes, scrambled eggs, pudding, custard, ice cream, ripe fruits); overcook foods until soft or blend foods into a puree. Dunk bread, sandwiches in teas or soup.
- Eat cool temperature foods; they may be more soothing. Cut food into small pieces.
- Avoid fried, spicy, hard (chips, seed, nuts, raw vegetables), salty, sticky (peanut butter candy), acidic foods (e.g., pickles, citrus fruits, juices), slippery foods (e.g., bologna, macaroni, Jello); and foods that stick to the palate (e.g., peanut butter, white bread).
- Drinking small amounts of fluids with meals may improve chewing and swallowing ability. Stimulate saliva production by eating sour candy, or gum. For persons having poor swallowing coordination, thicken liquids with ingredients such as powdered milk, mashed potato, corn starch, or oatmeal.

- Tilt head forward or backward to ease swallowing.

- Maintain good oral and dental hygiene. Keep mouth clean by rinsing often with a dilute solution of hydrogen peroxide and water, or a solution recommended by the dentist, at least three times a day, particularly after eating (do not swallow the solution).

- If tooth brushing is painful or causes bleeding, use a cotton swab for cleaning. Avoid oral irrigators (e.g., water shooting hygiene device) and commercial mouthwashes.

Taste Alterations

- Keep mouth clean by rinsing often and brushing with a soft toothbrush.

- Attempt to increase aroma in foods (smelling is a stronger sensor than tasting). Try using different spices (e.g., sugar, lemon, vinegar, salt, herbs) and wine in the recipes. Enhance the appearance of food by presenting it with different colors and textures.

- Experiment with foods to determine which are appealing and which not. Taste change is often temporary and if it recurs, the list of appealing and unappealing foods may change.

REFERENCES

1. Keusch GT, Thea DM. Clinical Nutrition. Med Clin North Am 1993;77(4):795–814.
2. Task Force on Nutrition Support in AIDS. Update: October 1989 Guidelines for Nutrition Support in AIDS. Nutrition 1989;5:39–46.
3. Bunce LV. Practical approaches to nutrition in AIDS patients. AIDS Clinical Care. 1993;5(11):88–89.
4. Wong G. HIV Disease Nutrition Guidelines Chicago: Physicians Association for AIDS Care 1993.
5. Tighe J. Nutritional guidelines for people with HIV infection. Focus 1990;5(2):3.

Health Promotion and Maintenance

Health promotion strategies pose few risks and may have a positive effect on the well-being of patients by increasing their participation in their own health care. Although unproven, some health promotion interventions may contribute to slowing disease progression (1–5). Three basic components to maintain health include good nutrition, regular exercise, and stress management (6).

Nutrition

Good nutrition ensures appropriate and adequate amounts of nutrients for the building, maintenance, and repair of cells and tissues, which are necessary to promote optimal functioning of the body (6). Nutrition is particularly important for people living with HIV since the body is prone to infections, and fighting infections requires calories. Several

HIV-associated infections affect the gastrointestinal tract, minimizing optimal nutrient intake and absorption, and altering metabolism (7–10). Significant weight loss commonly occurs during the progression of HIV disease (7–10). For persons living with HIV, early nutritional assessment and intervention may improve nutritional status and quality of life, slow weight loss, avoid nutritional complications, control nutrition-related symptoms, and lead to an increased ability to fight opportunistic infections seen in later stages of the disease (1,7,10,11,12).

NUTRITIONAL ASSESSMENT

Individuals living with HIV infection should have a baseline nutritional assessment and consult a registered dietician for dietary counseling to discuss nutrition and its importance in maintaining health (7,10,13). A nutritional assessment and intake analysis may reveal weight loss, altered body composition and micronutrient deficiencies. The objectives of nutritional interventions are to maintain (and if necessary replace) lean body mass, prevent nutrient deficiencies, and optimize nutritional stores (e.g., protein) (7,12,13). Topics which should be discussed with the dietician include maintaining lean body mass (as opposed to fat), weight management, food safety, vitamin and mineral supplements, nutritional supplements, food substitutes, nutritional complications and their management (6,7,13). The health care provider or dietician should calculate the daily caloric and protein requirements, as well as help develop a nutritional plan which incorporates the individual's food preferences. It may be necessary to modify requirements in the presence of conditions which may predispose one to malnutrition (e.g., infection, malabsorption, etc.). Elements in a complete nutritional assessment include: the medical profile, diet and weight history, laboratory and metabolic indices, and physical exam in conjunction with the nutritional parameters (e.g., mid-arm circumference) (12).

BALANCED DIET

A well-balanced diet consists of eating a variety of foods which contain an adequate intake of protein and calories. In a well-balanced diet, 50–55% of calories should be carbohydrates (mainly complex carbohydrates); 15–20% from protein; and 30% or less from fat (6). A diet high in protein and calories has been recommended to help retain lean body mass for persons living with HIV (7,10,14). In addition, adequate amounts of fluids should be included in the daily diet. A daily multivitamin/mineral can be taken. Megadoses of vitamins and minerals should be avoided since excessive amounts of nutrients can be harmful, interfering with effects of other vitamins and causing toxicity (6,7,13,14). Small, frequent meals or snacks (at least four times per day) are recommended. If weight is below ideal body weight range, calories from carbohydrate and proteins should be increased (6). Chemical stimulants such as caffeinated drinks (coffee, dark teas, soft drinks); alcoholic drinks or recreational drugs (cigarettes, cigars, cocaine, etc.) should be minimized and avoided if possible (6,14). Nontraditional dietary practices, such as macrobiotic and fad diets, or herbal powders, are not recommended if they cannot ensure an adequate and balanced intake of nutrients (7). Any nontraditional therapy considered should be discussed with the dietician to evaluate its nutritional benefits and/or potential deficiencies and toxicities (16).

RECORDING PROGRESS AND CHANGES

Any health changes that take place should be noted and mentioned to the health team at the next visit (6). In addition, a record of the daily diet, the amount, time of meal or snack, and side effects (if any) that are experienced should be kept (6). Side effects can occur from some medications, stress, or poor nutrition. A progress record can help the dietician evaluate food intake more precisely and provide individualized recommendations.

WEIGHT

Several factors affect weight, including caloric intake, physical activity, metabolism, and symptoms or side effects. Genetic make-up and overall health may also influence weight. To gain weight, food intake should be increased (i.e., high-calorie, high-protein diet) and regular exercise will help build and maintain muscle tissue. When there is more muscle mass in the body, the additional energy reserves in the muscles can be used when the food intake is low due to illness, which minimizes the length and severity of side effects and shortens recuperation time (6). A dietician should be consulted to determine desirable body weight range and a nutritional program. High-calorie, high-protein foods should be eaten when trying to gain weight or when experiencing poor appetite (6,15). Calories provide energy, and protein-rich foods help maintain muscle mass and rebuild muscle. High-calorie and high-protein foods are from the protein, dairy, starch and fat groups. Fat is a good source of calories but may not be tolerated if someone is experiencing diarrhea. Ideas to increase caloric intake (6,13,16) are shown in Table 10.3. In the event that dietary needs cannot be met by a regular well-balanced diet, nutritional supplements may be introduced.

NUTRITIONAL SUPPLEMENTS

When there is insufficient calorie or protein intake, or difficulty in maintaining or gaining weight, nutritional supplements may be introduced (7,10). Nutritional supplementation includes blended food products, commercial formulas, and intravenous solutions. Commercial drinks are usually high-protein and high-calorie; a homemade supplement can be concocted by blending some milk, ice cream or ice milk and/or fruits (noncitrus) (6). Flavor can be enhanced with chocolate, different types of essence and/or condiments. If milk cannot be tolerated, soy milk, tofu, honey and a small amount of oil can be used as a substitute for milk or ice cream. Commercial supplements are available with

Table 10.3.
Increasing Calories and Protein to Diet

- Enrich drinks, breads, cereals, desserts, soups, vegetables, and entrees with milk, milk powder, cheese, jelly, honey,* peanut butter, or other nuts, or other calorie-containing condiments.
- Increase protein (and calories) by adding cheese, milk, eggs, yogurt, peanut butter, beans, and nuts (if able to chew and swallow) to sauces, salads, soups, fruits, vegetables, and main dishes.
- Fortify drinking milk with powdered skim milk. Use soy formula or Lactaid brand milk, if there is a lactose intolerance.
- Substitute whole milk or half and half for water when making soup, instant cocoa, custards, puddings, etc.
- Use dressings, mayonnaise, butter, sour cream, sauces and gravies liberally for higher calories. Add high fat foods—sour cream, ice cream, half and half, whipped cream, mayonnaise, margarine, cream, salad dressing, sauce or gravy to meat, grains, pasta, potatoes, vegetables, and desserts (if tolerated).
- Eat between meals and have bedtime snacks (e.g., milkshakes, desserts, ice cream).
- Eat high calorie snacks: trail mix, nuts, peanut butter, bagel and cream cheese.
- If fatty foods reduce the appetite or if diarrhea develops when too many fatty foods are eaten, drink juices or nutritional supplements (e.g., Ensure, Isocal, Sustacal) and choose foods high in protein and carbohydrates but low in fat (e.g., pudding made with low/nonfat milk, hard-boiled eggs, lean meats, poultry or fish, eaten with a small amount of starchy foods).

*Raw honey should not be given to children and honey should not be given to infants under 1 year old.

lactose (a type of sugar found in dairy products) or lactose-free. Alternative feeding routes for nutritional support (e.g., enteral or parenteral feeding) should be discussed with the physician and/or dietician.

NUTRITIONAL MANAGEMENT OF SIDE EFFECTS

Inadequate dietary intake may result from medication side effects, infections and other diseases, or a lack of appetite. Anorexia, nausea, and vomiting may also lead to lowered intake, while symptoms such as mouth sores, swallowing problems and taste alterations can make eating difficult. Suggested interventions that may minimize these complications are outlined elsewhere (see Nutritional Management of Symptoms).

FOOD SAFETY

For persons living with HIV, food safety is important in order to avoid foodborne diseases. Recommendations for food safety are discussed under Precautions for Persons Living with HIV.

Exercise

Activity is required for maintenance of muscle mass. Periods of physical inactivity will lead to the inability to gain muscle mass and wasting (17). Decreased muscle mass also contributes to fatigue, making food preparation and even eating more difficult (17). The long-term effect of exercise on persons living with HIV is under investigation, and some preliminary studies have suggested that HIV-positive persons may experience psychological and immunological improvement from exercise (4,5,18). Benefits of regular exercise include: increased endurance and flexibility, increased lung capacity, increased muscle-to-fat ratio, increased stamina and energy, improved sleeping pattern, decreased stress, improved appetite, improved wound healing, and regular bowel activity (6). Guidelines for an exercise program for HIV-infected persons have been published and are outlined below (6,19).

- Before starting an exercise program, individuals should have a physical examination, and their exercise plan discussed with their physician.

- Novice exercisers should start exercising slowly, every other day for about 10–15 minutes each time (if possible). The length of workout session should be gradually increased up to 45 minutes at a time (and kept under one hour). Exercises should include the arms and legs, otherwise, other exercises should be incorporated to complement favorite activities. A variety of exercises tones and conditions different muscles. A good exercise program has 3 phases: 25% warm-up exercise, 50% conditioning, and 25% cooling down.

- Exercise should be done regularly. It may be helpful to have an exercise partner for both company and support and an exercise program that is enjoyable, and not painful or boring. For beginners, walking is a good exercise, with the eventual addition of wrist and/or ankle weights. Aerobic activities like walking, jogging, or cycling can be done every other day.

- Exercise should not be done to the point of exhaustion. After a workout, one should feel moderately tired but refreshed, with more energy and stamina after rest. Fatigue, sore muscles, or poor appetite, may indicate one is exercising too hard and the workout should be decreased. For more specific information, an exercise professional (e.g., exercise physiologist or physical therapist) should be consulted.

- Exercise should be stopped if one develops a cold or flu and resumed after feeling better. If temperature is elevated, one should not exercise until it returns to normal.

- Replenish the body with plenty of fluids (water, fruit juices, sport drinks) and eat enough calories to maintain body weight.

- Stretching exercises can be done daily. It is important to develop good breathing mechanics that involve deep regular breaths.

Stress Management

HIV infection is not only associated with physical illness, but psychological and social stresses. Changes in medical status, or personal and work relationships can trigger psychological distress. Psychosocial factors such as life stressors, social support and coping style have been associated with immune measures and physical symptoms in HIV-infected persons (20). In one longitudinal cohort study, CD4 cell count was inversely related with life stressors and passive coping (20). In another study, greater social participation (e.g., social activities, helping others in AIDS crisis) was associated with longer survival time of HIV-infected men (21). Specific interventions to address psychosocial needs include counseling, support groups, therapy, stress management techniques, and pharmacological treatment.

Stress management is an important aspect in managing HIV disease (22). It is important to understand and recognize which situations are not controllable (e.g., earthquake, traffic problems, etc.) (6,22). For controllable situations, recognizing the source of the stress, and determining what actions can be taken to remove or minimize stress is important (22). It is also necessary to recognize stress in order to implement stress reduction and management (22). Physical signs of stress include headaches, eye strain, upset stomach, rash, disrupted sleeping patterns. Psychological signs of stress include feeling depressed or anxious, being short-tempered, disoriented, and having a short concentration span (23). Other suggestions regarding the management of stress include the following (6,22,23):

- Try not to foresee future events; refocus on immediate plans or things that make you calm now.
- Avoid physically and/or mentally stressful situations whenever possible, avoiding "what if" situations.
- Talk to people who have shared the same experience. Discussing how they conquered their fears may be helpful.
- Have a sense of humor.
- Exercise regularly, relax, and pamper yourself.
- Engage in activities which relieve your mind, are fun and enjoyable.
- Get enough sleep, rest and/or naps; take breaks whenever needed.
- Reaffirm your self-worth often.
- Establish a good support system of friends and family.
- Avoid or limit the use of drugs, alcohol, coffee, tobacco, sweets, and chocolate.
- Deep breathing and mental exercises (e.g., meditation, visualization, relaxation techniques, self-hypnosis) may be helpful for some individuals. A person learning a stress reduction technique may not see any real benefits for 4 to 6 weeks, so be patient.
- Developing stress management and coping skills with a trained counselor.
- Other alternative options to reduce stress include hypnosis, imagery, and acupuncture.

- If anxieties cannot be managed, discuss the use of anti-anxiety medication with your physician.

Sleep

Getting enough sleep and rest is important. Difficulty sleeping may occur as a result of anxiety, depression and medical illness. If having difficulty falling asleep, the following has been suggested (14,24):

- Nap for 5 to 20 minutes during the day (more than 30 minutes may disturb night sleep).

- Avoid activities that make you mentally aroused in the hour before you sleep.

- Exercising during the day may improve sleep.

- Caffeine and alcohol have been shown to interfere with sleep. Reduce or avoid caffeine and alcohol as much as possible or at least a few hours before planning to sleep.

- Go to bed and get up at approximately the same time each day. An erratic sleeping schedule can make it difficult to sleep.

- A heavy meal should not be eaten late in the day. Honey has also been suggested to help put one to sleep *(Note: do not give honey to infants under 1 year of age)*.

Smoking

Studies on smoking and its effect on HIV disease progression have demonstrated contradictory results. Although there has been evidence which suggests that cigarette smoking is associated with greater declines in CD4 cells, and a greater incidence of opportunistic infections (3,5), there have also been studies showing no association between smoking and disease progression (25). However, since smoking in the general population has been shown to be associated with lung disease, smoking cessation should be considered to keep one's body as healthy as possible (24).

REFERENCES

1. McKinley MJ, Goodblock J, Salbe AD. Improved nutritional status as a result of nutrition intervention in adult HIV+ outpatients. IXth International Conference on AIDS. Berlin, June 1993 (PO B36-2365).
2. Moseson M, Zeleniuch-Jacquotte A, Belsito DY, et al. The potential role of nutritional factors in the induction of immunologic abnormalities in HIV positive homosexual men. J Acquir Immune Defic Syndr 1989;2:235–247.
3. Royce RA, Winkelstein W. HIV infection, cigarette smoking and CD4+ T-lymphocyte counts: preliminary results from the San Francisco Men's Health Study. AIDS 1990;4:327–333.
4. Schlenzig C, Wehrenberg, Poppinger J, et al. The role of physical exercise in the treatment of patients with HIV disease (abstr). Presented at the IXth International Conference on AIDS. 1993 (WS-B29-5 p72).
5. Jewett JF, Hecht FM, Preventive health care for adults with HIV. JAMA 1993;269:1144–1153.

6. Wong, G. HIV Disease Nutrition Guidelines (1993). Chicago: Physicians Association for AIDS Care.
7. Task Force on Nutrition Support in AIDS. Update: October 1989 Guidelines for Nutrition Support in AIDS Nutrition 1989;5(1):39–46.
8. Keusch GT, Thea DM. Clinical nutrition. Med Clin North Am 1993;77:795–814.
9. Kotler DP. Malnutrition in HIV infection and AIDS. AIDS 1989;3(suppl 1):S175–S180.
10. Mascioli E. Nutrition and HIV infection. AIDS Clinical Care 1993;5:1–3.
11. McKinley MJ, Goodman-Block J, Salbe AD. Improved nutritional status as a result of nutrition intervention in adult HIV+ outpatients. IXth International Conference on AIDS. Berlin, June 1993 (PO-B36–2365).
12. Kotler DP, Hellerstein MK, Fields-Gardner C, Smith J. Nutritional aspects of HIV. In: AIDS/HIV Treatment Directory. NY:AmFAR 1995;7:–11.
13. Bunce LV. Practical approaches to nutrition in AIDS patients. AIDS Clinical Care 1993;5(11):88–89.
14. Breuer NL. A Guide to Self Care for HIV Infection, 2nd ed. AIDS Project Los Angeles; Los Angeles. 1993.
15. Tighe J. Nutritional guidelines for people with HIV infection. Focus 1990;5(2):3.
16. Cowell C, Rubin KW. Children with AIDS living at home: a challenge for a community support team. Nutrition Focus 1989;4:1–5.
17. Grunfeld C, Kotler DP. Wasting in the acquired immunodeficiency syndrome. Seminars in Liver Disease 1992;12:175–187.
18. Laperriere AR, Antoni MH, Scheiderman N, et al. Exercise intervention attentuates emotional distress and natural killer cell decrements following notification of positive serologic status for HIV-1. Biofeedback Self Regul 1990;15:229–242.
19. Sullivan DJ. Fitness and a Healthy Body 1992. Burroughs Wellcome. Research Triangle Park.
20. Goodkin K, Blaney N, Feaster D, et al. Psychosocial variables predict long term changes in psychological distress and laboratory progression markers of HIV-1 infection. IXth International Conference on AIDS. Berlin, June 1993 (PO-D22-4074).
21. Caumartin SM, Joseph JG, Gillespie B. The relationship between social participation and AIDS survival in the Chicago MACS/CCS cohort. IXth International Conference on AIDS. Berlin, June 1993. (PO-D20-4008).
22. Hamilton J. Sherman S. Coping with stress. In: Moffatt B, Spiegel J, Parrish S, Helquist M, eds. AIDS: A Self-Care Manual. AIDS Project Los Angeles; Los Angeles.
23. McKusick L. The Power of Attitude. 1992 Burroughs Wellcome. Research Triangle Park.
24. Pinsky L, Douglas PH, Metroka C. The Essential HIV Treatment Fact Book. Pocket Books: NY, 1992.
25. Eskild A, Petersen G. Cigarette smoking is not associated with rapid progression to AIDS. IXth International Conference on AIDS. Berlin, June 1993 (PO-B02-0943).

Caring for Infants and Children Living with HIV

Until the diagnosis of HIV infection is established, parents or guardians should care for an infant with undetermined HIV status in a manner similar to that for an HIV-infected child. The following summarizes recommendations given for caring for HIV-infected children (1–6).

Health Care (1,2)

- The infant should be immunized with the recommended shots and boosters. These include: diphtheria, pertussis (whooping cough), and tetanus (DPT); polio (IPV); and mumps, measles, and rubella (MMR). Other immunizations may include: *Haemophilus influenzae* type B (HIb), hepatitis B (HepB), pneumococcal infection (after two years of age), and influenza (yearly). Oral polio should be avoided until the infant is known to be uninfected. It should also be avoided if the infant lives with other HIV-infected people. Injectable killed polio vaccine (IPV) should be substituted for live polio vaccine

- Avoid common illnesses by keeping the child away from people who are sick.
- A proper diet, regular exercise, and plenty of sleep is especially important for a child living with HIV.
- Regular medical follow-up and blood tests are important to assess whether a baby is HIV infected as well as to maintain the child's health. Medications should be given correctly and on time. Any unusual behavior or symptoms should be reported to the practitioner. The child should visit the dentist regularly (twice a year).
- Exposure to children with known infections (e.g., tuberculosis, chicken pox or measles) should be reported immediately to the practitioner.

SYMPTOMS WHICH SHOULD BE REPORTED PROMPTLY TO THE PHYSICIAN (1)

- Fever
- Cough
- Fast or difficult breathing
- Loss of appetite and poor weight gain
- White patches or sores in the mouth
- Persistent diaper rash
- Blood in the diaper or bowel movements
- Diarrhea (frequent loose, watery, bowel movements)
- Vomiting
- Contact with a person who has chicken pox, measles, tuberculosis (TB) or other contagious diseases

SIGNS AND SYMPTOMS OF HIV INFECTION IN BABIES (1)

- Swelling in the lymph glands in the neck, under the arms, and in the diaper area
- Swollen belly, sometimes with diarrhea
- Itchy skin rashes
- Frequent lung infections (pneumonia)
- Frequent ear and sinus infections
- Problems with gaining weight or growth
- Inability to do activities that healthy babies do (e.g., sitting alone, crawling, walking)

General Precautions

- HIV cannot be transmitted by casual contact. One cannot get infected by living in the same house, eating at the same table, using the same toilet or bathroom, kissing on the cheek.

- HIV has been found in saliva, but has not been shown to be a source of HIV transmission. To avoid the low possibility of HIV transmission, infants or toddlers who put things in their mouths frequently while playing together should be supervised by an adult.

- Hands should be washed before and after any diaper change. If there are any bloody secretions or severe and persistent diarrhea, gloves should be worn when changing the baby, and the diaper disposed in a plastic bag.

- Any open lesions on the infected person should be covered and gloves used for any contact with potentially infected secretions and excretions. Hands should be washed after exposure to blood and body fluids and before caring for a child. Gloves should be worn if lesions are present on the care taker's hands.

- Care should be taken when handling blood from an infected child (e.g., cuts, wounds). Cover any spilled blood with a solution of 1 part bleach and 9 parts water. Set 5 minutes and wipe using vinyl or latex gloves. Dispose in a plastic trash bag.

- Teach personal care habits (e.g., washing hands, brushing teeth) to the child as soon as he or she is able. Maintain dental hygiene, brushing the child's teeth until he or she is able.

- Toys should be washed periodically in hot soapy water. Toothbrushes, razors, or towels should not be shared. Other precautions for housekeeping and disinfection can be found in *Precautions for Persons Living with HIV*.

- Dishes and utensils should be washed in hot, soapy water after each use. A separate set of dishes and utensils is not necessary.

- Sheets and clothing that are stained with blood should be washed in hot water and household bleach.

- Child care providers do not need to be informed of a child's HIV status. In some jurisdictions, the child's diagnosis cannot be released without the written consent of the parent or legal guardian. However, parents may choose to inform child care providers of the child's HIV infection to ensure good hygiene practices are enforced, as well as to observe signs of illness that might require medical attention and assist meeting the child's special emotional and social needs (3). All families should be routinely informed by preschool child care programs whenever a highly infectious illness (e.g., measles, chickenpox) occurs in any child (3).

Helpful Hints When Giving Medications to Babies and Toddlers

- Use a soft plastic dropper or syringe for liquids.
- Mix medicine in food for spoon feeding.
- Sit in a firm comfortable chair.
- Put a bib or towel on the baby.
- Stay calm and use a soft voice (Do not allow the child to decide whether or not to take the medication).
- Reward the baby with juice or water to rinse the mouth.

REFERENCES

1. US Dept Health and Human Services. HIV and Your Child. AHCPR Publication no. 94-0576. January 1994.
2. Hauer LB, Dattel BJ. Management of the pregnant woman infected with human immunodeficiency virus. J Perinatology 1988;8:258–262.
3. Task Force on Pediatric AIDS. Guidelines for human immunodeficiency virus (HIV)-Infected children and their foster families. Pediatrics 1992:89:681–683.
4. Holman S, Berthaud M, Sunderland, et al. Women infected with human immunodeficiency virus: counseling and testing during pregnancy. Sem Perinatology 1989;13:7–15.
5. Children's Hospital of Los Angeles. Children with HIV infection, 2nd ed. Los Angeles, CA, 1989.
6. CDC. Education and Foster Care of Children Infected with HTLV-III/LAV. MMWR 1985;34:517–521.

Guidelines for the Care Giver

Persons infected with HIV and persons providing home care for those who are HIV infected should be fully educated and trained regarding appropriate infection control techniques. Training and education in infection control for HIV- infected persons and those who live with or provide care to them in the home should be an integral and ongoing part of the health care plan for every person with HIV infection. Recommendations have been made by the CDC for persons providing care for a person with AIDS in the home setting and are summarized below (1–3).

Infection Control

- Persons who provide nursing care for HIV-infected patients should employ precautions to reduce exposures to blood and other body fluids.
- Care should be taken when handling needles and sharp objects contaminated with blood. Needles should not be recapped by hand or removed from syringes. Needles and sharp objects should be disposed of in puncture-proof containers, and the containers kept out of reach from visitors and children.
- If handling a used needle and syringe, pick it up by the barrel of the syringe and carefully drop it into a puncture-proof container. Dispose of the container before it is overflowing with needles.

- If accidentally stuck with a used needle, wash the site of exposure thoroughly with soap and water; then contact your physician for further evaluation, advice, and perhaps treatment.

- Latex or rubber gloves should be worn if there is a possibility of direct contact with blood, blood-tinged body fluids or other body fluids, secretions, or excretions. Because urine and feces may contain a variety of pathogens, including HIV, persons providing nursing care to HIV-infected persons should wear gloves during contact with these substances.

- If large amounts of blood are present, in addition to wearing gloves, wear an apron or smock to prevent clothing from being soiled.

- Always wash hands after contact with blood and other body fluids, secretions, or excretions, and after removing gloves.

- Bandages should be used to cover cuts, sores, or breaks on exposed skin of persons with HIV infection and of persons providing care. Persons who provide such care should also wear gloves when there is a possibility of direct contact with HIV-infected blood.

- Cytomegalovirus (CMV) may be present in urine and saliva of the person with HIV. Wash hands carefully after touching saliva and urine. This is especially important for a pregnant woman who is not immune to CMV, since she can transmit CMV to her fetus.

Household Hygiene

- Remove blood from surfaces and containers with soap and water or a household cleaning solution, then disinfect the area with a solution made by mixing household bleach and water (e.g., 1 part bleach to 100 parts water, or 1¼ cup bleach to 1 gallon) for use on floors, showers, tubs, etc. (4). Discard bleach solution after 24 hours, since it is less effective when old.

- Flush all liquid waste containing blood down the toilet, being careful to avoid splashing. Tissues and other flushable items with blood, semen, or vaginal fluid should be flushed. Items which are soiled with blood, semen, or vaginal fluid which are not flushable should be disposed of in a plastic bag which is closed securely.

- Wash the clothes and linens used by the person with HIV in the usual way. Use soap or detergent and either cold or hot washing cycles, following instructions on package. Bleach may be used to remove stains, but it is not necessary to add bleach to washing machines to kill the virus. Clothes may also be dry-cleaned or hand-washed.

- Separate dishes or eating utensils are not required by persons with HIV and do not need special methods of cleaning. Wash as normal, with soap or detergent and hot water.

- A person with HIV should not prepare food when s/he has diarrhea.

- Do not share razors or toothbrushes.

Preventing Secondary Infection in the Person with HIV

- The person with HIV should avoid close contact with people who have contagious diseases (e.g., chicken pox, cold, flu, stomach flu) until symptoms have resolved.

- If the care giver has a cold or flu and there is no one else who can provide care, wear a surgical-type mask and wash your hands before touching the person with HIV.

- Persons with skin infections (e.g., boils, cold sores, fever blisters, shingles) should avoid contact with a person with HIV infection. If contact is unavoidable, keep skin sores covered and wash hands before contact. The care giver should wear gloves, if s/he has a rash or sores on his/her hands.

- See also Precautions for the Person Living with HIV

Precautions for the Care Giver When Persons with HIV Have the Following:

- *Hepatitis B virus / acute hepatitis.* The care giver should consult his/her physician about receiving treatment and/or vaccine to prevent hepatitis.

- *Chickenpox or shingles (zoster).* Care givers who have never had chickenpox should not be in the same room with an HIV-infected person who has chicken pox or shingles. If being in the same room is unavoidable, then surgical-type mask and gloves should be worn; hands should be washed before and after providing care. These precautions should be taken until the chickenpox or shingles have completely crusted over. The physician should also be consulted for consideration of prophylaxis or therapy.

- *Fever blisters or cold sores (herpes simplex).* They often appear around the mouth or nose. The care giver should avoid kissing or touching these sores. If sores must be touched with the hands, wear gloves and wash hands carefully afterwards. This is particularly important if the care giver has eczema or broken skin (allergic skin), since herpes simplex virus can cause severe skin disease in persons with eczema.

- *Coughing for more than one to two weeks.* The person with HIV should be tested for tuberculosis (TB). If diagnosed with TB, the care giver and other contacts who live or visit the home should also be tested. Discuss this with the physician, nurse, or local health department.

- *Diarrhea.* Diarrhea in a person with HIV may be caused by an infection. The care giver should wear gloves during contact with diarrheal discharge from the person with HIV. Any person with diarrhea should not prepare food for others.

Providing Emotional Support to the Person with HIV

- Encourage the person with HIV to become involved in his/her own care, determine a schedule, and make decisions when possible. These actions will provide a sense of control and independence.

- Include the person with HIV whenever possible. Keeping someone company is just as important as conversation. Allow for quiet time.

- Do not be afraid to talk about the disease. Offer to help find professional counseling if desired. Inform the health care team about your relationship to the person with HIV and your role as a care giver.

- Do not be afraid to touch a person with HIV. Holding a hand, giving a hug or back rub may be comforting. However, also be sensitive to people who do not want physical closeness.

- If the person with HIV shows changes in feelings and moods, and has difficulty in thinking clearly, speaking, concentrating, moving, or psychological problems develop, discuss these developments with the health care team.

Care for the Care Giver

To help cope with feelings of frustration, the care giver may need to share his/her feelings with others, including other care givers, counselors, clergy, or health professionals. Call the local AIDS service organizations for support. Backup help should be arranged, so the care giver has some free time. The care giver should not ignore his/her own needs. For more information, contact a physician, local health department, local AIDS organization or call the national AIDS hotline numbers. These can be found in the Resources section.

REFERENCES

1. CDC. Human immunodeficiency virus transmission in household settings—United States. MMWR 1994;43:347–356.
2. CDC. Recommendations for prevention of HIV transmission in health care settings. MMWR 1987;36 (no.2S).
3. U.S. Dept of Health and Human Services/CDC. Caring for Someone with AIDS. 5/94 Inv. #498
4. CDC. Use of bleach for disinfection of drug injection equipment. MMWR 1993;42:418–419.
5. CDC. Recommendations for the prevention of HIV transmission in health-care HIV settings. MMWR 1987;36 (Suppl 2S):9S–11S.

CHAPTER 11

Resources

INFORMATIONAL AND EDUCATIONAL AIDS RESOURCES

There are a wide range of HIV-related social, educational, and treatment resources available in the community. These services are important for the individual as they may provide a sampling of resources available to persons with HIV infection, their families and friends, and their health care providers. As organizations are continually developing, resource lists are often only current up until the time of publication. However, national information resources and hotlines, such as the National AIDS Information Clearinghouse, as well as state and local health departments can often provide additional and updated resources and referrals which may meet the individual's needs.

INTERNATIONAL RESOURCES

AIDS Clinical Trials Information Service
  PO Box 6421
  Rockville, MD 20849-6421
  USA
  Tel 1 (301) 217-0023
  FAX 1 (301) 738-6616
Global Network of People Living with HIV and AIDS
  PO Box 1AR
  London W1a 1AR
  United Kingdom
  Tel 44 71 935 0208
  FAX 44 71 935 0208

International Community of Women Living with HIV/AIDS
  PO Box 2338
  London W8 4ZG
  United Kingdom
  Tel 44 71 221 1316
  FAX 44 71 243 8481
International Council of AIDS Service Organisations (ICASO)
  Central Secretariat
  c/o Canadian AIDS Society
  100 Sparks Street, Suite 701
  Ottawa, Ontario K1P5B7
  Canada
  Tel 1 (613) 230 3580
  FAX 1 (613) 563 4998

International Federation of Red Cross and
Red Crescent Societies
  PO Box 372
  CH 1211 Geneva 19
  Switzerland
  Tel 41 22 734 5580
  FAX 41 22 733 0395
International Planned Parenthood
Federation (IPPF)
  PO Box 759
  Inner Circle, Regent's Park
  London NW1 4LQ
  United Kingdom
  Tel 44 71 486 0741
  FAX 44 71 487 7950
National Council for International
Health
  1701 K Street, North West, Suite 600
  Washington, DC 20005
  USA
  Tel 1 (202) 833-5905
  FAX 1 (202) 833-0075
UNAIDS (United Nations-WHO)
  633 3rd Ave, RM 2626
  New York, NY 10017
  Tel (212) 824-6643
United Nations Children Fund (UNICEF)
  3 United Nations Plaza
  New York, NY 10017
  USA
  Tel 1 (212) 236-7166
  FAX 1 (212) 326-7336
Women's International Network
  187 Grant Street
  Lexington, MA 02173-2140
  USA
The World Bank
  1818 H Street, North West
  Washington, DC 20433
  USA
  Tel 1 (202) 458-2381
  Fax 1 (202) 477-0645
World Health Organization
  Global Programme on AIDS
  CH 1211 Geneva 27
  Switzerland
  Tel 41 22 791 4652
  FAX 41 22 791 0317
  E-mail: (Internet) GPAINFO@WHO.CH

AFRICA

WHO Regional Office for Africa
  PO Box 6
  Brazzaville
  Congo
  Tel 242 83 38 69
  FAX 242 83 18 79
AIDS Counseling Trust
  PO Box 7225
  Harare
  Zimbabwe
  Tel 263 735 780
  FAX 263 792 340
African Medical Research and Education

Foundation (AMREF)
  PO Box 2773
  4 Pango Road
  Dar es Salaam
  Tanzania
  Tel 255 36 407
  FAX 255 46 440
ENDA
  BP 3370
  44 Rue Kleber
  Dakar, Senegal
  Tel 221 22 42 29
  FAX 221 22 26 95
UNICEF—Zimbabwe
  PO Box 1250
  Harare
  Zimbabwe

THE AMERICAS

WHO Regional Office for the Americas
  Pan American Health Organization
  525 23rd Street, North West
  Washington, DC 20037
  USA
  Tel 1 (202) 861-3200
  FAX 1 (202) 223-5971
Canadian Public Health Association
  AIDS Education and Awareness Program
  400-1565 Carling Avenue
  Ottawa, Ontario K1Z 8R1
  Canada
  Tel 1 (613) 725 3769
  FAX 1 (613) 725 9826
Inter-agency Coalition on AIDS and
Development
  1 Nicholas Street, Suite 300
  Ottawa, Ontario K1N7B7
  Canada
  Tel 1 613 241 7007
  FAX 1 613 241 5302
ABIBA (Associacao Brasileira
Interdisciplinar de AIDS)
  Rua Sete de Setembro, 48 1/2 andar
  20050-000
  Rio de Janiero-RJ
  Brazil
  Tel 55 21 224 16 54
  FAX 55 21 224 34 14
Conasida (Comision Nacional del Sida)
  Ministerio de Salud de Chile
  Moc-Iver 541, Oficina 68
  Santiago
  Chile

ASIA AND THE PACIFIC

WHO Regional Office for South-East Asia
  World Health House, Indraprastha
  Estate
  Mahatma Gandhi Road
  New Delhi 110002
  India
  Tel 91 331 78 04
  FAX 91 11 331 86 07
  Telex WHO NEW DELHI 3165095

WHO Regional Office for the Western
Pacific
    PO Box 2932
    1099 Manila
    The Philippines
    Tel 63 2 521 8421
    FAX 63 2 521 1036
    Telex UNISANTE MANILA 27652
United Nations Development Programme
(UNDP)
    Regional Project on HIV/AIDS
    55 Lodi Estate
    New Delhi 110 003
    India
AIDS Research Foundation of India
    124/1 GN Chetty Road
    T. Nagar
    Madras
    India
    Tel 91 44 8014
    FAX 91 44 825 6842
Empower
    Concrete House
    57/60 Tiwanont Road
    Tambon Talat Kwan
    Nonthaburi 11000
    Thailand
    Tel 66 2 234 3078
    FAX 66 2 234 3078
Thai Red Cross Society
    Programme on AIDS
    1871 Rama IV Road
    Bangkok 10330
    Thailand
Health Action Information Network
(HAIN)
    9 Cabanatuan Road
    Philam Homes
    Quezon City 1104
    The Philippines
    Tel 63 2 97 88 05
    FAX 63 2 721 8290
HIV/AIDS and Development
Programme
    ACFOA
    Private Mail Bag 3
    Deakin ACT 2600
    Australia
    Tel 61 6 285 1816
    FAX 61 6 285 1720
South Pacific Commission
    BP D5 Noumea Cedex
    New Caledonia
    Tel 687 26 38 18
    FAX 687 26 3818

EUROPE

WHO Regional Office for Europe
    8, Scherfigsvej
    DK-2100
    Copenhagen 0
    Denmark
    Tel 4531 29 01 11
    FAX 45 31 18 11 20

Appropriate Health Resources and
Technologies Action Group (AHRTAG)
    Farrington Point
    29-35 Farrington Road
    London EC1M3JB
    United Kingdom
    Tel 44 71 242 0606
    FAX 44 71 242 0041
    E-mail:(Internet) ahrtag@geo2.geonet.de
British Medical Association Foundation for
AIDS
    Tavistock Square
    London WC1H0JR
    United Kingdom
Centre Regional d'Information et de
Prevention du SIDA (CRIPS)
    192 rue Lecourbe
    75015 Paris
    France
    Tel 33 1 53 68 88 88
    FAX 52 5 606 7216
Dutch Centre for Health Promotion and
Health Education
    Unit of Library and Documentation
    PO Box 5104
    3502 JC Utrecht
    The Netherlands
    Tel 31 30 971 150
    FAX 31 30 964 082
STD Foundation
    PO Box 9074
    Kaap Hoorndreef 60
    Utrecht
    The Netherlands
    Tel 31 30 628 234
    FAX 31 30 611 457

AIDS HOTLINES AND INFORMATION RESOURCES

AIDS HOTLINES

National AIDS
    Hotline: 1 (800) 342-AIDS
Spanish AIDS
    Hotline: 1 (800) 344-SIDA
Hearing Impaired AIDS
    Hotline: (TDD Service)
    1 (800) 243-7889
Children of the Night
    Hotline: 1 (800) 551-1300
Consumer Nutrition
    Hotline: 1 (800) 366-1655
Drug Abuse
    Hotline: 1 (800) 662-HELP
National Gay/Lesbian Crisis Line
    1 (800) 767-4297
Pediatric and Pregnancy AIDS
    Hotline: 1 (212) 430-3333
PWA Coalition
    Hotline: 1 (800) 828-3280

STATE AIDS HOTLINES (800 AREA CODE USED WITHIN STATE)

Alabama 1 (800) 228-0469
Alaska 1 (800) 478-AIDS
Arizona 1 (800) 334-1540
Arkansas 1 (800) 445-7720
California (Northern) 1 (800) 367-AIDS
California (Southern) 1 (800) 922-AIDS
California (Spanish) 1 (800) 222-7432
Colorado 1 (800) 252-AIDS
  (Spanish) 1 (800) 333-4336
Connecticut 1 (800) 842-2220
Delaware 1 (800) 422-0429
DC 1 (202) 332-2437
  (Spanish) 1 (202) 328-0697
Florida 1 (800) 352-AIDS
  (Spanish) 1 (800) 545-SIDA
  (Haitian Creole) 1 (800) AIDS-101
Georgia 1 (800) 551-2728
Hawaii 1 (800) 321-1551
Idaho 1 (800) 833-2437
Illinois 1 (800) 243-AIDS
Indiana 1 (800) 848-AIDS
Iowa 1 (800) 445-AIDS
Kansas 1 (800) 232-0040
Kentucky 1 (800) 654-AIDS
Louisiana 1 (800) 992-4379
Maine 1 (800) 851-AIDS
Maryland 1 (800) 638-6252
Massachusetts 1 (800) 235-2331
  (Spanish) 1 (800) 262-7248
  (TYY) 1 (800) 272-2577
Michigan 1 (800) 872-AIDS
  (TYY) 1 (313) 547-3655
Minnesota 1 (800) 248-2437
Mississippi 1 (800) 826-2961
  (Spanish) 1 (800) 344-7432
Missouri 1 (800) 533-AIDS
Montana 1 (800) 233-6668
Nebraska 1 (800) 782-AIDS
Nevada 1 (800) 842-AIDS
New Hampshire 1 (800) 752-2437
New Jersey 1 (800) 624-2377
New Mexico 1 (800) 545-AIDS
New York 1 (800) 541-AIDS
  (Spanish) 1 (800) 233-7432
North Carolina 1 (800) 525-AIDS
North Dakota 1 (800) 472-2180
Ohio 1 (800) 332-AIDS
  (TYY) 1 (800) 332-3889
Oklahoma 1 (800) 522-9054
Oregon 1 (800) 777-AIDS
Pennsylvania 1 (800) 692-7254
Puerto Rico 1 (800) 981-5721
Rhode Island 1 (800) 726-3010
South Carolina 1 (800) 322-AIDS
South Dakota 1 (800) 592-1861
Tennessee 1 (800) 525-AIDS
Texas 1 (800) 299-2437
  (TYY) 1 (800) 252-8012
Utah 1 (800) 252-8012
Vermont 1 (800) 882-AIDS
Virgin Islands 1 (809) 773-2437
Virginia 1 (800) 533-4148

Washington 1 (800) 272-AIDS
West Virginia 1 (800) 642-8244
Wisconsin 1 (800) 334-AIDS
Wyoming 1 (800) 327-3577

AIDS NATIONAL INFORMATION RESOURCES

National AIDS Information Clearinghouse
  1 (800) 458-5231
AIDS Clinical Trials Information Service
  (ACTIS) 1 (800) TRIALS-A
For the Hearing Impaired TTY/TDD
  1 (800) 243-7012
AIDS Treatment Information Services
  1 (800) HIV-0440
AIDS Treatment News 1 (800) TREAT 12
American Foundation for AIDS Research
  (Treatment Info) 1 (800) 39 AMFAR
Maternal and Pediatric AIDS Vaccine
  Trials Info 1 (800) TRIALS-A
Mothers Initiative (Mothers of PWAs)
  1 (800) 828-3280
National Association of People with AIDS
  1 (202) 898-0414
National Hemophilia Foundation
  1 (212) 219-8180
National Hospicelink (Information on Local
  Facilities) 1 (800) 331-1620
National Institutes of Health (NIH)
  Clinical Center 1 (800) AIDS-NIH
(Information regarding new NIH drug
  studies)
National Library of Medicine
  1 (800) 638-8480
(Information regarding on-line AIDS
  databases)
National Native American AIDS Hotline
  1 (800) 283-2437
National Pediatric HIV Resource Center
  1 (800) 362-0071
National Sexually Transmitted Diseases
  1 (800) 227-8922
Project Inform (AIDS Experimental Drug
  Info) 1 (800) 822-7422
Teens Teaching AIDS Prevention Program
  (TTAP) 1 (800) 234-TEEN

RECORDED INFORMATION FROM THE CENTERS FOR DISEASE CONTROL

Current number of AIDS cases and deaths
  1 (404) 330-3020
Distribution of cases by transmission
  category 1 (404) 330-3021
Top ten cities and states with AIDS
  residents 1 (404) 330-3022
HIV Information 1 (404) 332-4555

GENERAL INFORMATION FOR HEALTH CARE PROVIDERS

HIV Telephone Consultation Service
  1 (800) 933-3413
Hospital Infection Control (CDC
  Information Service) 1 (404) 639-3406

NATIONAL ORGANIZATIONS

ADAPT (Association For Drug Abuse, Prevention & Treatment)
  552 Southern Blvd
  Bronx, NY 10455
  (718) 665-5421
Advocates For Youth (formerly *Center for Population Options*)
  1025 Vermont Avenue, North West, Suite 210
  Washington, DC 20005
  (202) 347-5700
AIDS Action Council
  1875 Connecticut Avenue, North West, Suite 700
  Washington, DC 20009
  (202) 986-1300
AIDS Coalition To Unleash Power (ACT-UP)
  496 A Hudson Street, Suite G4
  New York, NY 10014
  (212) 989-1114
AIDS National Interfaith Network
  110 Maryland Avenue, North East
  Washington, DC 20002
AIDS Treatment Data Network
  259 West 30th Street
  New York, NY 10001
  (212) 268-4196
  Hotline (212) 268-4196
American Association of Physicans for Human Rights (AAPHR)
  2940 16th Street, Suite 105
  San Francisco, CA 94103
  (415) 255-4547
American Civil Liberties Union
  AIDS and Civil Liberties Project
  132 West 43rd Street
  New York, NY 10036
  (212) 994-9800
American College of Obstetricians and Gynecologists (ACOG)
  409 12th Street
  Washington, DC 20024
  (202) 638-5577
American Foundation for AIDS Research (AmFAR)
  733 Third Avenue, 12th Floor
  New York, NY 10019
  (800) 39-AmFAR
American Hospital Association
  840 North Lake Shore
  Chicago, IL 60611
  (312) 280-6000
American Medical Association
  535 North Dearborn
  Chicago, IL 60610
  (312) 645-5000
American Public Health Association
  1051 15th Street, North West
  Washington, DC 20005
  (202) 789-5688
American Red Cross—National
AIDS Education Program

8111 Gatehouse Road
  Falls Church, VA
  (703) 206-7130
Centers for Disease Control
AIDS Information Office
  Atlanta, GA
  (404) 329-2891
Center For Interdisciplinary Research In Immunology And Disease (CIRID) at UCLA
  UCLA School of Medicine
  10833 Le Conte Avenue
  Los Angeles, CA 90024
  (310) 825-1510
Coalition of Hispanic Health & Human Services Organization (COSSMHO)
  1501 16th Street, North West
  Washington, DC 20036
  (202) 387-5000
National Hemophilia Foundation (HANDI)
  110 Greene Street, #303
  New York, NY 10012
  (212) 431-8541
  (800) 42-HANDI
Hispanic AIDS Forum
  121 Avenue of the Americas, Suite 505
  New York, NY 10013
  (212) 966-6336
  Hotline (212) 966-6336
Intergovernmental Health Policy Project
  AIDS Resource Center
  2021 K Street, North West, Suite 800
  Washington, DC 20006
  (202) 872-1445
Lambda Legal Defense & Education Fund
  666 Broadway, 12th Floor
  New York, NY 10012
  (212) 995-8585
National AIDS Minority Information and Education
  Howard University, Suite 3-B
  2139 Georgia Avenue, NW
  Washington, DC 20001
  (202) 865-3720
National Latino Lesbian Gay Organization
  PO Box 4483
  Washington, DC 20003
  (202) 544-0092
Midwest Hispanic AIDS Coalition
  PO Box 470859
  Chicago, IL 80647
  (312) 772-8195
National AIDS Clearinghouse
  AIDS Information Office
  PO Box 6003
  Rockville, MD 20850
  (800) 458-5231
National Association of People with AIDS (NAPWA)
  1413 K Street, North West, 8th Floor
  Washington, DC 20005
  (202) 898-0414
National Council of La Raza
  Union Station Plaza

810 First Street, North East, Suite 300
Washington, DC 20002
(202) 289-1380

National Black Women's Health Project
1237 Ralph Abernathy Boulevard
Atlanta, GA 30310
(404) 758-9590

National Gay and Lesbian Task Force
1734 14th Street, North West
Washington, DC 20009-4390
(202) 332-6483

National Institute of Allergy and Infectious
Diseases (NIAID)
National Institutes of Health
9000 Rockville Pike
Bethesda, MD 20892
(301) 496-0545

National Institute on Drug Abuse
5600 Fishers Lane
Rockville, MD 20857
(301) 443-0441

National Institutes of Health, Clinical
Center
Patient Referral Service
Building 10, Room 1C-255
Bethesda, MD 20892
(301) 496-4891

National Lawyer's Guild AIDS Network
558 Capp Street
San Francisco, CA 94102
(415) 824-8884

National Leadership Coalition on AIDS
1730 "M" Street, North West, Suite 905
Washington, DC 20036
(202) 429-0930

National Minority AIDS Council
300 Eye Street, North East
Washington, DC 20002
(202) 544-1076

National Network of Runaway & Youth
Services
1319 "F" Street, North West, Suite 401
Washington, DC 20004
(202) 783-7949
Hotline (202) 783-7954

National Pediatric HIV Resource Center
AIDS Program, 15 South Ninth Street
Newark, NJ 07107
(800) 362-0071

National Urban League
500 East 62nd Street
New York, NY 10021
(212) 310-9110

National Women's Health Network
514 10th Street, North West, Suite 400
Washington, DC 20004
(202) 347-1140

Office Of Disease Prevention And Health
Promotion
National Health Info Center
PO Box 1133
Washington, DC 20013
(800) 336-4797

Pediatric AIDS Foundation

1311 Colorado Avenue
Santa Monica, CA 90404
(310) 395-9051

Pharmaceutical Manufacturers Association
Communications Division
1100 15th Street North West
Washington, DC 20005
(202) 835-3400

Parents And Friends Of Lesbians And
Gays, Inc.
1101 14th Street, North West, Suite 1030
Washington, DC 20005
(202) 638-4200

Physicians Association for AIDS Care
101 West Grand Avenue, Suite 200
Chicago, IL 60610
(312) 222-1326

Planned Parenthood Federation of America
810 7th Avenue
New York, NY 10019
(212) 541-7800

Project Inform
1965 Market Street, Suite 220
San Francisco, CA 94103
(415) 558-8669
Hotline (800) 822-7422 (outside
California)
Hotline (800) 344-7422 (inside California)

PWA Coalition
50 West 17th Street, 8th Floor
New York, NY 10011
(800) 828-3280

Sex Information And Education Council Of
The United States (SIECUS)
130 West 42nd Street, Suite 2500
New York, NY, 10036
(212) 819-9770

The Names Project Foundation
AIDS Memorial Quilt
2362 Market Street
San Francisco, CA 94114
(415) 882-5500

U.S. Conference of Mayors
U.S. Conference of Local Health Officers
(USCLHO)
1620 Eye Street, North West
Washington, DC 20006
(202) 293-7330

U.S. Department of Health And Human
Services, AIDS Research
Building 31, Room 11-A-48
9000 Rockville Pike
Bethesda, MD 20892-0001
(301) 496-5615

STATE AND LOCAL ORGANIZATIONS

ALABAMA

Alabama Department of Public Health
HIV/AIDS Division
434 Monroe Street

Montgomery, AL 36130
(205) 613-5357 *Hotline:* (800) 228-0469

Birmingham

Jefferson County Department of Health
1400 6th Avenue, South
Birmingham, AL 35202-2648
(205) 933-9110 *Hotline:* (205) 591-4448
AIDS Task Force of Alabama (ATFA)
PO Box 55703
Birmingham, AL 35255
(205) 324-2437 *Hotline:* (205) 591-4448
Birmingham AIDS Outreach
PO Box 550070
Birmingham AL 35255
(205) 322-4197 *Hotline:* same

Decatur

Tri-County Health Department
PO Box 1628
Decatur, AL 35602
(205) 353-7021 *Hotline:* (800) 228-0469

Dothan

Houston County Health Department
PO Box 2087
Dothan, AL 36302
(205) 793-1911

Double Springs

Winston County Health Department
PO Box 1029
Double Springs, AL 35553
(205) 489-2101 *Hotline:* (800) 228-0469

Mobile

Mobile County Health Department
PO Box 2867
Mobile, AL 36652
(205) 690-8167
Mobile AIDS Coalition
Box 40051
Mobile, AL 36640
(205) 633-0400 *Hotline:* (205) 432-AIDS
Mobile AIDS Support Services
107 North Ann Street
Mobile, AL 36604
(205) 433-6277 *Hotline:* (205) 432-AIDS

Montgomery

Montgomery County Health Department
800 B West South Boulevard
Montgomery, AL 36105
(205) 284-3553
Montgomery AIDS Outreach.
PO Box 5213
Montgomery, AL 36103
(205) 284-2273 *Hotline:* (205) 284-CARE

Tuscaloosa

West Alabama AIDS Outreach
PO Box 031947
Tuscaloosa, AL 35403
(205) 758-2437 *Hotline:* (800) 228-0469

ALASKA

Alaska State Section of Epidemiology
AIDS/STD Program
PO Box 240249
Anchorage, AK 99524
(907) 561-4406 *Hotline:* (800) 478-AIDS

Anchorage

Alaska Health Project
1818 West Northern Lights
Anchorage, AK 99517
(907) 276-2864 *Hotline:* (800) 478-2864
Alaskan AIDS Assistance Association
730 "I" Street, Suite 100
Anchorage, AK 99501
(907) 276-1400 *Hotline:* (800) 478-2437
Municipality of Anchorage Health
Department
STD Clinic
825 "L" Street, Room 101
Anchorage, AK 99501
(907) 343-4611

Fairbanks

Fairbanks Health Center
800 Airport Way
Fairbanks, AK 99701
(907) 452-1776 *Hotline:* (800) 478-1777
Interior AIDS Association
PO Box 71248
Fairbanks, AK 99707
(907) 452-4222

Juneau

Juneau Pubic Health Center
3412 Glacier Highway
Juneau, AK 99801
(907) 465-3353
Shanti of Juneau
PO Box 22655
Juneau, AK 99802
(907) 463-5665 *Hotline:* (800) 478-2437

ARIZONA

Arizona Department of Health
Office of HIV/AIDS Services
3008 North Third Street
Phoenix, AZ 85012
(602) 230-5819
Arizona Department of Health
3815 North Black Canyon Highway
Phoenix, AZ 85012
(602) 230-5819 *Hotline:* (800) 334-1540

Flagstaff

Coconino County Department of Public
Health Services
2500 North Fort Valley Road
Flagstaff, AZ 86001
(602) 779-5164 *Hotline:* (602) 525-1199

Phoenix

Maricopa County Public Health Clinic
2225 North 16th Street

Phoenix, AZ 85006
(602) 258-1678
Arizona AIDS Information Line
PO Box 16423
Phoenix, AZ 85011
(602) 234-2753 *Hotline:* (602) 234-2752
Arizona AIDS Project
4460 North Central Avenue
Phoenix, AZ 85012
(602) 265-3300 *Hotline:* (602) 227-1927
Community AIDS Council
506 East Camelback Road
Phoenix, AZ 85012
(602) 265-2437 *Hotline:* (602) 265-AIDS
Concioio Latino de Salud
PO Box 1032
Phoenix, AZ 85001
(602) 606-6788
Phoenix Shanti Group/Phoenix Shanti
Living Center
1314 East McDowell
Phoenix, AZ 85006
(602) 271-0008 *Hotline:* (602) 271-0008

Tucson

Pima County Health Department-AIDS
Program
150 West Congress, Room 334
Tucson, AZ 85701
(602) 740-8554
People with AIDS Coalition of Tucson
801 West Congress
Tucson, AZ 85702
(602) 770-1710
Shanti Foundation of Tucson
602 North 4th Avenue
Tucson, AZ 85705
(602) 622-7107
Tucson AIDS Project
151 South Tucson Boulevard, Suite 252
Tucson, AZ 85716
(602) 322-6226 *Hotline:* (602) 326-AIDS

Yuma

Yuma County Health Department AIDS
Project
201 S. Second Ave
Yuma, AZ 85364
(602) 329-0751

ARKANSAS

Arkansas Department of Health
Division of AIDS/STD
4815 West Markham Street
Little Rock, AR 72205
(501) 661-2408

Little Rock

AIDS Support Group
210 Pulaski
Little Rock, AR 72201
(501) 374-3605
Arkansas AIDS Foundation
5911 "H" Street

Little Rock, AR 72205
(501) 663-7833

CALIFORNIA

California Department of Health Services
Office of AIDS
830 "S" Street
Sacramento, CA 94234-7320
(916) 445-0696
Computerized AIDS Information Network
(CAIN) & California AIDS Clearinghouse
1625 North Hudson Avenue
Los Angeles, CA 90028
(213) 993-7415

Auburn

Placer County Health and Medical Services
11484 B Avenue
Auburn, CA 95603
(916) 889-7141

Bakersfield

Kern County Health Department
Public Health Nursing
1700 Flower Street
Bakersfield, CA 93305
(805) 861-3644

Berkeley

Berkeley Health Department
2180 Milvia Street
Berkeley, CA 94704
(510) 644-6500
East Bay AIDS Center
3031 Telegraph Avenue, Suite 235
Berkeley, CA 94704
(510) 204-1870

Campbell

Aris Project
595 Millich Drive, Suite 104
Campbell, CA 95008
(408) 370-3272

Chico

Butte County Health Department
AIDS Education Project
695 Oleander Avenue
Chico, CA 95926
(916) 891-2865

El Cajon

El Cajon Health Department
113 East Douglas Avenue
El Cajon, CA 92020
(619) 479-4446

Eureka

Humboldt County Department of Public
Welfare
929 Koster Street
Eureka, CA 95501
(707) 445-6023
North Coast AIDS Project
529 I Street

Eureka, CA 95501
707-445-6200

Fremont

Tri-City Health Center
38355 Logan Drive
Fremont, CA 95035
(415) 794-8848

Fresno

Fresno County Health Department
1221 Fulton Mall
Fresno, CA 93775
(209) 445-3434
Central Valley AIDS Team
PO Box 4640, 606 East Blemont
Fresno, CA 93744
(209) 264-2437 *Hotline:* (209) 264-2436

Guerneville

Sonoma County AIDS Network (SCAN)
PO Box 1599
Guerneville, CA 95446
(707) 887-1581/(707) 544-1581

Long Beach

Long Beach Department of Health
AIDS Prevention and Clinic
2525 Grand Avenue
Long Beach, CA 98015
(310) 570-4000
Center for Community Research and
Services
1407 East 4th Street
Long Beach, CA 90802
(310) 436-4602
Families Who Care (FWC)
6475 East Pacific Coast Highway,
Suite 202
Long Beach, CA 90803
(310) 498-6366

Los Angeles

LA County Health Services
AIDS Programs, 6th Floor
600 South Commonwealth Avenue
Los Angeles, CA 90005
(213) 351-8000
Los Angeles County Drug Abuse Program
Office
8702 Santa Monica Boulevard
Los Angeles, CA 90069
(800) 564-6600
AIDS Clinic, County/University of
Southern California Medical Center
1175 North Cummings
5P21 Outpatient Building
Los Angeles, CA 90033
(213) 226-5028
AIDS Health Care Foundation
1800 North Argyle Avenue, Third Floor
Los Angeles, CA 90028
(800) AHF-2101

AIDS Project Los Angeles (APLA)
1313 North Vine Street
6721 Romaine Street
Los Angeles, CA 90038
(213) 962-1600/993-1533
Hotline: (800) 922-AIDS
AIDS Service Center
126 West Delmar Boulevard
Pasadena, CA 91105
(818) 796-5633 *Hotline:* (818) 449-8421
Asian Health Project
The Clinic For Women
3860 West MLK Boulevard
Los Angeles, CA 90008
(213) 295-6571
Avance Human Services
5350 East Beverly Boulevard
Los Angeles, CA 90022
(213) 726-2201 *Hotline:* (800) 432-7432
Being Alive/PWA Action Coalition
3626 Sunset Boulevard
Los Angeles, CA 90029
(213) 667-3262
Center for Interdisciplinary Research in
Immunology and Disease (CIRID) at UCLA
AIDS Education and Prevention
12-639 Factor Building
10833 Le Conte Avenue
UCLA School of Medicine
Los Angeles, CA 90024-1747
(310) 825-1510
Cara A Cara Latino AIDS Project
3324 Sunset Boulevard
Los Angeles, CA 90026
(213) 661-6752
Caring for Babies with AIDS
PO Box 351535
Los Angeles, CA 90035
(213) 931-9828
Community Outreach Risk/Reduction
Education Program CORE Program
6570 Santa Monica Boulevard
Los Angeles, CA 90038
(213) 460-4444
El Centro Human Services, Milagros AIDS
Project
1001 South Goodrich Boulevard
Los Angeles, CA 90022
(213) 721-1332
The Gay and Lesbian Community Services
Center
1625 North Hudson Avenue
Los Angeles, CA 90028
(213) 993-7400
Jewish AIDS Services of Los Angeles
6505 Wilshire Boulevard, #608
Los Angeles, CA 90048
(213) 732-5648
Minority AIDS Project/Los Angeles
5149 West Jefferson Boulevard
Los Angeles, CA 90016-3836
(213) 936-4949 *Hotline:* (213) 936-4949
Pediatric AIDS Network
6430 Sunset Boulevard, Suite 1003

Los Angeles, CA 90028
(213) 669-5616
T.H.E. Clinic for Women
3860 West Martin Luther King Boulevard
Los Angeles, CA 90008
(213) 295-6571
UCLA AIDS Institute
60-054 CHS
10833 Le Conte Avenue
Los Angeles, CA 90024-1678
(310) 794-7209
UCLA Center for AIDS Research and
Education (CARE)
BH-412 CHS
10833 Le Conte Avenue
Los Angeles, CA 90024-1793
(312) 206-6414
Women AIDS Project
8240 Santa Monica Boulevard
West Hollywood, CA 90046
(213) 650-1508

Modesto

Stanislaus Community AIDS Project
1620 North Carpenter
Modesto, CA 95359
(209) 572-2437 *Hotline:* (209) 577-2437

Oakland

AIDS Minority Health Initiative
1440 Broadway, Suite 403
Oakland, CA 94612
(510) 763-1872
AIDS Project of the East Bay
656 16th Street
Oakland, CA 94609
(510) 834-8181 *Hotline:* same
Asian Health Services
310 8th Street, #200
Oakland, CA 94607
(510) 444-AIDS
National Native American AIDS
Prevention Center
3515 Grand Avenue, Suite 100
Oakland, CA 94610
(415) 658-2051 *Hotline:* (800) 283-AIDS
The Center for AIDS Services
5720 Shattuck Avenue
Oakland, CA 94609
(510) 655-3435

Palm Springs

Desert AIDS Project, Community
Counseling and Consultation Center
750 South Vella Road
Palm Springs, CA 92262
(619) 323-2118
Hemophilia Foundation of Southern
California
33 South Catalina Avenue, #102
Pasadena, CA 91106
(818) 793-6192

Redding

Shasta County Health Department,
Community AIDS Education Program

2650 Breslaver Way
Redding, CA 96001
(916) 225-5591

Riverside

Riverside County Health Department
4065 County Circle Drive
Riverside, CA 92503
(909) 358-5209 *Hotline:* (800) 243-7275
Inland AIDS Project
1240 Palmyrita, Suite E
Riverside, CA 92507
(714) 784-2437 *Hotline:* (800) 499-AIDS

Sacramento

Sacramento County Health Department,
AIDS Education
3701 Branch Center Road
Sacramento, CA 95827
(916) 366-2922
CARES
2710 Capitol Avenue
Sacramento, CA 95816
(916) 443-3299
Hemophilia Council of California
1507 21st Street, Suite 300
Sacramento, CA 95814
(916) 448-7444
Sacramento AIDS Foundation
920 20th, 2nd Floor
Sacramento, CA 95814
(916) 448-2437
Sacramento Urban Indian Health Project
801 Broadway
Sacramento, CA 95818
(916) 441-0918

Salinas

Monterey County Health Department
1270 Natividad Road
Salinas, CA 93906
(408) 755-4529

San Bernardino

San Bernardino County Health Department
799 East Rialto Avenue
San Bernardino, CA 92415
(904) 383-3060

San Diego

San Diego County Health Services
1700 Pacific Highway
San Diego, CA 92101
(619) 236-2237
AIDS Foundation of San Diego
4080 Centre Street
San Diego, CA 92103
(619) 686-5050 *Hotline:* (619) 686-5000
Center for Social Services AIDS
PO Box 3357
San Diego, CA 92163
(619) 692-2077 *Hotline:* (619) 692-4297
Hemophilia Council of California Project
2350 6th Avenue, Suite 218
San Diego, CA 92103
(619) 543-1355

Logan Heights Family Health Center
1809 National Avenue
San Diego, CA 92113
(619) 234-8171
San Diego Hospice
4311 Third Avenue
San Diego, CA 92103
(619) 688-1600 *Hotline:* (619) 688-1600
Planned Parenthood
10737 Camino Ruiz
San Diego, CA 92126
(619) 566-4223

San Francisco

San Francisco Public Health Department
AIDS Activity Office
25 Van Ness Avenue, Suite 500
San Francisco, CA 94102
(415) 554-9000
AIDS/ARC Division Catholic Charities
1049 Market Street, Suite 200
San Francisco, CA 94103
(415) 864-7400
AIDS Project, Jewish Family and
Children's Service
1600 Scott Street
San Francisco, CA 94115
(415) 561-1241
AIDS Project/Jewish Family and Children's
Services
1600 Scott Street
San Francisco, CA 94115
(415) 567-8860
Asian American Communitites Against
AIDS
1596 Post Street, 1st floor
San Francisco, CA 94109
(415) 563-0553
Bayview-Hunter's Point Foundation
AIDS Service Program
150 Executive Park Boulevard, #3100
San Francisco, CA 94134
(415) 822-8200
Black Coalition on AIDS
1042 Divisadero Street
San Francisco, CA 94103
(415) 346-2364 *Hotline:* (415) 822-2437
California Nurses Association, AIDS
Education and Training
1855 Folsom Street, Suite 670
San Francisco, CA 94103
(415) 864-4141
Gay Asian Pacific Alliance
1841 Market Street
San Francisco, CA 94103
(415) 575-3939
Institute Familiar de La Raza
2639 24th Street
San Francisco, CA 94110
(415) 647-5450
Latino AIDS Project
2689 24th Street
San Francisco, CA 94110
(415) 647-5450
Mission Crisis Service
111 Potrero Avenue

San Francisco, CA 94103
(415) 558-2071
National Catholic AIDS Network
PO Box 422984
San Francisco, CA 94142
(415) 874-3031
Office for Civil Rights
Department of Health & Human Services
50 United Nations Plaza, Room 322
San Francisco, CA 94102
San Francisco General Hospital AIDS
Program
995 Potrero, Ward 84
San Francisco, CA 94110
(415) 476-0828
Project AWARE—Association for Women's
AIDS Research & Education
3180 18th Street, #205
San Francisco, CA 94110
(415) 476-4091
Project Inform
1965 Market Street, Suite 220
San Francisco, CA 94103
(415) 558-8669 CA *Hotline:* (800) 344-7422
San Francisco AIDS Foundation (SFAF)
25 Van Ness Avenue, Suite 660
San Francisco, CA 94103
(415) 864-5855
Shanti Project
525 Howard Street
San Francisco, CA 94105
(415) 777-2273
UC San Francisco AIDS Health Project
PO Box 0884
San Francisco, CA 94121
(415) 476-6430

San Jose

Santa Clara County Health Department
AIDS Services
976 Lenzen Avenue
San Jose, CA 95126
(408) 299-4151

San Luis Obispo

San Luis Obispo County Health Department
AIDS Program
285 South Street, Suite J
San Luis Obispo, CA 93401
(805) 781-5540 *Hotline:* same
San Luis Obispo AIDS Support Network
1817 B. Charro
San Luis Obispo, CA 93401
(805) 541-5752

San Mateo

San Mateo County AIDS Program
8700 Edison Street
San Mateo, CA 94403
(415) 573-2588

Santa Ana

Orange County Health Care Agency
1725 West 17th Street
Santa Ana, CA 92702
(714) 834-3129 *Hotline:* (800) 922-2437

Santa Barbara

Santa Barbara County Health Care Services
300 North San Antonio Road
Santa Barbara, CA 93105
(805) 681-5365
AIDS Counseling and Assistance Program
Gay and Lesbian Resource Center (GLRC)
417 Santa Barbara Street, Suite A18
Santa Barbara, CA 93101
(805) 963-3636 *Hotline:* (805) 965-2925
Westside Neighborhood Medical Clinic
628 West Michaeltorena Street
Santa Barbara, CA 93101
(805) 963-1546 *Hotline:* (805) 962-1058

Santa Cruz

Santa Cruz AIDS Project/Projecto Sida
Santa Cruz
911-A Center Street
Santa Cruz, CA 95060
(408) 427-3900 *Hotline:* (408) 458-4999

Santa Rosa

Sonoma County AIDS Project
3313 Chanate Road
Santa Rosa, CA 95404
(707) 576-4734 *Hotline:* (707) 576-4363

Stockton

San Joaquin County Public Health Services
1601 East Hazelton Avenue
Stockton, CA 95205
(209) 468-3820
San Joaquin County AIDS Program
4410 North Pershing, Suite C-4
Stockton, CA 95330
(209) 476-8533

Tarzana

Tarzana Treatment Center
18646 Oxnard Street
Tarzana, CA 91356
(818) 342-5897

Vallejo

Solano County Health Department, AIDS
Program
355 Tuolumne Street
Vallejo, CA 94590
(707) 553-5556 *Hotline:* (707) 553-5552

COLORADO

Colorado Department of Health
STD/AIDS Control/DCEED-
STDS-A3
4300 Cherry Creek Drive, South
Denver, CO 80220
(303) 692-2720

Boulder

Boulder County Health Department
3450 Broadway Boulevard
Boulder, CO 80304
(303) 441-1171
Boulder County AIDS Project
2118 14th Street

Boulder, CO 80302
(303) 444-6121

Colorado Springs

El Paso County Health Department
301 South Union Boulevard
Colorado Springs, CO 80910
(719) 578-3199 *Hotline:* (303) 578-9092

Denver

Denver Public Health Department
605 Bannock Street
Denver, CO 80204
(303) 436-7200
Colorado AIDS Project
PO Box 18529
Denver, CO 80218
(303) 837-0166 *Hotline:* (800) 333-AIDS
People with AIDS Coalition of Colorado
PO Box 300339
Denver, CO 80203
(303) 837-8214

Englewood

Tri-County Health Department
7000 East Belleview
Englewood, CO 80111
(303) 220-9200

Fort Collins

Larimer County Health Department
1525 Blue Spruce
Fort Collins, CO 80524
(303) 498-6700
Northern Colorado AIDS Project
Box 182
Fort Collins, CO 80522
(303) 223-6227

Grand Junction

Mesa County Health Department
515 Patterson Road
Grand Junction, CO 81501
(303) 244-1743
Western Colorado Health Network
513 Patterson Road
Grand Junction, CO 81506
(303) 248-6900 *Hotline:* (800) 765-8594

CONNECTICUT

Connecticut State Department of Health
Services
150 Washington Street
Hartford, CT 06105
(203) 566-1157

Bridgeport

Bridgeport Health Department
752 East Main Street
Bridgeport, CT 06608
(203) 576-7469

Greenwich

Greenwich Department of Health, Office of
HIV Information and Services
101 Field Point Road

Greenwich, CT 06836-2540
(203) 622-6496

Hartford

Hartford Health Department
AIDS/HIV Program
80 Coventry Street
Hartford, CT 06112
(203) 722-6742 *Hotline:* (203) 722-6742
AIDS Project/Hartford
30 Arbor Street
Hartford, CT 06105
(203) 523-7699 *Hotline:* (203) 247-AIDS
Hartford Gay and Lesbian Health
Collective
PO Box 2094
Hartford, CT 06145
(203) 278-4163
Hispanic Health Council
96 Cedar Street, Suite 3A
Hartford, CT 06106
(203) 527-0856
Info Line, North Central
900 Asylum Avenue
Hartford, CT 06105
(203) 522-4636 *Hotline:* same

Middletown

Middletown Department of Health
PO Box 1300
Middletown, CT 06457
(203) 344-3474
Community Health Center, Inc.
635 Main Street
Middletown, CT 06457
(203) 347-6971

New Britain

New Britain Health Department
HIV Counseling & Testing
31 High Street
New Britain, CT 06501
(203) 224-2420
AIDS Project/Greater New Britain
PO Box 1214
New Britain, CT 06053
(203) 225-6789 *Hotline:* same

New Haven

New Haven Health Department
One State Street
New Haven, CT 06511
(203) 787-6957 *Hotline:* (203) 787-6453
AIDS Project New Haven
PO Box 636
New Haven, CT 06503
(203) 624-0947 *Hotline:* (203) 624-2437
Fair Haven Community Health Center
374 Grand Avenue
New Haven, CT 06513
(203) 777-7411
Hispanos Unidos Contra El SIDA/AIDS
(HUCS)
PO Box 161, 263 Grand Avenue
New Haven, CT 06513
(203) 772-1777

Yale-New Haven Hospital
AIDS Care Program
20 York Street, Welch Center
New Haven, CT 06504
(203) 785-5303

New London

New London AIDS Educational, Counseling
and Testing Service
120 Broad Street, Health Department
New London, CT 06320
(203) 447-AIDS *Hotline:* same

Norwalk

Norwalk Health Department
137 East Avenue
Norwalk, CT 06851
(203) 854-7779 *Hotline:* (203) 854-7979
Mid-Fairfield County AIDS Project
83 East Avenue
Norwalk, CT 06851
(203) 855-9535 *Hotline:* (203) 854-7979

Stamford

Stamford Health Department, AIDS
Program
888 Washington Boulevard, 8th Floor
Stamford, CT 06904
(203) 977-4387 *Hotline:* (203) 967-AIDS
Liberation Programs
125 Main Street
Stamford, CT 06901
(203) 356-1980

Torrington

Torrington Area Health District
1116 Litchfield Street
Torrington, CT 06790
(203) 489-0436 *Hotline:* (203) 482-8141
North West Connecticut AIDS Project
100 Migeon Avenue
Torrington, CT 06790
(203) 482-1596

Waterbury

Waterbury AIDS Program
402 East Main Street
Waterbury, CT 06702
(203) 574-6883

DELAWARE

Delaware Department of Health and Social
Services, Public Health Division
PO Box 637
Dover, DE 19903
(302) 739-3032

Wilmington

HIV/ AIDS Program Office
3000 Newport Gap Pike, Building G
Wilmington, DE 19808
(302) 995-8422 *Hotline:* (800) 422-0429
Delaware Lesbian and Gay Health
Advocates
601 Delaware Avenue
Wilmington, DE 19801
(302) 652-6776 *Hotline:* (800) 422-0429

Public Health Clinic
  Porter State Service Center
  511 West 8th Street
  Wilmington, DE 19801
  (302) 571-3521

DISTRICT OF COLUMBIA

Washington

Agency for HIV/AIDS
  DC Commission of Public Health
  1660 "L" Street, North West, Suite 700
  Washington, DC 20036
  (202) 332-AIDS *Hotline:* same
DC Women's Council on AIDS
  715 8th Street, South East
  Washington, DC 20005
  (202) 544-8255
Damien Ministries
  PO Box 10202
  Washington, DC 20018-0202
  (202) 387-2926
  (800) 783-LIVE
Drug Abuse Institute
  Howard University Hospital
  2041 Georgia Avenue, North West
  Washington, DC 20060
  (202) 865-1456
Inner City AIDS Network
  912 Third Street, North West
  Washington, DC 20001
  (202) 789-4226
SALUD
  2701 Ontario Road, North West
  Washington, DC 20009
  (202) 483-6806 *Hotline:* (800) 322-5404
Washington Area Council on Alcohol and
  Drug Abuse
  1707 "L" Street, North West, Suite 200
  Washington, DC 20036
  (202) 682-1700 *Hotline:* (202) 783-1300
Whitman-Walker Clinic
  1407 South Street, North West
  Washington, DC 20009
  (202) 797-3500 *Hotline:* (202) 332-2437

FLORIDA

Florida State Department of Health
  2251 North Palafox Street
  Pensacola, FL 32501
  (904) 435-6500 *Hotline:* (800) FLA-AIDS

Bradenton

Manatee County Public Health Unit
  410 6th Avenue, East
  Bradenton, FL 34208
  (813) 748-0666

Daytona Beach

Volusia County Public Health Unit
  501 South Clyde Morris Boulevard
  Daytona Beach, FL 32115
  (904) 947-3400 *Hotline:* (904) 947-3416
Keech Street Clinic
  431 South Keech Street

Daytona Beach, FL 32114
  (904) 947-3587 *Hotline:* (904) 947-3416

Fort Lauderdale

Broward County Department of Health and
Rehabilitation Services (DHRS)
  2421 South West 6th Avenue
  Fort Lauderdale, FL 33315
  (305) 467-4774 *Hotline:* (800) FLA-AIDS
Center One/Anyone in Distress
  3015 North Ocean Boulevard, #111
  Fort Lauderdale, FL 33308
  (305) 537-4111

Fort Myers

Lee County AIDS Task Force
  2231-A McGregor Boulevard
  Fort Myers, FL 33901
  (813) 337-1441 *Hotline:* (813) 337-2437

Gainesville

Health and Rehabilitative Services (HRS)
AIDS Program
  1000 North East 16th Avenue
  Gainesville, FL 32601
  (904) 336-5776
North Florida AIDS Network
  PO Box 5755
  Gainesville, FL 32605
  Hotline: (904) 372-4370

Jacksonville

Duval County Public Health Unit
  HRS-HIV Main Street Clinic
  962 North Main Street
  Jacksonville, FL 32206
  (904) 630-3300
Mental Health and Welfare Services
  421 West Church Street, Suite 103
  Jacksonville, FL 32202
  (904) 630-4939
PWA Coalition/Jacksonville
  1628 San Marco Boulevard, Suite 5
  Jacksonville, FL 32207
  (904) 398-9292

Key West

AIDS Help
  PO Box 4374
  Key West, FL 33041
  (305) 296-6196
AIDS Prevention Center
  513 Whitehead Street
  Key West, FL 33040
  (305) 292-6701
PWA Coalition of Key West
  709 Olivia Street
  Key West, FL 33040
  (305) 296-5701

Kissimmee

Osceola County Public Health Unit
  1875 Boggy Creek Road
  Kissimmee, FL 34744
  (407) 870-1400

Lucha

   1200 Central Avenue, #111
   Kissimmee, FL 34741
   (407) 932-4482 *Hotline:* same

Miami

Dade County Public Health Unit
   AIDS Program Office
   401 North West 2nd Avenue, Suite 126
   Miami, FL 33128
   (305) 324-2491 *Hotline:* (800) FLA-AIDS
Body Positive Resource Center
   175 North East 6th Street
   Miami, FL 33137
   (305) 576-111
Center for Haitian Studies
   8325 North East 2nd Avenue
   Miami, FL 33138
   (305) 757-9555
Health Crisis Network
   5050 Biscayne Boulevard
   Miami, FL 33137
   (305) 751-7775 *Hotline:* (305) 751-7751
South Florida AIDS Network
   Jackson Memorial Hospital
   1611 North West 12th Avenue, Old M.E.
   Miami, FL 33136
   (305) 585-7744
Switchboard of Miami
   75 South West 8th Street, 4th Floor
   Miami, FL 33130
   (305) 358-1640 *Hotline:* (305) 358-HELP

Naples

HRS Collier County Public Health Unit
   3301 East Tamiami Trail
   Naples, FL 33942
   (813) 774-8226

Orlando

HRS Orange County Public Health Unit,
   832 West Central Boulevard, Office 218
   Orlando, FL 32805
   (407) 836-2680 *Hotline:* (407) 836-3680
Central Florida AIDS Unified Resources
   741 West Colonial
   Orlando, FL 32804
   (407) 849-1453 *Hotline:* (407) 849-1452

Panama City

Bay County Public Health Unit
   605 North MacArthur Avenue
   Panama City, FL 32401
   (904) 872-4455

Pensacola

Escambia AIDS Services & Education
   PO Box 13584
   Pensacola, FL 32591
   (904) 456-7079 *Hotline:* (904) 456-6997

Saint Petersburg

HRS Pinellas County Public Health Unit
   500 7th Avenue, South
   Saint Petersburg, FL 33733
   (813) 823-0401

Sarasota

HRS Sarasota County Public Health Unit
   PO Box 2658
   Sarasota, FL 34230
   (813) 954-2900
Sarasota AIDS Support
   3002 North Tamiami Trail, #4
   Sarasota, FL 34234
   (813) 351-1551 *Hotline:* (813) 351-AIDS

Tallahassee

Florida HRS HIV/STD/TB Program
   1317 Winewood Boulevard
   Tallahassee, FL 32399
   (904) 487-3684 *Hotline:* (800) FLA-AIDS
Leon County Public Health Unit
   2965 Municipal Way
   Tallahassee, FL 32304
   (904) 487-3186
Florida AIDS Hotline
   PO Box 20169
   Tallahassee, FL 32316
   (904) 681-9131 *Hotline:* (800) FLA-AIDS

Tampa

Hillsborough County Public Health Unit
   1105 East Kennedy Boulevard
   Tampa, FL 33602
   (813) 272-6200
HRS District VI Health Program Office
HIV/AIDS Program
   4000 Dr. Martin Luther King Jr.
   Boulevard
   Tampa, FL 33614
   (813) 871-7520
Tampa AIDS Network
   11215 North Nebraska, Suite B-3
   Tampa, FL 33612
   (813) 979-1919 *Hotline:* (813) 221-6420
Tampa Hillsborough Action Plan
   5015 North 22nd Street
   Tampa, FL 33610
   (813) 237-6800

West Palm Beach

Palm Beach County Public Health Unit
HIV Clinic
   3518 Broadway
   West Palm Beach, FL 33407
   (407) 845-4444
Comprehensive AIDS Program of Palm
Beach County
   2580 Metrocenter Boulevard, Suite 1&2
   West Palm Beach, FL 33416
   (407) 687-3400
PWA Coalition—West Palm Beach
   2580 Metrocenter Boulevard
   West Palm Beach, FL 33407
   (407) 697-8033

GEORGIA

Georgia Department of Human Resources
Division of Public Health
   868 Peachtree Street, Room 210
   Atlanta, GA 30309
   (404) 894-5307

Alamo

Wheeler County Health Department
  PO Box 669
  Alamo, GA 30411
  (912) 568-7161

Atlanta

Fulton County Health Department
  99 Butler Street, South East
  Atlanta, GA 30303
  (404) 730-1469
AIDS Program, Office of Infections
  2 Peachtree Street, North East, 6th Floor
  Atlanta, GA 30303
  (404) 657-2588
AID Atlanta
  1438 West Peachtree Street, North West
  Atlanta, GA 30309
  (404) 874-6517 *Hotline:* (800) 551-2728
AIDS Hotline for Women
  580 14th Street, North West
  Atlanta, GA 30318
  (404) 875-7115 *Hotline:* (404) 888-9991
National Association of PWAs-Atlanta
  PO Box 1018
  Atlanta, GA 30301
  (404) 874-7926
Outreach
  3030 Campbellton Road, South West
  Atlanta, GA 30311
  (404) 346-3922 *Hotline:* (800) 441-2437
  (404) 527-3994
St. Joseph's Hispanic Services
  5665 Peachtree–Dunwoody Road, North
  East
  Atlanta, GA 30342
  (404) 851-7776 *Hotline:* same

Augusta

East Central Health District, AIDS Projects
Office
  1001 Bailie Drive
  Augusta, GA 30910
  (404) 724-8802

Cochran

Bleckley County Health Department
  101 South East 8th Street
  Cochran, GA 31014
  (912) 934-6590

Columbus

West Central Health District
Communicable Diseases Office
  1315 DeLaunay Avenue, Suite 201
  Columbus, GA 31901
  (706) 323-2437

Decatur

DeKalb County Board of Health
  440 Winn Way
  Decatur, GA 30030
  (404) 294-3856

McRae

Telfair County Health Department
  PO Box 328
  McRae, GA 31055
  (912) 868-7404

Mount Vernon

Montgomery County Health Department
  PO Box 212
  Mount Vernon, GA 30445
  (912) 583-4602

Savannah

Chatham County Health Department
HIV Program
  2011 Eisenhower Drive
  Savannah, GA 31406
  (912) 356-2155 *Hotline:* (912) 356-2437

Waycross

Southeast Health Unit
  1101 Church Street
  Waycross, GA 31501
  (912) 285-9280

HAWAII

Hawaii State Department of Health
  1250 Punchbowl Street
  Honolulu, HI 96813
  (808) 586-4410 *Hotline:* (808) 922-1313
Hawaii State Department of Health,
STD/AIDS Prevention Program
  3627 Kilauea Avenue, Room 304
  Honolulu, HI 96816
  (808) 735-9280

Hilo

Big Island AIDS Project
  308 Kamehameha, Suite 214
  Hilo, HI 96721
  (808) 935-6711

Honolulu

Gay Community Center
  1820 University Avenue
  YWCA, 2nd Floor
  Honolulu, HI 96822
  (808) 926-6000 *Hotline:* (808) 926-1000
Life Foundation/The AIDS Foundation of
Hawaii
  PO Box 88980
  Honolulu, HI 96815
  (808) 971-2437

Kahului

Maui AIDS Foundation
  55 Kaahumanu Avenue
  Kahului, HI 96732
  (808) 871-2437 *Hotline:* 877-4856

Kapaa

Malama Pono, Kauai AIDS Project
  PO Box 1500
  Kapaa, HI 96746
  (808) 822-0878 *Hotline:* same

Lihue

Kauai District Health Office
  3040 Umi Street
  Lihue, HI 96766
  (808) 245-4495

IDAHO

Idaho Department of Health and Welfare
STD/AIDS Program
  450 West State Street
  Boise, ID 83720
  (208) 334-6526

Boise

Central District Health Department
  707 North Armstrong Place
  Boise, ID 83704
  (208) 375-5211
Idaho AIDS Foundation
  PO Box 421
  Boise, ID 8370
  (208) 345-2277 *Hotline:* (800) 677-2437

Coeur d'Alene

Panhandle Health District I
  2195 Ironwood Court
  Coeur d'Alene, ID 83814
  (208) 667-3481

Lewiston

North Central District Health Department
  215 10th Street
  Lewiston, ID 83501
  (208) 799-3100

Pocatello

Southeastern District Health Department
  465 Memorial Drive
  Pocatello, ID 83201
  (208) 233-9080

ILLINOIS

Illinois Department Public Health
  525 West Jefferson Street, 1st floor
  Chicago, IL 26761
  (217) 524-5983 *Hotline:* (800) AID-AIDS

Champaign

Gay Community AIDS Project GCAP
  PO Box 713
  Champaign, IL 61324
  (217) 351-AIDS *Hotline:* same

Chicago

Chicago Department of Health
STD/HIV Program
  50 West Washington, Room 233
  Chicago, IL 60602
  (312) 747-0120
AIDS Foundation of Chicago
  1332 North Halsted Street, Suite 303
  Chicago, IL 60622
  (312) 642-5454
AIDS Pastoral Care Network APCN
  4753 North Broadway, Suite 800

Chicago, IL 60640
  (312) 334-5333
Chicago House and Social Service Agency
  913 West Belmont Avenue
  Chicago, IL 60657
  (312) 248-5200
Cook County Hospital/HIV Primary Care
  1900 West Polk, Room 1011
  Chicago, IL 60612
  (312) 633-5182 *Hotline:* (312) 252-8833
Families' & Children's AIDS Network
  721 North LaSalle Street, Suite 301
  Chicago, IL 60610
  (312) 655-7360 *Hotline:* (312) 655-7360
Hemophilia Foundation of Illinois
  332 South Michigan Avenue, Suite 812
  Chicago, IL 60604
  (312) 427-1495
Howard Brown Memorial Clinic (HBMC)
  945 West George Street
  Chicago, IL 60657
  (312) 871-5777
Kupona Network
  4611 South Ellis
  Chicago, IL 60653
  (312) 536-3000 *Hotline:* (312) 536-3530
Midwest Hispanic AIDS Coalition
  PO Box 470859
  Chicago, IL 60647
  (312) 772-8195 *Hotline:* (800) 542-1984
Test Positive Aware Network
  1340 West Irving Park Boulevard,
  Suite 259
  Chicago, IL 60613
  (312) 404-8726 *Hotline:* (312) 404-8726

Effingham

Effingham County Health Department
  901 West Virginia
  Effingham, IL 62401
  (217) 342-9237

Elgin

Open Door Clinic
  164 Division Street, Suite 607
  Elgin, IL 60120
  (708) 695-1093 *Hotline:* (800) 339-1093

Granite City

Madison County AIDS Program
  1308-A Niedringhaus
  Granite City, IL 62040
  (618) 877-5110

Maywood

Cook County Department of Public Health
  1701 South 1st Avenue
  Maywood, IL 60153
  (312) 869-6110 *Hotline:* (312) 865-4875

Morrison

Whiteside County Health Department
  18929 Lincoln Road
  Morrison, IL 61270
  (815) 772-7411 *Hotline:* same

Peoria

Peoria City County Health Department
2116 North Sheridan Road
Peoria, IL 61604
(309) 679-6000
Central Illinois Friends of PWA
416 St. Mark's Court, Suite 403
Peoria, IL 61603
(309) 673-6722

Rockford

Winnebago County Public Health
Department
401 Division Street
Rockford, IL 61104
(815) 692-5092 *Hotline:* (800) AID-AIDS

Urbana

Carle Comprehesive HIV Clinic
602 West University Avenue
Urbana, IL 61801
(217) 337-3424

INDIANA

Indiana State Health Department
HIV/STD
1330 West Michigan Street, Room 232
Indianapolis, IN 46206
(317) 633-0851 *Hotline:* (800) 848-AIDS

Anderson

Shalico Center
1106 Meridian Plaza, Suite 640
Anderson, IN 46016
(317) 646-9206

Bloomington

Monroe County AIDS Community Action
645 South Rogers Street
Bloomington, IN 47403
(812) 339-1691

Elkhart

Elkhart County Health Department
315 South 2nd Street, Room 1116
Elkhart, IN 46516
(219) 523-2328 *Hotline:* (219) 293-8671
Elkhart County AIDS Community Action
Group
306 West High Street
Elkhart, IN 46516
(219) 293-6519

Fort Wayne

Fort Wayne Allen County Health
Department
1 Main Street, Room 505
Fort Wayne, IN 46802
(219) 428-7504
AIDS Task Force
2124 Fairfield Avenue
Fort Wayne, IN 46802
(219) 744-1144 *Hotline:* same

Gary

Gary Health Department
1145 West 5th Avenue

Gary, IN 46402
(219) 882-5567 *Hotline:* (219) 885-5475
Gary Neighborhood Services
300 West 21st Avenue
Gary, IN 46407
(219) 883-0431 *Hotline:* (219) 885-1133

Indianapolis

Marion County Health Department
3838 North Rural
Indianapolis, IN 46205
(317) 541-2000 *Hotline:* (317) 639-AIDS
El Centro Hispano/The Hispanic Center
617 East North Street
Indianapolis, IN 46204
(317) 636-6551
Damien Center
1350 North Pennsylvania
Indianapolis, IN 46202
(317) 632-0123
Indiana Community AIDS Action Network
3951 North Meridian, Suite 200
Indianapolis, IN 46208
(317) 920-3190 *Hotline:* (800) 659-7580

Lafayette

Project AIDS Lafayette
810 North Street
Lafayette, IN 47903
(317) 742-2305 *Hotline:* (800) 524-3229

South Bend

AIDS Assistance of North Indiana
PO Box 11582
South Bend, IN 46634
(219) 234-2870 *Hotline:* (800) 287-AIDS

IOWA

Iowa Department Public Health
AIDS Program
321 East 12th Street
Des Moines, IA 50319
(515) 281-5601 *Hotline:* (800) 445-AIDS

Davenport

Scott County Health Department
428 Western Avenue, 5th Floor
Davenport, IA 52801
(319) 326-8618
Quad Cities AIDS Coalition
605 Main Street, Suite 6A
Davenport, IA 52803
(319) 324-8638 *Hotline:* (319) 324-8638

Des Moines

Polk County Health Department
1907 Carpenter
Des Moines, IA 50314
(515) 286-3789

Dubuque

Dubuque Regional AIDS Coalition
1300 Main Street, City Hall Annex
Dubuque, IA 52001
(312) 589-4181 *Hotline:* (800) 637-2919

Iowa City

Johnson County Public Health Department
AIDS Project
    1105 Gilbert Court
    Iowa City, IA 52240
    (319) 356-6040
Crisis Center
    321 East 1st Street
    Iowa City, IA 52240
    (319) 351-2726 *Hotline:* (319) 351-0140
Iowa Center for AIDS/ARC Resources and
Education
    PO Box 2989
    Iowa City, IA 52244
    (319) 338-2135
Iowa City Free Medical Clinic
    120 North Dubuque Street
    Iowa City, IA 52245
    (319) 337-4459

Waterloo

Black Hawk County Health Department
    1407 Independence Avenue
    Waterloo, IA 50703
    (319) 291-2413
Peoples Community Health Clinic
    403 Sycamore Street
    Waterloo, IA 50703
    (319) 236-1332 (24 hours)

KANSAS

Kansas Health and Environment
Department
Bureau of Disease Control
    109 South West 9th Street
    Topeka, KS 66612
    (913) 296-1500 *Hotline:* (800) 232-0040

Kansas City

Wyandotte County Health Department
    619 Ann Avenue
    Kansas City, KS 66101
    (918) 321-4803 *Hotline:* (918) 573-6716

Lawrence

Lawrence-Douglas County Health
Department
    336 Missouri, Suite 201
    Lawrence, KS 66044
    (913) 843-0721

Topeka

Topeka-Shawnee County Health
Department
    1615 West 8th
    Topeka, KS 66601
    (913) 295-3636
Topeka AIDS Project
    1615 South West 6th Street
    Topeka, KS 66606
    (913) 232-3100

Wichita

Wichita-Sedgwick County Health
Department
    1900 East 9th Street

Wichita KS 67214
    (316) 268-8441 *Hotline:* same
AIDS Referral Services
    1809 North Broadway, Suite E
    Wichita, KS 67214
    (316) 264-2438 *Hotline:* (316) 264-2437

KENTUCKY

Department of Health Services
    275 East Main Street
    Frankfort, KY 40621
    (502) 564-3418

Bowling Green

Barren River District Health Department
    1109 State Street
    Bowling Green, KY 42102
    (502) 781-2490
AIDS Southern Kentucky
    PO Box 09733
    Bowling Green, KY 42102
    (502) 842-5833

Lexington

Lexington Fayette County Health
Department
    650 Newtown Pike
    Lexington, KY 40508
    (606) 288-AIDS
AIDS Volunteers of Lexington
    214 Maxwell Street
    Lexington, KY 40508
    (606) 275-2865 *Hotline:* (606) 231-7545
Lexington Gay Services Organization
    PO Box 11471
    Lexington, KY 40575
    (606) 231-0335 *Hotline:* same

Louisville

Jefferson County Health Department
HIV/AIDS Program
    400 East Gray Street, Room 323
    Louisville, KY 40202
    (502) 574-5600
Jefferson County Human Services
    810 Barrett Avenue
    Louisville, KY 40204
    (502) 574-6013
AIDS Services Center
    810 Barrett Avenue, #266B
    Louisville, KY 40204
    (502) 574-5490 *Hotline:* same
Community Health Trust
    PO Box 4277
    Louisville, KY 40204
    (502) 574-5496 (24 hrs)
HIV-AIDS Legal Project
    Urban County Government Center
    810 Barrett Avenue, Suite 652
    Louisville, KY 40204
Kentuckiana PWA Coalition
    810 Barrett Avenue
    Louisville, KY 40204
    (502) 574-5493 *Hotline:* (800) 676-5490

Richmond

Madison County Health Department
  PO Box 906
  Richmond, KY 40475
  (606) 623-7312

Winchester

Clark County Health Department
  400 Professional Avenue
  Winchester, KY 40391
  (606) 744-4482 *Hotline:* (800) 654-6539

LOUISIANA

Louisiana State Office of Public Health
HIV/AIDS Services
  325 Loyola Avenue
  New Orleans, LA 70112
  (504) 568-7524 *Hotline:* (504) 944-2437

Alexandria

Central Louisiana AIDS Support Services
  824 16th Street
  Alexandria, LA 71301
  (318) 442-1010 *Hotline:* (800) 444-7993

Baton Rouge

East Baton Rouge Parish Health Unit
  353 North 12th Street
  Baton Rouge, LA 70821
  (504) 342-1711
OHH/OPH Clinic
Leo Butler Community Center
  950 East Washington Street
  Baton Rouge, LA 70802
  (504) 342-1799
St. Anthony's Home
  PO Box 749
  Baton Rouge, LA 70821
  (504) 765-8917

Lafayette

Lafayette Parish Health Unit
  2100 Jefferson Street, Building B
  Lafayette, LA 70501
  (318) 262-5616

New Orleans

New Orleans Health Department
AIDS Prevention Program
  2105 Banks Street
  New Orleans, LA 70112
  (504) 565-7437
New Orleans Health Department
  1300 Perdido Street, Room 8E13
  New Orleans, LA 70012
  (504) 565-6900 *Hotline:* (504) 524-7837
New Orleans AIDS Task Force
  1407 Decatur Street
  New Orleans, LA 70116
  (504) 945-4000 *Hotline:* (594) 944-AIDS
Northern AIDS Task Force
  Box 2616
  New Orleans, LA 70176
  (504) 944-2437 *Hotline:* (504) 522-AIDS
Project Lazarus

PO Box 3906
New Orleans, LA 70177
(504) 949-3609

MAINE

Maine Department of Human Services
Office on AIDS
  State House Station 11
  Augusta, ME 04333
  (207) 289-3747

Bangor

Bangor STD Clinic
  103 Texas Avenue
  Bangor, ME 04401
  (207) 947-0700

Lewiston

The STD Clinic
  239 Main Street Lewiston, ME 04240
  (207) 795-4019

Portland

Portland-Public Health Division
  389 Congress Street, Room 307
  Portland, ME 04101
  (207) 874-8300 ext. 8784
The AIDS Project, Inc. (TAP)
  22 Monument Square, 5th Floor
  Portland, ME 04101
  (207) 774-6877 *Hotline:* (800) 851-AIDS
Maine Health Foundation, Inc.
  222 St. John St
  Portland, ME 04102

MARYLAND

Maryland Department of Health and
Mental Hygiene
  201 West Preston Street
  Baltimore, MD 21201
  (301) 333-2273

Annapolis

Anne Arundel County Health Department
  3 Harry S. Truman Parkway
  Annapolis, MD 21401
  (301) 224-7109
Love and Action
  3 Church Street
  Annapolis, MD 21401
  (301) 268-3442 *Hotline:* same

Baltimore

Baltimore City Health Department
Preventive Medicine and Epidemiology
Bureau of Sexually Transmitted Diseases
  303 East Fayette Street, 5th Floor
  Baltimore, MD 21202
  (301) 396-4448
AIDS Action Baltimore
  2105 North Charles Street
  Baltimore, MD 21218
  (410) 837-2437
Baltimore Community Research Initiative
  22 South Greene Street

Baltimore, MD 21201
(410) 328-3588
Center For AIDS Education
201 West Preston Street, Room 308
Baltimore, MD 21201
(410) 225-5013 *Hotline:* (800) 638-6252
Chara House/St. Vincent's
4203 Belvieu Avenue
Baltimore, MD 21215
(410) 367-1191 (24 hrs)
Franciscan Center AIDS Outreach
2212 Maryland Avenue
Baltimore, MD 21218
(301) 467-5340
Health Education Resource Organization
101 West Read Street, #825
Baltimore, MD 21201
(410) 685-1180 *Hotline:* (410) 545-4774
PWA Coalition of Baltimore, Inc
101 West Read Street, #808
Baltimore, MD 21201
(410) 625-1677

Cambridge
Dorchester County Health Department
751 Woods Road
Cambridge, MD 21613
(410) 228-3223

Columbia
AIDS Alliance of Howard County
5537 Twin Knolls Road, #433
Columbia, MD 21045
(410) 995-4976
Howard County Health Department
10630 Little Patuxent Parkway
Century Plaza Building, #400
Columbia, MD 21044
(410) 313-7500

Elkton
Cecil County Health Department
401 Bow Street
Elkton, MD 21921
(410) 996-5100

Silver Spring
Montgomery County Health Department
2000 Dennis Avenue
Silver Spring, MD 20902
(301) 217-7681

MASSACHUSETTS
Massachusetts Department of Public
Health
150 Tremont Street
Boston, MA 02111
(617) 727-2700

Boston
AIDS Action Committee
131 Clarendon Street
Boston, MA 02116
(617) 437-6200 *Hotline:* (800) 235-2331

Boston City Hospital
818 Harris Avenue
Thorndike Building, Room 311
Boston, MA 02118
(617) 424-5160 *Hotline:* (617) 424-5916
Fenway Community Health Center
7 Haviland Street
Boston, MA 02115
(617) 267-0900 *Hotline:* (617) 267-9001

Cambridge
Cambridge Cares About AIDS, Inc
678 Massachusetts Avenue, #402
Cambridge, MA 02139
(617) 661-3040

Mattapan
Haitian American Public Health
Initiatives, Inc.
10 Fairway Street, #225
Mattapan, MA 02126
(617) 298-8076

New Bedford
New Bedford Health Department
100 Brock Avenue
New Bedford, MA 02744
(508) 991-6174
Project CARE AIDS Advocacy Center
PO Box 2097
New Bedford, MA 02741
(508) 990-8280

Provincetown
Provincetown AIDS Support Group
96-98 Bradford Street
PO Box 1522
Provincetown, MA 02657
(508) 487-9445

Rocksbury
Project Star
The Foundation for Children
1800 Columbus Avenue
Rocksbury, MA 02119
(617) 442-7442

Springfield
River Valley AIDS Project
120 Maple Street
Springfield, MA 01103
(413) 737-AIDS

Worcester
AIDS Project Worcester, Inc.
305 Shrewsbury Street
Worcester, MA 01604
(508) 755-3773

MICHIGAN
Michigan Department of Public Health
3500 North Logan Street
Lansing, MI 48909
(517) 335-8022

Ann Arbor

Hemophilia Foundation of Michigan
    411 Huron View Boulevard, #101
    Ann Arbor, MI 48103
    (313) 761-2535 *Hotline:* (800) 482-3041
Washtenaw Bounty AIDS/STD Program
    555 Towner, #121
    Ann Arbor, MI 48104
    (313) 484-6760

Detroit

AIDS Care Connection
    4221 Cass Avenue
    Detroit, MI 48071
    (313) 993-1320
CareGivers
    2111 Woodward Avenue, #700
    Detroit, MI 48201
    (313) 964-5070
La Casa Family Services
    3815 West Fort
    Detroit, MI 48216
    (313) 841-7380

Flint

Genesee County Health Department
    630 South Saginaw Street
    Flint, MI 48502
    (313) 257-3585 *Hotline:* (313) 257-1014
Wellness HIV/AIDS Services
    311 East Court Street
    Flint, MI 48502
    (313) 232-0888

Grand Rapids

Grand Rapids AIDS Resource Center
    1414 Robinson Road, South East
    Grand Rapids, MI 49516
    (616) 459-9177

Kalamazoo

Kalamazoo County Human Services
    113 West Kalamazoo Avenue
    Kalamazo, MI, 49007
    (616) 383-8881 *Hotline:* same
Kalamazoo AIDS Resource and Education
Services
    628 South Park Street
    Kalamazoo, MI 49007
    (616) 381-2437

Lansing

Ingham County Health Department
    PO Box 30161
    Lansing, MI 48909
    (517) 887-4308
Lansing Area AIDS Network
    855 Grove Street, #207
    Lansing, MI 48823
    (517) 487-0077

Muskegon

Muskegon County Health Department
    1611 East Oak
    Muskegon, MI 49442
    (616) 724-6311
Muskegon Area AIDS Resource Services

928 West Norton, Box 617
Muskegon, MI
(616) 722-2437 *Hotline:* (616) 722 AIDS

Pontiac

Oakland County Health Division
    1200 North Telegraph Road
    Ponitac, MI 48341
    (810) 858-5476
Care Givers
    1030 Featherston, #267
    Ponitac, MI 48342
    (313) 334-5100
Pontiac Urban League
    295 West Huron
    Ponitac, MI 48341
    (810) 338-4581

MINNESOTA

Minnesota Department of Health
AIDS/STD Prevention Services
    717 Delaware Street South East
    Minneapolis, MN 55440
    (612) 623-5000 *Hotline:* (612) 870-0700

Duluth

Duluth Community Health Center
    2 East 5th Street
    Duluth, MN 55805
    (218) 722-1497

Elk River

Sherburn County Public Health
Department
Government Center
    Elk River, MN 55330
    (612) 241-2750 *Hotline:* (800) 433-5237

Minneapolis

Minneapolis Health Department
    250 South 4th Street
    Minneapolis, MN 55415
    (612) 673-2301
Aliveness Project/PWA Coalition
    730 East 38th Street
    Minneapolis, MN 55427
    (612) 822-7846 (24 hours)
    Hotline: (612) 822-3016
Minnesota AIDS Project
    2025 Nicolet Avenue
    Minneapolis, MN 55404
    (507) 282-8771
    TTD/TTY (612) 870-0700
    Hotline: (800) 248-2437
Red Door Clinic
    525 Portland Avenue, South
    Minneapolis, MN 55415
    (612) 348-3238

St. Paul

American Indian Health Care Association
    245 East 6th Street, #499
    St, Paul, MN 55404
    (612) 293-0233
Family Tree Clinic

1619 Dayton Avenue
St. Paul, MN 55104
(612) 645-0478 *Hotline:* (800) 783-2287
St. Paul Public Health
555 Cedar Street
St. Paul, MN 55101
(612) 292-7735 *Hotline:* (612) 292-7735

Worthington
Nobles Rock Health Service
    Box 757
    Worthington, MN 65156
    (507) 372-8256

MISSISSIPPI
Mississippi State Department of Health
HIV/AIDS Prevention Program
    2423 North State Street, Box 1700
    Jackson, MS 39215
    (601) 960-7723 *Hotline:* (800) 826-2961

Biloxi
South Mississippi AIDS Task Force
    478 Caillavet
    Biloxi, MS 25520
    (601) 435-1234 *Hotline:* (601) 435-1234

Jackson
Mississippi Gay/Lesbian Alliance
    PO Box 8342
    Jackson, MS 39284
    (601) 371-1318 (24 hours)
    Hotline: (800) 537-0851

MISSOURI
Missouri Department of Health
Bureau of AIDS Prevention
    1730 East Elm
    Jefferson City, MO 65102
    (314) 751-6438 *Hotline:* (800) 533-AIDS

Charleston
Mississippi County Health Department
    1200 East Marshall
    Charleston, MO 63834
    (314) 683-2191

Columbia
Columbia/Boone County Health
Department
    PO Box N
    Columbia, MO 65205
    (314) 874-7335
Mid Missouri AIDS Project
    811 East Cherry Street
    Columbia, MO 65201
    (314) 875-2437

Hillsboro
Jefferson County Health Department
    405 Second Street
    Hillsboro, MO 63050
    (314) 296-1844

Joplin
Joplin City Health Department
    513 Kentucky

Joplin, MO 64801
    (417) 623-6122
Four State Community AIDS Project
    726 Illinois
    Joplin, MO 64803
    (417) 624-1250 *Hotline:* Same

Kansas City
Kansas City Missouri Health Department
HIV/AIDS Program
    1423 East Linwood
    Kansas City, MO 64109
    (816) 923-2600 *Hotline:* (816) 923-AIDS
Good Samaritan Project
    3030 Walnut Street
    Kansas City, MO 64108
    (816) 561-8784 *Hotline:* (800) 234-TEEN
Guadelupe Center
    2641 Belleview
    Kansas City, MO 64108
    (816) 561-6885
Peer to Peer
KC Youth AIDS Project
    706 West 42nd Street, #106
    Kansas City, MO 64111
    (816) 531-1787 *Hotline:* (800) 767-1787
Swope Parkway Health Center
    4900 Swope Parkway
    Kansas City, MO 64130
    (816) 923-5800 *Hotline:* (816) 923-5800
The AIDS Council
    2801 Wyandotte, #167
    Kansas City, MO 64108
    (816) 751-5166

Springfield
AIDS Project of the Ozarks
    1722-LL South Glenstone Avenue
    Springfield, MO 65804
    (417) 881-1900 *Hotline:* (800) 743-5767

St. Louis
St. Louis County Health Department
    6065 Helen Avenue
    St. Louis, MO 63134
    (314) 522-6410
Missouri HIV/AIDS Education Network
    4050 Lindell Boulevard
    St. Louis, MO 63108
    (314) 658-2019
St. Louis Effort for AIDS
    5622 Delmar Boulevard, #104E
    St. Louis, MO 63112
    (314) 367-2382 *Hotline:* (314) 367-8400
St. Louis Metropolitan AIDS Program
    634 North Grant
    St. Louis, MO 63103
    (314) 658-1159

MONTANA
Montana Department of Health and
Environmental Control
AIDS/STD Program
    Cogswell Building
    Helena, MT 59620
    (406) 444-2457

Montana Department of Health
Montana AIDS Program
Preventive Health Services Bureau
  1400 Broadway
  Helena, MT 59620
  (406) 444-3565

Billings

Yellowstone City/County Health
Department
  217 North 27th Street
  Billings, MT 59101
  (406) 256-6821
Yellowstone AIDS Project
  3308 Second Avenue, North
  Billings, MT 59601
  (406) 245-2029 *Hotline* (800) 233-6668

Helena

Lewis & Clark City/County Health
Department
  1930 9th Avenue
  Helena, MT 59601
  406-443-2584
Helena Family Planning
  1930 9th Avenue, #201
  Helena, MT 59601
  (406) 442-3830
Lewis & Clark County AIDS Project
  631 Helena Avenue
  Helena, MT 59624
  (406) 449-1357

Missoula

Missoula City/County Health Department
  301 West Alder
  Missoula, MT 59802
  (406) 523-4775
Missoula AIDS Council
  PO Box 9102
  Missoula, MT 59802
  (406) 543-4770 *Hotline:* (800) 662-9002

NEBRASKA

Nebraska Department of Health
  301 Centennial Mall, South
  Lincoln, NE 68509
  (402) 471-2937
  Hotline: (800) 782-AIDS

Lincoln

Lincoln-Lancaster County Health
Department
  2200 St. Mary's Avenue
  Lincoln, NE 68502
  (402) 441-8056
Minority AIDS Education Task Force
  2300 "O" Street
  Lincoln, NE 68510
  (402) 474-3950

Omaha

Douglas County Health Department
  1819 Farnam Street, #401
  Omaha, NE 68183
  (402) 444-7475

Nebraska AIDS Project
  3624 Leavenworth Street
  Omaha, NE 68105
  (402) 484 8100 *Hotline:* (800) 782-2437

NEVADA

Nevada Department of Human Resources
Division of Health
HIV/AIDS Program
  505 East King Street, Room 304
  Carson City, NV 89710
  (702) 687-4800 *Hotline:* (800) 842-2437

Las Vegas

Clark County Health District
  625 Shadow Lane
  Las Vegas, NV 89128
  (702) 383-1393 *Hotline:* (702) 383-1303
Aid for AIDS of Nevada
  1111 Desert Lane
  Las Vegas, NV 89102
  (702) 382-2326 *Hotline:* (702) 474-2437
Nevada Association of Latin Americans
AIDS Outreach Center
  2346 East Bonanza
  Las Vegas, NV 89102
  (702) 384-6002

Reno

Washoe County District Health
Department
  1001 East 9th Street
  Reno, NV 89512
  (702) 328-2400
Nevada AIDS Foundation
  1225 Westfield Avenue, #8
  Reno, NV 89504
  (702) 329-2437 *Hotline:* same
Nevada Hispanic Services
  190 East Liberty Street
  Reno, NV 89501
  (702) 786-6003

NEW HAMPSHIRE

New Hampshire Division of Public Health
Services
STD/HIV Program
Health and Welfare Building
  6 Hazen Drive
  Concord, NH 03301
  (603) 271-4576 *Hotline:* (800) 752-AIDS

Concord

Concord Regional Visiting Nurse Association
  250 Pleasant Street
  Concord, NH 03302
  (603) 224-4093 *Hotline:* same

Keene

AIDS Services for the Monadnock Region
  331 Main Street
  Keene, NH 03431
  (603) 357-6855 24 hours
  Hotline: (800) 693-7903

Manchester

Manchester Health Department
795 Elm Street, #302
Manchester, NH 03101
(603) 624-6466

NEW JERSEY

New Jersey Department of Health
AIDS Prevention and Control
50 East State Street
Trenton, NJ 08625
(609) 984-6000

Atlantic City

Atlantic City Division of Health
35 South Martin Luther King Boulevard
Atlantic City, NJ 08401
(609) 347-6547 *Hotline:* (609) 347-6456
Sencit-Baltic Family Practice Center
1325 Baltic Avenue
Atlantic City, NJ 08401
(609) 347-5200 *Hotline:* (609) 347-6456
South Jersey AIDS Alliance
1301 Atlantic Avenue
Atlantic City, NJ 08401
(609) 347-1085 *Hotline:* (800) 281-2437

Camden

Camden County Health Department
AIDS Program
2101 Ferry Avenue
Camden, NJ 08104
(609) 757-8606 *Hotline:* (609) 365-AIDS

Collingswood

AIDS Coalition of Southern New Hampshire
900 Haddon Avenue, #201
Collingswood, NJ 08108
(609) 854-7578 *Hotline:* (800) 229-2437

Dover

The AIDS Center/Hope House
19-21 Belmont Avenue
Dover, NJ 07802
(201) 361-7443 *Hotline:* (201) 361-7232

East Orange

Caribbean Haitian Council
26 Ashland Avenue
East Orange, NJ 07017
(201) 678-5059
HIV Counseling & Testing Site
143 New Street
East Orange, NJ
(201) 266-5498 *Hotline:* (201) 266-5454

Middletown

Middletown Township Health Department
1 Kings Highway
Middletown, NJ 07748
(908) 615-2096 *Hotline:* (201) 615-2095

New Brunswick

Hyacinth AIDS Foundation
103 Bayard Street, Third Floor
New Brunswick, NJ 08901
(908) 246-0204 *Hotline:* (800) 433-0254

New Jersey Women and AIDS Network
5 Elm Row, #112
New Brunswick, NJ 08901
(908) 846-4462

Newark

AIDS Resource Foundation for Children
182 Roseville Avenue
Newark, NJ 07107
(201) 483-4250

Trenton

New Horizon Treatment Services
132 Perry Street
Trenton, NJ 08618
(609) 394-8988

NEW MEXICO

New Mexico Department of Health and
Environment
AIDS Prevention Program
1190 St. Francis Drive
Sante Fe, NM 87503
(505) 827-0086
New Mexico Department of Health
HIV/AIDS/STD Services & Prevention
715 East Idaho, #4A
Las Cruces, NM 88001
(505) 524-6006 *Hotline:* (800) 545-AIDS

Albuquerque

New Mexico AIDS Servvices
4200 Silver Avenue, South East, #D
Albuquerque, NM 87108
(505) 266-0911
New Mexico Association of PLWA
111 Mont Claire, South East
Albuquerque, NM 87108
(505) 266-0342
Youth Development/AIDS Education
2929 Barcelona, South West
Albuquerque, NM 87105
(505) 877-0371

Las Cruces

Southern New Mexico Human Development
PO Box 2285
Las Cruces, NM 88001
(505) 523-6360 *Hotline:* 505-523-6360

Sante Fe

AIDS Wellness Program
811 St. Michael Drive
Sante Fe, NM 87501
(505) 983-1822
AIDS/ARC Home Care Program
Human Services Department
Pera Building Room 524
Sante Fe, NM 87504
(505) 827-4332

NEW YORK

New York State Department of Health
Empire State Plaza
Corning Tower Building, 14th Floor
Albany, NY 12237
(518) 474-7542 *Hotline:* (800) 541-AIDS

New York State Department of Health
AIDS Institute
   5 Penn Plaza
   New York, NY 10001
   (212) 613-2492

Albany

AIDS Council of North East New York
   88 4th Avenue
   Albany, NY 12202
   (518) 434-4686 *Hotline:* (518) 445-2437
Albany Medical College/AIDS Program
   47 New Scotland Avenue
   Albany, NY 12208
   (518) 262-4399

Bath

Steuben County Public Health
   3 Pulteney Square
   Bath, NY 14810
   (607) 776-9631 *Hotline:* (800) 346-2211

Bronx

Albert Einstein College of Medicine
Family Care Center
   1300 Morris Park Avenue, #401
   Bronx, NY 10461
   (212) 430-4227 *Hotline:* (212) 430-3333
Bronx-Lebanon Hospital Center
AIDS Program Office
   1650 Grand Concourse
   Bronx, NY 10457
   (718) 590-1820
Montefiore Adolescent AIDS Program
   111 East 210th Street
   Bronx, NY 10467
   (212) 882-0232

Brooklyn

Brooklyn AIDS Task Force
   465 Dean Street
   Brooklyn, NY 11217
   (718) 783-0883 *Hotline:* (718) 485-8111
Caribbean Women's Health Association
   2725 Church Avenue
   Brooklyn, NY 11226
   (718) 826-2942
Haitian Coalition on AIDS
   50 Court Street, #605
   Brooklyn, NY 11201
   (718) 855-7275 *Hotline:* (718) 855-0972
People of Color in Crisis
Support and Referral
   462 Bergen Street
   Brooklyn, NY 11217
   (718) 596-7979

Buffalo

Erie County Department of Health
   95 Franklin Street
   Buffalo, NY 14202
   (716) 858-7687
AIDS Alliance of West New York
   367 Delaware Avenue
   Buffalo, NY 14202
   (716) 852-6778

AIDS Community Services of West New
York
   121 West Tupper Street
   Buffalo, NY 14201
   (716) 847-AIDS *Hotline:* (716) 847 AIDS
Benedict House of West New York
   124 Plymouth Avenue
   Buffalo, NY 14401
   (716) 881-3082 24 hours
La Alternativa/Hispanic AIDS
   176 Jersey Street
   Buffalo, NY 14201
   (716) 881-0732

Dutchess County

AIDS-related Community Services
   89 Market Street
   Poughkeepsie
   Dutchess County, NY 12601
   (914) 471-992-1442 *Hotline:* same

Hawthorne

Westchester County Health Department
   19 Bradhurst Avenue
   Hawthorne, NY 10532
   (914) 593-5067 *Hotline:* (914)-593-AIDS

Ithaca

Tompkins County Health Department
   401 Dates Drive
   Ithaca NY 14850
   (607) 274-6674 *Hotline:* (800) 562-9423

Liberty

AIDS-related Community Service
   PO Box 5999920
   Infirmary Road
   Liberty, NY 12754
   (914) 292-0100 *Hotline:* (800) 992-1442

Mayville

Chautaugua County Health Department
   Hall R. Clothier Building
   7 North Erie Street, 4th Floor
   Mayvill, NY 14757
   (716) 753-4314 *Hotline:* (716) 753-4314

New York

AIDS Resource Center
   275 7th Avenue, 12th Floor
   New York, NY 10001
   (212) 633-2500
Body Positive
   2095 Broadway, Suite 306
   New York, NY 10023
   (212) 721-1346
Bureau of HIV Education Outreach &
Community Development
   311 Broadway, 4th Floor
   New York, NY 10007
   (212) 285-4625
Community Family Planning Council
   184 Fifth Avenue
   New York, NY 10010
   (718) 991-9250 *Hotline:* (718) 991-9498
Gay Men's Health Clinic

129 West 20th Street
New York, NY 10011
(212) 337-1950 *Hotline:* (212) 807-6655
Men of Color AIDS Prevention Program
NYC Department of Health
New York, NY 10013
(212) 239-1796
PWA Health Group
150 West 26th Street, Suite 201
New York, NY 10001
(212) 255-0520
PWA Coalition of NY
50 West 17th Street, 8th Floor
New York, NY 10011
(212) 647-1415 *Hotline:* (800) 828-3280
Spellman Center for HIV-Related Disease
St. Clares Hospital
415 West 51st Street
New York, NY 10019
(212) 459-8130 *Hotline:* (212) 454-8092
The Streetwork Project
545 8th Avenue, 22nd Floor
New York, NY 10018
(212) 695-2220
Upper Manhattan AIDS Task Force
55 West 125th Street, #1103
New York, NY 10027
(212) 369-5800 (24 hours)

Rochester

AIDS Rochester
1350 University Avenue, #C
Rochester, NY 14607
(716) 442-4440 *Hotline:* (716) 232-4430
Baden Street Settlement
152 Baden Street
Rochester, NY 14605
(716) 325-4910 *Hotline:* (716) 262-3168
Community Health Network
758 South Avenue
Rochester, NY 14620
(716) 244-9000
Puerto Rican Youth Development
997 Clinton Avenue
Rochester, NY 14621
(716) 325-3570
University of Rochester AIDS Center
601 Elmwood Avenue
Rochester, NY 14642
(716) 275-0528

Schenectady

Schenectady County Public Health Services
1 Broadway Center, Room 840
Schenectady, NY 12305
(518) 386-2824
Schenectady Family Health Services
602-608 Craig Street
Schenectady, NY 12307
(518) 370-1441

Syracuse

Onodaga County Health Department
421 Montgomery Street

Syracuse NY 13202
(315) 435-3648
AIDS Community Resources
627 West Genesee Street
Syracuse, NY 13204
(315) 475-2430

Warsaw

Wyoming County Health Department
338 North Main Street
Warsaw, NY 14569
(716) 786-8890 *Hotline:* (716) 786-2233

NORTH CAROLINA

North Carolina Department of
Environment, Health, & Natural
Resources
Division of Adult Health
PO Box 27687
Raleigh, NC 27611-7687
(919) 733-7081
North Carolina HIV/STD Control Branch
PO Box 27687
Raleigh, NC 27611
(919) 733-7301

Asheville

Western North Carolina AIDS Project
PO Box 2411
Asheville, NC 28802
(704) 252-7489

Brevard

Transylvania County Health Department
Community Services Building
Brevard, NC 28712
(704) 884-3135

Charlotte

Mecklenburg County Health Department
249 Billingsley Road
Charlotte, NC 28211
(704) 336-4700
Metrolina AIDS Project
Box 32662
Charlotte, NC 28232
(704) 333-1435 *Hotline:* (800) 289-AIDS

Durham

Durham County Health Department
414 East Main Street
Durham, NC 27701
(919) 560-7600
AIDS Service Project
Box 3203
Durham, NC 27715
(919) 286-7475 *Hotline:* (919) 286-4107
North Carolina Lesbian/Gay Health Project
PO Box 3203
Durham, NC 27715
(919) 286-4107 *Hotline:* (919) 286-4107

Greensboro

Guilford County Public Health Department
301 North Eugene Street
Greensboro, NC 27401
(919) 373-3899

TRIAD Health Project
313 South Greene Street, #200
Greensboro, NC 27401
(919) 275-1654

Raleigh

North Carolina HIV/STD Control
PO Box 27687
Raleigh, NC 27611
(919) 733-7301
AIDS Service Agency
PO Box 12583
Raleigh, NC 27605
(919) 834-2437

Wilmington

New Hanover County Health Department
2029 South 17th Street
Wilmington, NC 28401
(919) 343-6500 *Hotline:* (919) 251-3232

NORTH DAKOTA

State Department of Health
State Capitol Building
Bismarck, ND 58505
(701) 224-2372

Grand Forks

Grand Forks Public Health
Box 1518
Grand Forks, ND 58201
(701) 746-2525

Williston

Upper Missouri District Health Unit
512 4th Avenue, East
Williston, ND 58801
(701) 572-5471 *Hotline:* (800) 472-2180

OHIO

Ohio Department of Health
AIDS Activities Unit
PO Box 118
Columbus, OH 43266
(614) 466-5480
Hotline: (800) 332-AIDS

Akron

Akron Health Department
177 South Broadway
Akron, OH 44308
(216) 375-2960
Northeast Ohio Task Force on AIDS
655 North Main Street
Akron, OH 44310
(216) 375-2000 *Hotline:* (216) 375-AIDS

Canton

Canton City Health Department
420 North Market Avenue
Canton, OH 44702
(216) 489-3322 *Hotline:* (216) 489-3243

Cincinnati

Cincinnati Health Department
3101 Burnet Avenue
Cincinnati OH 45229

(513) 357-7300 *Hotline:* (513) 357-7300
AIDS Volunteers of Cincinnati
2183 Central Parkway
Cincinnati, OH 45214
(513) 421-2437
Hotline: (513) 421-2437

Cleveland

Cleveland Health Department
1925 St. Clair Avenue
Cleveland, OH 44104
(216) 664-2324
Cleveland Clinic Foundation
9500 Euclid Avenue
Cleveland, OH 44195
(216) 444-0175
Cleveland Neighborhood Health Services
12800 Shaker Boulevard
Cleveland, OH 44120
(216) 991-3000
Health Issues Task Force
2250 Euclid Avenue
Cleveland, OH 44115
(216) 621-0766
University Hospital of Cleveland
Immunology Unit
2074 Abington Road
Cleveland, OH 44106
(216) 844-7890

Columbus

Columbus Health Department
181 Washington Boulevard
Columbus, OH 43215
(614) 645-6446
FACES
Children's Hospital HIV Program
700 Children's Drive
Columbus, OH 43205
(614) 461-2248 *Hotline:* (614) 461-2000
Columbus AIDS Task Force
1500 West Third Street, Third Floor
Columbus, OH 43212
(614) 488-2437 *Hotline:* (800) 488-2437

Dayton

Combined Health District/Montgomery
County
451 West Third Street
Dayton, OH 45422
(513) 225-5984 *Hotline:* (513) 225-4507
AIDS Foundation Miami Valley
PO Box 3539
Dayton, OH 45401
(513) 277-2437 *Hotline:* (513) 223-2437

Toledo

Toledo Health Department
635 North Erie Street
Toledo, OH 43624
(419) 245-1700
David's House Compassion
Nova Program
PO Box 391
Toledo, OH 43697

(419) 244-6682
Good Samaritan Parish
PO Box 4907
Toledo, OH 43620
(419) 244-2124
Hotline: (419) 244-2124
Medical College Hospital
HIV Counseling & Testing
Ruppert Health Center
3000 Arlington Avenue
Box 0008
Toledo, OH 43699
(419) 381-3741

Youngstown

Youngstown Health Department
AIDS Unit
City Hall Building, 7th Floor
26 South Phelps Street
Youngstown, OH 33402
(216) 742-8811 *Hotline:* (216) 742-8811
Mahoning County Area AIDS Task Force
PO Box 1143
Youngstown, OH 44501
(216) 742-8811 *Hotline:* (216) 742-8811

OKLAHOMA

Oklahoma State Department of Health
1000 Northeast 10th Street
Oklahoma City, OK 73152
405-271-4636

Oklahoma City

City County Health Department/Oklahoma
City
921 Northeast 23rd Street
Oklahoma City, OK 73105
(405) 425-4451
AIDS Support Program
PO Box 12185
Oklahoma City, OK 73112
(405) 525-6277
Drug Recovery
415 Northwest 7th Street
Oklahoma City, OK 73101
(405) 232-9804 *Hotline:* (405) 424-4347
Oasis Foundation
PO Box 57754
Oklahoma City, OK 73157
(405) 525-2437

Tulsa

Tulsa City County Health Department
4616 East 15th
Tulsa, OK 74114
(918) 744-1000
HIV Resource Consortium
4154 South Harvard, Suite H-1
Tulsa, OK 74135
(918) 749-3455
Indian Health Care Resource Center/Tulsa
915 South Cincinnati
Tulsa, OK 74119
(918) 582-7225

OREGON

Department of Human Resources
1400 South West Fifth Avenue, Room 811
Portland, OR 97201
(503) 229-5032
Oregon Health Division
HIV Program
800 North East Oregon Street, Suite 745
Portland, OR 97232
(503) 731-4029 *Hotline:* (800) 777-2437

Eugene

Lane County Public Health
135 East 6th Street
Eugene, OR 97401
(503) 687-4013
HIV/AIDS Resources
3477 East Amazon Drive
Eugene, OR 97405
(503) 342-5088

Medford

Jackson County Public Health Services
1005 East Main
Medford, OR 97501
(503) 776-7335

Portland

Multnomah County Health Division
426 South West Stark Street, 3rd Floor
Portland, OR 97204
(503) 248-5020
Cascade AIDS Project
620 South West 5th, Suite 300
Portland, OR 97204
(503) 223-5907 *Hotline:* (800) 777-AIDS
Waverly Children's Home
3550 South East Woodward Street
Portland, OR 97202
(503) 234-7532

PENNSYLVANIA

Pennsylvania Department of Health
AIDS/HIV Factline
2A Kline Village
Harrisburg, PA 17104
(717) 238-2437 *Hotline:* (800) 662-6080

Bethlehem

Bethlehem Health Bureau
10 East Church Street
Bethlehem, PA 18018
(215) 865-7057
AIDS Service Center
557 East Broad Street
PO Box 1800
Bethlehem, PA 18016
(215) 974-8701 *Hotline:* (215) 974-8700

Harrisburg

South Central AIDS Assistance Network
2A Kline Village, Suite A
Harrisburg, PA 17104
(717) 238-2437 *Hotline:* (800) 662-6080

Philadelphia

AIDS Activities Coordinating Office
  1220 Sansom Street, 7th Floor
  Philadelphia, PA 19107
  (215) 686-1800 *Hotline:* (215) 985-AIDS
AIDS Information Network
  32 North 3rd Street
  Philadelphia, PA 19119
  (215) 922-5120
AIDS Task Force/ Philadelphia
  1642 Pine Street
  Philadelphia, PA 19103
  (215) 545-8686 *Hotline:* (215) 732-AIDS
Action AIDS
  1216 Arch Street, 4th Floor
  Philadelphia, PA 19107
  (215) 981-0088
Asociacion de Puertorriquenos en Marcha
  2147 B 6th Street
  Philadelphia, PA 19122
  (215) 236-8885
Bebashi North
  5205 North Broad Street
  Philadelphia, PA 19141
  (215) 457-9050
Congreso De Latinos Unidos
  713 West Thompson Street
  Philadelphia, PA 19123
  (215) 763-8870
Philadelphia FIGHT
  419 South 19th Street, #201
  Philadelphia, PA 19146
  (215) 893-2672

Pittsburgh

Allegheny County Health Department
  3441 Forbes Avenue
  Pittsburgh, PA 15213
  (412) 578-8332
Pittsburgh AIDS Task Force
  905 West Street, 4th Floor
  Pittsburgh, PA 15221
  (412) 242-2500

Reading

Berks AIDS Health Crisis
  429 Walnut Street
  Reading, PA 19603
  (215) 375-6523 *Hotline:* (215) 375-2242

Williamsport

AIDS Resource Alliance/North Central
  Lycoming County
  507 West 4th Street
  Williamsport, PA 17701
  (717) 332-8448

York

York City Bureau of Health
  1 Market Way West, 3rd Floor
  York, PA 17405
  (717) 849-2252
YHESSI
  101 East Market Street
  York, PA 17401
  (717) 846-6776

RHODE ISLAND

Rhode Island Department of Health
Office of AIDS
  105 Cannon Building
  3 Capitol Street
  Providence, RI 02908
  (401) 277-2320

Providence

Family AIDS Center for Treatment &
Support (FACTS)
  18 Parris Avenue
  Providence, RI 02907
  (401) 521-3603
Rhode Island Project/AIDS
  95 Chestnut Street, 3rd Floor
  Providence, RI 02903
  (401) 831-5522 *Hotline:* (800) 726-3010

SOUTH CAROLINA

South Carolina Department of Health and
Environmental Control
  2600 Bull Street
  Columbia, SC 29201
  (803) 758-5445

Charleston

Charleston County Health Department
  334 Calhoun Street
  Charleston, SC 29401
  (803) 724-5815
Low Country AIDS Services
  PO Box 207C
  Charleston, SC 29402
  (803) 577-2437

Columbia

SC AIDS Education Network
  2768 Decker Boulevard, #98
  Columbia, SC 29206
  (803) 736-1171

SOUTH DAKOTA

State Department of Health
  Joe Foss Building
  325 East Capitol Avenue
  Pierre, SD 57501
  (605) 773-3361

Fort Thompson

Indian Health Service
  PO Box 200
  Fort Thompson, SD 57339
  (605) 245-2288

Pierre

South Dakota Urban Indian Health
  122 East Dakota
  Pierre, SD 57501
  (605) 224-8841

Rapid City

Rapid City Indian Health Advisory
  Box 1608
  Rapid City, SD 57701
  (605) 343-2368

TENNESSEE

Tennessee Department of Health
AIDS Program
　C2-221 Cordell Hall Building
　Nashville, TN 37247
　(615) 741-7500 *Hotline:* (800) 525-AIDS

Chattanooga

Chattanooga-Hamilton County
Health Department
　921 East 3rd Street
　Chattanooga, TN 37403
　(615) 757-2009 *Hotline:* (615-267)-AIDS
Chattanooga CARES
　701 Cherokee Road
　Chattanooga, TN 37405
　(615) 267-AIDS

Knoxville

Knox County Health Department
　925 Cleveland Place
　Knoxville, TN 37917
　(615) 544-4156 *Hotline:* (615) 544 4162
East Tennessee Regional Health Office
　1522 Cherokee Trail
　Knoxville, TN 37920
　(615) 546-9221
AIDS Response Knowxville
　PO Box 6069
　Knoxville, TN 37914
　(616) 523-2437

Memphis

Memphis/Shelby County Health
Department
　814 Jefferson Avenue, Room 227
　Memphis, TN 38105
　(901) 576-7742 *Hotline:* (901) 576-7575
Friends for Life HIV Resources
　321 Bellevue
　Memphis, TN 38174
　(901) 272-0855 *Hotline:* (901) 278-AIDS
Memphis Health Center
　360 EH Crump Boulevard
　Memphis, TN 38126
　(901) 947-1647

Nashville

Metropolitan Health Department
　311 23rd Avenue
　Nashville, TN 37203
　(615) 862-5900
Nashville CARES
　700 Craighead, #200
　Nashville, TN 37202
　(615) 385-1510 *Hotline:* (615) 385-AIDS
Project COPE
　Meharry Medical College
　2701 Jefferson Street
　Nashville, TN 37208
　(615) 327-1220 *Hotline:* (615) 327-1220
Vanderbilt AIDS Project
　A-2215 Medical Center North
　Nashville, TN 37232
　(615) 322-2237 *Hotline:* (615) 322-2437

TEXAS

Texas Department of Health
　1100 West 49th Street
　Austin, TX 78756
　(512) 458-7375

Amarillo

NWTH-Public Health Service
　411 South Austin Street
　Amarillo, TX 79106
　(806) 371-1100
Panhandle AIDS Support Organization
(PASO)
　604 West 8th Street
　Amarillo, TX 79101
　(806) 372-1050

Austin

Austin Travus County Health Department
　HIV Services
　15 Waller Street
　Austin, TX 78702
　(512) 469-2123 *Hotline:* (512) 469-2169
AIDS Services of Austin
　PO Box 4874
　Austin, TX 78765
　(512) 451-2273 *Hotline:* (512) 458-AIDS
ALLGO
　Informe SIDA
　PO Box 13501
　Austin, TX 78702
　(512) 474-2001
HIV Wellness Center
　302B Oakland Street
　Austin, TX 78763
　(512) 472-2753 *Hotline:* (512) 472-2753
People's Community Clinic
　2909 North Interstate 35
　Austin, TX 78722
　(512) 478-4939
Project Transition
　PO Box 4826
　Austin, TX 78765
　(512) 454-8646

Corpus Christi

Corpus Christi-Nueces County Health
Department
　HIV Clinic
　1702 Horne Road, Room 28
　Corpus Christi, TX 78416
　(512) 851-7239
Coastal Bend AIDS Foundation
　1118 Third Street
　Corpus Christi, TX 78463
　(512) 883-5815 *Hotline:* (512) 883-CARE
Corpus Christi Drug Abuse Council
　405 John Sartain
　Corpus Christi, TX 78403
　(512) 882-9979

Dallas

Dallas County Health Department
　1936 Amelia Court, Room 205
　Dallas, TX 75235
　(214) 920-7916 *Hotline:* (214) 351-4335

AIDS Resource Center
2701 Reagan
Dallas, TX 75219
(214) 521-5124 *Hotline:* (214) 522-2290
DARCO Drug Services
2608 Inwood Road
Dallas, TX 75235
(214) 956-7181 (24 hours)
AIDS Services of Dallas
PWA Coalition of Dallas
PO Box 4338
Dallas, TX 75208
(214) 941-0523
Oak Lawn Community Services
3434 Fairmont
Dallas, TX 75219
(214) 520-8108 *Hotline:* (214) 351-4335
Open Arms/Bryans House
Box 191402
Dallas, TX 75219
(214) 559-3946 (24 hours)

El Paso

El Paso City/County Health Department
22 South Campbell
El Paso, TX 79901
(915) 543-3509 *Hotline:* (915) 543-3574
Centro de Salud Familiar La Fe
700 South Ochoa Street
El Paso, TX 79901
(915) 545-4550
South West AIDS Committee
1505 Mescalero
El Paso, TX 79925
(915) 772-3366

Fort Worth

Tarrant County Public Health
180 University Drive
Fort Worth, TX 76107
(817) 871-7341
AIDS Outreach Center
1125 West Peter Smith
Fort Worth, TX 76104
(817) 335-1994 *Hotline:* (817) 336-0066
American Institute for Teen AIDS
Prevention
6032 Jacksboro Highway, Suite 100
Fort Worth, TX 76136
(817) 237-0230

Houston

Houston Department Health and Human
Services
8000 North Stadium Drive
Houston, TX 77054
(713) 794-9092 *Hotlines:* (713) 794-9020,
(713) 794-AIDS
Harris County Health Department
2501 Dunstan
Houston, TX 77005
(713) 620-6883
AIDS Foundation Houston
3202 Wesleyan Annex
Houston, TX 77027
(713) 623-6796 *Hotline:* (713) 524-AIDS

Amigos Volunteers in Education and
Service
2510 Broad Street, Suite 100
Houston, TX 77087
(713) 640-2837
Baylor Population Program
One Baylor Plaza
Houston, TX 77030
(713) 798-7581 *Hotline:* (713) 798-7567
Bering Community Service Foundation
PO Box 540517
Houston, TX 77254
(713) 526-6071
Chicano Family Center
7524 Avenue East
Houston, TX 77012
(713) 923-2316
Covenant House Texas
1111 Lovett Boulevard
Houston, TX 77006
(713) 523-2231 (24 hours)
Hotline (800) 999-9999
Crisis Intervention of Houston
Box 130866
Houston, TX 77219
(713) 527-9864 *Hotline:* (713) 228-1505
Montrose Clinic
1200 Richmon
Houston, TX 77006
(713) 520-2080 *Hotline:* (713) 520-2000
Omega House
602 Branard
Houston, TX 77006
(713) 523-7110 (24 hours)
Over the Hill
3402 Dowling
Houston, TX 77004
(713) 520-9554

Laredo

City of Laredo Health Department
2600 Cedar Avenue
Laredo, TX 78044
(210) 723-2051 *Hotline:* (210) 722-2437

Lubbock

Lubbock Health Department
1902 Texas Avenue
Lubbock, TX 79408
(806) 767-2593
South Plains AIDS Resource Center
4204 B 50th Street
Lubbock, TX 79493
Texas Tech University-HSC
Lubbock General Hospital/Infectious
Disease
Lubbock, TX 74430
(806) 743-3150

Midland

Permian Basin Community Centers
401 East Illinois Avenue
Midland, TX 79702
(915) 570-3300 *Hotline:* (915) 570-3300

San Antonio

BEAT AIDS
  3923 IH 10 East
  San Antonio, TX 78219
  (210) 333-3709
Black Efforts Against the Threat
  3060 East Commerce Street
  San Antonio, TX 78220
  (512) 271-3877
Community Clinic
  210 West Olmos
  San Antonio, TX 78212
  (210) 821-5522
FFACTS Project
  Brady/Green Community Health Center
  527 North Leona
  San Antonio, TX
  (210) 270-3710
San Antonio AIDS Foundation
  818 East Grayson Street
  San Antonio, TX 78208
San Antonio Metropolitan Health
  827 North Frio
  San Antonio, TX 78207
  (512) 224-2437

Tyler

Tyler-Smith County Health District
  P.O. Box 2039
  Tyler, TX 75702
  (215) 597-7091
East Texas Crisis Center
  3027 South East, Loop 323
  Tyler, TX 75701
  (903) 595-3199 *Hotline:* (214) 595-5591
Tyler AIDS Services
  PO Box 131293
  Tyler, TX 75713
  (903) 592-0757

Waco

Waco-McLennan County Public Health
District
  225 West Waco Drive
  Waco, TX 76707
  (817) 756-AIDS

Wichita Falls

Wichita County Public Health District
  1700 Third Street
  Wichita Falls, TX 76301
  (817) 761-7837

UTAH

Utah Department of Health
  288 North 1460 West
  Salt Lake City, UT 84116
  (801) 538-6191 *Hotline:* (800) 537-1046

Ogden

Weber-Morgan Health Department
  2570 Grant Avenue
  Ogden, UT 84401
  (801) 399-8854

Provo

City-County Health Department
  Utah County
  589 South State Street
  Provo, UT 84604
  (801) 370-8798

Salt Lake City

PWA Coalition of Utah
  1406 South 1100 East
  Salt Lake City, UT 84105
  (801) 484-2205
Utah AIDS Foundation
  1408 South 110 East
  Salt Lake City, UT 84105
  (801) 487-2323 *Hotline:* (800) FON-AIDS

Vernal

Unitah Basin Health Distric
  Unitah County Courthouse
  152 East, 100 North
  Vernal, UT 84078
  (801) 781-0770

VERMONT

Vermont Department of Health
  108 Cherry Street
  Burlington, VT 05402
  (802) 863-7245 *Hotline:* (802) 882-AIDS

Brattleboro

Brattleboro AIDS Project
  67 Main Street
  Brattleboro, VT 05346
  (802) 254-8263 *Hotline:* (802) 254-4444

Burlington

Vermont CARES
  30 Elmwood Avenue
  Burlington, VT
  (802) 863-AIDS

VIRGINIA

VA Health State Department
Bureau STD/HIV
  Main Street Station
  Room 112
  Richmond, VA 23218
  (804) 786-6267

Alexandria

Alexandria Health Department
  517 North St. Asaph Street
  Alexandria, VA 22314
  (703) 838-4389
Northern Virginia AIDS Ministry
  413 Duke Street
  Alexandria, VA 22314
  (703) 739-2437

Arlington

Whitman-Walker Clinic-Northern Virginia
  3426 Washington Boulevard, #102
  Arlington, VA 22201
  (703) 358-9550

Charlottesville

Thomas Jefferson District Health
Department
   11389 Rose Hill Drive
   Charlottesville, VA 22906
   (804) 972-6229
AIDS Support Group
   214 Rugby Road
   Charlottesville, VA 22902
   (804) 979-7714 *Hotline:* (800) 752-6862

Fredericksburg

Fredericksburg Area HIV/AIDS Support
Services
   415 Elm Street
   Fredericksburg, VA 22401
   (703) 371-7532

Kinsale

Three Rivers AIDS Coalition (TRAC)
   369-A Highway 604
   Kinsale, VA 22488
   (804) 472-3075 *Hotline:* (800) 738-8722

Lynchburg

Lynchburg Health Department
   1900 Thomson Drive
   Lynchburg, VA 24505
   (804) 947-6783

Newport News

Peninsula AIDS Foundation
   326 Main Street
   Newport News, VA 23601
   (804) 591-0971 *Hotline:* (800) 533-4148

Norfolk

Norfolk Public Health Department
   401 Colley Avenue
   Norfolk, VA 23507
   (804) 683-2700
Children's AIDS Network Interfaith
Involvement
   222 West 21st Street, Suite F-116
   Norfolk, VA 23517
   (804) 640-0929
The AIDS Fund
   Tidewater AIDS Crisis Task Force
   740 Duke Street, #520
   Norfolk, VA 23510
   (804) 626-0127
Urban League-Hampton Roads
   840 Church Street, Suite I
   Norfolk, VA 23510
   (804) 627-0864

Petersburg

Petersburg Health Department
   301 Halifax Street
   Petersburg, VA 23803
   (804) 861-6582
Crater AIDS Action Program
   32 East Wythe Street
   Petersburg, VA 23803
   (804) 733-5711 *Hotline:* (804) 862-3100

Richmond

Richmond City Health Department
   500 North 10th Street, Room 114
   Richmond, VA 23219
   (804) 780-4211
Central Virgina AIDS Services & Education
   1627 Monument Avenue
   Richmond, VA 23220
   (804) 359-4783
Family and Children's Service
   Family Friends Project
   1518 Willow Lawn Drive
   Richmond, VA 23230
   (804) 282-4255
Fan Free Clinic
   1721 Hanover Avenue
   Richmond, VA 23220
   (804) 358-6343 *Hotline:* (804) 358-AIDS
HEAL
   2800 Third Avenue
   Richmond, VA 2322
   (804) 321-0287
Medical College of Virginia Hospital
   Division of Pediatrics & Emergency
   Box 514
   Richmond, VA 23298
   (804) 786-6493

Roanoke

AIDS Council of Western Virginia
   Council of Community Services
   PO Box 598
   Roanoke, VA 24004
   (703) 985-3131 *Hotline:* 703-985-3131
Roanoke AIDS Project
   PO Box 4367
   Roanoke, VA 24015
   (703) 857-7653 *Hotline:* 703-982-AIDS

WASHINGTON

Department of Health
   HIV/AIDS Prevention
   PO Box 47840
   Olympia, WA 98504
   (206) 586-0426

Bellingham

HIV/AIDS/STD Program
   Whatcom County Health Department
   Bellingham WA 98227
   (206) 676-4593

Everett

Snohomish Health District
   3020 Rucker Avenue, Room 206
   Everett, WA 98271
   (206) 339-5251 *Hotline:* (800) 344-AIDS
Helpers of People with AIDS
   1918 Everett Avenue
   Everett, WA 98201
   (206) 388-0236

Longview

Cowlitz-Wahkiakum Health District
   1516 Hudson Street

Longview, WA 98263
(206) 425-7400 *Hotline:* (206) 577-0272

Olympia

Thurston County Health Department
HIV/AIDS Program
329 West 4th Avenue
Olympia, WA 98501
(206) 786-5277 *Hotline:* (800) 272-AIDS

Seattle

Seattle/King County Health Department
  AIDS Prevention Project
  2124 4th Avenue, 4th Floor
  Seattle, WA 98121
  (206) 296-4999 *Hotline:* (206) 296-4999
El Centro de La Raza
  2524 16th Avenue, South
  Seattle, WA 98144
  (206) 329-7960
Health Information Network
  PO Box 30762
  Seattle, WA 98103
  (206) 784-5655
Northwest AIDS Foundation
  127 Broadway, East
  Seattle, WA 98102
  (206) 329-6963 *Hotline:* (206) 329-6963
People of Color Against AIDS Network
  1200 South Jackson, Suite 25
  Seattle, WA 98144
  (206) 322-7061
Seattle AIDS Support Group
  303 17th Avenue, East
  Seattle, WA 98112
  (206) 322-2437 *Hotline:* (206) 322-2437
Seattle Treatment Education Project
  127 Broadway East, #200
  Seattle, WA 98102
  (206) 329-4857 *Hotline:* (800) 869-7837
Shanti-Seattle
  PO Box 20698
  Seattle, WA 98102
  (206) 322-0279 *Hotline:* (206) 329-6963

Tacoma

Tacoma-Pierce County Health Department
  3629 South D Street
  Tacoma, WA 98408
  (206) 591-6060 *Hotline:* (206) 591-6060
Pierce County AIDS Foundation
  625 Commerce Street, Suite 370
  Tacoma, WA 98406
  (206) 383-2565
Tacoma Urban League
  2550 South Yakima Avenue
  Tacoma, WA 98405
  (206) 383-2006

Yakima

Yakima Health District
  104 North First Street
  Yakima, WA 98902
  (505) 575-7959 *Hotline:* (800) 535-2771
New Hope Clinic

PO Box 2546
Yakima, WA 98907
(509) 453-7144

WEST VIRGINIA

West Virginia Department of Health
  1800 Washington Street East, Room 206
  Charleston, WV 25305
  (304) 348-2971

Charleston

Kanawha Charleston Health Department
  108 Lee Street East
  Charleston, WV 25301
  (304) 348-0700
Charleston AIDS Network
  Box 1024
  Charleston, WV 25324
  (304) 345-4673

Clarksburg

Clarksburg-Harrison Health Department
  Courthouse/Correctional Center
  306B Washington Avenue
  Clarksburg, WV 26301
  (304) 624-8570

Morgantown

Monongalia County Health Department
  453 Van Voorhis Road
  Morgantown, WV 26505
  (304) 598-5100
Mountain State AIDS Network
  235 High Street, #306
  Morgantown, WV 26505
  (304) 292-9000 *Hotline:* (800) 585-444

Parkersburg

Mid-Ohio Valley AIDS Task Force
  PO Box 1274
  Parkersburg, WV 26102
  Hotline: (800) 642-8244

Wheeling

Wheeling-Ohio County Health Department
  1500 Chapline Street, Room 106
  Wheeling, WV 26003
  (304) 234-3720
AIDS Task Force—Upper Ohio Valley
  PO Box 6360
  Wheeling, WV 26003
  (304) 232-6822 *Hotline:* (304) 234-8161

WISCONSIN

Wisconsin Division of Health
  AIDS/HIV Program, Room 96
  1414 East Washington Avenue
  Madison, WI 53711
  (608) 267-1808 *Hotline:* (800) 334-2437

Green Bay

Center Project
  824 South Broadway Street
  Green Bay, WI 54304
  (414) 437-7400 *Hotline:* (800) 675-9400

Hurley

Iron County Public Health
Courthouse, 300 Taconite
Hurley, WI 54534
(715) 561-2191

Kenosha

South East Wisconsin AIDS Project
6927 39th Avenue
Kenosha, WI 53141
(414) 657-6644 *Hotline:* (800) 924-6601

Madison

Madison Department of Public Health
210 MLK Jr Boulevard, Room 507
City County Building
Madison WI 53710
(608) 266-4821 *Hotline:* (608) 246-4858
Madison AIDS Support Network
303 Lathrop Street
Madison, WI 53705
(603) 238-6276 *Hotline:* (800) 486-6276

Milwaukee

Milwaukee Health Department
841 North Broadway, Room 228
Milwaukee, WI 53202
(414) 278-3521
AIDS Resource Center of Wisconsin
PO Box 92505
Milwaukee, WI 53202
(414) 273-1991 *Hotline:* (414) 273-2437
Milwaukee Indian Health Board
930 North 27th Street
Milwaukee, WI 53208
(414) 931-8111
The Wisconsin AIDS Line
PO Box 92505
Milwaukee, WI 53202
(414) 273-2437

Stevens Point

Portage County Human Services
817 Whiting Avenue
Stevens Point, WI 54481
(715) 345-5350 *Hotline:* (715) 344-2140

Wausau

Central Wisconsin AIDS Network
1200 Lakeview Drive, #200
Wausau, WI 54403
(715) 848-9060

WYOMING

Division of Health and Medical Services
Wyoming Department of Health and Social
Services
Hathaway Building, 4th Floor
Cheyenne, WY 82002
(307) 777-7121

Casper

Casper Natron County Health Department
1200 East Third Street, Room 280
Casper, WY 82601
(307) 235-9280

Wyoming AIDS Project
Box 9353
Casper, WY 82609
(307) 237-7833 24 hours
Hotline: (800) 675-2698

UNITED STATES TERRITORIES

American Samoa

Department of Health
Government of American Samoa
LBJ Tropical Medical Center
Pago Pago, American Samoa 96799
(011) 684-663-4590 (overseas)

Guam

Department of Public Health and Social
Services
Government of Guam
PO Box 2816
Agana, Guam 96910
(0110-671) 734-2944 (overseas)

Mariana Islands

Department of Health Services
Commonwealth of the Northern Mariana
Islands
Office of the Governor
Saipan, Mariana Islands 96950
(011-670) 6111, 6112 (overseas)

Trust Territory of the Pacific Islands

Bureau of Health Services
Office of the High Commissioner
Trust Territory of the Pacific Islands
Saipan, Mariana Islands 96950
Cable Address: HICOTT Saipan
011-670-9854 (overseas)

Puerto Rico

Puerto Rico Department of Health
Edificio A Hospital de Psiquiatria
Rio Piedras, Puerto Rico 02908
(401) 277-2231
Commonwealth of Puerto Rico
STD-HIV Prevention Program
PO Box 71423
(809) 754-8118
Hotline: (809) 765-1010

San Juan

San Juan Health Department
AIDS Task Force
PO Box 367156
San Juan, PR 00936
(809) 751-6075
Hotline: (809) 751-5858
Fundacion AIDS de Puerto Rico
Box 36-4842
San Juan, PR 00936
(809) 782-9600
Iniciativa Communitaria de Investigacion
Old San Juan Station
PO Box 774

San Juan, PR 00917
(809) 250-8629

Virgin Islands
Commissioner of Health
Virgin Islands Department of Health
PO Box 7309
St. Thomas, U.S. Virgin Islands 00801
(809) 774-6097

SELECTED NEWSLETTERS AND PUBLISHED RESOURCES

The following are just a sample of AIDS resource publications available and do not represent an endorsement.

AIDS/HIV Clinical Trial Handbook for patients (English and Spanish)
AmFAR
  733 Third Avenue, 12th Floor
  New York, NY 10017-3204
  (800) 39-AmFAR
AIDS Clinical Care
  Massachusetts Medical Society
  1440 Main Street
  Waltham, Mass. 02154-1649
  (800) 843-6356
AIDS Medicine in Development
Pharmaceutical Manufacturers
Association, Communications Division
  1100 15th Street North West,
  Washington, DC 20005
  (202) 835-3400
AIDS Treatment Data Network
  The Experimental Treatment Guide
  259 West 30th Street, 9th Floor
  New York, NY 10001
  (212) 268-4196
  (212) 643-0820 (Spanish)
  (212) 4199 (FAX)
AIDS Treatment News
  ATN, PO Box 411256
  San Francisco, CA 94141
  (800) 873-2812
  (415) 255-0588
Association for the Care of Children's
Health Needs (ACCH)
  7910 Woodmont Avenue, Suite 300
  Bethesda, MD 20814
  (301) 654-6549
BETA (Bulletin of Experimental
Treatments for AIDS)
  San Francisco AIDS Foundation
  PO Box 2189
  Berkeley, CA 94702
  (510) 549-4300
  (800) 959-1059
Body Positive
  2095 Broadway, Suite 306
  New York, NY 10023
  (212) 721-1346
Clinical Trials: Talking It Over

National Institute of Allergy and
Infectious Disease (NIAID)
Office of Communications
National Institutes of Health, Building 31,
Room 7A32
Bethesda, MD 20892
FAACTS (Facts on Alternate AIDS
Compounds and Treatments)
  111 Gates Street
  San Francisco, CA 94110
  (415) 648-1357
FOCUS Newsletter
  UC San Francisco AIDS Health Project
  Box 0884
  San Francisco, CA 94143-0084
  (415) 476-6430
Just Kids Newsletter
  (for HIV-infected kids, teens, and their
  parents)
  c/o 3 Corners, Inc.
  PO Box 42
  Village Station, New York, NY 10014
Medical Alert, The Active Voice
  NAPWA-Link (National Association of
  People with AIDS)
  1413 K Street, North West
  Washington, DC, 2005
  (703) 998-3144
NIAID AIDS Agenda and Dateline: NIAID
NIAID
  NIH, Building 31 7A.50
  Bethesda, MD 20892
Notes from the Underground
  People with AIDS Health Group
  150 West 26th Street, Suite 201
  New York, NY 10001
  (212) 255-0520
PAAC NOTES
  Physicians Association for AIDS Care
  101 West Grand Avenue, Suite 200
  Chicago, IL 60610
  (312) 222-1326
PLUS Voice: The Magazine About Life and
HIV
  PLUS Magazine, Inc.
  945 West George Street
  Chicago, IL 60657-9974
  (312) 929-9761
Positive Directions News
  140 Clarendon Street, Suite 805
  Boston, MA 02115
  (617) 262-3456
Positive Social Support Newsletter
  Lambda Center
  PO Box 163654
  Sacramento, CA 95816
  (916) 442-0185
P.I. Perspectives
  Project Inform, San Francisco
  1965 Market Street, Suite 220
  San Francisco, CA 94103
  (800) 822-7422, outside California
  (800) 344-7422, inside California
Someone at School Has AIDS: A Guide to
Developing Policies for Students and School

Staff Members Who Are Infected with HIV
National Association of State Boards of
Education (NASBE), Publications
Department
   1012 Cameron Street
   Alexandria, VA 22314
   (703) 684-4000
Treatment and Data Digest
   ALT-UP/NY
   135 West 29th Street, 10th Floor
   New York, NY 10001
Treatment Issues
Gay Men's Health Crisis (GMHC)
   Department Medical Information
   129 West 20th Street
   New York, NY 10011
   (212) 337-1950
Up Front Drug Information
   Street Pharmacologists Update
   5701 Biscayne Boulevard, Suite 9PH
   Miami, FL 33137
   (305) 757-2566
World newsletter (for HIV-positive
women)—English or Spanish
   PO Box 11535
   Oakland, CA 94611
   (415) 658-6930

AIDS RESOURCE DIRECTORIES

The AIDS/HIV Treatment Directory
   AmFAR
   733 Third Avenue, 12th Floor
   New York, NY 10017-3204
   1 (800) 39-AmFAR
Local AIDS Services: The National
Directory
   US Conference of Mayors AIDS Programs
   1620 Eye Street, New York, 4th Floor
   Washington, DC 20006
   (202) 293-7330
Women and AIDS: Living with HIV/AIDS
   Nat'l Women's Health Network
   514 10th Street, North West
   Washington, DC 20004
   (202) 347-1140
North American Syringe Exchange
Network
   Point Defrance AIDS Project
   535 Dock Street, Suite 112
   Tacoma, WA 98402
   (206) 272-4857
Alabama Directory of AIDS Education and
Service Programs
   Department of Pathology
   University of South Alabama
   2451 Fillingim Street
   Mobile, AL 26617
   (205) 471-7322
Alaska AIDS Resource Directory
   Alaska AIDS Assistance Association
   3601 "C" Street
   Anchorage, AK 99524
   (907) 276-1400
Arizona HIV/AIDS Resource Matrik
   Office of Health Promotion & Education

Department of Public Health
   1825 East Roosevelt Street
   Phoenix, AZ 85006
AIDS Information and Sources in Arkansas
   Arkansas Medical Society
   PO Box 5776
   Little Rock, AR 77205-5776
   (501) 224-6489
Arkansas AIDS/STD Resource Guide
   Arkansas Department of Health
   AIDS/STD Program
   4815 West Markham
   Little Rock, AR 77205-3867
   (501) 661-2408
California Directory of Agencies
Conducting AIDS Education & Prevention
Projects
   California AIDS Clearinghouse
   PO Box 1830
   Santa Cruz, CA 95061-1830
   (408) 438-4822
Directory of HIV Clinical Research in the
Bay Area
   San Francisco Community Consortium
   3180 18th Street, Suite 201
   San Francisco, CA 94110
   (415) 476-9554
Southern California Treatment Directory
   COMBAT
   1800 North Highland, Suite 610
   Los Angeles, CA 90028
   (213) 469-5888
Colorado HIV/AIDS Resource Directory
   Colorado Department of Health
   DCEED-STD-A3
   4300 Cherry Creek Drive South
   Denver, CO 80222-1530
   (303) 331-8320
The Metro Washington Directory of HIV
Related Services
   Metropolitan Washington Council of
   Governments
   1875 "I" Street, North West, Suite 200
   Washington, DC 20006-5454
   (202) 223-6800
Directory of HIV/AIDS Organizations in
Hawaii
   Hawaii State Department of Health
   STD/AIDS Prevention Branch
   3627 Kilauea Avenue, Suite 304
   Honolulu, HI 96816
   (808) 735-5303
Illinois AIDS Resource Directory
   Illinois Department of Public Health
   100 West Randolph #6-600
   Chicago, IL 60601
   (312) 917-4846
Iowa AIDS Resource Manual
   Iowa Department of Public Health
   Lucas Building, 3rd Floor
   Des Moines, IA 50319
   (515) 242-5899
Kansas AIDS Referral List
   Kansas Department of Health &
   Environment

Bureau of Disease Control
Mills Building #605
109 South West 9th
Topeka, KS 66612-1271
(913) 296-0022

HIV/AIDS Service Programs in Louisiana
Louisiana State Health Department
325 Loyola Avenue, Room 615
New Orleans, LA 70012-5508

Louisiana HIV/AIDS Service Directory
Louisiana State University, AETC
1542 Tulane Avenue
New Orleans, LA 70112
(504) 568-3855

List of Resources in the State of Maine
Maine HIV Prevention Program
Department of Human Services
State House Station 11
Augusta, ME 04333
(207) 287-3747

AIDS Resources in Maryland
Maryland Department of Health &
Mental Hygiene
201 West Preston Street
Baltimore, MD 21201-2399
(301) 225-1255

AIDS Resource Directory of Michigan
United Community Services of
Metropolitan Detroit
1212 Griswold
Detroit, MI 48226-1899

Michigan AIDS Resource Guide
Michigan Department of Public Health
AIDS Prevention
3423 North Logan & MLK Jr Boulevard
Lansing, MI 48909
(517) 335-8371

Minnesota AIDS Related Resources for
Referral
Minnesota AIDS Project
2025 Micollat Avenue, #2000
Minneapolis, MN 55204
(612) 870-7773

Montana AIDS Resource Directory
Montana Department of Health &
Environment
AIDS/STD Program
Cogswell Building
Helena, MT 29360
(406) 444-4740

Nevada HIV/AIDS Resource Directory
Nevada State Health Division
HIV/AIDS Program
Capitol Complex
505 East King Street, Room 304
Carson Ctiy, NV 89701
(702) 885-4800

New Jersey AIDS Resource Guide
New Jersey Department of Health, Office
of Asst. Commissioner
Division of AIDS Prevention and Control
CN 363 50 East State Street
Capitol Center Trenton, NJ 08625-0363
(609) 984-5874

New Hampshire AIDS Resource Guide

New Hampshire Division of Public
Health Services, Bureau of Disease
Control
HIV/AIDS Program
Concord, NH 03301
(603) 271-4469

NY AIDS Service Directory
New York Department of Social Services,
Materials Resource Center
40 North Pearl Street
Albany, NY 12243
(518) 473-8320

North Carolina AIDS Resource Directory
North Carolina Health Department
Box 2091
Raleigh, NC 27602
(919) 733-7301

Directory of Philadelphia Area AIDS/HIV
Clinical Trials
Philadelphia Fight
201 North Broad Street, 6th Floor
Philadelphia, PA 19107
(215) 557-8265

Texas HIV/AIDS Community Resource
Directory
Texas Department of Health
Public Health Promotion Divison
1100 West 49th
Austin, TX 78756-3199
(512) 252-8012

AIDS Resources in Utah
Utah Health Department
Box 16660
Sal Lake City, UT 84116-0660
(801) 538-6191

AIDS Resources in West Virginia
West Virginia Department of Health and
Human Services
151 11th Avenue
South Charleston, WV 25303
(304) 348-2950

Wisconsin AIDS Update
Wisconsin AIDS/HIV Program
Department of Health
PO Box 309
Madison, WI 53701

Wyoming AIDS Resource Manual
Wyoming AIDS Prevention Program
Hathaway Building #475
Cheyenne, WY 82002
(307) 777-5800

ADDITIONAL PATIENT RESOURCES

PATIENT ASSISTANCE/DRUG REIMBURSEMENT PROGRAMS

Call the Department of Health in your
state or county for more information on
AIDS drug reimbursement programs and
eligibility criteria. Other direct sources of
information are listed below:

US Health Resources and Services Agency
AIDS Drug Reimbursement Program
(301) 443-9086
NY State AIDS Drug Assistance Program
(ADAP) (800) 542-2437

State Drug Assistance Program

Alabama (205) 613-5364
Arkansas (501) 661-2315
Arizona (602) 230-5819
California (916) 324-8429
Colorado (303) 866-2445
Connecticut (203) 566-2550
District of Columbia (202) 724-5206
Delaware (302) 995-8422
Florida (904) 487-2478
Georgia (404) 894-5307
Hawaii (808) 732-0315
Iowa (515) 281-4938
Idaho (208) 334-6526
Indiana (317) 633-8476
Kansas (913) 633-8476
Kentucky (502) 564-6539
Louisiana (504) 568-5508
Massachusetts (617) 566-8358
Maine (207) 289-5060
Maryland (410) 366-1717
Michigan (517) 335-8468
Minnesota (612) 297-3344
Missouri (314) 751-6438
Mississippi (601) 960-7723
Montana (406) 444-3565
Nebraska (402) 559-4637
New Hampshire (603) 271-4576
New Jersey (609) 588-7038
New Mexico (505) 827-8426
New York (518) 473-2873
Nevada (702) 687-4804
North Carolina (919) 733-3091
North Dakota (701) 224-2378
Ohio (614) 466-4693
Oklahoma (405) 271-4636
Oregon (503) 731-4000
Pennsylvania (717) 782-6057
Rhode Island (401) 464-2183
South Carolina (803) 737-4040
South Dakota (605) 773-3364
Tennessee (615) 741-7500
Texas (512) 458-7357
Utah (801) 538-6496
Virginia (804) 225-4844
Virgin Islands (809) 776-8311
Vermont (802) 241-2880

Washington (206) 586-4979
Wisconsin (608) 267-3583
West Virginia (304) 348-8990
Wyoming (307) 777-5800

Pharmaceutical Patient Assistance Programs

Abbott Laboratories (800) 688-9118
(Physician calls only)
Amgen, Inc. (800) 272-9376
Astra Pharmaceutical Products, Inc.
(800) 488-3247
Bristol Myers Squibb (800) 788-0123
Burroughs Wellcome (800) 722-9294
Ciba Pharmaceuticals (800) 257-3272
Fujisawa Pharmaceuticals (800) 366-6323
Hoechst Roussel Pharmaceuticals
(800) 422-4779
Hoffman-La Roche, Inc. (800) 443-6676
Immunnex Corp. (800) 334-6273 (Physician
calls only)
Janssen Pharmaceutica (800) 544-2987
Lederle Laboratories (800) 533-2273
Miles Pharmaceuticals (800) 998-9180
Ortho Biotech (800) 447-3437/(800) 411-
1366
Pfizer (800) 869-9979/800-254-4445
Sandoz Pharmaceuticals Corp (800) 447-
6673
Schering-Plough Corp (800) 521-7157
Smith Kline Beecham (800) 546-0420
Syntex Corporation (800) 444-4200
(Physician calls only)
Upjohn Co. (800) 253-8600/36004
Vestar, Inc. (800) 247-3303
US Bioscience (808) 8-USBIOS

BUYERS' CLUBS

AIDS Manasota. Sarosota, FL
(813) 954-6011
Atlanta Buyers' Club, Atlanta, GA
(404) 874-4845
Carl Vogel Foundation, Washington, DC
(202) 232-4898
DC Buyers' Club, Washington, DC
(202) 232-5954
Denver Buyers' Club, Denver, CO
(303) 837-8214
Healing Alternatives, San Francisco, CA
(415) 626-4053
PWA Health Group, New York, NY
(212) 255-0520
PWA Health Link, Ft. Lauderdale, FL
(800) 456-4792

GLOSSARY

Abstinence—Refraining from participating in something, e.g., not engaging in sexual intercourse or drug activities.

Acid-Fast Bacillus (AFB)—Any bacillus that is resistant to decolorization with acidified organic solvents after staining with a dye. Used in a test to identify *Mycobacterium tuberculosis* and other mycobacteria.

Advocacy—Action taken on behalf of individuals by themselves, their families, health care providers, or others to ensure appropriate access to, and availability of, health care services.

Aerosolized Pentamidine—A drug used for *Pneumocystis carinii* pneumonia (PCP) prophylaxis that is dispersed through a nebulizer in a mist. It is inhaled and goes directly to the lungs.

AFB Isolation—A specific type of hospital isolation for persons with acute *M. tuberculosis* used to prevent the spread of infection during the infectious phase of the disease.

Agency for Health Care Policy and Research (AHCPR)—Agency within the Public Health Service, U.S. Department of Health and Human Services. It sponsors research on the effectiveness and cost-effectiveness of medical care.

AIDS—Acquired Immune Deficiency Syndrome (AIDS) is an infectious, viral disease resulting in suppression of the immune system in otherwise healthy individuals. AIDS is caused by the human immunodeficiency virus (HIV) infection and is characterized by the presence of one or more disease as defined by the Centers for Disease Control (CDC).

HIV (AIDS) Antibody Test—A test to determine if an individual has antibodies to HIV, the virus that causes AIDS. Presence of HIV-specific antibodies indicates that the person has been exposed to HIV.

AIDS Clinical Trials Group (ACTG)—A network of over 50 medical centers nationwide that participate in the evaluation of treatments for HIV-related infections. Sponsored by the National Institute of Allergy and Infectious Diseases.

Airborne Transmission—Mode of transmission in which an infectious agent passes through the air to infect susceptible individuals by droplet infection (e.g., sneezing, coughing).

Americans with Disabilities Act—(Public Law 101-336) This legislation was passed in July 1990, and established equal opportunity for persons with disabilities regarding employment, public accommodation, transportation, state and local government services, and telecommunications.

Anal Sex—a type of sexual intercourse in which a man's penis enters his partner's anus.

Anergy—Inability to react immunologically to an antigenic stimulus. Usually used to denote lack of response to specific antigens injected into the skin of the forearm.

Antibody—A protein produced by a B-lymphocyte that specifically binds a particular antigen which leads to attack by the immune system. Proteins in the blood or secretory fluids that tags, destroys, or neutralize bacteria, viruses, and other harmful toxins. It is a member of a class of proteins named immunoglobulins, which are produced and secreted by B-lymphocytes in response to stimulation by antigens.

Antigen—A foreign molecule or substance which raises a specific immune response (against these substances).

Antiretroviral Drug—A drug that reduces the replication rate of HIV. Used to treat HIV-infected persons, the most common are zidovudine, didanosine, and zalcitabine.

Anti-viral—A compound or process which destroys a virus or supresses its replication.

Aphthous Ulcers—Single or multiple recurrent, well-circumscribed painful ulcers that develop on nonkeratinized oral mucosa.

Asymptomatic HIV Infection—An early stage of HIV infection, when no physical symptoms are present.

Atypical Cells of Undetermined Significance (ACUS)—Abnormal cells with certain characteristics that are revealed on Pap smear.

Attenuated Virus—A weakened virus that has a reduced ability to infect or produce disease.

Autologous—Refers to the same organism or one of its parts; originates from within the organism itself.

Azidothymidine (AZT)—Also called Retrovir or Zidovudine. An antiviral that is effective in treating HIV infection and AIDS. It works by preferentially inhibiting the action of reverse transcriptase during HIV replication.

3′azido-2′, 3′dideoxythymidine (see azidothymidine).

Bacille Calmette-Guerin (BCG)—A vaccine containing a bovine-derived, live, attenuated strain of mycobacterium that has been used in countries other than the United States as immunization against tuberculosis.

Beta-2-microglobulin (β2M)—A protein that is tightly bound to the surface of all cells with a nucleus. β2M is released into the blood when a cell dies. Elevated β2M levels occur in a variety of diseases and cancers. Although β2M is nonspecific for HIV infection, elevated β2M levels are correlated with progression of HIV disease.

Body Fluids—The various liquids found in the human body. Only blood, semen, vaginal secretions, and breast milk have been found to contain concentrations of HIV that are high enough to infect another person. Saliva, sweat, tears, and urine have not been shown to transmit HIV.

Candidiasis—An infection with a fungus of the *Candida* family, generally *C. albicans,* that most commonly involves the skin (dermatocandidiasis), oral mucosa (thrush), respiratory tract (bronchocandidiasis), and vagina (vaginitis). Candidiasis of the esophagus, trachea, bronchi, or lungs is an indicator disease for AIDS.

Carcinoma In Situ—An early, curable stage of cancer in which the tumor has not spread beyond a defined superficial site.

Case Management—The coordination of a patient's health care and social services by one or more individuals familiar with both the patient's needs and community resources.

Casual Contact—Refers to nonintimate behaviors such as working, eating, playing, studying, hugging, or holding hands. Casual contact does not transmit HIV.

CD4 Cell Count (T4 Count)—The number of CD4 (T4 helper) cells in a cubic millimeter of blood, it is a surrogate marker of immunodeficiency. As the CD4 cells decline, the risk of developing opportunistic infections increases. The trend of several consecutive CD4 counts is more important than any one measurement.

CD4 Percentage—The number of CD4 cells in relation to the total number of lymphocytes. As HIV infection progresses, the percentage of CD4 cells decreases.

Cellular Immunity—The part of the immune system that relies primarily upon specific defense cells.

Centers for Disease Control and Prevention (CDC)—Federal agency that is responsible for monitoring the AIDS/HIV epidemic and carrying out efforts to prevent HIV infection.

Central Nervous System (CNS)—The brain, spinal cord, and its coverings (meninges).

Cervical Dysplasia—An abnormality in the size, shape, or organization of the cells lining the cervix that can be detected on a Pap smear. Prompts further examination.

Cervical Intraepithelial Lesion (CIN)—A condition revealed by Pap smear which necessitates further evaluation.

Clinical Trials—Scientifically governed investigations of medications in volunteer subjects. Their purpose is to seek information regarding the products' safety (Phase I) and efficacy (Phase II/III).

Cohort Studies—A form of analytical epidemiology in which a group of individuals who share a particular risk factor for a disease are studied.

Colposcopy—A procedure examining the surface of the uterine cervix through a flexible fiberoptic tube.

Community Based—Describes services delivered at a local level.

Compassionate Use—A way of providing experimental drugs to sick persons who have no other treatment options. "Compassionate use" of a drug must be approved by the FDA, often on a case-by-case basis.

Condom—A sheath that fits over a man's penis or into a woman's vagina to prevent semen from entering the partner's body after ejaculation. Condoms also prevent a man's penis from coming in contact with his partner's body fluids. The correct use of a latex condom during every act of intercourse can greatly reduce the risk of HIV infection. Also called rubbers.

Confidentiality—The right inherent in the contract between the health care provider and patient that ensures that information on the patient's medical conditions will be released to a third party only after explicit permission is obtained from the patient or guardian.

Cotton-wool Spots/Patches—White deposits on the retina that represent small areas that have lost their blood supply due to blockage of local vessels.

Cross-sectional/Prevalence Studies—Monitoring of a population for occurrence of diseases, noting the time and kind of diseases. A form of descriptive epidemiology.

Cunnilingus—Oral female genital contact.

Cytomegalovirus (CMV)—A member of the herpes virus family that can cause fever, fatigue, enlarged lymph glands, aching, and mild sore throat. CMV infections can produce hepatitis, pneumonia, retinitis, and colitis in persons living with AIDS. CMV infection may lead to blindness, chronic diarrhea, or death.

Cytopenia—A reduction in the number of cells found in a clinical specimen.

Dapsone—A drug used for PCP prophylaxis. In persons who have the hereditary condition glucose-6-phosphate dehydrogenase (G6PD) deficiency, dapsone can cause destruction of red blood cells (hemolysis).

Dementia—Loss of mental function due to damaged brain cells and brain inflammation in AIDS-afflicted patients.

Descriptive Epidemiology—Epidemiological studies that describe the occurrence of disease by person, place and time.

Developmentally Oriented—Care that is based on the individual's functional level and chronologic age. Functional level includes physical, cognitive, psychosocial, and communicative development.

Didanosine (ddI; Trade Name, Videx; Also Called Dideoxyinosine)—One of the nucleoside analog drugs currently approved by the Food and Drug Administration that inhibits the reverse transcriptase enzyme of HIV. Its major toxicities are pancreatitis and peripheral neuropathy.

Dideoxycytidine (ddC)—2′,3′-dideoxycytine; see zalcitabine.

Dideoxyinosine (ddI)—2′,3′-dideoxyinosine; see didanosine.

Direct Fluorescent Antibody Staining for *Treponema pallidum* (DFA-TP)—A specific test (direct fluorescent antibody staining on a biopsy sample) for *T. pallidum,* the organism that causes syphilis. The presence of *T. pallidum* organisms in lesions of early acquired or congenital syphilis in this test definitively makes a diagnosis of syphilis.

Directly Observed Therapy (DOT)—A process in which a patient takes a medication while under direct observation by another individual. Usually used in antituberculous treatment.

Dyspnea—Difficult or labored breathing.

Early HIV Infection—No major physical health symptoms are yet present at this stage of infection, though psychological symptoms may be present.

EIA—See ELISA.

Empiric Therapy—Treatment based on the clinician's judgement and the patient's symptoms and signs and offered before a diagnosis has been confirmed.

Encephalopathy—Injury or damage to the brain.

Endemic Pattern—Patterns of continuous infection that allow epidemic diseases to remain present in populations.

Enzyme-linked Immunosorbent Assay (ELISA)—The most common assay for HIV antibodies. Used for screening donated blood, it is usually the first clinical screening test used to detect HIV infection. A positive ELISA or EIA test result should be confirmed with a Western blot or an immunofluorescent assay test in order to conclusively diagnose HIV infection.

Epidemic—An outbreak of contagious disease, such as HIV infection, that spreads rapidly within a population.

Epidemiology—The study of patterns of disease occurrence in populations and the factors affecting them.

Expanded Access—Refers to the concept of making experimental drugs more widely available to patients with life-threatening diseases prior to marketing approval. Mechanisms include parallel track, Treatment IND, and compassionate use. Information available through the FDA.

False-negative—A negative test result for a person who is actually infected.

Family Centered—Care that recognizes and respects the pivotal role of the family in the lives of children and other members.

False-positive—A positive test result for a person who is actually not infected

Fellatio—Oral—male genital contact.

Fisting—Penetration of the anus with the hand.

Floaters—"Spots before the eyes"; semitransparent bodies perceived to be floating in the field of vision that move rapidly with eye movement but drift slightly when the eyes are still.

Fluorescent Treponemal Antibody Absorption Test (FTA-ABS)—A treponemal test to detect antibodies against *Treponema pallidum.*

Food and Drug Administration (FDA)—Federal agency responsible for approving new pharmaceutical products and medical devices and for monitoring drug performance following approval.

Funduscopy—Visual examination of the retina with an ophthalmoscope.

Glucose-6-phosphate Dehydrogenase (G6PD) Deficiency—An inherited enzyme deficiency that can lead to hemolysis of red blood cells (RBCs) when an affected individual is exposed to drugs with oxidant properties.

Hairy Leukoplakia—A white lesion seen in the oral cavity of HIV-infected individuals, most commonly on the lateral margins of the tongue. It may be flat or raised with vertical corrugations and is not removable.

Helper T-lymphocytes—T-Lymphocytes that "help" T-killer and B-lymphocytes respond to antigens. Destruction of the helper lymphocytes is the major problem in AIDS.

Hemoptysis—The coughing up of blood from the lungs; may be a symptom of tuberculosis.

HIV (Human Immunodeficiency Virus)—The virus that causes AIDS; Previously called HTLV-III, LAV and ARV. HIV is classified as a lentivirus in a subgroup of the retroviruses. It infects and destroys a class of lymphocytes, CD4 cells, which cause progressive damage to the immune system. This family of retroviruses has RNA as its genetic material and makes an enzyme, reverse transcriptase, that converts viral RNA into viral DNA. The viral DNA then is incorporated into the host cell's DNA and is replicated along with it. The predominant form of HIV in North America, Europe and Central Africa is called HIV-1. A closely related retrovirus found in Western Africa is called HIV-2.

HIV Antibody (HIV-Ab)—The antibody to HIV, which usually appears within six weeks after infection. Antibody testing early in the infection process may not produce accurate results, since some recently infected people have not yet begun producing antibodies and test negative even though they are infected. Therefore, a single negative antibody test result is not a guarantee that a person is free from infection.

HIV Counseling—Information provided to an individual before and after HIV testing (pre- and posttest counseling) regarding the implications and impact of testing, HIV infection care, and prevention of HIV transmission.

HIV-infected—Infected with the human immunodeficiency virus, with or without evidence of illness.

HIV-negative—Not infected with HIV, as determined by a negative test for antibody to HIV or for the presence of the virus.

HIV-positive—Infected with HIV, as determined by a positive test for antibody to HIV or for the presence of the virus.

HIV-positive Test—A blood sample is determined to be positive for HIV, if the blood is reactive on an initial ELISA test, repeatedly reactive on a second ELISA run on the same specimen, and confirmed positive on Western blot or other supplemental test.

Hospice—A health facility in which medical and mental health care are provided to a terminally ill patient. The hospice philosophy emphasizes alleviating the patient's discomfort and supporting the family in the grieving process.

Human Papilloma Virus (HPV)—The virus that causes genital warts. Certain types of HPV (types 16 and 18) are associated with cervical cancer.

Humoral Immunity—Branch of immune system which primarily relies on antibodies.

Immune System—The circulating cells and plasma fluids in the blood that provide continuous protection from foreign infectious agents, activate wound repair, and eliminate toxins and waste products. The mechanism of the body that recognizes foreign agents or substances, neutralizes them, and recalls the response later when confronted with the same challenge.

Immunity—Natural or acquired resistance to a specific disease. Immunity may be partial or complete, long lasting or temporary.

Immunization—Administration of antigenic components of an infectious agent to stimulate a protective immune response.

Immunocompromised—Describes the condition that exists when the body's immune system defenses are lowered and the ability to resist infections and tumors weakens.

Immunodeficiency—A breakdown or an inability of certain parts of the immune system to function that renders a person susceptible to certain diseases that he or she ordinarily would not develop.

Immunofluorescence Antibody (IFA)—A serologic assay using antibody tagged by a fluorescent molecule. There is an HIV-specific IFA assay available to confirm the results of a positive HIV ELISA test.

Immunoglobulin (Ig)—Protein produced by plasma cells derived from B-lymphocytes and found in the blood and other body tissues. Increased levels of two types of immunoglobulins, IgA and IgG, are usually seen in patients with HIV infection are related to the HIV-induced activation of B-lymphocytes. Immunoglobulin A is found in high concentrations in mucous membranes and in secretions such as saliva. It does not cross the placenta. Immunoglobulin G is found in the serum and does cross the placenta.

Incidence—The proportion of a population that develops new cases of a disease during a particular time period.

Incubation Period—Asymptomatic HIV incubation in otherwise healthy individuals during which time the disease may be unwittingly transmitted. The interval between initial infection and appearance of the first symptom or sign of disease.

Informed Consent—Process by which individuals considering participation in an investigational drug trial are informed by an investigator in simple terms of the risks and benefits of the proposed treatment and voluntarily agree to participate in the trial. The consent form is a written document that attests to the fact that the person signing understands the purposes and risks of the study. Also refers to the process in which an individual voluntarily consents to diagnostic testing and release of information (disclosure) after appropriate counseling.

Investigational New Drug (IND)—See Treatment IND.

In Vitro—Testing and experiments conducted in a laboratory setting.

In Vivo—Testing and experiments conducted in animals or humans.

Isoniazid (INH)—An antibiotic that has activity against *M. tuberculosis*, the micro-organism that causes tuberculosis.

Kaposi's Sarcoma—A normally rare cancer that develops frequently in AIDS-afflicted patients. A painless tumor of the wall of blood vessels or the lymphatic system that usually appears on the skin as pink-to-purple spots. It may also occur internally, independent of skin lesions.

Killer or Cytotoxic T-lymphocytes—T-lymphocytes that kill target cells that they bind to.

Latency—A state of virus infection when the virus genetic material remains hidden in the cell but no virus is produced. The latent virus may become reactivated at a later time.

Lentiviruses—A subclass of retroviruses to which HIV belongs. There are lentiviruses that infect other species, including old world monkeys, sheep and cats.

Lumbar Puncture (LP)—Insertion of a needle into the spinal canal to obtain a sample of cerebrospinal fluid.

Lymphadenopathy Syndrome (LAS)—Persistently enlarged lymph nodes or "swollen glands," sometimes an early sign of HIV infection that is progressing. Also called PGL (persistent generalized lymphadenopathy).

Lymphocytes—Cells of the immune system that respond specifically to foreign substances, secreting specific antibodies. There are several kinds of lymphocytes—B-lymphocytes and T-lymphocytes. During infection, B-lymphocytes are transformed into plasma cells that produce antibodies specific to the pathogen. This transformation occurs through interactions with various types of T-cells and other components of the immune system. T-lymphocytes are derived from the thymus and participate in a variety of cell-mediated immune reactions. Three fundamentally different types of T-cells are recognized: helper, killer, and suppressor.

Lymphoma—Cancer of the lymph tissue.

Lytic Infection—Viral infection of a cell that results in death of the cell.

Macrophages—Mononuclear phagocytes derived from monocytes that occur in the blood vessel walls and in connective tissue.

Mandatory Reporting—System under which a physician is required by law to inform health authorities when a specified illness is diagnosed.

Microhemagglutination Assay for *T. pallidum* (MATP)—A treponemal test for syphilis.

Multidrug-resistant tuberculosis (MDR-TB)—Tuberculosis caused by a strain of the organism *Mycobacterium tuberculosis* that is resistant to more than one of the major antituberculous drugs.

***Mycobacterium Avium-Intracellular* Complex (MAC)**—An acid-fast microorganism that causes lung and other organ system infections in individuals whose immune systems are severely damaged.

Mycobacterium Tuberculosis—The micro-organism that causes tuberculosis.

Myopathy—Inflammation of muscle tissue due to infection or adverse reaction to a medication.

Neopterin—A molecule produced by macrophages in response to gamma interferon and found in serum, urine, and cerebrospinal fluid. Elevated neopterin levels have been reported in individuals in all phases of HIV disease. According to some studies, high neopterin levels have been associated with a poor prognosis; low levels have correlated with a better prognosis.

Neurodevelopmental Delays—Changes in the level of functioning of the central nervous system that lead to the loss of skills that a child has developed or would have developed over time.

Neuropathy—An abnormal, degenerative, or inflammatory condition of the peripheral nervous system.

Neuropsychological Defects—Alterations in behavior that are related to a central nervous system illness and interfere with an individual's ability to function in an age-appropriate fashion.

Neurosyphilis—A form of advanced syphilis in which the infection has spread to the central nervous system.

Nondirective Counseling—Describes a type of counseling in which the counselor supplies information and helps the client to arrive at a decision that reflects the client's needs and wishes.

Non-lytic Infection—Viral infection of a cell that results in virus production, but survival of the cell. Most retroviruses normally carry out non-lytic infections. HIV infection of macrophages is non-lytic.

Nucleoside Analog—A synthetic compound similar to one of the components of DNA or RNA; a general type of anti-retroviral drug (e.g., acyclovir, zidovudine, lamivudine (3TC), didanosine, zalcitabine).

Opportunistic Infections—Infections by common micro-organisms that usually do not cause problems in healthy individuals, however may cause serious, possibly life-threatening illness when an individual's immune system is compromised.

Oral-genital Sex—See cunnilingus and fellatio. Also called oral sex.

p24 Antigen Test (p24 Antigen Capture Assay)—Laboratory test that measures p24, the protein found in the viral core of HIV. This test can sometimes detect HIV infection before seroconversion. p24 is consistently present in only about 25 percent of HIV-infected persons. Persistent p24 antigenemia has been associated with an increased risk of progression to AIDS in HIV-infected individuals.

Papanicolaou (Pap) Smear—A microscopic examination of the surface cells of the cervix, usually conducted on scrapings from the opening of the cervix. A staining procedure is used to detect various abnormal conditions of the female genital tract.

Parenteral—Intravenous or intramuscular administration of substances such as therapeutic drugs or nutritive solutions.

Partner Notification—The process of informing sexual or needle-sharing partners of an HIV-infected person that they have been or are at risk of contracting HIV infection. May be done by the HIV-infected person, a health care provider, or a public health worker.

Pentamidine—A drug used for PCP prophylaxis and treatment.

Perinatal Transmission—Transmission of HIV from mother to infant by blood or body fluids. May occur in utero, at the time of delivery, and possibly by breast-feeding. Also known as vertical, and maternal-fetal transmission.

Phagocytes—Cells of the immune system that "eat" foreign cells or infected cells. There are two kinds of phagocytes: macrophages and neutrophils (granulocytes).

Phase I Clinical Trial—Typically involves 20 to 100 patients and lasts several months. The major purpose is to determine safety and dose. Approximately 70% of drugs successfully complete phase I.

Phase II Clinical Trial—Typically involves up to several hundred patients and usually lasts from several months to two years. The major purposes are to continue to determine short-term safety and, primarily, effectiveness. Approximately 33 percent of drugs successfully complete phase II.

Phase III Clinical Trial—Typically involves from several hundred to several thousand patients and may last from one to four years. The major purposes are to study safety, effectiveness, and dosage. Approximately 25 to 30 percent of drugs successfully complete phase III.

***Pneumocystis Carinii* Pneumonia (PCP)**—Form of pneumonia seen in persons with HIV. The leading cause of death in patients with AIDS, PCP is caused by the opportunistic pathogen, *P. carinii,* which can infect the eyes, skin, spleen, liver, and heart, as well as the lungs.

Polymerase Chain Reaction (PCR)—A laboratory technique employing molecular biology technology to identify the nucleic acid sequence of HIV in the cells of an infected individual. This technique is sensitive and can detect a single copy of viral DNA in one cell out of 10,000. It is useful for early detection of perinatally infected infants and monitoring patients on clinical trials.

Pregnancy Counseling—Process of discussing with a woman of childbearing age her options regarding whether to become pregnant or, if she is already pregnant, whether to continue or terminate the pregnancy.

Prevalence—The fraction of individuals in a population who have a disease or infection at a particular time.

Primary Immune Response—The immune response that follows exposure to an infection or an antigen for the first time. There is a lag period before antibodies are produced.

Primary Prevention—Aimed to promote good health and protection from becoming infected with HIV

Prophylaxis—Intervention intended to preserve health and prevent the initial occurrence of a disease (primary prophylaxis) or to prevent the recurrence of a disease (secondary prophylaxis).

Protease Inhibitors—A class of drugs to treat HIV infection. Targets an enzyme needed at a later stage of HIV's life cycle, for assembling new virus particles. Protease Inhibitors are to be used in combination with nucleoside analogs (e.g., saquinavir).

Protected Sex—Refers to the use of a condom during sexual intercourse.

Pruritus—The symptom of itching.

Purified Protein Derivative (PPD)—Protein-rich material derived from the microorganism *M. tuberculosis.* Used as a skin-test reagent to detect current or prior infection with that organism.

Pyrazinamide—An antibiotic used as part of multidrug combinations to treat tuberculosis.

Rapid Plasma Reagin (RPR)—A nontreponemal test for detection of syphilis, the basis of which is agglutination.

Red Blood Cell (Erythrocytes)—Blood cells that are responsible for carrying oxygen and carbon dioxide to and from the tissues.

Retinitis—Inflammation of the retina; linked to cytomegalovirus infection in persons with AIDS. Untreated, it can cause blindness.

Reverse Transcriptase—An enzyme that is unique to all retroviruses. It reads the genetic information of the retrovirus, which is RNA, and makes a DNA copy.

Risk Reduction—Behavior change by an individual to decrease the likelihood of acquiring an infection.

Safe Sex—Sexual activity conducted in such a way that there is no risk of transmission or acquisition of the infection.

Safer Sex—Sexual activity which minimizes the risk of HIV transmission, by reducing the exchange of body fluids (e.g., consistent use of condoms, avoiding unprotected anal intercourse).

Secondary Immune Response—An immune response that follows exposure to an infection or an antigen that the immune system has already encountered. The strength of the response is greater, it occurs more rapidly, and it lasts longer.

Secondary Prevention—Prevention efforts directed toward preventing the further spread of HIV transmission among those who are HIV infected.

Sensitivity—The ability of a test to correctly identify an individual who is infected.

Seroconversion—The change from HIV-negative to HIV-positive antibody status.

Serologic Test—Any of a number of tests that are performed on the clear, liquid portion of blood (serum). Often refers to a test that determines the presence of antibodies to antigens such as viruses.

Seronegative—Having a negative test for antibodies to a substance or organism, such as HIV.

Seropositive—Having a positive test for antibodies to a substance or organism, such as HIV.

Seroreverter—A person whose antibody status has changed from positive to negative. Used to describe perinatally exposed infants who are not truly infected and become HIV antibody negative as they lose maternal HIV antibody.

Shooting Galleries—Sites where drugs are sold and injection equipment rented and shared by customers.

Shooting Up—Slang term which refers to injecting drugs.

Side Effect—Action or effect of a drug other than that desired (e.g., headache, liver damage).

Sign—An indication of a disease or disorder that is observed by the health care provider.

Squamous Intraepithelial Lesion (SIL)—Findings in cells revealed by Pap smear that indicate changes requiring further evaluation.

Specificity—The ability of a test to correctly identify an individual who is not infected.

Sterilization—A procedure killing all micro-organisms, where the probability of a microorganism surviving on an item is less than 1 in a million. Can be accomplished by heat, ethylene oxide gas, and a number of liquid chemical germicides.

Stomatitis—Any of numerous inflammatory diseases of the mouth having various causes (e.g., mechanical traumas, irritants, allergy, vitamin deficiency, infection).

Surrogate Markers—Levels of cells or proteins that indirectly indicate HIV activity. CD4 cell counts are surrogate markers of the progression of HIV disease.

Symptom—Any perceptible, subjective change in the body or its functions that indicates disease or phases of disease, as reported by the patient. Should be distinguished from a sign.

Syndrome—A group of symptoms and diseases that together are characteristic of a specific condition.

Teratogenicity—The ability to cause malformations in a fetus.

Thrush—Oral candidiasis; infection of the mouth or pharynx with the yeast candida. Frequently occurs in persons with a severely damaged immune system; may appear as discrete or confluent white patches on the mucous membranes.

T-lymphocytes—T-lymphocytes do not release antibodies, (unlike B-lymphocytes), but they specifically recognize and bind foreign antigens. Three fundamentally different types of T-lymphocytes exist: killer, helper, and suppressor.

Treatment Investigational New Drug (IND)—Application for the FDA's authorization to use an investigational drug that appears to be safe, and may be effective, in a defined group of patients with serious or life-threatening conditions, and who have no satisfactory alternatives. The purpose is to facilitate availability of promising new drugs as early in the drug development process as possible.

Treponema Pallidum—The micro-organism that causes syphilis; sometimes referred to as a spirochete because of its shape.

Trimethoprim-sulfamethoxazole (TMP-SMX)—A first-line combination drug for PCP prophylaxis and treatment. Possible side effects include rash, pruritus, cytopenia, liver abnormalities, and gastrointestinal upset.

Tuberculin Unit (TU)—Term used to describe doses of purified protein derivative.

Tuberculosis (TB)—Disease caused by the organism *M. Tuberculosis.*

Vaccine—A killed or harmless microorganism that can induce an immune response to a disease-causing agent and confers protection against the disease-causing agent in uninfected people. Vaccines stimulate an immune response and may protect or modify subsequent infection by that organism.

VDRL Test—A screening test for syphilis developed at the Venereal Disease Research Laboratories.

Vertical Transmission—Transmission of virus from mother to fetus. See perinatal transmission.

Viral Envelopes—Structures that surround some virus particles, resembling membranes around cells. Viral envelopes contain virus-specified proteins that are important in binding cell receptors. Viral envelope proteins are major targets for the immune system.

Wasting Syndrome—Weight loss that is involuntary and progressive; associated with advanced HIV infection.

Water Sports—Contact with urine during sex, i.e., urination on or in the partner's body.

Western Blot (WB)—A test for the presence of antibodies to multiple antigens of HIV; used to confirm HIV infection following a positive ELISA test. The Western Blot displays antibodies to specific HIV viral proteins in a separate, well-defined band. A positive result shows stripes at the locations for two or more viral proteins. A negative result is blank at these locations.

White Blood Cells (Leukocytes)—All blood cells except red blood cells. Leukocytes consist of a variety of blood cells including lymphocytes, neutrophils, eosinophils, macrophages, and megakaryocytes.

Window Period—The period of time before antibody to HIV becomes detectable in the blood but after exposure and infection with HIV

Works—Slang for drug-injecting equipment.

Zalcitabine (ddC; Trade Name HIVID; Also Called Dideoxycytidine)—One of the FDA-approved nucleoside analog drugs that inhibits the reverse transcriptase enzyme of HIV. Its major limiting toxicity is peripheral neuropathy. It has the advantage of being 10% more potent than ZDV and has been used in combination therapy with ZDV in patients with advanced disease.

INDEX

Page numbers followed by *t* or *f* indicate tables or figures, respectively